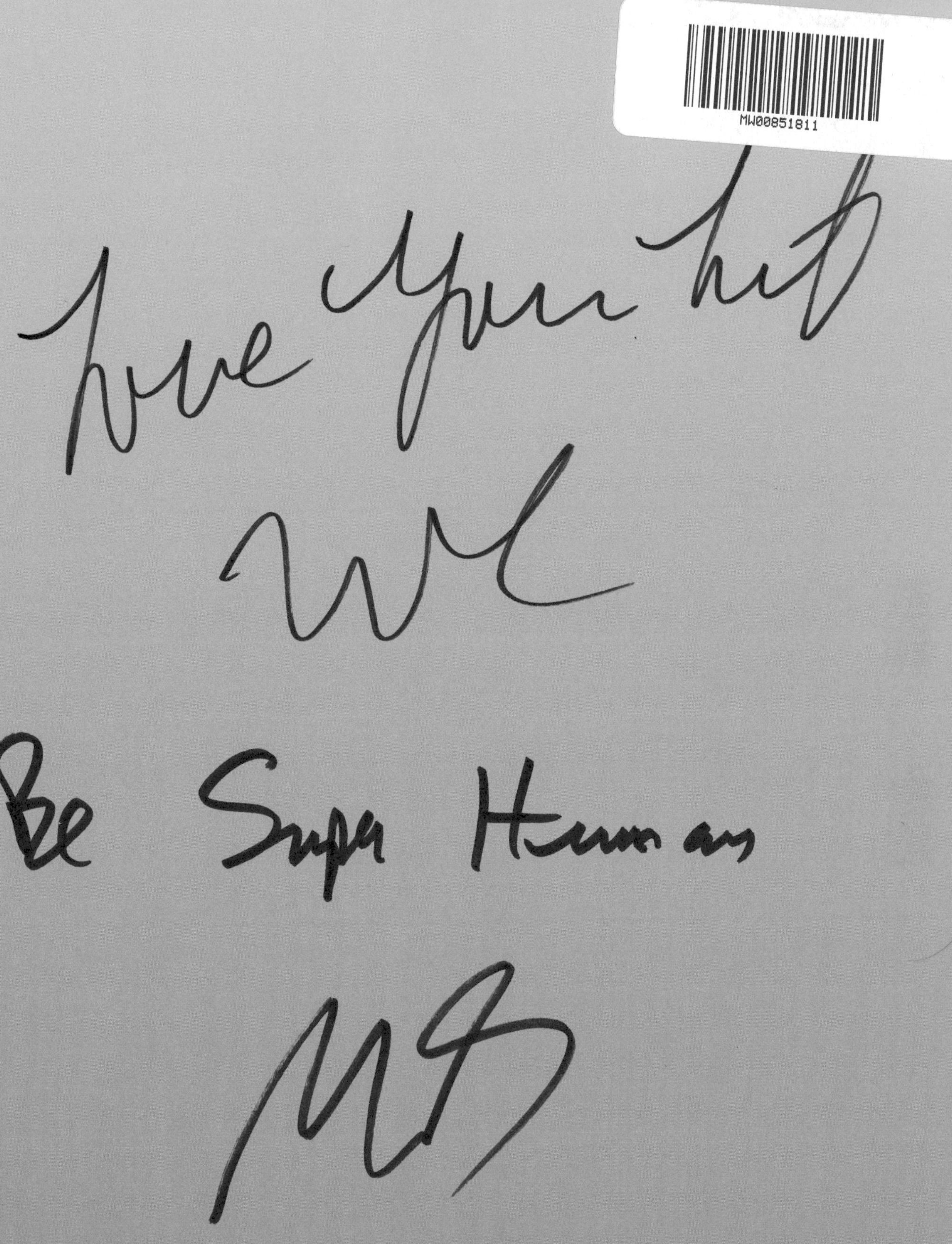
Love your life
Be Super Human

THE ULTIMATE NUTRITION BIBLE

THE ULTIMATE NUTRITION BIBLE

EASILY CREATE THE PERFECT DIET THAT FITS YOUR LIFESTYLE, GOALS, AND GENETICS

MATT GALLANT AND
WADE T. LIGHTHEART

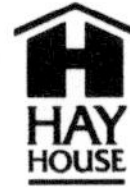

HAY HOUSE, INC.
Carlsbad, California • New York City
London • Sydney • New Delhi

Published in the United States by: Hay House, Inc.: www.hayhouse.com® • ***Published in Australia by:*** Hay House Australia Pty. Ltd.: www.hayhouse.com.au • ***Published in the United Kingdom by:*** Hay House UK, Ltd.: www.hayhouse.co.uk • ***Published in India by:*** Hay House Publishers India: www.hayhouse.co.in

Indexer: Joan Shapiro • *Cover design:* Julie Davison
Interior design: Nick C. Welch • *Interior photos/illustrations:* Quentin Matheson
Photos of the authors: Rachel Megan and Kyle Jones, Tasha Cooney

Cataloging-in-Publication Data is on file at the Library of Congress

Hardcover ISBN: 978-1-4019-7454-1
E-book ISBN: 978-1-4019-7455-8
Audiobook ISBN: 978-1-4019-7456-5

10 9 8 7 6 5 4 3 2 1
1st edition, September 2023

Printed in the United States of America

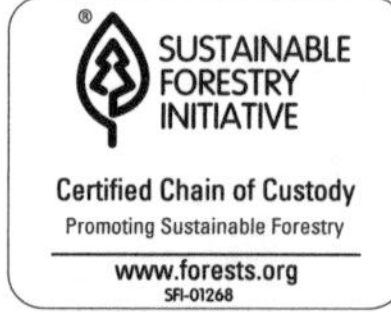

SFI label applies to the text stock

This product uses paper and materials from responsibly sourced forests. For more information, please go to: bookchainproject.com/home.

We would like to dedicate this book to our parents, our mentors, everyone at BIOptimizers, everyone who has ever trusted BIOptimizers with their health—past, present, and future—and to everyone who is on the same mission of bringing biological optimization to the world.

THANK YOU.

CONTENTS

Every Diet Decoded

Universal Nutritional Optimizers

PREFACE

Things were getting heated. Matt and Wade were sitting on the deck of a Vancouver health food store eating their lunch, and the argument continued . . .

Matt said, with total conviction, "Dude, keto is the greatest diet ever. The results are undeniable. Look at my clients' transformations. It's how our bodies evolved."

Wade replied, "Oh yeah? Bro, I just won a national natural bodybuilding championship on a plant-based diet. We don't need meat."

This argument raged on for years. We were two zealots battling for the Dietary Championship. We were more focused on being right than finding the truth. This book is the resolution of these conflicts as we found common ground and discovered universal nutritional principles.

BUILD YOUR OWN ADVENTURE

Please don't be intimidated by the size and scope of this book. This book is designed to help you build your own adventure. You can jump around and read the chapters that are the most important to you today. Apply the strategies and reap the rewards.

This book is designed to be your guide for the rest of your life. It's the opposite of the latest fad diet. It's a reference guide that you can use to help you accomplish all your goals. As your goals change, open it up, read the relevant chapter, and achieve your next goal.

ENDING THE DIETARY MADNESS

If you have any interest in nutrition, you've no doubt asked yourself some of these questions:

- What's the best diet for weight loss?
- What's the healthiest way to eat?
- What's the hottest diet in Hollywood?
- Are fats bad? Are fats good?
- Are carbs evil?
- What about keto? Paleo? Raw food? Intermittent fasting? Is eating plants the way?

If you're confused when it comes to nutrition, you're not alone. Over 78 percent of people are lost.[1] In the world of weight loss, people continue to fail. Long-term failure rates are at 97 percent. Based on our multiple decades of experience, we've found that the remaining 3 percent are usually extremely driven people.

THE DIET INDUSTRY'S ILLUSION OF SUCCESS

Twelve-week transformation pictures provoke your emotional reactions and are used to sell to your desires for faster results. Most people can sustain willpower for a few weeks with very little consideration of what works for them psychologically, emotionally, or spiritually. They grit it out and "do what it takes" without any awareness of the price they will pay in the future.

Expert marketers will prey on your desires for magic bullets and miracle fat loss solutions. They tell you that one magic potion or diet is all you need to make all your fat loss dreams come true.

Dieters finish each 12-week transformation and take glorious "after" pictures, only to regain everything within a year.

Eventually, the majority of diet followers hit a wall (or multiple walls). The weight loss stops, health problems start, the dieter doesn't feel good, the dieter gets psychologically tired of it, and the dieter quits.

Who can consider it a victory if 97 percent of dieters regain all of the weight back, and more, within three years?[2]

Then the dieters look for their next dieting tribe to join, and they rinse and repeat. Very few people find a dietary approach that works for them for life. This book solves that problem. It ends the group-diet-hopping madness.

Why do we use the word *tribe*? The answer is that tribal dynamics are hardwired into our DNA and psyche. Tribal dynamics helped keep us alive back when tribes were critical to survival.[3] Just like our starvation self-defense mechanisms, this ancient programming is still a part of us. The potential pitfall is when people join the wrong tribe and it leads them to bad health decisions. And this is what we've seen for the last few decades in nutrition.

Rarely are diets designed for lifelong results; neither do they take into account the root causes that led you to gain weight or become unhealthy in the first place. The failed results are never advertised.

Every diet that creates caloric deficits will produce some results, at least in the short term. Can people lose weight eating Twinkies and McDonald's? The answer will surprise you. Find out in Chapter 2, Why Every Diet Works . . . (for a While).

Every diet typically produces results across a bell curve. Its marketers will focus on and showcase the small minority of elite success stories at the end of the bell curve and avoid discussing the failures.

The top 3 percent of dieters who achieve extraordinary results become the loudest advocates of the new "magic" diet, and this is used to advertise it. They believe this diet is the answer for everyone and become strongly biased against all other diet philosophies. People on social media want to look like these "influencers" and get sold on trying whatever this latest diet philosophy is, hoping for a miracle.

Social media algorithms are designed to show users more of what they're interested in, which forms an echo chamber that reinforces messages. Thus, it creates the illusion that everyone is getting results from a given diet. People get their dietary beliefs validated by algorithms that feed them articles and social media posts related to their tribe. This reaffirms their biases and strengthens their tribal mentality.

TRIBAL DIET WARS

The nature of the human psyche is to want to belong to a group, such as a family or other tribe.

Throughout human existence, being part of a group was essential to survival. Getting kicked out of one meant almost certain death. The survival instinct to stay connected is baked into our nervous system, identity, and our social bonding. It's wired into our very DNA.

In the modern world, we could argue that our highly digitalized society has led many people to feel less connected and even chronically depressed because of the loss of real-life personal connections. This is true even though our lives—for the most part—are easier and more abundant than ever. People often overeat as part of a stress response while they deplete their motivation and connection neurochemicals further by scrolling on their phones in search of deeper relationships.

The need to belong to a group is a powerful driver of our behaviors, and it's no less prevalent in the many diet tribes that have emerged in the last few decades. Diet philosophies have become a new reason to join groups. The so-called diet wars have become the norm in the nutrition world as people strongly identify themselves with one faction or another.

It is a natural tendency to be attracted to others who share uncommon commonalities, whether these are belief systems, philosophies, religions, or diets . . . It could even be said that diets have become a new form of religion. People adhering to a diet are respected, while those falling off the wagon are deemed sinners. Dietary zealots attack other dietary factions on social media. Diet leaders gaslight other diet leaders and try to convince everyone that their way is the "one true way." Sound like a cult yet?

Keto zealots attack vegetarians, vegan zealots attack paleo, and carnivores attack plant eaters. Dietary warfare is waged on the web, and group members get caught in the drama.

Groups are no longer local thanks to the power of the Internet. People join communities of fellow diet devotees that give them a sense of group belonging and something to fight for. Social media strengthens these group bonds.

It's no surprise, as the battle for nutritional "supremacy" among dietary group leaders is worth a fortune. Every diet leader wants to convince you that their way is the *only way*. Dietary group leaders take advantage of the human need to be a part of a tribe.

THE PATHWAY TO SUCCESS: TRANSCENDING DIETARY DOGMA

Our first important message is: we shouldn't be building groups around diets and food. The dogmatic approaches that groups encourage can lead to many unhealthy decisions—both physical and psychological.

To achieve long-term success, you need to transcend these group drives by using the Bruce Lee principle: "Absorb what is useful, discard what is useless, and add what is specifically your own."

In real-world fights, if you stick to only one dogmatic fighting tradition—be it judo, tae kwon do, jiujitsu, or anything else—you will be beaten. Bruce Lee shattered thousands of years of dogmatic martial arts thinking by adopting what worked from each philosophy and discarding anything that didn't work.

Eventually, this evolved to what we know today as mixed martial arts (MMA). In MMA, you develop a fighting style that is best for your body's natural strengths. We believe you should do the same thing with your nutrition.

In other words: extract what works, stop what doesn't, avoid committing to one opinion, and consider all options. Then use data, experts, and your own biofeedback to refine and optimize a more effective dietary strategy that works best for you.

DIET VS. NUTRITIONAL STRATEGIES

Dieting refers to a short-term eating strategy to achieve a given objective (for example, "I need to lose 20 pounds before my sister's wedding"). Most diets are rigid, structured, cookie-cutter, and dogmatic approaches that leave little room for flexibility or individualization. They tend not to address what happens after you achieve your goals.

Study after study confirms that people who diet end up regaining most of the weight, regardless of diet type.[4, 5] Worse yet, yo-yo dieters develop more health risks and body fat than if they had never dieted at all.[6]

Despite how convincing the illusion of its success is, the diet mentality sets people up for a lifetime of failures.

Instead, we suggest applying a flexible mindset and tailoring your nutritional strategies based on your goals, your genetics, and your personality.

THE GRAND UNIFIED THEORY OF NUTRITION

We (Matt and Wade) have a combined 60-plus years of real-world experience in the fitness and nutrition industry. We've been coached by some of the most successful bodybuilding coaches of all time. If we add the experience our mentors have in these fields, we end up with a couple hundred years of experience. We've built a Jedi Council of health geniuses that have helped us transcend our own dogmatic beliefs.

We spent years debating with each other. Matt was a keto zealot trying to convince Wade that this was "the ultimate diet," while Wade tried to convince Matt that plants were the way. As young guys, we were extremely dogmatic about our respective diets. We were the most popular trainers at World's Gym in Vancouver, and we constantly butted heads over which diet was best. We were both achieving world-class results with our respective clients.

Wade was a three-time national bodybuilding champion and Mr. Universe entirely on a plant-based diet with 85 grams of protein a day. Although his choice to do bodybuilding on a plant-based diet was highly controversial, he thought being plant-based was the answer for everyone.

Matt performed best on a high-meat ketogenic diet. He had been able to lose up to 64 pounds in 14 weeks on it (which was a massive mistake that we will get into in Chapter 2) and build almost 50 pounds of lean muscle mass in three years naturally. Plus, a few of his clients had achieved phenomenal results (such as losing 191 pounds in 18 months). He was getting world-class results from pro athletes. He thought everyone should be on a ketogenic diet.

To some extent, we both achieved our health, aesthetic, and performance goals with our respective diets. And the diets fit into our life philosophies.

Yet, after a decade, we realized that it's pointless to try to change each other's minds. We realized that neither person was interested in hearing the other. We were more interested in proving our points and our own biases, because we truly enjoyed the diets we had.

It took us a long time, but we realized that we had a lot to learn from each other, citing data and research, and observing our clients' responses. By keeping our minds open, staying up-to-date with the latest diet research, and comparing our real-world experiences, we've worked on removing our biases and dogmatic beliefs. We both realized that every diet could work—from keto to vegan to paleo—and that what matters is individualization.

We've been exposed to the rise and fall of virtually every dietary strategy available—not to mention that we've been blessed to work with some of the smartest experts in the world of health, fitness, and nutrition.

We've spent the last couple of years boiling down our knowledge into essential nutritional principles and strategies that you can apply to virtually any diet system. You can mix and match these specific nutritional strategies and principles to create the ultimate nutritional game plan that works *for you*.

The Grand Unifying Theory of Nutrition will help you filter through the barrage of people pounding their fists and shouting, "My way is the only way!" You'll never be suckered into another diet scam again.

THE END OF DIET WARS

The purpose of this book is simple: to end diet wars by giving *you* the entire picture . . . all of the data, proven strategies, and hard-earned insights that you need to find the nutritional strategy that will work for you now and for the rest of your life.

The key is to follow a program where you're highly attracted to the positives, and in which the negatives don't feel like sacrifices to you. In other words, you're really attracted to your plan's upside and are okay with its downsides.

In making choices, you want to take into account your:

- Spiritual beliefs
- Psychological needs
- Emotional tendencies
- Goals
- Gut biome
- Genes
- Lifestyle

Unlike a cookie-cutter diet, your nutritional strategy is an evolving way of eating. Therefore, it needs to be customized for you and for any given time, including how to address nutritional deficiencies that contribute to symptoms or cravings.

More important, nutritional strategies should be flexible and adaptable. You can stack multiple strategies and switch between them based on what you're trying to achieve, depending on your goal (which side of the BIOptimization Triangle you're working on).

There are numerous nutritional strategies that we will cover in this book. Every strategy has pros and cons. Remember, follow the ones for which you're really attracted to the benefits and are at peace with the downsides. A good example is fasting. Some people *psychologically love* fasting, which makes it a viable strategy for them. Others fear fasting, so for them it's not a good option.

BE WARY OF "GAME-CHANGING" DOCUMENTARIES

Marketers are masters of grabbing your attention and convincing you of what they want you to believe. They use testimonials from professional athletes and public figures to demonstrate credibility. They cherry-pick evidence that supports their views. These documentaries show that you can build a case for virtually any diet.

N=1 vs. Clinical Research Study

Some nutritional experts use research as if it's the gospel written in granite by God himself. Others cherry-pick research that suits their marketing agenda. Others ignore science, spinning their own good-sounding theories and presenting them as truth.

We love science and research, and that's why we fund a lot of it ourselves. However, we're also aware of its limitations.

When you try things on yourself, it's an experiment with a sample size of one. You're dealing with your own genetics and epigenetics. In the end, the only person who matters is *you;* that's why we call this strategy the "Me Diet." That's why this book is designed to help you build your personal "Me Diet." Some key questions to ask are:

- Is this diet strategy right for me?
- Is it right for me, right now?
- What's the best way to succeed?

This book will provide you with those answers.

We're going to do our best to be as scientifically grounded as possible throughout this book. Some of our theories and approaches haven't been proven by science yet, but they work in the real world. And when we have far-out theories about things, we will frame them as such. Our goal is to update this book every few years with the latest research. Nutritional science is constantly evolving, and many things we believe are true today will be proven obsolete tomorrow.

This book puts an end to diet approaches that are guaranteed to fail. Instead, we give you the latest breakthroughs in strategies that work. We give you universal approaches that can work for everyone; plus, we give you the key factors that you need to personalize one for you.

We've based this book on nutritional research, training research, and psychological science as it applies to nutrition and dietary success. This book isn't for people who want to keep believing in magic when it comes to their bodies.

Here are our eight promises if you read this book from start to finish:

1. You will never be confused about nutrition and diets again. You will have the understanding you need to build the best diets for you, and evolve them based on your goals, for the rest of your life.
2. You will never fall prey to diet marketing lies again.
3. You will have a wide variety of effective nutritional strategies that you need to lose excess body fat and reach your ideal weight.
4. You will know how to avoid regaining weight and stay slim forever.
5. You will know how to build as much lean muscle as you want.
6. You will know how to optimize your nutrition to maximize your life span and health span (we call it your "BioSpan").
7. You will know how to eat for maximum athletic performance.
8. You will know the best nutritional strategies to optimize your mental performance.

Of course, this book isn't a compendium of magic bullets either. Knowledge by itself isn't power. When it comes to nutrition and health, *consistently applied* knowledge is power.

The key is to take total responsibility for your body. That starts with educating yourself with the highest-quality information possible, and that's what we offer in this book. The rest is up to you.

We're a little biased, but we consider this the most powerful nutrition book ever created. Why? Because we've unified every seemingly conflicting dietary approach into a cohesive system that you can make your own.

Are there things we got wrong in this book? Almost certainly. Will there be new discoveries that make some of this information obsolete in a few years? Yes. And that's why we will update this book every few years with the latest breakthroughs. We are excited to learn, grow, and evolve as nutritional educators to keep sharing what works with you.

This is the end of the diet wars and the beginning of your journey to what we call Biologically Optimized Health. This is a dynamic, ongoing journey. By continually going through the BIOptimization Process—assess, test, and optimize—God willing, you can optimize your aesthetics, performance, and health and live a great life to 100 years and beyond.

This book's philosophy can be summarized this way:

> "The biggest enemy we have to fight against right now is our tribal past. What served us so well for thousands of years is now an obsolete concept. It's no more about the survival of this tribe or that one, but about *Homo sapiens* as a species. For the first time in our collective history, we must think of ourselves as a single tribe on a single planet. We are a single tribe, the tribe of humans."
>
> — Marcelo Gleiser in ***The Trouble with Tribalism***

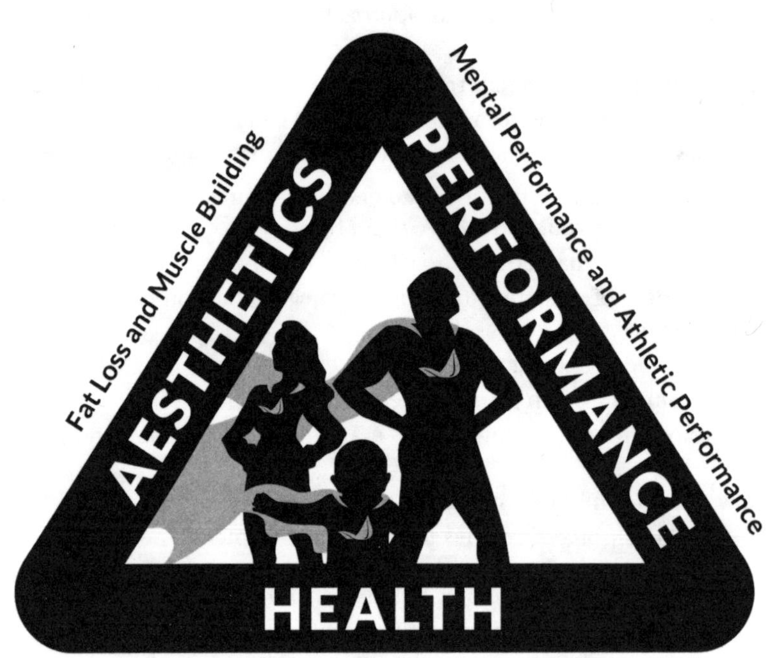

Life Span and Health Span

Optimizing Health Since 2004

CHAPTER 1

THE REAL REASON 97 PERCENT FAIL WITH THEIR WEIGHT LOSS

We sincerely hope that this chapter changes everything in your mind—and in the industry's—when it comes to dieting. Once you understand the core message here, you'll never see dieting the same way again . . . *ever.*

THE SHOCKING TRUTHS ABOUT CALORIES AND METABOLISM

Calories and *metabolism* are by far the most obsessed-over words and concepts in the world of dieting. In this chapter, we're going to reveal the surprising truths about calories and metabolism based on science and some shocking experiments. More important, we're going to give you some new breakthrough strategies that you need to focus on to achieve short-term and long-term success.

In this chapter, you'll learn:

- The actual reason why 97 percent of dieters regain most of their weight in the long run, and how to become part of the elite top 3 percent who consistently keep weight off without sacrifices or compromises.
- How to maximize the calories you burn and start consistently achieving your aesthetic goals without going overboard or jeopardizing your health and wellness.
- How emotional eating can interfere with your dieting goals—and the key to unlocking the underlying emotions and/or traumas so you can defeat overeating and unhealthy eating habits for good.
- Why formulating your own personal strategy to combat your genetics is critical for achieving lifelong victory with your health, performance, and aesthetic goals.
- Discover the undeniable evidence for how to attain true, successful, long-term weight loss, and how three critical tools allow you to lose body fat permanently and safely (without making you go through the yo-yo diet insanity).
- Three cautionary tales of the common mistakes people make that destroy their metabolism, and how to ensure that your body feels safe throughout your weight loss journey.

Metabolism

The chemical reactions in the body's cells that change food into energy and building blocks.
Our bodies use this energy and building blocks to do everything from moving to thinking to growing to healing.

Let's start with the bottom line. The real reason we struggle with our weight and keeping it off is one thing: genetics. And we're not talking about the "I have bad genetics" narrative.

First, we still have the same fundamental genetic programming that kept our ancestors alive in tough times. Our ancient, hard-wired biological nature has not adapted to today's challenges. Our modern sedentary lifestyles, combined with readily available, cheap, hyper-palatable calorie-loaded foods, have led us to an obesity pandemic.

Second, the real reason that weight loss is so challenging is because starvation survival mechanisms are built into your DNA. Your body has one core primary objective: to survive.

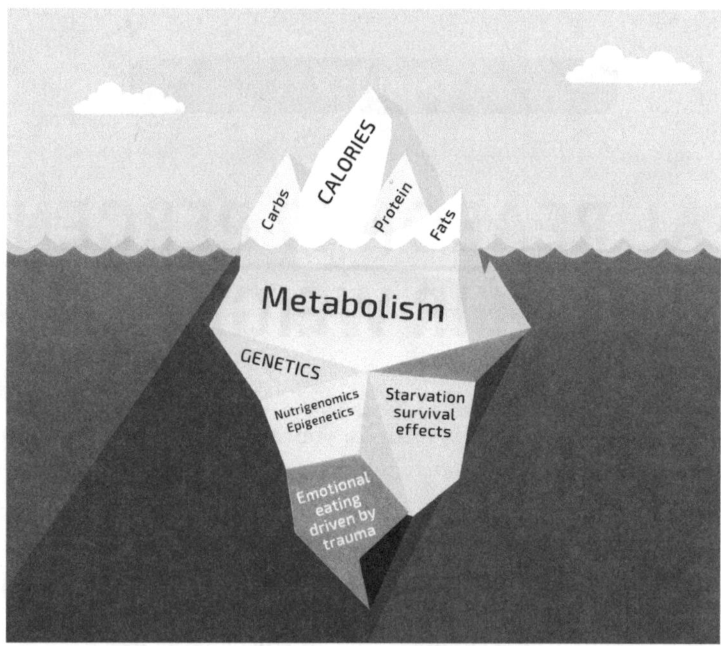

Diagram: the essence of obesity vs. the perception of obesity

The human body has evolved over millions of years to maximize its chances of survival. Understanding this undeniable fact and creating smart strategies around biological reality is the key to lifelong victory.

Let's take a time machine back to the caveman days.

There aren't any convenience stores or fast-food restaurants around. Food has to be hunted or gathered. There are no fruits or vegetables to pick during the long, hard winter months. You might go days or weeks without any food.

To maximize the odds of survival, the body has created many self-defense mechanisms. And these mechanisms are why people fail with their weight loss objectives in the long term. Ignoring this and activating these starvation survival mechanisms is the formula for guaranteed continuous failure.

The male body will start shutting down and potentially die at around 3 percent body fat. Imagine a 150-pound caveman named Carl with 10 percent body fat. This means he has about 7 percent body fat he can lose before he's in serious trouble. The math is: 7 percent of 150 pounds equals 10.5 pounds of fat. This means he has around 35,750 "survival calories" left (3,500 calories per pound of fat multiplied by 10.5 pounds of fat).

Testosterone

A steroid hormone that stimulates development of male secondary sexual characteristics, produced mainly in the testes, but also in the ovaries and adrenal cortex.

Leptin

A protein produced by fat cells that is a hormone acting mainly in the regulation of appetite and fat storage.

Thyroid

A gland that makes and stores hormones that help regulate the heart rate, blood pressure, body temperature, and the rate at which food is converted into energy.

Ghrelin

A hormone that is produced and released mainly by the stomach with small amounts also released by the small intestine, pancreas, and brain.

Assuming Carl is burning 2,500 calories a day as he walks for hours to gather or hunt food, he has about 14 days left of survival, which *is not* very long in the winter months. It might take him a few weeks to find and kill another animal. Looking at it from this perspective, Carl's situation seems pretty dire.

Fortunately for Carl, his body evolved to protect him in this situation. It will lower his metabolism to burn fewer calories. At 1,250 calories burned per day, Carl the Caveman could survive for double the amount of time. But the "bad" news for dieters is, we still possess these starvation survival mechanisms.

Here's a short list of the starvation survival strategies the body activates in extended calorie deprivation:

1. Lowers leptin
2. Lowers testosterone
3. Lowers thyroid function
4. Lowers non-exercise activity thermogenesis (NEAT)
5. Increases ghrelin (which increases hunger)
6. Prompts shrunken fat cells to store more fat
7. Increases the number of fat cells
8. Burns lean muscle mass

It's almost like a *Star Trek* episode wherein the Starship *Enterprise* starts shutting down nonessential systems to preserve its energy. The body works the same way. We'll delve deeper into the effects of these processes later in the chapter.

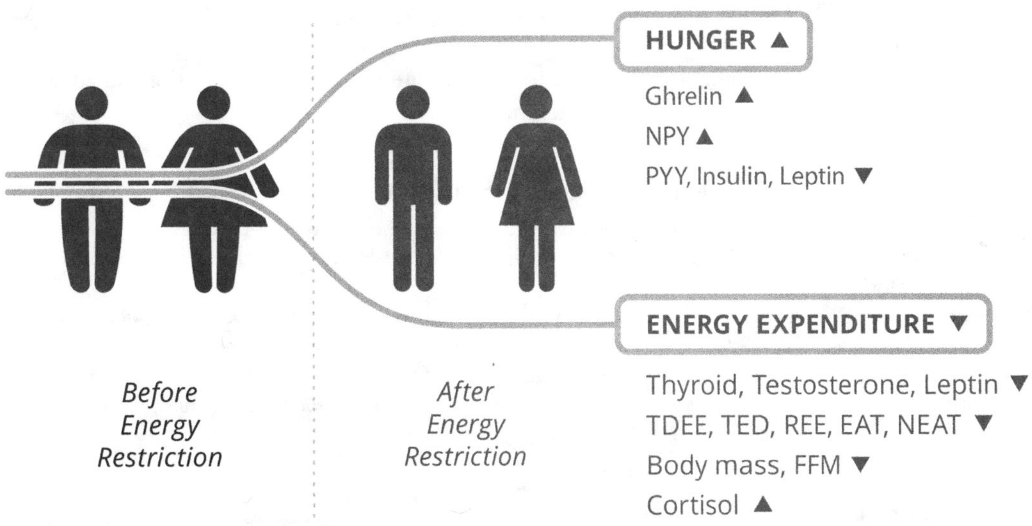

WE DIDN'T EVOLVE TO HANDLE DONUTS, DINERS, OR DIETS

The fundamental weight loss challenge, as we've noted, is that we still have the same genetic programming as Carl the Caveman.

Nowadays, we are surrounded by limitless food options that are engineered for overeating 24/7. We can literally push a button in an app and get almost anything our taste buds desire. These hyper-palatable foods are seasoned with hyper-intense flavorings, high-fructose corn syrup, salt, and fat.

Food companies engineer their products for specific combinations of sweet, salty, fatty, and pleasurable mouthfeel to hijack your brain's reward mechanisms. And master marketers know how to present it to you and create cravings in your mind.

FOOD IS LIKE HEROIN?

Studies show that the same area of the brain that is activated with heroin and other drugs is also activated with certain types of food, making those foods just as addictive as heroin.[1]

Salt, sugar, and fat increase our likelihood of survival, but in prehistoric days they weren't as easy to come by. Therefore, we naturally find these foods delicious, and when we eat them, our brains flood with dopamine, the reward neurotransmitter.[2]

A study found that 94 percent of rats would choose a sweetener over cocaine, suggesting that the sweet taste is intensely rewarding and addictive.[3]

Sugary foods also trigger the release of serotonin, the calm, happy, and antidepressant neurotransmitter.[4] Worse yet, the fructose in high-fructose corn syrup can reduce your satiety response,[5] so you can finish a tub of ice cream without feeling full.

Certain foods can trigger a huge insulin response, which can trigger a blood sugar crash. You will then feel hungry and irritable as you reach for more sugary foods to bring your blood sugar back up.[6] Sugary foods and beverages that are without fiber or proteins can spike your insulin, but so can dairy proteins that are high in branched-chain amino acids.[7, 8]

Like drugs, these foods can downregulate your dopamine receptors so that you need more of the same foods to hit the same high. Also, once you try to quit eating them, you may experience some withdrawal symptoms.

Most diets tend to work as a good short-term antidote to some of the problems above by making you eat less, creating a temporary caloric deficit.

However, your innate survival desires and the desire to fit in will cause you to eat more. Imagine if Carl the Caveman found a donut shop next to his cave—to maximize his chances of survival, he would eat until he was sick.

The Hunger is a self-defense mechanism that encourages you to eat more and regain lost body fat. Your body doesn't care about looking good on Instagram; it cares about survival. We believe The Hunger is driven either by chronically elevated ghrelin (the hunger hormone) or elevated levels of the peptide NPY in the brain. Many fitness competitors have reported this experience.

If you decide to do an aggressive weight loss program and activate your body's starvation survival mechanisms, your odds of success are close to zero. And we aren't different from you.

Matt Was Hungry for Two Years

Matt had already lost more than 30 pounds over two years. Then, when he was getting ready for his wedding, he wanted to lose an additional 15 pounds to look his best. Matt pushed *hard.* He was doing sprints up hills in the jungle of Panama and cut his calories aggressively.

Matt did lose the final 15 pounds, but then came the *hunger.* Hunger appears when your body chronically elevates ghrelin (the hunger hormone) as a self-defense mechanism to encourage you to eat more and regain some body fat. Your body doesn't care about looking good on Instagram; it cares about survival.

Matt felt hungry for two years after his wedding and regained most of the lost weight. The hunger only subsided after his weight rebounded back to its old level.

After Wade dieted for 11 months and pushed his body fat down near its genetic limit, it fought back, and Wade regained 42 pounds in the following weeks (read the entire story later in this chapter).

These were huge learning lessons for Matt and Wade. Their bodies fought back to make them eat more and maximize their odds of survival.

Since that time, we've dived into the research, and the evidence for long-term weight success is undeniable: we need to make the body feel safe throughout the journey.

Cutting-edge weight loss coaches have developed new strategies to help deal with this hardwiring. They include refeeds, diet breaks, and reverse dieting. These are three critical tools for people wanting to lose body fat permanently and safely—without going through the yo-yo diet insanity. We will discuss these later in the book.

HOW THEY SET UP THE BIGGEST LOSERS FOR EPIC LOSSES

The popular TV show *The Biggest Loser* placed morbidly obese participants on a diet of 1,200 calories per day and a regimen of six intense 90-minute workouts each week. Of course, everyone lost a tremendous amount of weight and fat. They looked like major successes; however, they were unknowingly set up to fail.

Afterward, the participants went back to their normal lives without understanding the starvation survival mechanisms that set them up to regain their weight. A 2016 follow-up study measured the basal metabolic rate (BMR), body composition, and weight of 14 of the participants six years after season eight of the show.[9]

The participants had regained 70 percent of the weight they'd lost. Their average BMR had dropped from 2,607 calories preshow to 1,996 postshow. At the six-year follow-up, their average BMR had dropped to 1,903, and they'd regained about half of the lean mass they'd lost, so more of the regained weight was fat.

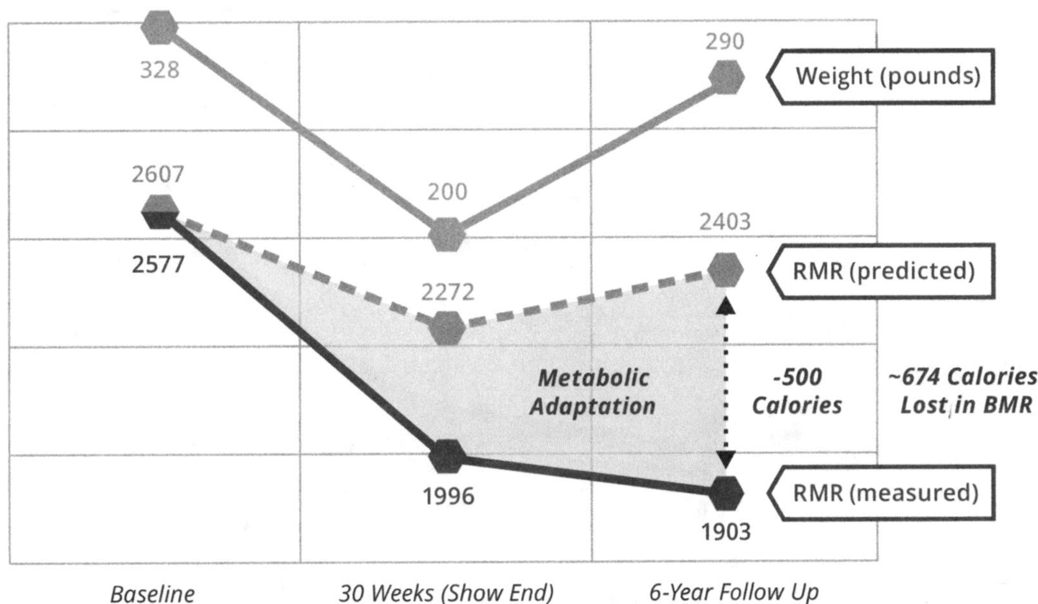

As the participants regained the fat, their leptin increased. However, their BMR remained significantly suppressed. Their metabolism burned 700 fewer calories a day, which is *a lot* less.

So, the short-term "lose weight at any cost" approach of *The Biggest Loser* TV show came at the expense of the participants' long-term success. This is a good example of what's wrong with the dieting world.

THE TERRIFYING PRICE OF METABOLIC DESTRUCTION: LESSONS FROM THE MINNESOTA STARVATION EXPERIMENT

Toward the end of World War II, the famous nutrition physiologist Ancel Keys conducted the Minnesota Starvation Experiment. Its purpose was to better understand the effects of famine on human physiology and ways to rehab people from wartime famine states.

The study enrolled 36 men with good mental and physical health. They went through 12 weeks of eating 3,200-calorie diets before six months of semi-starvation at 1,560 calories, split into two meals per day.

In the subsequent 12 weeks, the participants were divided into four groups, each fed at different levels of restricted refeeding calories. Then, in the final eight weeks, the participants were allowed to eat as much as they wanted as the researchers recorded and monitored food intake. The men in the study lived in a controlled environment, were assigned work tasks, and had to walk 22 miles each week.

Over the starvation period, participants lost 20 to 26 percent of their initial bodyweight. They experienced decreases in sex drive, cognitive function, strength, vitality, body temperature, respiration, and heart rate.

Interestingly, they also became apathetic and developed mental health problems such as depression and hysteria. They became obsessed with food and started to collect and exchange recipes, which they hadn't done before.

They also developed disordered eating patterns. Some of the men started self-mutilating, and one of them even cut off three of his fingers during the rehab phase.

During the refeeding phase, the men experienced an insatiable hunger that lasted for months no matter how much they ate. They consumed, on average, over 5,000 calories a day, and some ate over 11,500 calories. The starvation survival effects were in full swing.

In 2003, 19 of the 36 participants who were still alive were interviewed about the experiment. They admitted that they still had some lingering fear of starvation and food obsession decades after the study had ended. In other words, they had been traumatized by starvation.

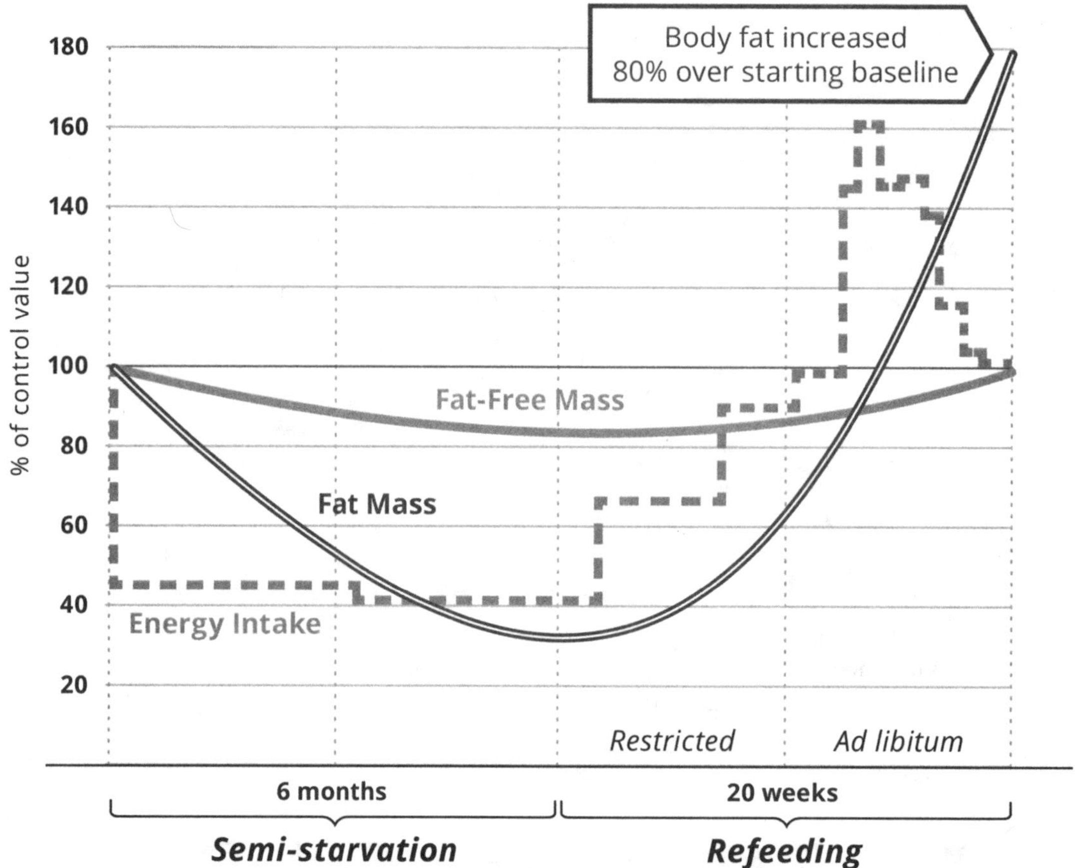

Although this study occurred in 1945, countless physique competitors and dieters still trigger the same responses with their diet and exercise programs. They push their metabolism too far, triggering the wrath of the body's starvation survival mechanisms. The damages are typically much more severe than weight regain.

PAINFUL LESSONS FROM ELITE BODYBUILDERS

We've both personally experienced metabolism backlash—Wade with his Mr. Universe show prep, and Matt as he dieted for his wedding. Wade's coach, Scott Abel, also overstretched his metabolic slingshot as a physique competitor before observing the effect thousands of times with his clients and followers. Scott's book *Understanding Metabolism* helped us understand the fundamental nature of metabolism. We owe massive kudos to Scott for sharing his genius with the world.

According to Scott, physique competitors go through even more severe starvation and intense training, and for longer, than participants in the Minnesota experiment did. If the body reaches such a low body fat too fast, this can trigger the starvation survival effects.

"I Gained 42 Pounds of Fat and Water in 11 Weeks," by Wade T. Lightheart

I spent 11 months eating 1,500 calories per day while training twice a day for the Mr. Universe contest. I didn't care what it took. I was going to achieve the mission. I didn't have much energy to think or do much else outside the gym. I lost my sex drive and felt very irritable.

After the show, I gained 42 pounds of fat and water in 11 weeks. I was constantly ravenous and couldn't stop eating. I had wrecked my digestive system and gut biome.

At the time, genetic testing wasn't available, so I worked with a naturopathic doctor and microbiome expert to reoptimize my hormones and digestive system. It took about a year to squash the ghrelin response and reboot my metabolism before reintroducing fasting and diet strategies.

It took a full two years and tens of thousands of dollars to bring my overall health back into the optimal zone and to wake up feeling *good* in the morning. It was a painful, valuable lesson.

Stories like this are hardly unique to bodybuilding. Every year, tens of millions of people embark on 12-week transformations only to later regain all their weight and then some. Afterward, they spend months or years in shame, feeling like failures before returning to the dieting bandwagon. Then they repeat the same tumultuous process, only to further damage their metabolism and do it all over again. And many just give up completely.

The health effects of such extreme dieting and show prep can be even more catastrophic for women. Their menstrual cycles are more sensitive to caloric restrictions. Women are genetically designed to carry more body fat than men; they also suffer more from body image issues and disordered eating, which can make them more obsessed with their physical imperfections.

In Scott Abel's book *Understanding Metabolism,* he shares numerous pictures of female physique competitors. The women started off around 140 pounds before the show and dieted down to 100 pounds for the show before ballooning to over 200 pounds afterward. Then they went into more extreme dieting, used drugs, and did excessive cardio for their next shows. The damage to their bodies, mental health, and relationships often led to psychological traumas.

When your body goes into energy-preservation mode, it shuts off the reproductive axis, which can cause irregular menstrual cycles or stop them altogether, and cause infertility.[10] Low estrogen in women and low testosterone in men can reduce bone density.[11] The physical demand of intense training in caloric deficit can overstress the body, driving nutrient deficiencies, and it may trigger chronic illnesses in people who have a genetic predisposition—as happened to Molly Galbraith.

Molly Galbraith's Show Prep Story

After four years of physique competition, Molly Galbraith developed extreme fatigue, and her body stopped responding to diet and exercise. It took a year for her to get diagnosed with Hashimoto's thyroiditis, polycystic ovarian syndrome, and adrenal dysfunction. She spent the next three years and over $20,000 on different practitioners to get her health back on track.

Usually, when original body fat levels are restored, leptin goes up and ghrelin goes down. However, for people who push their metabolism to the breaking point, such as these physique competitors, their ghrelin and NPY levels (more on this later in the chapter) may stay elevated for months or years. They often experience an insatiable appetite that eventually breaks their willpower and leads to weight gain.

We're not saying that it's impossible to get into great shape without metabolic destruction. However, very few people should enter physique competitions. Scott Abel believes that about 5 percent of the population has the genetics to get lean enough for a bodybuilding show without destroying metabolism. He often talks prospective clients out of competing if they are in it for the wrong reasons.

The other 95 percent of you can still get into fantastic shape, and this book has the strategies you need. You just won't be "peeled and shredded," as we say it in the bodybuilding world, with low, single-digit body fat (and most people don't even find it visually appealing).

These stories should serve as cautionary tales. The message is simple: you must ensure that your body feels safe throughout your weight loss journey, or it will fight back, because survival is its #1 objective.

The good news is that once you understand how to hack and optimize metabolic adaptation and avoid the starvation survival mechanisms, you can get into your dream shape without suffering negative health consequences. This is what we do with our private VIP clients.

WHY 97 PERCENT FAIL WITH THEIR LONG-TERM WEIGHT LOSS

Your body is an adaptation machine. The less you eat, the more your body reduces the energy it expends. And, the more you exercise, the more efficient the body becomes at that exercise (especially cardio). Thus, you will burn fewer calories as you repeat the same activities.

Cut your calories too far and too fast, and your body will activate its starvation survival mechanisms. These starvation survival effects are the reasons most dieters eventually regain the weight (like *The Biggest Loser* participants). Statistically, dieters regain over half of their lost weight within two years, and more than 80 percent within five years.[12]

Without an understanding of proper dieting and metabolism rebuilding, it's nearly impossible to maintain long-term results.

METABOLIC ADAPTATION: THE STARVATION SURVIVAL EFFECTS

Metabolic adaptation is your body's starvation survival mechanisms kicking in. This natural adaptation kept our ancient ancestors alive in times of famine. It's also what creates weight loss plateaus and drives weight regain.

Our physiology evolved for survival as hunter-gatherers when food was scarce. When the body undergoes metabolic adaptation, the following processes happen:

Leptin Drops

- Leptin is a hormone released by your fat cells; it sends signals to an area in the brain called the hypothalamus. It regulates food intake (by making you feel satiated) and energy expenditure. When you lose fat, your fat cells release less leptin. Your hypothalamus is the command center for sex hormones, cortisol, thyroid, and hunger hormones.
- Lowered leptin dials down sex and thyroid hormones while turning up your stress response and hunger hormones.

Testosterone Goes Down

- Many extreme dieters suffer from low testosterone and other hormone imbalances that lead to low sex drive and a major drop in anabolism (which lowers metabolism even further).[13, 14] It's not unusual for the natural testosterone in men to drop 70 to 80 percent during extreme dieting phases.[15] Anabolism is when your body is in a resourceful state for growth. When you're anabolic, it's easier to build and protect your precious lean muscle tissue. It's one of the most powerful layers of the Optimized Metabolism System (see Chapter 7).

Thyroid Activity Lowers

- Basal metabolic rate plummets as active thyroid hormone (T3) decreases.[16] A person can eat the same things and exercise the same way but still regain weight, because now baseline calorie expenditure has decreased. They may feel colder and more lethargic.

Movement (NEAT) Slows Down

- One of the most interesting discoveries in the last few years has been that most people with "faster" metabolism burn more calories via non-exercise activity thermogenesis (NEAT). This activity accounts for the calories people burn all day long as they live their lives: with restless legs, being animated with their arms, blinking, facial expressions, etc.
- One of the starvation survival effects is that your body slows down your NEAT. Most people aren't aware of it either. They just move less. Their body is preserving energy.[17, 18]

Hunger Hormones Increase

- Your body wants to store fat to prepare for future starvation periods by making you hungrier. Ghrelin—the opposite hormone to leptin—rises, so you will find that it takes monumental effort to resist the hunger and cravings that arise if you trigger the survival mechanisms. We call ghrelin the unbeatable hormone because eventually everyone succumbs to it. (Even Michael Jordan, who competed at around 3 percent body fat, famously said he wanted nothing more in retirement than to play golf and *grow a pot belly*.)
- Being hungry drains willpower. Ghrelin increases impulsivity and reward behavior.[19] It sensitizes neurons to dopamine.[20] As a result, you'll be more likely to consume hyper-palatable comfort foods and sugar just to get that potent dopamine hit. Fighting those impulses and cravings for these foods can drain a tremendous amount of willpower.
- An interesting experiment compared underweight, anorexic women to healthy women. Subjects were asked to choose between taking $20 immediately or $80 in 14 days. Both the anorexic and healthy women with higher ghrelin were more likely to choose the immediate $20 rather than to wait to get the $80.[21] In other words, ghrelin drives shortsighted decisions, which is how most people blow their diets.
- Key insight: ghrelin and hunger must be managed in order to succeed.

More of the Hungry (Shrunken) Fat Cells

- Compared to people who have always been the same size, previously fat people burn fewer calories and accumulate fat more easily.
- Weight loss shrinks fat cells, but the fat cells are still there, primed to store more fat and produce less overall leptin. In contrast, people who have always been at the same size have fewer fat cells, which are fuller and stable, and are less inclined to store more fat.[22]

The Number of Fat Cells Increases

- This is one of the most shocking recent discoveries. It was believed for decades that the only time the body created new fat cells was during phases of extended weight gain. The theory was that once existing fat cells were filled, new ones were created. It turns out that one way that the body fights back during deep weight *loss* cycles is to create *more* fat cells. Why? Because fat cells send *signals* to the brain and body. More fat cells mean more signals, maximizing odds of survival. Bidirectional communication exists between adipocytes (fat cells) and other tissues.[23] For example, fat cells produce peptides that can drive insulin resistance.
- The body produces fat cell precursors (preadipocytes) that can easily develop into fat cells once a calorie surplus becomes available.[24, 25] As soon as you start to eat more food, these cells quickly mature into small fat cells. This is the body priming itself for a weight rebound.
- With more small fat cells along with the other fat cells that you have just shrunken by losing weight, your body fat set point shifts as your fat cells—both new and old—strive to be as big as they were before all the weight loss.[26]
- Your brain also produces other hunger-stimulating signals, including neuropeptide Y (NPY). NPY is the most potent appetite-stimulating hormone known, sending signals of constant hunger. Researchers have discovered that NPY is what stimulates the replication of fat cell precursors that evolve into fat cells.
- Researcher Yaiping Yang says, "This may lead to a vicious cycle where NPY produced in the brain causes you to eat more and therefore gain more fat around your middle, and then that fat produces more NYP hormone which leads to even more fat cells."[27] This is believed to be one of the main reasons why many people gain *more* weight than they lost. They have more fat cells than they did before they started their weight loss journey.

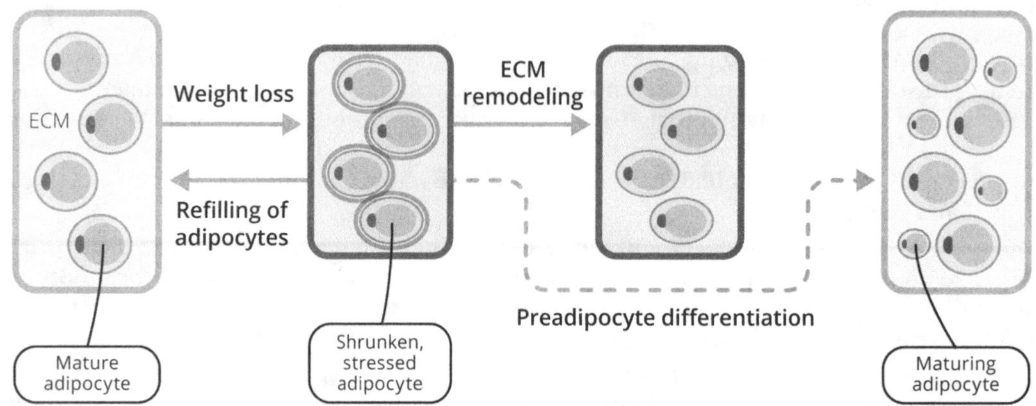

Fat loss stresses out the fat cells, which can cause them to trigger preadipocytes to develop into more new, small fat cells.[28]

Loss of Lean Muscle

- One of the body's self-defense mechanisms is to get rid of lean muscle. Why? Because lean muscle burns more energy. On average, for most dieters, 25 percent of the weight they lose is lean muscle tissue.[29] This is bad in many ways:
  - Your metabolism drops even further (muscle burns more calories).
  - You'll feel worse (being catabolic doesn't feel good). Catabolism is when your body is breaking down. You're losing valuable lean muscle tissue. You feel physically weak.
  - It can increase the amount of "weight" you need to lose to reach your goal.
  - It can harm your aesthetics (meaning you won't look as good). This appearance is also known as "the skinny-fat look."
- The aggressiveness of weight loss also impacts the loss of muscle. In one experiment, aggressive dieters lost more than double the amount of muscle than the less aggressive group.[30]
- It's worth noting that the best results have come from high-protein diets, which only had 11 percent lean muscle loss. This is why protein is the king macro when it comes to dieting (and muscle building). That's why we built several versions of Protein Breakthrough (including plant-based and keto versions) to help you with your weight loss journey.

SUMMARY

If you feel a bit unsettled by this chapter, then we did our job. If you feel lost and confused about what the solution is, don't worry. We've got you. The book will give you all the strategies you need to maximize your odds of success and win the Me Diet game.

We noted that 97 percent of people fail in their weight loss attempts because *starvation survival mechanisms* are built into our DNA.

The extended calorie deprivation that most people undergo to lose weight activates many self-defense mechanisms, and it's the reason many people fail with their weight loss objectives in the long term. Here's a list of the starvation survival effects the body activates:

- Lower leptin: Your fat cells release less of this hormone, which results in more hunger, more stress, less energy spent, and reduced thyroid and sex hormones.
- Lower testosterone: Natural testosterone can drop 70 to 80 percent during extreme dieting, which leads to lower sex drive and a huge drop in anabolism (muscle building) and slower metabolism.
- Lower thyroid function: Baseline calorie expenditure decreases, resulting in weight regain even while consuming the same calories and exercising. You'll feel cold and sluggish.
- Lower NEAT: To preserve more energy, your body moves less without you even noticing this change, resulting in fewer calories burned.

- Increased ghrelin (which increases hunger): This is the opposite hormone to leptin (the satiety hormone). Your cravings go up and you feel hungry all the time. It eventually breaks your willpower. This is your body attempting to store fat for future calorie-deprivation periods.
- Shrunken fat cells that store more fat: During weight loss, fat cells don't disappear; they simply shrink. And then they respond by producing less leptin and storing more fat.
- More fat cells: Your body fights back and prepares for survival by creating more fat cell precursors. And as soon as there's a surplus of calories, these mature and store fat.
- Loss of lean muscle mass: Lean muscle burns more energy, so the body destroys muscle to reduce energy expenditure. This results in a slower metabolism, negatively impacting the way you look. And it can lead to emotional issues. For most dieters, 25 percent of weight loss is lean muscle tissue.

These starvation survival effects are why progress slows down or completely stops. Extreme dieting and excessive exercise lead to metabolic destruction. And after the weight loss, the weight is regained.

Metabolic adaptation is our body's starvation survival mechanisms kicking in. It's what has kept humanity alive for thousands of years, but it's also why weight loss attempts fail. When our body undergoes metabolic adaptation, the less we eat, the less energy the body will spend. The more we exercise, the more efficient it will become and burn fewer calories.

The breakthrough strategy to achieve short- and long-term success is to *make the body feel safe throughout the journey* with refeeds, diet breaks, and reverse dieting. With these three tools, you can safely lose body fat permanently and avoid the yo-yo effect.

CHAPTER 2

WHY EVERY DIET WORKS . . . (FOR A WHILE)

This chapter is going to shatter some key diet myths and open your mind to some shocking facts about weight loss—and why every diet works (in the short term).

In this chapter you will learn:

- Only a few, coveted diets truly work for weight loss, right? *Wrong!* Learn the secret behind why every diet works for weight loss, at least for a short time.
- Some foods are evil, right? *Wrong!* Learn why it's critical for you to remove *junk food* from your vocabulary.
- Why focusing only on lowering your calories can lead to devastating results if not done properly.
- You can lose weight even by just eating Twinkies, Oreos, and Cheez-Its? We'll reveal more in this chapter.

WHY EVERY DIET WORKS

Let's start with some fundamentals.

There is one simple reason why every diet works.

Nutritional Truth Bomb #1: Every Diet with a Caloric Deficit Works

Every diet works because the laws of thermodynamics are immutable. Weight loss happens when you burn more calories than you eat. Obesity and the associated modern lifestyle diseases are a result of overconsumption. If "calories in" are less than "calories out," you will lose weight—at least in the short term.

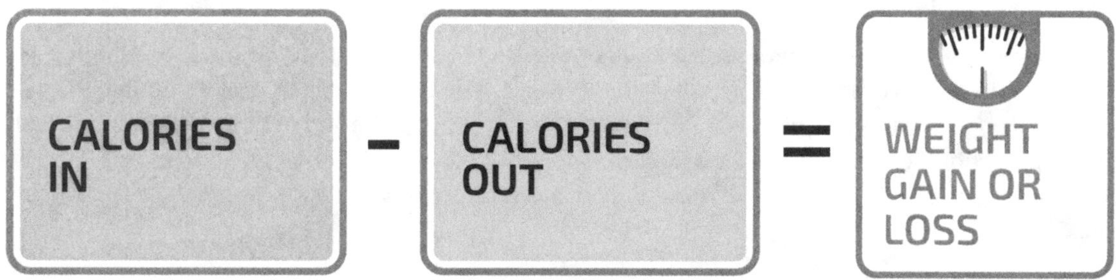

There are two camps when it comes to "calories in, calories out" (CICO).

The first camp preaches CICO as if that's all anyone needs to know to succeed with their diets. CICO has been marketed as "the" solution for decades; yet the majority of people are getting fatter. Focusing on CICO exclusively has epically failed the masses.

The second camp fights with the CICO camp. It wants to believe in magic. There has to be an ethereal weight loss factor somewhere: insulin, glucagon, hormones, ketones . . . *something*!

This fight is nonsensical (as most diet wars are), because they're both correct. CICO is an immutable law, *and* yes, many variables impact calorie expenditure (such as hormones, anabolism, etc.). We will cover those in depth in Chapter 7, The Optimized Metabolism.

A New Metabolic Model

As you see in the diagram below, there are several layers to "calories out." This book dives deep into a variety of ways that you can increase your calorie expenditure, because just focusing on lowering your calories can lead to devastating results if not done properly.

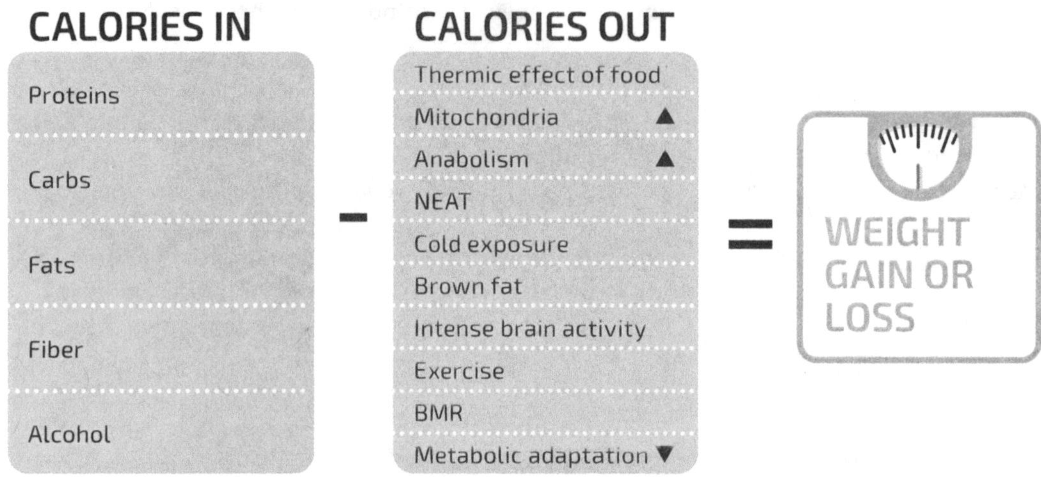

A few scientists and biohackers have done some extreme experiments to showcase the truth of CICO. We're not advocating any of the below activities. We're only sharing them to highlight the simple fact that when it comes to losing weight, *every diet works*.

Here are a few fascinating examples:

The Twinkie Diet Experiment

Mark Haub, an overweight nutrition professor at Kansas State University, tried the Twinkie Diet experiment. He ate only junk foods—Twinkies, Oreos, and Cheez-Its—for 10 weeks. The only catch was that he limited his calories to 1,800 calories a day, which was a significant caloric restriction for him. At the end of his experiment, he had lost 27 pounds. His "bad" cholesterol (LDL) and triglycerides also went down significantly.

The Twinkie Diet showed that caloric restriction *is* more important than food itself for weight loss in the short term.

The McDonald's Snake Diet

The *Super Size Me* documentary may have you thinking that fast foods like McDonald's will kill you. In the documentary, Morgan Spurlock ate 5,000 calories of McDonald's for 30 days. He gained 24 pounds, increased his cholesterol to 230 mg/dL, and developed fatty liver and sexual dysfunction.

Cole Robinson, a powerlifter and personal trainer, discovered that he felt great on alternate-day fasting and one meal a day. According to him, when he went from six meals a day to this fasting regimen, his training recovery accelerated and strength went up, even at the same macronutrient (protein, fat, and carbohydrate) content and caloric intake (around 3,000 calories per day).

He then decided to experiment with eating only McDonald's on a fasting regimen for 30 days. Again, he made sure to have the same macronutrient composition and calories as before.

Keep in mind, however, that he did this diet in a relatively healthy way. He ate a lot of salads and skipped the fries and soda. He also continued to work out and might have expended more calories by working out harder.

Fatty liver

Too much fat buildup in liver cells

At the end of 30 days, Robinson had gained bone density and lost a negligible amount of muscle mass while staying lean at 11 percent body fat. His inflammatory marker proteins (hs-CRP) even went down.

Robinson's story shows that junk food causes obesity if, and only if, you overeat it. It also shows that many health problems come from a surplus of calories. This leads to a critical point: there are no "evil" foods.

It's important to stop demonizing foods. Demonizing dietary choices leads to guilt and can lead to more serious psychological conditions. An unhealthy psychological relationship with "junk foods" creates stressful experiences when you eat them. It often leads to a binge and diet cycle driven by guilt, shame, and remorse.

A core goal of writing this book is that we want to help you remove all guilt and shame associated with eating, including enjoying junk food. Even the term *junk* should probably be eliminated from our vocabulary.

Are there foods that are healthier than others? Of course. However, if you want to enjoy a burger, a slice of pizza, an ice cream, or a cronut once in a while, you can, as long as it works within your overall dietary strategy. Even if you "fall off the wagon" and indulge, it's crucial to avoid beating yourself up.

There is an entire dietary group dedicated to this approach called If It Fits Your Macros (IIFYM), and many people report great success with it. You'll find more on this in Chapter 25.

Again, let's be clear: we are not advocating that you follow the Twinkie Diet or the McDonald's Snake Diet. These are just great examples of the point we're trying to make about weight loss here: we can't escape the laws of thermodynamics—that calories consumed minus calories burned equals weight gain or weight loss.

However, most CICO zealots aren't being very helpful by focusing on the physics of weight loss. People need a lot more than that to succeed. And we're going to give you *everything* you need to succeed.

We've Made Every Diet Work, by Matt Gallant

Between Wade and me, there aren't many diets we haven't done.

The first time I dieted at the age of 16, I used the Atkins Diet (a ketogenic approach) to go from 190 pounds to 147 pounds.

Then the bodybuilding bug bit me, and my goal was to build as much mass as possible. First, I used If It Fits Your Macros (IIFYM) to go from 147 to 175 pounds in one year. Then I switched to the Anabolic Diet (a cyclical ketogenic diet) and went from 147 pounds to 235 pounds. Then, I ate carnivore (a strict, meat-only form of keto) and lost 64 pounds in 14 weeks. In the last two decades, I've gone back and forth between keto and including carbs. Every diet worked. Some just worked better than others for me.

Over the years, Wade has gone from IIFYM to vegan to vegetarian to raw food and made every diet work.

We've done virtually every type of fasting.

We've made every diet work—some better than others. The question is: Which one is the best *for you*?

Nutritional Truth Bomb #2: Every Diet Is a Short-Term Antidote to the Standard American Diet

Going from the standard American diet (or the SAD, as it's affectionately known) to any other structured diet usually means an instant massive reduction in calories. Europe and North America consumed the most calories last year at 3,540 per day.[1] This is way beyond most people's calorie-burning capacity and thus why many are gaining weight.

Aside from its humongous portions, the standard American diet sets people up for overeating and obesity with:

- Hyper-palatable (sweet, salty, and fatty) foods that are engineered for overeating and comfort eating[2]
- Hunger-generating foods[3]
- Limitless food options around the clock[4]
- Mindless eating[5]
- Foods that are too high in toxins[6]
- Foods that are too low in some nutrients (such as omega-3 fats, vitamins, and minerals)[7]
- Promotion of fat-storing gut bacteria[8]
- Food engineered to activate serotonin and dopamine, which can create strong, hard-to-break food addictions[9,10]

Neurotransmitter

Any of a group of chemical agents released by neurons (nerve cells) to stimulate neighboring neurons or muscle or gland cells, thus allowing impulses to be passed from one cell to the next throughout the nervous system.

Serotonin

Is a monoamine neurotransmitter (aka 5-hydroxytryptamine). Its biological function is complex and multifaceted, modulating mood, cognition, reward, learning, memory, and numerous physiological processes such as vomiting and vasoconstriction.

Dopamine

A compound present in the body as a neurotransmitter and a precursor of other substances, including epinephrine. It's the molecule of motivation, drive and anticipation.

Nutritional Truth Bomb #3: New Diets Fix Deficiencies

Almost every diet is high in certain nutrients and low in micronutrients. For example, keto is naturally low in vitamin C but can be very high in other vitamins and minerals.

Micronutrient

These are vitamins and minerals required in trace amounts for the normal growth and development of living organisms. They are important co-factors in many critical biological functions.

Vegetarians and vegans have potential amino acid deficiencies, plus vitamin and mineral deficiencies such as those in vitamin B_{12}, vitamin A, and iron.

When people go on a new diet, they typically shift to a new and extreme way of eating. As an example, it's not uncommon for a vegan to experience an amino acid deficiency, feel bad, and then switch over to a keto or carnivore diet. Then they feel awesome because they now feed their body the aminos it has craved, experiencing an improvement in energy, overall well-being, and health.

But, as they stay on the new keto diet, they may develop a new set of nutrient deficiencies, and that's when their bodies might develop cravings and a drive to stop the diet.

Such deficiencies and toxicities usually take a few months to show up experientially. It can show up much earlier in blood tests and other biomarkers; however, it can take longer for people to start feeling ill.

When devising a nutritional strategy, it is important to test for and address your deficiencies. Your genetics also have a massive impact on this factor. If your body has certain genetic mutations (virtually everyone has a variety of nutrigenomic mutations), then you can be susceptible to certain deficiencies and toxicities. We strongly suggest you do our Nutritional Genetic test to learn incredibly valuable things about yourself. Go to: www.BIOptimizers.com/book/genes.

Nowadays, thanks to state-of-the-art tests such as SpectraCell, bloodwork, and genetic and microbiome testing, you can easily identify suboptimal nutrient levels.

The key is to intelligently design your diet to patch those deficiencies, plus use the right supplements. By doing that, you can make virtually every diet work long term.

Other Factors for Why Every Diet Works

- They usually increase protein, which increases "calories out" in two ways: the thermic effect of food intake, plus anabolism (muscle increase). Plus, protein increases satiety, which makes it easier to stay in a calorie deficit.
- They give people structure (vs. just eating what they "feel like").
- They give people *new* hope, bringing a temporary boost in motivation and drive.

SUMMARY

- Every diet works, as long as you're in a calorie deficit. So, what matters is to find one that works for you psychologically to maximize your odds of success. That's why this book explores the pros and cons of every fundamental diet—so you can choose the best one for you.
- Yes, "calories in, calories out" is a fundamental truth about how weight changes; however, the best approach is to focus on increasing "calories out" (and not just with exercise). To succeed, we need to understand much more than just the basic physics of weight loss.
- There are no evil foods. Let's stop beating ourselves up with shame, guilt, and fear when it comes to enjoying certain foods once in a while.
- Most health consequences from "junk food" come from simply overeating calories.
- Modern lifestyle diseases and obesity are a result of overconsumption.
- The standard American diet (SAD) leads to overeating and obesity with hyper-palatable foods (sweet, salty, and fatty), hunger-generating food, limitless food options, mindless eating, high toxins, low nutrients, more fat-storing gut bacteria, and food engineered to create hard-to-break addictions.
- Virtually every diet is a massive improvement compared to the standard American diet.
- Increased protein helps with weight loss by increasing anabolism, which burns more calories, lowers net calorie intake, and increases satiety. For these reasons, it's one of the main reasons that diets are improvements on the SAD.
- New diets create hope, which boosts motivation and drive.
- In the next chapter, we explore something even more valuable: why every diet fails.

CHAPTER 3

TOP 17 REASONS WHY MOST DIETS FAIL

The smartest path to success is to understand other people's mistakes and learn from them. Ignoring them and repeating the same mistakes over and over again is a form of insanity.

In this chapter, we're going to cover the 17 most common errors people make with diets in general (not just weight loss).

In the rest of the book, we're going to give you the antidotes to these mistakes, as well as all the strategies, tactics, and knowledge that you need to succeed.

In this chapter you'll learn:

- Diet breaks are evil, right? *Wrong!* Learn why diet breaks and refeeds are essential to keeping your goals on track by signaling to your body that it is *not* being threatened with starvation.
- Why the real challenge isn't the weight loss but rather the lifelong maintenance—and the five questions you need to ask yourself before starting an unsustainable diet.
- The four conditions that lead to trauma and how unprocessed traumas drive reactivity, escapism, resentments, fear, anger, and other destructive behaviors that impede your weight loss goals. The best tool for solving unresolved traumas that lead to subconscious and emotional eating.
- Two of the *most important* tools you can use to make your body *feel safe* when dieting so your starvation self-defense mechanisms don't kick in.
- The best tool for solving the unresolved traumas that lead to subconscious and emotional eating.

Studies have confirmed that long-term weight loss maintenance is extremely rare.[1, 2, 3] For the last few decades, only 3 percent have been able to achieve their weight loss goals long term. In our observation, that 3 percent is made up of extremely driven people who usually go "all in." This usually includes hiring coaches, trainers, nutritionists, and psychologists to maximize the odds of success.

By avoiding the 17 most common weight loss mistakes in this chapter and doing the opposite of each one, you will multiply your odds of success.

Let's dive in.

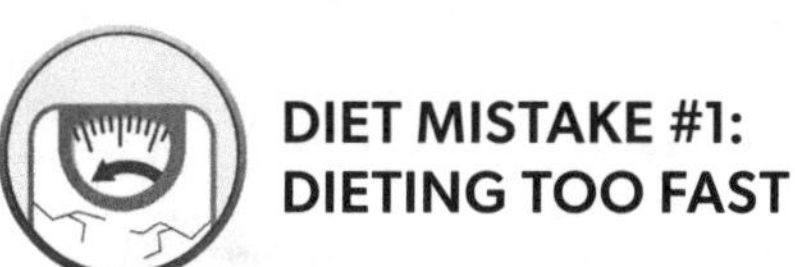

DIET MISTAKE #1: DIETING TOO FAST

Let's start with *the* fundamental reason for almost all weight loss failures: dieting too quickly.

So-called 12-week transformations and other short-term diet goals are some of the main culprits for these weight loss failures.

The faster you lose body fat and the more fat you lose, the harder your body fights back. The speed of weight loss seems to be the main trigger. As we saw in Carl the Caveman's example, losing too much body fat too fast activates your starvation self-defense mechanisms, and that's when you're basically screwed.

Can you lose body fat quickly? Yes, to a certain point. However, diet breaks should be incorporated strategically every few weeks to let the body know that *it's safe* (meaning that it won't starve to death).

Do not sacrifice your future for short-term gains. As an example, if you've got 50 pounds to lose, give yourself a year—even two. It will make the journey more enjoyable and maximize your odds of success.

The key is to develop long-term vision. Playing the tape forward is a valuable mental process that you can use in a variety of ways to get you out of your short-term desires.

Imagine two futures:

Future #1: You go all in and cut your calories severely, train like a pro athlete, and lose a bunch of weight over the next three months. Then you experience the starvation survival effects: Your metabolism drops, your hunger goes out of control, and you quit. Fast-forward a few months: you've regained all the weight you dropped, and you've given up on your aesthetic goals.

Future #2: You lose weight intelligently and take a bit more time to do it. You actually get to enjoy a better lifestyle than the hardcore dieter. Your body feels safe, and you get to your dream goal and stay there for the rest of your life.

Which future sounds better? Choose carefully.

In summary, avoid:

- The latest Hollywood diet fad and the "12-week transformations." These set you up for a brutal weight regain.
- Intense, massive training programs. These set you up for injuries and quitting.

DIET MISTAKE #2: NO DIET BREAKS OR REFEEDS

Diet breaks and refeeds are two of the most important tools to prevent starvation survival effects from kicking in. They help the body feel safe by giving it enough calories and avoid the fast track to metabolic adaptation. When your body eats at maintenance or above, it's no longer threatened by starvation.

Strategically using these tools makes all the difference in the world for extended fat loss journeys.

Diet breaks are when you eat at maintenance (usually for a week or two). They help keep your metabolism running faster during weight loss cycles.

Refeeds are when you consume higher calories for one or two days a week. As long as your weekly calories are in a deficit, you'll lose body fat. Make sure to track your overall calories and not to overeat on the weekends. You can easily blow five days of progress in a day or two.

Refeeds are also known as *cheat days* or *cheat meals*, but we don't like those terms. They imply that you're off track and breaking the rules. When they're well designed and an intentional part of your game plan, you're *not* cheating. You're just refeeding your body.

Many diets that have shown good results have incorporated weekly refeeds: Scott Abel's Cycle Diet, Dr. Mauro DiPasquale's Anabolic Diet, Bill Phillips's Body for Life, and Tim Ferriss's Slow Carb diet. There are many benefits to these, and we will cover them in Chapter 32.

The 11-Month Zombie Lifestyle, by Wade T. Lightheart

One of the most intense, focused times in my life was when I was preparing for the Mr. Universe contest. I ate an incredibly strict diet of rice cakes, potatoes, whey protein, and salad for 11 straight months. I experienced constant digestive distress, felt lethargic, and just thought, "It's normal. I'm dieting."

After a few months, my brain function started to decline. I remember walking into the gym and Matt asking me, "How's it going, bro?" All I could muster was, "Another day in paradise, man!"

My brain was on autopilot, and my ability to focus and think was severely compromised. The main mistakes I made were not taking any diet breaks and taking almost zero refeeds. This set me up for the massive 42-pound rebound after the show.

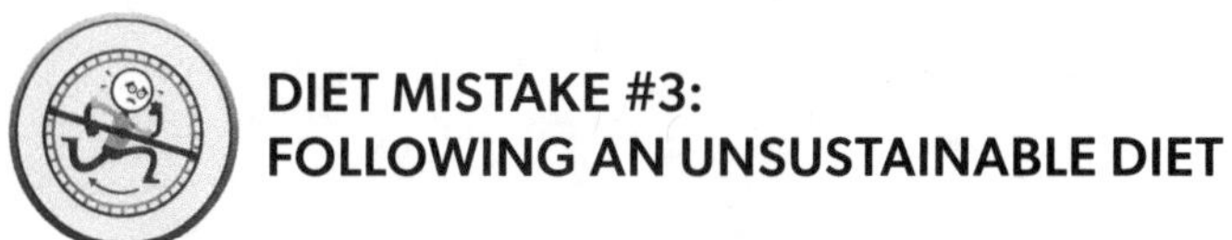

DIET MISTAKE #3: FOLLOWING AN UNSUSTAINABLE DIET

Unsustainable diets take many shapes and forms.

- Are you giving up foods that you love?
- Are you forcing yourself to eat foods you don't enjoy?
- Are you too hungry?
- Are you nutrient deficient?
- Is the diet psychologically or spiritually misaligned with your core values?

Can you follow a strict, unsustainable diet for a short time and achieve great results? Yes! Anyone with a bit of willpower can cut calories using drastic measures, but the real question is: What's next? What are you going to do after that?

If you choose to do an unsustainable diet, just make sure that you've got another dietary strategy lined up after it. Otherwise, you're setting yourself up for guaranteed failure. To be successful *for life*, you must find a nutritional philosophy that you can follow *for life*.

One important factor to keep in mind is: what is unsustainable today might become your favorite way to eat tomorrow.

This book is going to give you virtually every viable possibility and the best practices so that you can consciously choose and build the best diet for you.

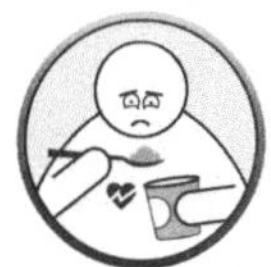

DIET MISTAKE #4: NOT RESOLVING UNDERLYING EMOTIONAL TRAUMAS AND ISSUES

Most people who are overweight use food as a drug. People with food issues use food to escape the emotional pain or boredom they're feeling. This is because food has druglike effects on both dopamine and serotonin.

Healing traumas that affect your nervous system is just as important as eliminating the Ben & Jerry's from your freezer.

When most people hear the word *trauma*, they imagine horrific experiences. However, many experts in the field call such horrific experiences "big-T" Trauma. Not everyone has had those. But virtually everyone carries what experts call "little-t" trauma.

There are four conditions that lead us to feel traumatized:

- We experience a painful event
- We experience an unexpected event
- We feel alone
- We don't have the resources to process emotional pain

Most people keep accumulating traumas for their entire lives because they don't learn to process pain as it happens. They just keep suppressing it.

We cannot escape our traumas. We can only suppress them for so long. Unprocessed trauma drives reactivity, escapism, resentments, fear, anger, and other destructive behaviors. This is because trauma embeds itself in the body. Bessel van der Kolk's *The Body Keeps the Score* is probably the best book on this topic.

Matt and Wade have spent weeks of their lives using a variety of processes and technologies to permanently eliminate the traumas from their nervous systems; their peace and happiness rose exponentially as a result.

The key is to do a deep inventory of emotional issues and systematically clear them using tools such as the Emotional Freedom Techniques (EFT; also known as "tapping"), forgiveness work, neurofeedback, eye movement desensitization and reprocessing (EMDR), or other modalities.

Does healing trauma really help with weight loss? Yes, it does.

In a one-year trial conducted by Dawson Church, one of the world's leading EFT researchers, people lost between 11 and 22 pounds in the year using tapping. More importantly, they kept it off. The emotional impulses to escape with food had been removed.

DIET MISTAKE #5: NOT TRACKING FOOD CALORIES, MACROS, SLEEP, AND EXERCISE

This one is a mixed bag. Can you lose weight without measuring food and tracking calories? Yes, especially early on. As we covered in the previous chapter, just going from a standard American diet to any kind of structured diet usually leads to a significant calorie deficit (and therefore weight loss).

Most people underestimate the calories they're eating by 40 percent.[4] And then they wonder why they're not losing weight.

They unconsciously sneak in calories in a variety of ways: a handful of nuts here, a tablespoon of peanut butter there, a piece of chocolate after dinner, etc. (Note: unconscious eating is one of the body's starvation survival effects.) There's nothing wrong with those little snacks if they're part of your plan, but they can be the difference between losing weight and becoming stuck.

You can't improve what you don't measure. It's critical to create feedback loops (more on this in Chapter 32).

It's easy to lose weight in the beginning by making a few simple diet or exercise changes. However, this won't last forever. As you go further down the path, precise changes and decisions need to be made. It becomes a guessing game if you don't track inputs and outputs.

That said, many people *can* lose a significant amount of weight without calculating every calorie. Wade prefers eyeballing portion management with weekly weight tracking to see if he's losing or gaining body fat. Keep in mind that Wade has decades of experience and did spend many years weighing and measuring. Getting down to a world-class level of body fat is rarely possible without getting hyper precise.

Just as all Fortune 500 companies have world-class accounting practices, all high-performance athletes apply world-class tracking to their physiology. If you want to be in the 3 percent of people who manage their weight easily for life, putting accountability in place will shorten the time you take to get there. In fact, it might be the only way to get there and stay there.

The good news is that you may only have to measure for a few days. Then, if you're applying the Simplest Diet Secret (Chapter 9), it's easy to tweak portion sizes without measuring. Another option is to employ meal-prep companies that do all the measuring for you.

However, if your goal is to move to a superhuman level of aesthetics, we strongly suggest outsourcing the design of your diet to an expert and then tracking your calories. Hire a coach or nutritionist who does the math for you and simply tells you what to eat. Read on.

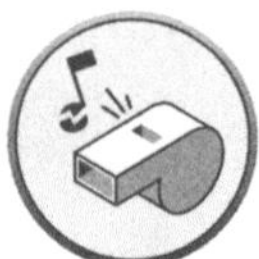

DIET MISTAKE #6: NO COACHING OR ACCOUNTABILITY IN PLACE

This might sound surprising, but you can't trust yourself when it comes to keeping yourself accountable in your weight loss journey. Why?

There are two primary reasons:

- The odds of you creating the right strategy are low unless you're a deep expert.
- Your starvation self-defense mechanisms can easily override your conscious mind. This is the big one, even for people like us.

Even though we *are* deep experts, we don't even trust ourselves to stay accountable like an outside authority can. Why?

Because:

- We can simply slack off with easier training plans (like not including things like squats and deadlifts).
- We can resist cutting calories when we should cut them.

- We can fail to add new things that we need to keep results flowing (like adding in a second workout).
- We can slide totally off course after one "slip"—if we have a bad day, or a bad week, we need a coach to get us refocused.

So, we're no exceptions to the rule.

Despite being experts in this field, we hire coaches to help us design our diets. Why? Because we know we can't trust our own minds—we're aware of all the starvation self-defense mechanisms and the tricks they can play. The diet boogeyman is real.

The starvation survival effects are numerous, and each of us can trigger a different set. But our point is universal: Get a coach! Preferably, find a good one that you bond with, who supports you and knows what they're doing.

One of the most powerful principles of success is to stack every advantage you can. Coaching and accountability are the most powerful advantages anyone can have. A great coach will help motivate you, solve your problems, and create a winning strategy.

We go into great depth on this in the "Jedi Council" appendix in our *From Sick to Superhuman* book.

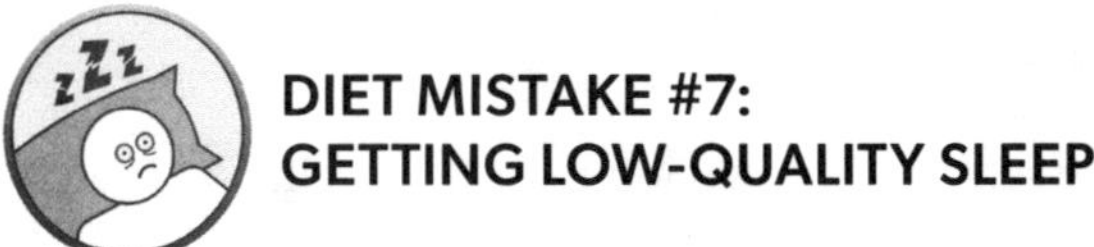

DIET MISTAKE #7: GETTING LOW-QUALITY SLEEP

What are the consequences of bad sleep for dieting?

The short answer is that you're going to get fatter, lose muscle, destroy your willpower, be in a horrible mood, and crash your immune system.[5]

Low-quality sleep makes losing weight many times harder. Your hunger hormones go up, your cravings increase, you start burning lean muscle mass instead of body fat, your willpower goes down, and your fat-burning hormones (HGH and testosterone) go down.

HGH

Human growth hormone is a peptide hormone that stimulates growth, cell reproduction, and cell regeneration in humans.

The groups who consistently had *less* sleep had higher levels of catabolic (muscle-destroying) hormones such as cortisol, and they also had lower levels of anabolic (muscle-building) hormones such as testosterone and insulin-like growth factor (IGF-1). There's more on this in point #17 at the end of this chapter.

Research has shown that low levels of sleep (5.5 hours nightly) significantly raise your body's respiratory exchange ratio (RER). This means your weight loss is going to be more muscle and less fat. This is the last thing you want.

The short-sleep research study referred to above was done on 10 overweight adults.[6] Over two weeks, the group getting 5.5 hours of sleep per night lost 55 percent less fat and 60 percent more muscle than the group getting 8.5 hours. Beyond this, the group getting 5.5 hours also reported greater cravings than the group getting 8.5 hours. *Cravings kill diets.* Levels of the hunger hormone, ghrelin, increased by 28 percent.[7] Our goal in any intelligently designed diet is to manage ghrelin and ideally lower it, not increase it.

If you can't manage hunger and cravings, your odds of success with any diet are close to zero. Sleep deprivation can easily lead to out-of-control food cravings.

We could write an entire book on the consequences of bad sleep. The point is that optimizing your sleep is one of the greatest investments you'll ever make. Great sleep levels you up in virtually every area of your life.

We repeat: great sleep is one of the biggest make-or-break factors for anyone trying to lose weight. Tackling your weight while sleeping poorly is like entering an ass-kicking contest with a broken leg. It's tough.

We suggest reading our in-depth chapter on optimizing your sleep in our book *From Sick to Superhuman.*

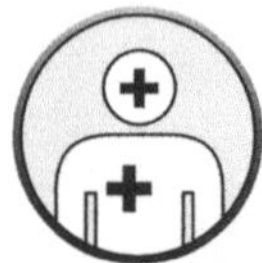

DIET MISTAKE #8: NOT ADDRESSING OTHER HEALTH PROBLEMS

You could call ignoring other health problems an indirect cause of diet failure. But the right diet will make you *healthier.* Underlying problems such as hormonal issues, thyroid issues, gut issues, fatty liver, and much more can make losing body fat and getting healthy a tough journey.

If your thyroid function drops too much, weight loss will become extremely difficult, if not impossible.

If your body isn't producing enough testosterone and growth hormones, your metabolism will slow down and your athletic performance will drop.

The point here is to make being *healthy* a primary goal and a guiding light for your "Me Diet."

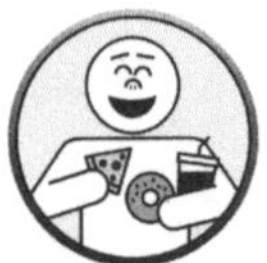

DIET MISTAKE #9: LOSING MENTAL VIGILANCE

Loss of mental vigilance is one of the main causes of long-term dietary failure. Once you lose mental vigilance, it's usually the beginning of the end.

People stop paying attention to their weight. They stop tracking calories and macros and unconsciously start increasing calories. It's easy to drop exercise habits and default to old eating habits. Food quality selection goes down.

Maybe the most fatal of all is that people get rid of their coaches. Great coaches help maintain your mental vigilance. They call you out when they see your behavior slipping. They help bring back awareness when it starts drifting away.

Do you know when you need the most mental vigilance around weight loss? *After* you've achieved your goal. Why?

First, that is the most dangerous point at which starvation survival effects start kicking in. Hunger usually goes into overdrive. Your motivation can drop massively after you achieve a significant goal.

Your body releases dopamine—a neurotransmitter responsible for happiness and motivation—when you're working toward a goal and any time you hit a milestone along the way. It's the chemical release that keeps you moving forward. But when your goal is reached, the neurotransmitter drops.[8, 9]

The Price of Losing Mental Vigilance, by Matt Gallant

Something I've learned one too many times is the cost of losing mental vigilance. I remember dieting for months, losing 30 pounds, and thinking, *Boom, baby! I did it!* Fast-forward a few weeks post diet, and the weight climb began. Fast-forward a few months, and I had regained almost all of it.

Even losing mental vigilance for a week has set me back *months.* I had been dieting for months to lose about 20 pounds. I went to visit my parents, stopped being mindful about calories, and gained back 10 pounds in 10 days. Yes, some of that was water, but there was definitely some fat in there. It took me eight weeks to get back to where I had been.

At this point in our journey, Wade and I have accepted and embraced mental vigilance for life. We don't want to have to do extended, arduous diets ever again.

As we've noted, in our opinion, the most important part of your weight loss journey starts *after* you've achieved your goal. This is when you need a great strategy to:

- Intelligently reverse diet out of your deficit practice without regaining weight.
- Find the ultimate sustainable lifestyle.
- Create new goals that will keep you focused.

Again, a great coach will help you with all of the above.

The point is never to drop your guard. Weigh yourself every day. Studies on people who have lost weight confirm that those who keep it off weigh themselves daily.[10, 11]

Get a body fat scan once or twice a year. Take pictures regularly. Join health communities. Get bloodwork twice a year. Hire coaches. Get accountability buddies. Find fun workout partners. Stack the odds of success in your favor.

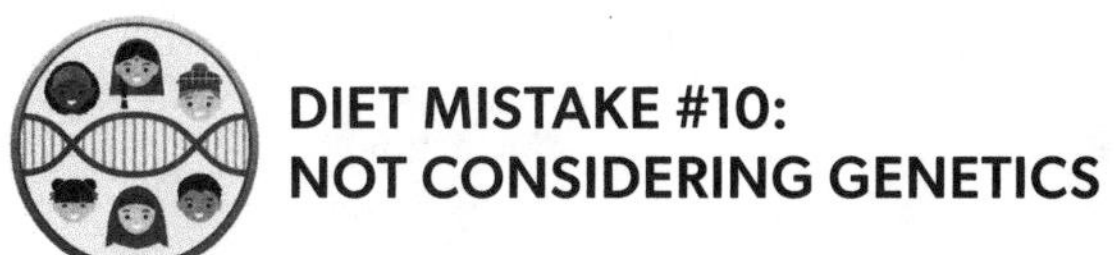

DIET MISTAKE #10: NOT CONSIDERING GENETICS

Diet fanatics are often so dogmatic about the diet that works for them that they force it on all their clients and social media followers. There is little to no consideration of individual genetics.

Nutrigenomics is the science of nutrition and genes. This is one of the most exciting new fields of health and nutrition. It's still early; however, massive amounts of research and discoveries are coming out at an accelerated rate.

Some people are genetically superior fat-burners, so they feel great with a ketogenic diet. Others who don't have the same genes struggle to enter ketosis and feel stressed on that system.

Some people feel amazing while they're fasting. Others become stressed, their HRV crashes, their cortisol goes up, and they enter a catabolic state (meaning that they're losing precious lean muscle tissue).

Your genetics and constitution also affect your body shape and tendency to store fat, which you should take into account when you set your aesthetic goals.

Without individualization, the one-diet-fits-all method can end up forcing square pegs into round holes. Working against your genes will always be an uphill battle.

We will go in depth on how you can use nutrigenomics to maximize your odds of success in Chapter 33. To learn more about your personal nutrigenomics, go to: www.BIOptimizers.com/book/genes.

Genetics

The science of heredity, dealing with resemblances and differences of related organisms resulting from the interaction of their genes and the environment.

Ketosis

A metabolic state characterized by raised levels of ketone bodies in the body tissues, which is typically pathological in conditions such as diabetes, or may be the consequence of a diet that is very low in carbohydrates.

Endocrine disruptor

A natural or synthetic chemical that mimics or blocks the action of a natural hormone and that may disrupt the body's endocrine system.

Obesogenic

Tends to cause obesity.

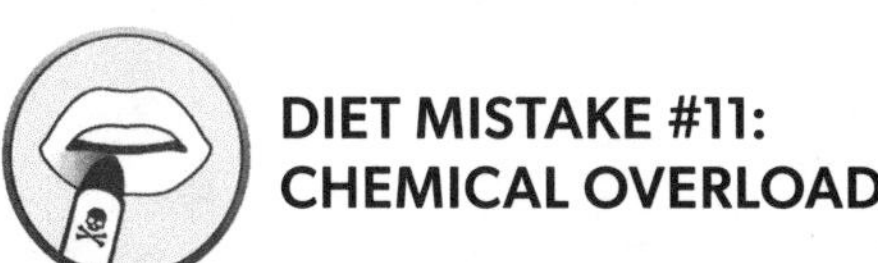

DIET MISTAKE #11: CHEMICAL OVERLOAD

Another indirect (but crucial) health factor is an overload of chemicals, which can negatively impact a variety of organs and systems in the body. This can lead to loss of energy, affecting metabolism.

Enzyme

A substance produced by a living organism, which acts as a catalyst to bring about a specific biochemical reaction.

Biome

A major ecological community of organisms adapted to a particular climatic or environmental condition on a large geographic area in which they occur.

Protein

Any of a class of nitrogenous organic compounds that consist of large molecules composed of one or more long chains of amino acids and are an essential part of all living organisms, especially as structural components of body tissues such as muscle, hair, collagen, etc., and as enzymes and antibodies.

Amino acid

The building block of muscles, neuro transmitters, peptides, and organs.
A simple organic compound containing both a carboxyl (—COOH) and an amino ($—NH_2$) group.

Metabolites

Any substance produced during metabolism (digestion or other bodily chemical processes). The term *metabolite* may also refer to the product that remains after a drug is broken down (metabolized) by the body.

Leaky gut

Also known as increased intestinal permeability, is a digestive condition in which bacteria and toxins can "leak" through the intestinal wall.

An average human in 2020 was being exposed to over 80,000 man-made chemicals.

A 2009 study by the Environmental Working Group found more than 200 toxic chemicals in cord blood samples from newborns. A woman who uses body care and beauty products could be exposed to more than 500 toxic chemicals before she leaves the house in the morning.

Studies of lab rodents have shown that it takes only one endocrine disruptor to cause obesity, even if the animals eat the same amount of food.[12]

Thousands of obesogenic chemicals are lurking in your home, office, air, food, and products you put on your skin. Studies have found these substances in human blood, sweat, urine, and fat cells.

These man-made chemicals can elevate your metabolic set point by:

- Disrupting the functions of sex hormones, thyroid, leptin, and insulin[13]
- Causing prolonged, low-grade chronic inflammation[14]
- Increasing micronutrient use and excretion, which may cause or worsen deficiencies
- Inhibiting digestive and cellular enzyme activity
- Throwing off your gut biome

These changes can lead to obesity, metabolic syndrome, autoimmune disorders, autism, infertility, and even mental health disorders.

Therefore, if your goal is to be biologically optimized and achieve long-term results, you must actively work on detoxifying your body and lowering your toxic burden, including in your food, your body, and your environment.

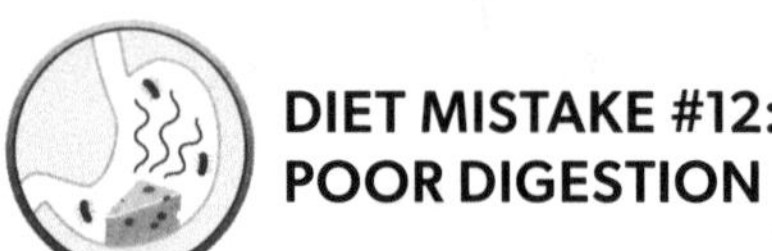

DIET MISTAKE #12: POOR DIGESTION

Poor digestion is another indirect contributor to dietary failures.

One of the keys to finding the right nutritional approach for you is to look for what makes you feel *great*. Feeling great helps you have more energy, drive, and motivation. Poor digestion can make it hard or impossible to feel awesome and thus impact your results. Not feeling great can easily lead you to quit a diet.

Suboptimal digestion—such as from enzyme deficiencies, low stomach acid, and an unhealthy gut biome—leaves more undigested food particles that can stimulate the immune system and feed bad gut bacteria. This condition can also lead to food allergies and sensitivities, and allow yeasts and parasites to grow.

Poor digestion can also lead to inflammation, which can impact your entire body.

Undigested proteins can lead to negative immune system responses (this is what allergies are). Protein and amino acid fermentation can often generate inflammatory or toxic metabolites.[15] You'll find more on this in the next point.

Our approach to solving these problems is simple:

Optimize your digestion with enzymes, probiotics, and HCl (included in many BIOptimizers digestive formulas). We will cover the process in great depth in Chapter 28.

When your digestion is optimized, you feel great, you have more energy, and you'll be more excited to keep going.

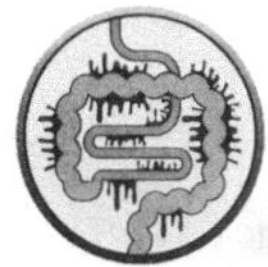

DIET MISTAKE #13: LEAKY GUT, FOOD SENSITIVITIES, AND FOOD ALLERGIES

This point is an extension of the previous one. Being biologically optimized is critical for feeling your best. That's why it's important to remove foods that are toxic and stressful to your body.

One person's "superfood" is another person's toxin. There are some powerful tests that will reveal your own personal superfoods. We will cover those in Chapter 31.

Perhaps one of the biggest drivers of chronic diseases is *metabolic endotoxemia*—being poisoned by toxins in bacterial cell walls. A leaky gut, caused by the typical modern diet and lifestyle—along with *dysbiosis* (bad bacteria causing gut issues)—can lead to metabolic endotoxemia.

Gluten
A general name for the proteins found in wheat, rye, barley, and triticale.

Zonulin pathway
Also known as haptoglobin 2 precursor, this is a protein that modulates the permeability of tight junctions between cells of the wall of the digestive tract.

Non-celiac
A clinical entity induced by the ingestion of gluten leading to intestinal and/or extraintestinal symptoms.

Casein
A protein found in milk and other dairy products.

Peptides
Short chains of between two and fifty amino acids, linked by peptide bonds.

Hypothalamus
A region of the brain, between the thalamus and the midbrain, that functions as the main control center for the autonomic nervous system by regulating sleep cycles, body temperature, appetite, etc. It also acts as an endocrine gland by producing hormones, including the releasing factors that control the hormonal secretions of the pituitary gland.

Many common foods in the modern diet can open up the gut barrier, such as:

- Gluten, which can activate the zonulin pathway and open up the gut barrier, even in people without celiac
- Industrial food additives, such as food texturizers
- Excess amounts of sugar or salt[16]
- Casein from A1 milk causing digestive issues and partially digested peptides being absorbed into the blood[17]

If you are healthy, your gut should be able to recover from these just fine.

However, for those with low-grade inflammation and dysbiosis, a leaky gut can expose undigested food and bacteria toxins to the immune system. They then develop food sensitivities, food allergies, and metabolic endotoxemia, causing more inflammation.

The inflammation leads to leptin resistance and many modern ailments. A leptin-resistant brain is a starved brain in a fat body. It cannot sense that your body is well fed, so you continue to be hungry while your hypothalamus reduces all nonessential energy expenditures.

In other words, diets that don't remove sources of inflammation and repair leaky guts tend to not produce sustainable results for these people.

Biome

A complex biotic community characterized by distinctive plant and animal species and maintained under the climatic conditions of the region, especially such a community that has developed to climax.

Fiber

Also known as bulk and roughage, this is made up of plant components that are not broken down by human digestive enzymes.

Polyphenol

Any of a group of naturally occurring compounds found significantly in fruits, vegetables, cereals, coffee, tea, and wine, and widely studied for properties believed to promote health and fight disease.

In Chapter 29, we cover gut biome BIOptimization, which studies have shown to strengthen your gut barrier and fix metabolic endotoxemia.[18] In Chapter 31, we cover tests for leaky gut and food sensitivities.

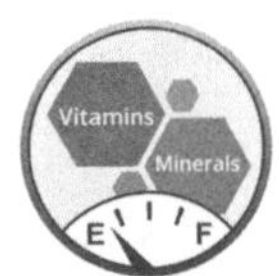

DIET MISTAKE #14: VITAMIN, MINERAL, AND NUTRIENT DEFICIENCIES

Many diets can lead to a variety of nutrient deficiencies unless they're properly designed. We will cover those in great depth as we review each type of diet and outline its potential pitfalls.

Nutrient deficiencies can affect the body in multiple ways, but the two most significant ones are:

- Systems in the body can become compromised. For example, your thyroid can become less active and thus lower your metabolism if you're deficient in iodine.
- You just quit.

There are two ways that nutrient deficiencies can cause people to quit. First, a deficiency can cause the body to produce certain cravings because it wants you to patch the problem. You may crave minerals and grab a bag of salty, high-calorie snacks. You might crave amino acids and go eat a burger. A key focus for any successful diet is to minimize cravings.

Second, when people don't feel good on a diet, they quit. If you don't feel great on yours, you're on the wrong diet or you're doing the diet wrong. Your personal, subjective feedback of how you feel on a diet is crucial. Trust your biofeedback. Once you find your Me Diet that is optimized for your mind and body, you will feel awesome.

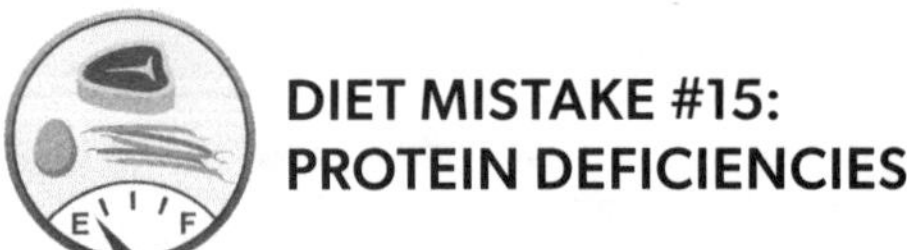

DIET MISTAKE #15: PROTEIN DEFICIENCIES

Amino acids—and therefore protein—are literally the building blocks of life. Many scientists believe that around 4 billion years ago, a miraculous dance of molecules came together into amino acids, which made life as we know it possible.[19]

Your body needs amino acids to thrive. When you eat protein, your body breaks it down into amino acids using enzymes.

Amino acids rebuild muscle tissue, peptides, neurotransmitters, organs, and much more. When it comes to dieting for weight loss, muscle building, or athletic performance, protein is the king macronutrient.

Most effective diets are higher in protein because protein is more satiating and has a higher thermogenic effect. The standard American diet is too high in fat and carbohydrates and too low in quality protein.

Calorie for calorie, protein breakdown takes 30 percent more energy to digest and assimilate than carbs and fats. In other words, if you replaced 1,000 calories of carbs and fats with the same number of protein calories, you'd be burning an additional 300 calories a day. That's an extra deficit of 300 calories a day just by eating a different macronutrient. That's a lot.

Carbohydrate

Any of a large group of organic compounds occurring in foods and living tissues and including sugars, starch, and cellulose. Carbohydrates contain hydrogen and oxygen in the same ratio as water (2:1) and typically can be broken down to release energy in the animal body.

Protein is also muscle-sparing if you are in a caloric deficit. The importance of this cannot be overstated. When you're losing body fat, protecting your lean muscle tissue is one of your top priorities.

And if you are trying to *gain* lean muscle mass, protein is essentially the main macronutrient you want. Protein feedings stimulate muscle growth.

When you shift from protein deficiency to optimal protein consumption, you'll get significant results, both in terms of fat loss and muscle building.

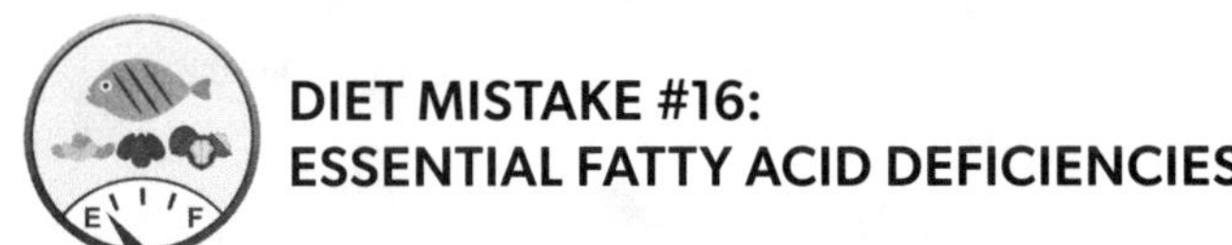

DIET MISTAKE #16: ESSENTIAL FATTY ACID DEFICIENCIES

There's one more essential macro: fat. Most people are overconsuming the wrong type of fats and are extremely deficient in essential fatty acids (EFAs). EFAs are the most important type of fats to focus on.

The standard American diet, and even most weight loss diets, are too high in omega-6 and too low in omega-3. This imbalance increases inflammation and reduces insulin sensitivity. Your health can improve radically when you balance inflammatory omega-6s with anti-inflammatory omega-3s.

Fats are another building block of the body—they literally become part of you. Hormones, brain, hair, skin, organs, and other tissues all use fats to build themselves. That's why selecting high-quality fats and minimizing bad fats tends to create a big improvement in lipid profiles and brain function.

The two primary fat factors to focus on are:

1. Optimizing your fats based on the diet you choose
2. Being mindful of your genetic mutation related to fat metabolism

When Wade dieted for 11 months straight on an extremely fat-deficient diet, his brain function tanked. He walked around like a zombie, operating on fumes and willpower.

Genetics are crucial in selecting the best fats for your body. Generic statements like "coconut oil is the best fat" and "saturated fats are evil" are uninformed opinions. Analyze your nutrigenomics to help find the best fats for your body. This can have a massive impact on your results.

For example, vegetarians and vegans need to be more vigilant to make sure they're getting enough docosahexaenoic acid (DHA, one of the EFAs). DHA is critical for brain function, eyes, reproductive function, and much more. Yes, the body can convert some of the alpha-linolenic acid (ALA) from seeds into DHA and EPA, but not efficiently. Microalgae is a much better source because it can help prevent cardiovascular, inflammatory, and nervous system conditions.[20]

Bottom line: optimize the fats based on your chosen diet and genetics. To learn more about your fat-burning genetics, go to: www.BIOptimizers.com/book/genes.

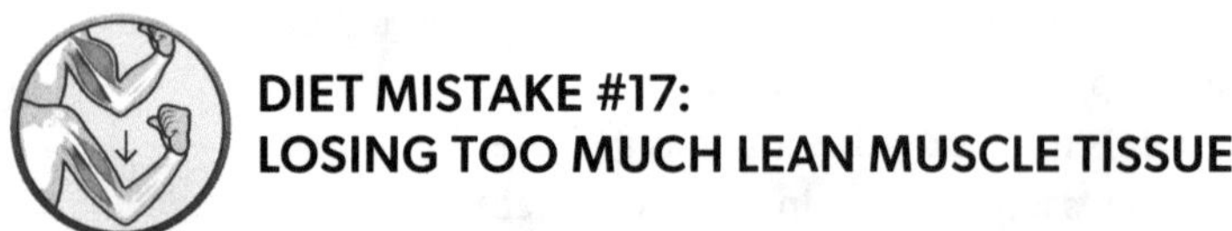

DIET MISTAKE #17: LOSING TOO MUCH LEAN MUSCLE TISSUE

This is absolutely one of the biggest problems with many people's overall approach to weight loss. They don't have the right strategy to preserve their vital lean muscle tissue as they lose weight.

Why is that so important?

Because lean muscle tissue has the following key benefits:

- It improves aesthetics. Virtually everyone looks better carrying more lean muscle mass. Their proportions are more attractive. That being said, how someone's body looks is 100 percent their own personal preference. Only a fraction of the population wants to look like a professional bodybuilder. We suggest becoming conscious of what your *ultimate* aesthetics are. Does a certain celebrity, athlete, or bodybuilder inspire you with their body aesthetic?
- It helps to store glucose. Muscles are fantastic carb storage units. The more muscles you carry, the more glycogen (carbs that have been broken down) you can store. This helps prevent blood-sugar-related health problems.
- It increases your basal metabolic rate. This means you have a faster metabolism. Each pound of fat-free weight has been calculated to use about 8 to 15 calories per day.[21]
- Muscles are vital for movement. Whether you're a professional athlete or an elderly person, muscles are what allow you to move in the world. And when you get older, they're a lifesaver.

Professor Claudio Gil Araújo followed 3,878 people for 6.5 years. The participants in the weakest quartile had a risk of dying that was 10 to 13 times higher than that of those in the top 3rd or 4th quartile. As you get older, the quality of your life becomes highly correlated with your lean muscle mass and strength.[22]

Leg strength is what determines whether you:

- Fall down easily
- Cross the street quickly
- Can carry your groceries
- Can go up and down stairs easily

One of our unique approaches with VIP clients that helps create world-class results is to focus on anabolism even when their goal is to lose body fat.

Don't confuse anabolism with anabolic steroids. Anabolism is simply the process of using the energy from food—after it has been broken down—to carry out other actions within the body. More anabolism means your body has increased protein turnover. It means it's building more lean muscle tissue. And the more anabolic you are, the more calories you're going to burn all day long.

SUMMARY

Only 3 percent of dieters achieve their weight loss goals long term. Here are 17 of the most common reasons 97 percent of people fail:

1. *Dieting too fast.* If you lose too much body fat too fast, it will activate the starvation survival effects that make your metabolism drop, increase hunger, and overthrow your willpower.
2. *No diet breaks or refeeds.* These strategies help your body feel safe and prevent the starvation survival effects.
3. *Following an unsustainable diet.* You can follow any diet for a short time, but you'll eventually quit if it's not one you can follow for life.
4. *Not resolving underlying emotional traumas and issues.* Food has druglike effects on both dopamine and serotonin receptors. People with food issues use food to escape the emotional pain or boredom they're feeling.

5. *Not tracking calories, macros, sleep, or exercise.* If your goal is to move to a superhuman level of aesthetics, we strongly suggest outsourcing the design of your diet to an expert and tracking your calories.
6. *No coaching or accountability in place.* You can't trust yourself when it comes to keeping yourself accountable in your weight loss journey.
7. *Low-quality sleep.* The consequences of bad sleep on dieting include getting fatter, losing muscle, destroyed willpower, horrible moods, and a crashed immune system.
8. *Not addressing other health problems.* For your weight loss journey to be optimized, your health needs to be optimized.
9. *Losing mental vigilance.* Loss of mental vigilance is one of the main causes of long-term weight loss failures.
10. *Not considering genetics.* Diet fanatics are often so dogmatic about the diet that works for them that they force it on all their clients and social media followers. There's little to no consideration for individual genetics.
11. *Chemical overload.* An overload of chemicals can negatively impact a variety of organs and systems in the body. This can lead to loss of energy and has effects on metabolism.
12. *Poor digestion.* Poor digestion can make it hard or impossible to feel awesome and thus impacts your results. It can easily lead to you quitting a diet.
13. *Leaky gut, food sensitivities, and food allergies.* Being biologically optimized is critical for feeling your best. That's why it's important to remove foods that are toxic and stressful to your body.
14. *Vitamin, mineral, and nutrient deficiencies.* Many diets can lead to a variety of nutrient deficiencies unless they're properly designed.
15. *Protein deficiencies.* When people shift from protein deficiencies to optimal protein consumption, they experience significant results both in terms of fat loss and muscle building.
16. *Essential fatty acid deficiencies.* Most people overconsume the wrong type of fats and are extremely deficient in essential fatty acids (EFAs). EFAs are the most important type of fats to focus on.
17. *Losing too much lean muscle tissue.* This is absolutely one of the biggest problems with many people's overall weight loss approach. They don't have the right strategy to preserve their vital lean muscle tissue as they lose weight.

This book sets out to burst the diet industry's bubble and equip you with the right tools and strategies for lifelong biological optimization (which we call BIOptimization). BIOptimization is the process of giving your body all of the nutrients it needs in optimal quantities and qualities. BIOptimization is about optimizing all of your body's organs and biological systems. The 17 mistakes listed above will essentially move you away from biological optimization.

CHAPTER 4

THE FIVE EPIC GOALS YOU CAN ACHIEVE WITH YOUR BODY

In this chapter, you will learn:

- The five epic biological goals. Discover what you can learn from bodybuilders for your aesthetic goals, CEOs and athletes for your performance goals, and even your ancestors for your health goals.
- How low your body fat should be. Learn how to transform body fat ranges from the unhealthy danger zone to the optimal athletic range, without tipping over the edge and landing yourself in the dangerous maximization zone.
- The magic ratios for building an attractive body.
- The secret to pushing your brain to superhuman levels in both intensity and duration. How CEOs and entrepreneurs are able to work 80-plus-hour weeks, reverse cognitive decline, and increase their creativity and concentration.
- Normal health is good, right? *Wrong!* Discover why a lack of disease or diagnosis is not necessarily an indicator of good health (and definitely not an indication of BIOptimized health).
- The difference between health span and life span, why both are critical in achieving optimal health, and how to use easy hacks for improving both, despite genetics.
- How to gain clarity on your diet goals to provide the focus necessary for succeeding in your journey.
- What it means to be a truly BIOptimized human, and how to get there.
- How much muscle mass you should have, and the various health ranges for body fat.
- The dark health secret of the world's most fit individuals.
- Why our definition of health is so much more than just the absence of disease.
- The 20 percent lock-in rule to achieve maximum results from your health journey.

Let's dive in . . .

Your goals are the destination around which everything is designed. This chapter dives into the five epic goals you can set for your body.

HOW GOALS EVOLVE

Getting clarity on your goals is critical. They provide the focus that helps you to create your life's journey. And in diet design, goals define which diet structure, diet type, calories, macros, and supplements you choose.

Most people start diets because they have aesthetic goals. They want to lose weight, and some want to gain lean muscle mass. Their pants are too tight. They don't like how they look in the holiday family picture.

It doesn't matter which goals get you inspired and motivated, as long as you start and take action. Just be mindful that your goals will evolve with time. In fact, for you to be successful long term, they need to evolve (more on this later in the chapter). Why? Because you need a never-ending stream of dopamine loops. Both Wade's and Matt's goals have evolved and continue to evolve with time. Our current goal is to do the following . . .

BECOME A BIOPTIMIZED HUMAN

Our definition of a *BIOptimized human* is someone who maximizes all three sides of the BIOptimization Triangle equally.

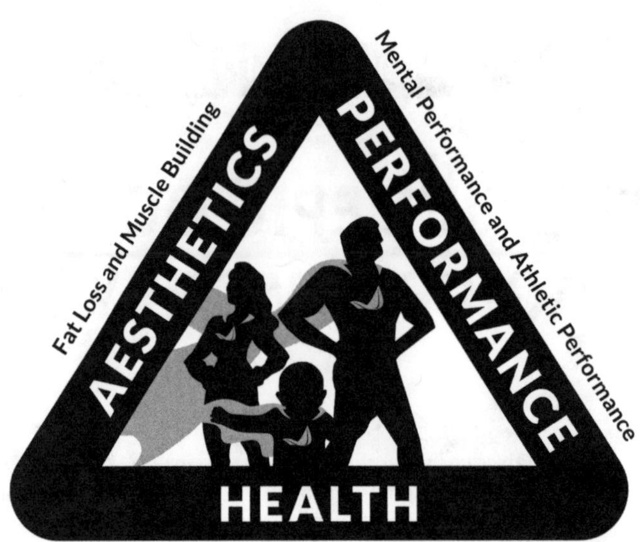

Optimizing Health Since 2004

BIOptimization means maximizing all three sides of the BIOptimization Triangle: aesthetics, performance, and health. Sometimes, you will need to prioritize one while balancing the others; however, trying to fully maximize a single side typically endangers the other two. For example, pushing aesthetics or athletic performance to a world-class level has detrimental impacts on health.

The BIOptimization Triangle can be broken down into five exciting journeys.

THE 5 EPIC BIOLOGICAL GOALS

Aesthetics:

1. Building lean muscle
2. Burning excess body fat

Performance:

3. Maximizing your athletic performance
4. Optimizing your mental performance

Health:

5. Maximizing your BioSpan (life span and health span)

EPIC AESTHETICS

Most people start a health and fitness journey with aesthetic goals. They want to look better. It ranges from guys who want to look like superheroes to guys who just want to look lean and fit. Some women want to hop on stage with bikinis, while others want to build thunderous booties—and some just want to look and feel good in their clothes.

We are not here to tell you how you should or shouldn't look. What you consider sexy and attractive is a highly personal choice. It's up to you. Whatever look you choose, we're here to give you the keys to make it happen.

That being said, research on attractiveness has shown that there are certain "magic ratios" that considerably increase attractiveness in the eyes of other people. So, if your goal is to become as attractive as possible, then this is useful information.

Men can optimize their physiques for the Adonis ratio, which is considered the golden ratio for the perfect male body:

- Shoulder 1.618 times larger than the waist
- Chest 6.5 times that of the wrist
- Upper legs 1.75 times that of the knee
- Go to www.BIOptimizers.com/book/dietapp to download our app and assess your current stats.

Based on the research, women can optimize their aesthetics by striving for the following ratios:

- Waist-to-hip between 0.67 and 0.8.

The good news is that women can increase the size of their glutes and hips with weight training (especially doing squats and deadlifts).

Until genetic engineering is available, you have two primary tools you can use to improve how you look: increase lean muscle and lower body fat. Note: plastic surgery is also an option to modify aesthetics (and we're not here to judge those who choose it).

The essence of bodybuilding is to shape your body like an artist sculpts a statue. Even if you don't want to look like a freakish bodybuilder, the process is the same. Bodybuilders change their ratios by increasing shoulder width and shrinking their waistline. Even a 65-year-old grandmother can use the same process to improve her health and how she looks.

Let's dive into the two aesthetic shapers . . .

QUEST #1: BUILD LEAN MUSCLE MASS

The benefits of having more lean muscle mass don't end there, because muscle mass increases longevity, health span, and functionality (see our book *From Sick to Superhuman* to learn more). Optimal levels of strength and lean muscle mass is one of the main determinants of health span and life span.

The benefits of building muscle mass include:

- Promoting a healthy metabolism and better blood sugar control
- Preventing or slowing down age-related fatigue, loss of function, disability, fall risk, frailty, and death
- Increasing mobility and balance, reducing falls and all-cause mortality[1]

How Much Muscle Mass Should You Have?

Here are the various health ranges for body fat and the fat-free mass index (FFMI). To calculate it, divide your fat-free lean body mass by your height in inches. Go to www.BIOptimizers.com/book/dietapp to download our app and assess your current stats.

Ideal FFMI Ranges

Range	Men's FFMI	Women's FFMI
Unhealthy Danger Zone	Below 14	Below 11
Unhealthy	15–17	12–14
Average/Healthy	18–19	15–17
Optimal/Athletic	20–27	18–22
Maximization Zone (Danger)	Over 28	Over 23

A couple of key points here:

- This chart was created by examining the stats of fitness competitors, as well as female pro bodybuilders.
- Past a 27 FFMI, you're entering the maximization zone. For 99.9 percent of the population, getting there almost certainly requires steroids, testosterone, and other performance-enhancing drugs.[2]

QUEST #2: LOSE EXCESS BODY FAT

Excess body fat hides your natural shape. Losing the fat reveals your natural shape and gets you closer to the optimal aesthetic ratios. We're not here to fat shame anyone; however, after working with hundreds of people, we hear that most do *not* feel comfortable when they carry excess body fat. Most people suppress their emotions about their obesity. Self-esteem and confidence go down as body fat goes up.

Less body fat also improves health conditions, including but not limited to:

- Insulin resistance issues
- Type 2 diabetes
- High blood pressure
- Poor immune function
- Heart disease and strokes
- Sleep apnea
- Joint pain and immobility
- Fatty liver
- Kidney disease

Virtually everyone on earth would choose to press a magic button to lower their body fat if it were that simple. Unfortunately, it isn't.

How Low Should Your Body Fat Be?

This is a critical question. Less is better until it becomes detrimental. Very few people have the genetics to get shredded. In this chapter, we will discuss the dark price that many people pay when they pursue aesthetic extremes.

Ideal Body Fat Ranges

Range	Men's Body Fat Levels	Women's Body Fat Levels
Unhealthy Danger Zone	35%+	40%+
Unhealthy	25–34%	30–39%
Average/Healthy	18–25%	23–29%
Optimal/Athletic	8–18%	11–22%
Maximization Zone (Danger)	7% or less	10% or less

- Less body fat typically translates to better health and performance.
- Every person has an optimal body fat range depending on their genetics and life history. The body has a set point. When you try to push past it too aggressively, expect your body to fight back and trigger the starvation survival effect and other health problems.
- Percentage-wise, less body fat is better up to a point. Once men get below 7 percent, and women get below 10 percent, the body goes into fight-flight-freeze mode, unless you're a genetic anomaly.

The lowest healthy level of body fat varies from person to person. Some are naturally thin, while others need more body fat to function optimally.

For men, body fat that's too low can result in the following:

- Severe metabolic damage, which can take months to recover from.
- Low testosterone, which can result in depression, low sex drive, and overall low quality of life.

Women need more body fat than men. For women, body fat that's too low can result in the following:

- Severe metabolic damage.
- Shutdown of reproductive hormones, causing loss of menstrual cycles and infertility. In some cases, it can induce early menopause or make menopausal symptoms worse.
- Loss of bone mass due to low estrogen.
- Starvation survival effects, which can cause fatigue, depression, low sex drive, lowered immunity, and overall reduced quality of life. Sometimes, this leads to a major chronic health problem.
- You can see how good your genes are for fat loss by taking this genetic test. Go to: www.BIOptimizers.com/book/genes.

You want just the right levels of fat to keep you warm and hormonally balanced.

Excess fat, especially visceral fat between your internal organs, can promote inflammation and metabolic derangements that contribute to declining health.

It is a great health goal to have close to zero visceral fat.[3, 4]

The Dark Secret of the World's "Fittest": The High Cost of Aesthetic Maximization

We want to be clear that we aren't advocating for you to become a bodybuilder or a bikini model. As we stated, very few people have the natural genetics to achieve these ideals without suffering dire consequences. This is why we want to warn you of the cost of pursuing aesthetic extremes.

Most people can achieve an optimal level of muscle mass by adding 10 to 20 pounds of lean muscle and maintaining it. Ideal body fat differs based on genetics and life history. To push past your natural genetic potential, you often make major sacrifices in health and performance. These usually involve using a wide array of performance-enhancing drugs.

For example, during the 10 months that Wade cut his body fat to single digits for a bodybuilding show, he continuously experienced a terrible mood, brain fog, horrible sleep, fatigue, joint pain, low sex drive, low energy, and constant cravings. He took extreme measures on competition day. He cut all water intake to look as shredded as possible, which hurt his kidneys. In other words, he sacrificed months of health and performance for one single day of competition. That is the price of competitive bodybuilding.

Despite all of these sacrifices, Wade placed sixth at a national bodybuilding championship. His coach told him he would have to go on a massive stack of drugs to be competitive enough to progress to the next level. This is the moment that Wade decided to become a natural bodybuilder. He was unwilling to sacrifice his health to achieve results.

Performance

"Food for fuel" is the motto of those who pursue performance, which has two aspects: mental and physical.

QUEST #3: MAXIMUM ATHLETIC PERFORMANCE

Dedicated athletes have one goal: to maximize their performance on the field. Optimizing athletic performance includes maximizing:

- Strength
- Speed
- Endurance
- Movement and balance skills
- Energy levels

You may think of physical performance in terms of what you can do in the gym. However, food is also vital in order for you to optimize recovery and energy. Food and supplements can also enhance athletic performance.

We will cover how to optimize your nutrition for maximum athletic performance in Chapter 17.

The Price of Athletic Performance Maximization

Similar to pro bodybuilders, pro athletes often shorten their lives.[5] Extreme training generates a lot of oxidative stress, which can quickly deplete nutrients and promote aging.

Many pro athletes use a variety of performance-enhancing drugs to gain an edge and become the best. If you ever choose this route, we suggest working with professionals who can help minimize the risks and damage that can happen with certain substances.

Die for a Gold Medal?

In the '90s, Dr. Robert Goldman asked elite athletes if they would be willing to take a drug that guaranteed their success in sports but would kill them within five years. Half the athletes said yes.

There is no doubt that abusive steroid use and water-cutting regimens are harmful and can shorten the life spans of athletes who use them.

QUEST #4: MAXIMUM COGNITIVE PERFORMANCE

Cognitive performance refers to:

- Cognitive function (the ability to learn, think, reason, and make decisions)
- Focus
- Memory
- Mood regulation
- Mental endurance
- Mental and cognitive resilience to stress

This is the realm of high performers, including CEOs, executives, marketers, entrepreneurs, artists, salespeople, and so on—in other words, people who use their minds to achieve their goals and objectives.

The top people in these realms are world-class mental athletes. They push their brains to superhuman levels both in intensity and duration. It's not unusual for entrepreneurs to work more than 80 hours a week while they pursue their dreams; their goal is to maximize their brain's functioning capabilities.

Age-related cognitive decline may start as early as 18 years old before accelerating as people reach old age.[6] Fortunately, there is a lot you can do about it, through both lifestyle and nutrition. Nootropics (such as the ones you can find at www.Nootopia.com) are the keys to optimizing your mental performance. We will cover them in greater depth in Chapter 18.

QUEST #5: MAXIMIZING BIOSPAN

BioSpan is composed of two factors: life span and health span. Life span is how long we live. Health span is our quality of life.

Life span capped out around our 40s for most of human history. Thanks to modern science, we have already made tremendous progress in this area in the last two centuries, and we're just getting started. Now, we're living up to the 70s and climbing. Contributors to this improvement came from advances in the medical system, antibiotics, improvements in economic prosperity, and more.

We live in exciting times. We understand the body at a level we never have before. New breakthroughs in health technology are happening at an exponential rate. We have more tools at our disposal. We have new ways of testing and optimizing our bodies: DNA, blood tests, sleep monitors, food allergy and gut biome tests, and many more.

Eventually, advances in health technology will allow humans to live well into their 100s, maybe even 200s, and beyond. Some people are shooting for biological immortality. Google's chief futurist, Ray Kurzweil, says humans will have eternal life by 2029.[7] Kurzweil has built an amazing track record of accurate predictions in the last few decades. Whether he's right about this prediction remains to be seen.

Using simple induction and deduction, it stands to reason that we can live for a much longer life span than our ancestors who didn't have the knowledge, health tech, or supplements we do now. Armed with this knowledge, you can positively impact your life span. Maybe you'll be one of the first great-great-grandparents.

We are certain that by building the right habits with the Power Moves in this book (and our book *From Sick to Superhuman*), you can extend your life span significantly. There is already tremendous scientific evidence showing major reductions in all-cause mortality with several of the solutions we share in our books.

Health Span

Health span is the length of *quality* health. Your health span is how long you remain healthy, functional, and vital. How long are you going to rock and roll?

For most people, health span is far more important than life span. When we tell someone, "We think you could live to be 150 years old," most people cringe and reply with, "I don't want to be decrepit." No one wants to spend 50 years unable to enjoy life.

In the typical aging pattern, people's health span starts to decline after 27, but goes down dramatically in the last few decades of life. We're living longer thanks to life-extending medical innovations. The problem is, it's at a lower quality of life.

"Average" health means aging into sickness and disability. This is not limited to the elderly—millennials are developing chronic illnesses as early as their thirties.

But here's the great news: you are in control of your health span. It's up to you to make the unbreakable commitment to yourself to optimize your health to maximize your health span. You can live an incredible life filled with energy, vitality, and joy right until the day you pass on to the other side.

Following the right diet for your body and optimizing it will have an enormous effect on your health span.

THE BIOPTIMIZATION HEALTH SPECTRUM: FROM SICK TO SUPERHUMAN

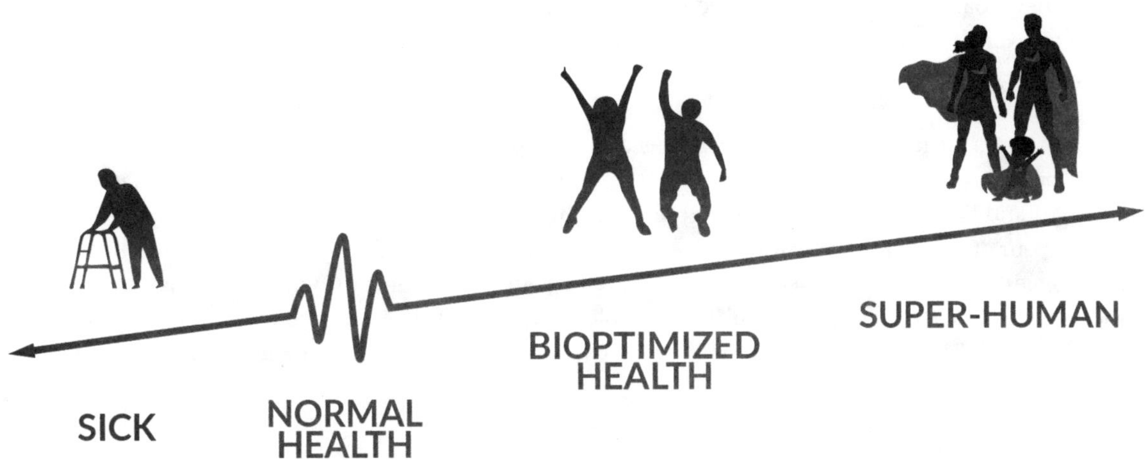

Beware of "Normal"

The medical definition of health is the absence of disease. This is when you have normal lab tests and an overall lack of diagnosis. A lack of disease is not necessarily a good indicator of health, and it's certainly no indication of BIOptimized health either. When doctors look at your biomarkers, they rarely care about you being "optimized." They just look for abnormally bad results and prescribe drugs to try to get you out of the danger zone.

Unfortunately, the mainstream system is designed to help sick people get to neutral health (at best)—and even then, they struggle. Two-thirds of Americans have now been diagnosed with chronic diseases, and they've become dependent on medication to stay alive and make life manageable.[8]

At the age of 17, Wade realized the importance of health when he observed his sister, Betsy, tragically die of cancer. He watched her go from literally near-superhuman to sick—and ultimately dead—all in a span of four years.

At the age of 16, she was the second-best Air Cadet in all of Canada. She had exceptional performance and strength and was on track toward a career in the military. Then she was diagnosed with cancer, which brought her and the entire family through four years of hell. No doctor, drug, or surgery could save her.

Our purpose is to help people go from sick to normal, and then from normal to superhuman. That's what our first book, *From Sick to Superhuman*, is about.

We're not interested in simply returning people to "normal"—instead, we set our sights on extraordinary levels of health, which we call "BIOptimized health." We define someone who is BIOptimized as someone whose body is functioning near its best and optimized on every major level.

BIOptimization's number one enemy is our genetic programming and psychological beliefs. Genetically, we're programmed to peak at age 27 and then start decaying as we age.[9] This can be combated, slowed down, and even reversed by using the information in this book. If you change your beliefs about what's possible for you—yes, you—then you can become BIOptimized by implementing the strategies in this book.

How to Be a World-Class Goal-Setter

Yes, we believe you can have it all! However, you can't build it all at once. We suggest having one core focus at a time. Then you move on to the next goal, and the next, and the next.

Use these three critical strategies for setting goals:

1. Always have a goal
2. Set one goal at a time
3. Build a multiyear road map of goals

For example, you may start with the goal of losing excess body fat. Once you've achieved your fat loss goals, you can choose a new goal. It could be building your ideal level of lean muscle, for example.

Some men want to focus on building lean muscle first. Then maybe they want to maximize their athletic performance.

For people who want to accomplish incredible feats in their careers, optimizing their brains for long-term performance may be the primary goal. Then health becomes the prize.

As most people get into their 50s and beyond, they start thinking about their mortality. This is when focusing on health span and life span can become the core focus. In our opinion, health span and life span should become your focus in your 40s. Why? Because it's much easier to maintain your health than it is to reverse health problems.

We do suggest building a multiyear goal road map for your body. Constantly having goals is one of the major keys to long-term success. This creates an unstoppable multilayered dopamine loop. If you only have one goal and you achieve it, then your motivation will drop. Creating a never-ending journey is the answer for life-long fulfillment.

The 20 Percent Lock-In Rule

Here's a very important concept: to lock in results, it takes 20 percent of the energy you spend to achieve the results.

This means that to maintain your fat loss, you spend 20 percent of the energy that it took you to lose the fat. To maintain lean muscle mass, it takes 20 percent of the energy you spent to build it, and so on.

This is how you can have it all. Achieve one goal, then lock in the results. Achieve the next goal and lock that one in, and keep going.

SUMMARY

To become a superhuman, you need to become BIOptimized. BIOptimization means maximizing all sides of the BIOptimization Triangle. There are five epic biological goals you can take with your body. These are:

Epic Aesthetics

Quest #1: Building lean muscle, which not only makes you look your best, but also increases longevity, health span, and resilience.
Quest #2: Burning excess body fat, which reveals your natural body shape, helps you get closer to the perfect body ratio, improves your self-esteem, and translates into better health and performance.

Epic Performance

Quest #3: Maximizing your athletic performance, which improves your speed, strength, endurance, movement, and even your energy.
Quest #4: Optimizing your mental performance, which improves your ability to think, reason, and focus; it also boosts your memory, mood, and ability to make decisions that can impact your life.

Epic Health

Quest #5: Maximizing your BioSpan, which is your life span plus your health span, is maximizing how long you live while maximizing quality of life. Yes, you can enjoy living far longer and at a higher quality of life than your ancestors did.

CONCLUSION

Now is an exciting time in which we have an unprecedented level of knowledge about the body. New breakthroughs in health technologies are happening at a record pace. We have more tests and tools at our disposal. This book is about systematically applying this knowledge and tools to maximize all three sides of the BIOptimization Triangle.

CHAPTER 5

HOW TO WIN ON ANY DIET

This chapter will teach you how to hack your mind and spirit to create the habits, systems, processes, and accountability that maximize the odds of success for any diet.

Achieving long-term success on any diet isn't easy (see that 97 percent fail rate in Chapter 1). Hopefully, after reading the first part of this book, you now understand why. To achieve your dream, you need every advantage possible. Just understanding biology isn't enough. Your mind controls your behavior and ultimately shapes your body.

This chapter is a compendium of psychological, behavioral, and spiritual edges. The more of them you use, the higher your odds of success. Stack as many as you can. Start with the ones that appeal to you the most and then progressively add more over time. This is how you win *big*.

In this chapter, you'll learn:

- How to hack your neurochemistry for diet success
- How to harness the power of habits, systems, processes, and accountability for maximum success on any diet
- How you can use the winning strategies that casinos in Las Vegas use to stack edges to your advantage and become unbeatable at any diet
- The 27 edges you can use to win at any and all diets you try
- The power of creating your own dopamine-driven loops to make winning feel effortless
- The secret to superhuman toughness
- How your diet success is truly in *your* hands
- How to upgrade from the worst habits that can potentially sabotage your diet

DECODING THE MULTI-BILLION-DOLLAR MACHINE

When Matt went to Las Vegas for the first time, he walked around with a casino marketing expert who decoded everything around them.

First, the casino buildings are epic attractions. They are billion-dollar investments that dazzle your mind as you witness their magnificent architecture and designs.

Then, they create magnetic attractions, like the water show in front of the Bellagio. This $40 million investment draws a third of onlookers to go inside when they hadn't planned to. These people then spend money in the casinos.

As you walk into the Bellagio, your mind is blown away by the $25 million's worth of beautiful glass creations on the ceiling. The beauty and opulence make you feel as though you're winning by just being there.

Then, everything is optimized to extract as much money out of you as possible:

- The carpets are busy and unattractive because they're designed to lift your eyes up to the level of the slot machines.
- The slot machines play C major chords because they're the most pleasant to the ear.
- They pump extra oxygen into the air to keep you alert and not want to go home to bed. The longer you play, the more of an advantage this gives the house.
- They leave out clocks and windows to disorient you from time.
- The bathrooms, buffets, and restaurants are really deep inside the building so you have to walk past the machines and tables to get there, increasing the odds you'll play.
- Sexy waitresses help keep the men distracted and playing.

- And, of course, there's free liquor, which is a huge part of the equation because it causes people to become less inhibited and make stupid decisions.
- And finally, the games are all rigged in the house's favor.

Casinos win by getting people buzzed and overstimulated so they keep gambling until all their money is gone. The casinos have stacked so many edges against you that the odds of you walking out of Las Vegas a winner are 5 to 10 percent.[1]

The applicable principle for you is to use this winning strategy of stacking edges to your advantage and become unbeatable. There's a massive array of biological, psychological, and societal forces that work against you, so you need every edge you can get your hands on.

HACK YOUR NEUROCHEMISTRY

Neurochemistry is one of the greatest drivers of human behavior. When your neurochemistry is stacked against you, success can seem impossible. When your neurochemistry is optimized, you will feel indomitable.

Thanks to the modern understanding of how these neurochemicals affect our brains and our actions, we can hack them in our favor. We've seen this work countless times with our clients and even ourselves. The story below illustrates this.

Ending the Yo-Yo Dieting Cycle, by Wade T. Lightheart

My longtime friend and client, Joanne, had struggled with her weight since her early teen years. She was the classic yo-yo dieter. On top of that, she had been receiving psychological counseling and medications for neurochemical imbalances.

It seemed like every year (sometimes several times a year), Joanne would cycle between a lean, motivated fitness that was dialed in perfectly with her diet, only to spiral into an uncontrollable pattern of bingeing and weight gain. This came with the associated feelings of shame, guilt, and depression.

She would switch diets, get more counseling, switch medications, and get on another routine, only to repeat the cycle six months later.

Approximately 15 percent of the population receives treatment for neurochemical conditions. Many neurochemicals are made in our guts by bacteria that are essential for our survival. Science has now proven that unoptimized guts wreak havoc on our health and emotions. That's why we invested in our BioLab in Europe, which carries out our research and development on probiotics.

Joanne transformed her gut health with our Cognibiotics, which is a formula that contains probiotics that produce various neurotransmitters. Joanne swears by the effects and has stabilized her weight and mood. She used EFT and customized nootropics from Nootopia to wean off her medication. Today she's happier than ever.

The moral of the story is, your struggles are real—but they often lead to breakthroughs and gifts. The key to maximizing success is to look at your body from all angles. We've seen incredible results by creating the right personalized diet strategies for our genetics, optimizing our gut health, improving our hormones, and adjusting for our lifestyle.

Without further ado, let's start stacking edges.

EDGE #1: CREATE YOUR OWN DOPAMINE-DRIVEN REWARD LOOPS

What if I told you that you're in control of your dopamine? You have far more power to hack it than you ever thought possible.

Knowing how to hack your dopamine system is one of the most powerful things ever. Dopamine is the molecule of drive, anticipation, and achievement. If you know how to multiply the dopamine levels in your mind, your ability to succeed will multiply with it.

How do you do this? You create your own layer cake of dopamine loops. You start by asking yourself, "What's important to me?" You create your own rules and decide what's a win. This may sound too simple to be a game changer, but we assure you that this is the edge of all edges for creating a set of winning rules for yourself.

As soon as you decide that something is important and you take action toward achieving it, you get a dopamine boost. As you move toward it and anticipate its outcome, your dopamine levels get elevated. Because dopamine is enjoyable, you'll continue to take that action over and over again. Why? Because humans want to feel better. Dopamine feels good.

The challenge is that most people don't consciously commit to new decisions and directions. Their core values are mostly unconscious, and their dopamine loops haven't been consciously crafted. Or they make the mistake of creating dopamine loops that are too far out into the distance. They aren't setting themselves up with a constant stream of dopamine hits.

This technique is the mental process that the world's toughest people have used to forge their unbreakable spirit.

The Secret to Superhuman Toughness

Why are some people able to do what seem to be superhuman feats of mental toughness and endurance? The answer is the dance between dopamine and noradrenaline.

Noradrenaline is the effort molecule that gets us started, but it also makes us quit when it gets elevated too much. When noradrenaline gets too high, we feel overwhelmed and it breaks our will. However, there is a hack that counters the noradrenaline.

Neuroscientist and Stanford researcher Dr. Andrew Huberman shines light on this topic: "When noradrenaline gets too high, animals quit. When it gets too high in animals in lab experiments, this is when they stop. The molecule that attenuates noradrenaline is dopamine."

This means if we can increase our dopamine levels while facing tough situations (which raises our noradrenaline levels), then we can give ourselves the ability to keep going. Huberman is saying that if we have enough dopamine, we can keep going and going and going.

This is one of the biggest revelations ever when it comes to pushing ourselves to superhuman levels of effort and success. It gives us an understanding of people like David Goggins, who has:

- Run more than 200 miles nonstop in 39 hours, and placed third in the toughest foot race on the planet—the Badwater 135, which takes place in Death Valley during the summer
- Set a Guinness World Record with 4,030 pull-ups
- Lost 110 pounds

People with superhuman mental toughness, like David Goggins, create incredibly strong dopamine loops that make them enjoy extreme things. He's determined, and he's decided that extreme effort equals winning. By making that decision, he's set up his brain for strong dopamine responses as he pushes himself. This allows him—and, potentially, all of us—to endure extremely challenging situations.

Because of this, he wakes up at 3 A.M. to go run in freezing-cold weather for three hours and films it on YouTube. He feels awesome, he loves it, and this edge is how he does it. This strategy is one that we used by choosing to believe in the saying, "no pain, no gain." It's a classic bodybuilding cliché that rewired our brains and allowed us to push ourselves in the gym.

EDGE #2: LAYER YOUR DOPAMINE LOOPS

The key is to layer multiple dopamine loops into micro loops, daily loops, weekly loops, multi-month loops, multi-year loops, and lifetime loops. It's a major mistake to have only one, main source of dopamine, like visualizing your "final form" weight. You're robbing yourself of so much dopamine when you do this.

Multi-Year Wins: The Ultimate Vision

Ask yourself, what's the ultimate dream? What do you want to look like? Don't let past mistakes and challenges stop you. You've got the tools now in this book, and you're getting them by reading about and integrating them into your life.

By creating a huge long-term vision, you give yourself a very strong, solid foundation of dopamine to ride on for years or even decades. This is what every kid who dreamt of being a professional athlete did. They had a vision and made the decision to go for it. The drive from the dopamine allowed them to overcome all of the challenges. This is how Wade became a three-time national natural bodybuilding champion.

Multi-Month Wins: Chop the Journey into Smaller Goals

As we mentioned earlier, your brain rewards you with a burst of dopamine when you achieve your goals. This is why 12-week programs work well psychologically. As neuroscientist Andrew Huberman says, "Your brain is always trying to assess the duration, path, and outcome to every decision."

- Duration: How long is this journey going to take?
- Path: What does it take to get there?
- Outcome: What am I going to get from it?

If the path feels too long, many people break before the journey even begins.

A powerful technique is to break the bigger vision into medium-size goals. When Matt went for his final form, his goals were:

- 242 pounds to 220 pounds
- 220 pounds to 210 pounds
- 210 pounds to 199 pounds
- Reverse diet back to maintenance without going over 205 pounds
- Stay between 205 and 212 pounds for more than two years

Doing this helped him to accomplish multiple things. First, he felt like it was a massive win when he hit 220 pounds, and then again at 210. Second, his brain already had the next goal cued up.

Weekly Reward Cycles

With fat loss, muscle gain, and athletic performance, a week is the key time window to focus on. Many people make the mistake of using a daily window for tracking calories, which is not a great approach because you can fast and feast a bit. In the end, what really matters is your weekly energy balance. If you achieve your weekly deficit, you're winning.

For example, when Wade works on dropping 30 pounds for a bodybuilding show, he breaks down the goal into weekly cycles. Over the 15 weeks, that's two pounds per week. So, the first week, he's got to make sure he's two pounds down. If he's there by the end of that week, he gets the reward of success, and he's got the next week cued up in his mind.

Daily Wins: Acknowledge All the Micro Wins

The goal is to live in a state of perpetual gratitude. You want to feel like you're *always winning,* even when you face difficult challenges. Looking at all the wins of your day is a powerful process. Maybe this is the most important dopamine loop creator of them all.

One of the best ways to accomplish this is to do a daily gratitude list. At the end of every day, take a couple of minutes and count *all* your blessings. Some people love to write them out by hand in a journal. Some people create digital gratitude spaces where they share their gratitude lists with a small group of friends. Not only do they feel that they're winning with their own list, but they feel inspired by others' lists.

How can you apply this idea in your journey?

Here's a small list of wins:

- Every workout is a win
- Every good meal is a win
- Every pound lost is a win
- Not gaining weight on vacation is a win
- Every successful week is a win
- Finding a training partner is a win
- Dropping a dress size is a win
- Looking better in your clothes is a win
- Completing a training program is a win
- Finishing a diet phase is a win
- Starting a new phase is a win
- Starting a new training program is a win
- Trying a new form of exercise is a win
- Staying at the same weight but losing body fat and gaining muscle is a win
- Hiring a coach is a win
- Learning from failure is a huge win
- Creating a new healthy habit is a win
- Stopping an old bad habit is a win
- Five more reps is a win
- A great night's sleep is a major win
- Every time you use a biohacking device, it's a win
- Every quarter-inch loss on the measuring tape is a win
- Create your own wins: Every time I________, it's a win

Tom Platz: The King of Intensity and Micro Dopamine Loops

When it comes to extremely difficult physical effort, micro dopamine loops are the solution. Tom Platz, a bodybuilder who built the most freakish legs of all time in his era, achieved feats of training intensity that perhaps no other human will ever repeat. He's considered by his peers to be the king of intensity when it comes to weight lifting. No one has been able to match many of his feats.

Here are some of the massive things Tom did:

- He squatted his bodyweight (225 pounds) for 10 minutes straight. He ended up doing over 100 reps and had to be driven to the hospital with oxygen deprivation. He said his legs grew for three weeks from that one single workout.
- He was famous for pushing one single set to the deepest levels of muscular failure—from concentric failure, to eccentric failure, to partial rep failure, to static rep failure.

He would hack his mind by just focusing on "five more reps." Not only that, he built a dopamine loop in his mind by deciding that every five additional reps was a win. Creating continuous micro dopamine loops within the set allowed him to push his body to superhuman levels of effort.

This mind hack is available to everyone. You just have to choose it. The first key choice is deciding that your health is your most valuable asset. If you lose that, what do you have left?

Remember: You're in control of your dopamine. You choose what's a win. Those simple decisions will create your dopamine loops. The point is to clearly celebrate every victory. Every win, no matter how small, matters! Be grateful for every little thing and every little win.

These wins help lower your noradrenaline, and the dopamine propels you into action. This is one of the most powerful psychological techniques ever.

EDGE #3: ALWAYS HAVE THE NEXT GOAL

Dopamine helps drive us to do things and achieve goals. But there's a very important aspect of dopamine that, if unmanaged, sets people up for failure and depression: it goes down massively once a goal is achieved.

As Dr. Andrew Huberman eloquently states, "Dopamine is the molecule of anticipation." This is why the moment of achievement can be so disappointing sometimes. People have this massive goal in their minds and finally hit it. The anticipation is gone.

There's a key process that Matt always used with all his clients: create the next goal before your current goal ends. You always need a series of goals. Having just one sets you up for failure.

Wade did the same thing on his own journey from farm boy to Mr. Universe. He created an epic vision and chopped it into dozens and dozens of goals for two decades. This fueled his dopamine and allowed him to endure extremely difficult diets and training regimens.

We've all heard the cliché "enjoy the journey." There's a lot of truth and power to that saying, because the journey to the goal is what fuels the dopamine. Once you achieve a goal, your dopamine drops unless you have the next goal set up. This is how our brains are hardwired. The solution is simple: create endless sets of goals.

EDGE #4: TAKE ACTION EVEN IF YOU DON'T FEEL LIKE IT

When Matt was 12 years old, he received his first weight set for Christmas. With it came a booklet from Joe Weider, and there was a key lesson in it: never miss a workout—because that's how you reprogram your brain to do the right action, no matter what. Matt recalls a day in college when a girlfriend he loved broke his heart. The last thing he wanted to do was go train. But he knew that it was a key moment.

As the legendary Tom Platz says, "Any problems you have in life, the iron always saves you." Matt trained and felt better, and more important, he knew he had rewired his mind to train even when it didn't feel like it.

This edge is one of the biggest make or breaks when it comes to success. Do you program your brain to "just do it!" when you don't feel like exercising or eating the next right meal? Or do you program your brain to "just F-it!"?

You must take the right action, *especially* when you don't feel like it. Why? Because it's a critical brain-programming moment. This is the moment in which you either break the cycle of failure or strengthen it.

Failure begins with missing just once. It's like they say in recovery, "Just don't have the first drink." The first drink leads to the second and to the third and to another, and next thing you know, people have lost years of their lives.

Hack your mind. Make the decision right now to take action even when you don't feel like it. It's how you hard-wire your brain to win, no matter what.

EDGE #5: VALUE LONG-TERM WINS OVER SHORT-TERM GRATIFICATIONS

Unless you plan on dying soon, life is a long game—so play it accordingly.

Throughout our careers, we've done and seen our fair share of 12-to-16-week transformations. Marketers know that it's much easier to sell those than multi-yearlong programs because people gravitate toward instant gratification. The problem is, the majority of people who go through the program do achieve results by the end, only to end up back where they started.

These short-term shred programs set you up for massive rebounds because of the body's starvation survival effects. The diets and workouts are so aggressive that they prime your body to fight back with a vengeance as soon as you're done with your bodybuilding show, photo shoot, or wedding that you lost weight for. Also, because the programs don't fit with your lifestyle, the chance of you maintaining them for life is very slim.

Both of us have made these mistakes. Matt regained 40 pounds after dieting for his wedding. Wade went from Mr. Universe to Mr. Marshmallow and gained 42 pounds in 16 weeks after aggressively preparing for the competition. Speaking of marshmallows . . .

One of the most revealing long-term experiments concerning this edge is known as "the marshmallow experiment."[2] Researchers took groups of young kids and gave them the following challenge: "We're giving you one marshmallow now. We're going to leave the room and come back later. If you didn't eat the marshmallow, we'll give you a second one. If you did eat it, you won't get any more."

Then they divided the kids into the following categories:

- Group A, the kids who ate the first marshmallow
- Group B, the kids who didn't eat it

The researchers followed the study subjects for years, and they found that Group B was far more successful in almost all aspects of life. Why? Because they valued long-term wins over instant gratification. This mindset carried over to virtually every part of their lives.

In our guided programs, we focus on the long term. This involves stacking and sequencing mental and nutritional strategies to maximize your odds of success without triggering your starvation self-defense response.

EDGE #6: SUCCESS IS A PROGRAM OF ACTION

You can't *think* your way to health. It's important to realize that achieving any health-related goal is a program of action, because you can't read books on running and become fit. You can't read books on squatting and become strong. The number-one key to success is the right actions consistently applied over time.

Obviously, belief and mindset are important, because if you believe you can be successful, you'll prioritize your program over other things in your life. One of our problems today is that we live in a voyeuristic world where people equate learning and listening to actually doing the work. Social media has hacked our neurochemistry by hacking our dopamine system with views, likes, shares, and comments. Taking action is the way to win.

EDGE #7: FIND THE GIFTS IN YOUR SETBACKS AND CHALLENGES

Another thing that might be even more important is to make sure that your challenges and most painful losses are reframed as wins.

For example, it's totally normal for weight loss to slow down, hit plateaus, or even sometimes reverse a little bit. Sadly, many quit on the spot when they experience these little setbacks, but a coach can help you find the wind and get back on the path.

Some perfectionists mess up one meal and then feel like catastrophic failures. Or they've lost two pounds every week, and this week they've only lost one, so they feel like they're failing. These experiences are 100 percent normal. They are the monsters on your hero's journey.

Here's a powerful technique to use in those moments: retroframing gratitude.

By expanding the time frame in your mind and looking back at how far you've come since the beginning of your journey, you can feel a deep sense of win. You can feel grateful that you've lost 50 pounds in the last year, even if you've gained 2 pounds this week. Your long-term progress is more important than the short-term mistakes or setbacks.

Look back and feel gratitude for what has happened, whether it's a net loss or gain. There's a gift there waiting to be unwrapped. Even when things don't go as planned, the learning is a win.

We're huge believers in running experiments and then unpacking what happened, including learning from things that didn't work. We can usually extract some gold from those experiences and use it in the future.

When we look back on our lives, we can see that many of our greatest leaps forward started from our biggest losses. The things that hit the hardest hurt the most, and they made us feel the worst or appeared to be the biggest failures at the time, but they led to course adjustments that steered us in the right direction.

Transform your losses into wins. Don't stop—adjust, adapt, move forward. And when in doubt, zoom out.

UPGRADE YOUR HABITS

Your life is dominated by habits so you might as well insert good habits.

— Paramahansa Yogananda

Ultimately, the quality of our life is a byproduct of our habits. Because our brains want to minimize energy expenditure at all times, 95 percent of your daily actions are on auto-pilot. Typically, only 5 percent of our actions are new, because new things are energetically expensive to figure out, understand, and practice. Winners have simply put in the effort to overcome this challenge and spend the energy to *hardwire* their new, healthy habits.

Building the right set of habits inevitably produces great results. The habits that we're laying out in this book are going to lead you to your dream body. This section gives you the keystone habits that maximize the odds of your success.

EDGE #8: UPGRADE YOUR WORST HABITS

Eliminating your favorite foods can be tough psychologically. It can be scary to give up your favorite things; nobody likes to feel deprived. It's not a good feeling. We all have food items we love, whether it's cereal, chocolate, ice cream, or chips.

One of the best approaches is to upgrade our favorite treats. This is usually far more appealing than the elimination process.

The great news is that you've got zero excuses for not upgrading. Countless companies are constantly creating healthier versions of all the popular vices.

Options include upgrading:

- Highly caloric and sugary breakfast cereals to lower-sugar, high-protein cereals
- High-sugar milk chocolate to organic dark chocolates
- High-sugar treats to sugar-free versions
- White-flour pancakes to keto pancakes
- "Weed" to CBD, CBG, or CBN (for better cannabinoids)
- Brain-destroying alcohol to brain-enhancing nootropics (like Nootopia)

These upgrades can make massive differences, helping to lower your calories and improve your health at the same time.

For example, you can go from Froot Loops to a high-protein, low-sugar cereal. If you're a chocoholic, you can go from sugary milk chocolate to 70-percent-cacao organic dark chocolate. Go from Ben & Jerry's to Halo Top. There's ice cream for every type of diet. You can always improve your choices and your satisfaction from enjoying these foods. Over time, your cravings will change, and you'll start loving the better versions. And eventually, you might transcend those cravings altogether.

Get healthier condiments too. Paleo Kitchen, for example, has done a great job at eliminating hyper-palatable ingredients, such as high-fructose corn syrup, that make bland food taste great but cause people to eat more. Almost every condiment in North America tastes very sweet, and people have normalized it.

Keep in mind, however, that these foods still have calories—but the good brands have half (or a quarter) of the calories of the original. Plus, many brands increase protein levels, which reduces net calories even further and boosts satiety. They allow you to satisfy your cravings and work with your existing food patterns without breaking your diet.

You can also find recipes and make your own healthier, less calorie-dense substitutions at home. For example, instead of frying everything in butter, you can use an olive oil spray. You can go from french fries to baked fries.

And when you're experienced with all these modifications, you can create healthy refeed meals with replacement recipe cooking. Make the healthier version of your favorite comfort food. Go check out our YouTube show, *Healthy Recreations*, to find hundreds of healthy versions of your favorite foods.

These swaps are transformative because you can get the rewarding effect of the meals, along with the emotions and memories, without feeling guilty about going off your diet. Whatever dietary philosophy you're into, you can get cookbooks that bring you these meals without the guilt or side effects. It's really powerful. You can also download our Me Diet app, which has thousands of world-class recipes for every kind of diet.

EDGE #9: CONTROL YOUR ENVIRONMENT

You want to limit cravings as much as possible. The key is to construct your environment to minimize temptations. They're going to happen, but you can reduce them significantly by getting them out of your house.

Recovering alcoholics can't have alcohol in their homes. Why create unnecessary temptation? Willpower is a finite resource. If you're constantly fighting your temptations, you'll eventually break and succumb to them. So, you can't have the wrong foods around the house, and you can't have easy outs.

You have to manage your environment. You'll be battling your brain and will most likely lose when the ghrelin goblins start tickling your tummy with hunger.

Eliminating unnecessary temptations makes it far easier to create new healthy habits.

EDGE #10: AVOID FOOD ADVERTISING

The food conglomerates hire some of the best marketers in the world to hijack your lizard brain with neuromarketing. These ads present food and drinks in ways that literally make you salivate. They know exactly how to push the hunger buttons in your brain. They make you hungry and crave their latest creation. *They install cravings that weren't there before the ad!*

We're not immune to this. Matt, being an experienced marketer, realized that when he saw food advertising, he'd start craving that food. He would feel the desire build up. The next thing he knew, he was going for it. One of his strategies was to build a "desire list" and have those foods on refeed days. He's structured his life so that he can go for it one or two days a week. Instead of blowing his plan, he makes it work with his overall plan and lifestyle. Over the years, Matt's cravings for a lot of the high-calorie, hyper-palatable foods have decreased (but he still loves a great burger).

Wade has noticed that it's easier for him to stay lean in rural areas, because in cities, he's exposed to much more food advertising.

If you can completely eliminate your exposure to food advertising, it will make sticking to your diet tremendously easier. However, it's everywhere now—cutting into your YouTube ads and social media content, for example. Our suggestion is not to follow those YouTube channels and Instagram pages.

EDGE #11: THE UNIVERSAL SECRET OF PHYSIQUE CHAMPIONS: FOOD PREP

Unless you can afford a private chef or meal prep, this is perhaps one of the most powerful habits anyone can develop.

Every top bodybuilder, fitness competitor, athlete, and person who has successfully achieved their health goals did so because they were prepared. We don't know of any pros that don't use one form of meal prep or another.

With your cooking, time is always a factor. The eating never ends, and you end up eating the same foods, so you want to batch your cooking and food prep. It allows you to follow your diet plan on autopilot every week, saving several hours while stacking the odds in your favor.

Cook and prepare as many meals as possible for your diet once or twice a week. If you've got potatoes, rice, lean meats, or whatever is on your diet philosophy, make five or six servings instead of one or two. Pack the other ones in containers and make them easy to get to. That way, if you've extended past your eating time, you can reach into your fridge or carry a portion with you anywhere.

If you're not into food prep, find a catering company or pay someone to prepare food for you.

If you're a variety person, it can be harder to stick to a plan, but it's possible if you have help preparing your foods. You might need to structure by having someone prepare a variety of foods that fit your calorie and macro totals.

If you do cook, pick out a rotation of meals that you pre-dial to fit your diet parameters, and then just cook the meals you like to cook.

EDGE #12: ALWAYS HAVE A BACKUP PLAN

Preparation is critical for winning the diet war. You've got to be almost like a Navy SEAL—always ready for any situation. When Wade wasn't a vegetarian, he used to carry a can of tuna, a fork, and a can opener in his jacket at all times. Today, he keeps packages of nuts with him when he travels. It might sound weird, but that's how you get to single-digit body fat levels. Virtually everyone in fitness, without exception, gets into supraphysiological low levels of body fat by doing these types of food prep. It's a recipe for success.

If you're traveling, commuting, or going to work, always bring along one or two more meals than you need. That way, if you get caught in traffic, you're late to work, or something happens with the kids, you don't get screwed. Have optimized backup meals everywhere. This is where protein bars, protein shakes, and well-designed snack packs can be diet savers.

Winners embrace accountability. Losers fear it. The more levels of accountability you can add to your life, the more successful you're going to be. This is true for business, and it's true for your body.

EDGE #13: HANG WITH THE WINNERS

The adage "you're the average of the five people you spend the most time with" also applies to health and fitness. The people who surround you provide an environment that is much stronger than your will alone.

When Matt committed to sobriety, he sat down with the five closest friends he used to drink and do drugs with and said, "Listen, I can't hang out with you if you're high. You guys can get high. I'm not telling you not to get high. But if you do, I'm just going to leave." To become sober, Matt was willing to move away from those relationships.

Envy is prevalent in human nature. And it's common for friends to become jealous of someone who transforms themselves. For example, if you're in a group of overweight people who bond over food and going to restaurants and you decide to lose 100 pounds, expect the rest of the group to feel threatened.

In these situations, it's very common for jealous friends to try to sabotage you. Sometimes, this even happens between spouses. We've heard this story many times from our private clients. Unfortunately, very few people transcend that, so you have to prepare yourself mentally. Don't get caught off guard.

Making an unbreakable commitment to your journey may require adjusting whom you spend your time with. While you won't necessarily have to sever ties with people, you're probably not going to the same restaurants with the same people and eating the same foods as before. You may see your friends a little less and under different circumstances, such as meeting them for coffee instead of at a bar or buffet.

These changes can be extremely uncomfortable for both you and your old friends. Sometimes the changes can be extraordinarily positive, though. Over time, you may inspire them to get healthy.

Eventually, four of Matt's old friends became inspired by his transformation and wanted to become sober as well. Matt became the anchor for them, as he had already transitioned and become rock-solid in his habits, mindset, and level of consciousness. They decided they wanted that too. This is something that you can look forward to once you become BIOptimized.

EDGE #14: GET A COACH

Working with a coach at any point in your journey is always a wise move. Most people don't have the willpower, the discipline, the habits, the drive, the knowledge, or the wisdom to get started and follow through. You want to hire the guy who's been successful with hundreds of clients.

Even coaches have coaches. We're no exceptions. Both of us have almost always had coaches throughout our journey. We were *far* more successful with coaches than when we didn't have them. Wade's physique made a quantum leap when he hired Scott Abel. We both constantly hire coaches to help keep us accountable. We still hire them today in our 40s and 50s. That's how much we believe in them.

Choose a coach with the right temperament for you. Find someone with whom you can create a deep bond. The key is to know yourself. Some people like to be intimidated and have their butts kicked (Matt was a good trainer for those types), while others do better with a coach who pumps their tires a little bit.

As coaches, we hold you to a standard that most people around you won't. Your circle of friends could be holding you back. For example, some families might believe they're genetically doomed to be obese. This is a lie. Such self-destructive stories impair your ability to reach your goals.

A good coach takes apart your lies and mirrors the truth back to you. Everyone hits roadblocks on their journey. A great coach will help you overcome your personal struggles and *win!* Go to www.BIOptimizers.com/book/coaching to have one of our coaches guide you through your journey.

EDGE #15: GET A PERSONAL TRAINER

If you can afford it, hire a personal trainer. We were both trainers for over a decade, and we can attest that a great trainer can take your results to another dimension. Our success rate at taking people to the next level was nearly 100 percent.

First, you'll learn proper form and technique. This can double or triple your results over time. Even if you can afford training for just a dozen sessions to teach you proper form, it's a great investment.

Next, you'll learn how to push your body. Most people have never pushed themselves physically, so they don't know what they're really capable of. A good trainer takes you beyond your comfort zone, and then they progressively expand your comfort zone to new levels.

Third, they supply motivation on "down" days. You might not feel like going to the gym, but just paying for your coach's time means you're losing money if you don't go. That's a very strong incentive to show up. As coaches, we supply the drive until people find it within themselves to become hooked and stay on this journey for life.

EDGE #16: BUILD AN EMOTIONAL SUPPORT TEAM

There are hard days ahead for all of us. Life's greatest pains are emotional—from big things like the heartbreak of losing a loved one, to the guilt stemming from the disappointment of missing a goal because you didn't follow instructions, to feeling like giving up. If someone doesn't have the right toolbox to process those challenging emotions, they're setting themselves up for failure. If someone has the right toolbox, their quality of life goes up as their happiness levels rise.

When it comes to emotional support and safety, at least 60 percent of men and 50 percent of women have experienced trauma.[3] They may not manifest as post-traumatic stress disorder (PTSD), but they are common reasons that people engage in emotional eating, sabotage themselves, or can't stay on diets. Some people are not even aware of what happened to them in the past, but they keep repeating their self-sabotaging patterns.

Matt shares his experience doing this work:

> I hit rock bottom at 32 from years of out-of-control alcoholism and drug addiction, and I was desperate for a solution. I stopped drinking. However, I was still me. I had stopped maturing emotionally from the time I started drinking, which was 20 years prior. I had no tools to cope with life's curveballs.
>
> Fortunately, I worked with multiple mentors in recovery as well as experts in Emotional Freedom Techniques (EFT) and have spent about eight weeks of my life working on cleaning my limbic system by combining neurofeedback with forgiveness. The result?

> "My reactivity to things is down 99 percent. Bad days with my wife went from two or three days a month to zero in years. I've become a much better business leader, since I stay calm no matter what. However, the best part is . . . I just feel at peace inside. I live in serenity. It's become a baseline that I protect by using the tools we are sharing with you in this book."

Coaches are not therapists, and it's outside their scope of practice to treat your traumas. Many people need both. However, a great coach needs to be trauma informed so they respond appropriately and avoid making the problem worse.

In Chapter 11, we discuss effective tools for cleaning emotional traumas, which can often be the limiting success factor for many.

EDGE #17: TRAINING AND ACCOUNTABILITY PARTNERS

Your ideal training partner is someone who's been working out for a long time. You know they're going to show up because it's ingrained in their habits, and they're unlikely to drop off.

There's power in partnering with friends.

Some people just go work out with their friends, which is better than going alone, especially if you're an obliger or an oxytocin type. Obligers find it easier to follow through with the expectations of others rather than their own. Therefore, they're more likely to succeed with external accountability. It can be fun, and you can bond. There's fellowship and friendship. These groups or partnerships can be another really powerful tool in stacking your odds.

There's also danger in partnering with friends.

If your friend doesn't have it locked in, your odds of success go down dramatically. Usually, if two people who haven't fully made the shift into the BIOptimized lifestyle are working together and one of them drops off, the other will drop off as well.

One way to further stack the odds is by creating a trifecta or quad of committed people. That way, if one person drops off, they get social pressure from the group. Also, the rest of the group will continue on with you if that person never comes back again. Our point is that a two-friend team of inexperienced participants is a weak system of accountability.

EDGE #18: FOCUS ON AVOIDING THE PAIN

Research has shown that people are more apt to succeed at something if they focus on avoiding some kind of pain, as opposed to striving for a goal. In other words, the negative has more power than the positive.

We are big fans of using both sides. However, we agree from experience that the fear of failure and embarrassment is a strong motivator. It's a great tool to embrace.

Make going off your program more painful than showing up to the gym and following your diet. For Wade, as a bodybuilder, the pain of walking onstage in front of a crowd with excess body fat on him was so great that he couldn't even consider deviating from his plan. Matt likes to use trips, events, and film shoots as motivators to stay on track. Some people use vacations. In Panama, people want to look good for Carnivale.

The best strategy is to layer dopamine loops. Stack the odds in your favor with a series of events that are always ahead that you can look forward to. A way to amplify the effectiveness of this edge is to use deadlines.

EDGE #19: CREATE REASONABLE, HIGH-PRESSURE DEADLINES

Many people, including Wade, do better with deadlines, especially when it comes to bodybuilding. Wade would set a show date and then work backward from there. The ticking clock is a powerful form of pressure.

Set a Reasonable Deadline

For example, if Wade starts at 205 pounds and needs to be 185 by May 15th, with an average weight loss of two pounds per week, he'll need 10 weeks to get there. But he adds 20 to 30 percent more time as a buffer. Sometimes he's given himself as many as 20 weeks to allow for things he can't control, because seldom do we have a perfect world.

EDGE #20 ACCOUNTABILITY GROUPS

There's a lot of power in working with others, as demonstrated by 12-step groups. The right group can be an extremely powerful transformation tool. When you find a sense of belonging with the right people, you're probably in the right group. We naturally bond deepest with people with uncommon commonalities that have experienced the same struggles in their journeys.

Such empowering groups create environments for new friendships and fellowship to flourish.

Digital versions of these groups can also be very helpful. That's why we built that functionality into our dieting app. Go to www.BIOptimizers.com/book/dietapp to download our app to make your Me Diet journey simple and easy to follow.

EDGE #21: FOOD JOURNALING

Many studies have confirmed that food journaling correlates with better weight loss outcomes.[4] For example, a Kaiser Permanente study involving 1,685 people found that the more subjects journaled their foods, the more weight they were likely to lose. In addition, those who journaled six days a week lost twice as much weight as those who journaled only one or two.[5]

The reason is that journaling increases self-awareness. It helps prevent us from slipping into an unconscious, downward spiral. Journaling creates a mirror, influencing people's food choices and compliance to a diet. Sharing your journals with your coach can take your results to the next dimension when you provide full transparency and record everything.

However, writing things down is less convenient and less accurate than taking pictures. Often, people write food records based on memory and estimated portion sizes. Remember, people underestimate their calories by 40 percent, so taking photos of everything you eat and sharing all of them with your coach is another way to stack your odds. The pain of sharing pics of a McDonald's Happy Meal and M&M's with your coach can be a powerful deterrent.

We've all had those moments when we broke down and indulged. The problem starts when we stop being self-aware and slip back into an unconscious weight-gaining mode.

You need to expose these habits, but only in an environment where you won't be judged about it. It's normal to fear being vulnerable, but a great coach will make you feel safe to share your relapses, which helps you achieve emotional freedom. We discuss this in Chapter 10.

EDGE #22: TRACKING PROGRESS

Most people cannot trust the mirror, because their perception, mood, and emotions affect how they see themselves. One day it's "I look goooood!" and the next day it's "I look bad!" Fluctuations in neurochemistry and mood can completely alter our self-perception. This is why we need objective measurements. We recommend taking all of the following:

1. Monthly photos
2. Monthly body fat measurements
3. Weekly tape measurements
4. Daily morning weigh-ins

Take pictures of yourself monthly. A lot of people start their weight loss journeys looking at their pictures and thinking, *Oh my God, do I really look like that?* People go through long phases of unconscious weight-gaining mode, and they lose the awareness that they're gaining weight. They don't see themselves accurately in the mirror. We understand that facing oneself after a multi-year or multi-decade weight gain cycle is hard. The key is to face the pain, clear it, and turn it into motivational fuel.

For body fat measurement, a DEXA scan is the best, but you can also use BodPods and skinfold calipers. For more on body composition measurements, refer to Chapter 13.

Measuring tape is one of the best tools. Why? Because it's cheap and easy. If your diet is working, you'll see the results. We strongly recommend measuring weekly. When you're losing bodyfat, measuring tapes provide a steady flow of wins and a solid source of dopamine.

Clothing fit can also be a good measurement. Some people use progressive clothing rewards, while others just have a pair of skinny jeans in the target size that they want. Or they track holes on a belt. Whatever reward system leads to that progress for you, do it. It's another way to create a dopamine loop.

Weigh yourself first thing in the morning, *every day.* However, make peace with the scale. Be aware of natural fluctuations and don't let them discourage you. Most of the time, small weight changes are just little shifts in water and intestinal bulk. What matters is the direction of your bodyweight *on a weekly basis.*

EDGE #23: CHOOSE SELF-ACCEPTANCE RATHER THAN SELF-JUDGMENT AND SHAME

Self-judgment and shame are two of the most common reasons people engage in emotional eating or quit a diet altogether. Once you make an unbreakable, lifelong commitment and reprogram your identity as a healthy person, you also have to commit to absolute self-acceptance.

Many people beat themselves up for missing their short-term goals or deviating from their diets. This usually leads to a spirally descent into the "F-its." Matt shares his experience: "Being raised as a perfectionist, I learned how to beat myself up. When I finally learned to truly accept and love who I am, no matter what, the suffering stopped. I don't beat myself up anymore."

Quite often, the beginning of a spiraling descent begins with, "Oh, I went off my diet during breakfast, so I might as well go to McDonald's for lunch." And this can often lead to, "I've already blown my diet, so F this!"

There are zero benefits from beating yourself up. It's all downside. Instead, identify the growth opportunity and focus on that. Focus on the lessons, the gifts, and the wins.

EDGE #24: EMBRACE EXTREME OWNERSHIP

There are two types of people in this world: those who take extreme ownership for everything in their lives, and those who blame everyone else. If you want to be successful, the following truth must be embraced: you are responsible for everything in your life.

You are responsible for every piece of food that enters your mouth. You are responsible for moving your body. You are responsible for activating the right genes in your body. You are responsible for your health.

Retired Navy SEAL Jocko Willink wrote the protocol manual for this edge: *Extreme Ownership.*

Yes, maybe you were born into a family that didn't value health and influenced you to become unhealthy. However, you are responsible for transcending that mindset *today* and reprogramming your mind for success *now.*

Take extreme ownership right here, right now. Turn on the switch. You have the power!

HACK YOUR SPIRIT.

There is no driver more powerful than being fueled by purpose.

EDGE #25: IDENTIFY YOUR WHY

Your "why," also known as your purpose, is the ultimate driver. A strong purpose pushes people to take actions over decades. Elon Musk is unstoppable because of his purpose, which is to save earth and help humans become a multi-planetary species. Money and wealth aren't the primary drivers anymore. In our experience, the compelling power of purpose is far stronger than any motivation or inspiration. Matt has experienced this with BIOptimizers. "The drive to help redefine and transform the world's health propels me into action. I just do what I need to do. I have endless energy and drive."

Wade became unstoppable in his quest for bodybuilding success, because he was driven by purpose. Matt is unstoppable in making biological optimization affordable and available to the entire world. The drive becomes limitless when you find your purpose and align your life to it.

Use the "Seven Levels Deep" exercise: ask, "Why?" seven times to identify your most compelling purpose. For example:

1. Why do you want to get healthy and lean out?
   → I want to look good in the mirror.
2. Why do you want to look good in the mirror?
   → Because I want to feel more confident and comfortable in my own skin.
3. Why do you want to be more confident and comfortable in your own skin?
   → Because I was made fun of as a kid and want to improve my body image.
4. Why do you want to improve your body image?
   → So that I have better self-esteem and confidence.
5. Why do you want to have better self-esteem and confidence?
   → So that I can get back to dating.
6. Why do you want to get back to dating?
   → So that I can find myself a great partner.
7. Why do you want to find yourself a great partner?
   → Because it's my life goal to start a family and be a great dad.

Recognize what your "whys" are, and then dig deeper.

Level Up Your Why

People start their health and fitness journey for different reasons. When Wade saw Troy Zuccolotto on the cover of *Muscle & Fitness* with a couple of beautiful women, that's all he needed. He decided right there: *This is the way.* His hormone-driven desires to impress the opposite sex got switched on, which is normal for most young men.

When Matt saw a couple of jacked bodybuilders at the beach at the age of 16, he felt small and weak, and he was inspired to start training. His fear of getting bullied again got activated. Matt wanted muscle to feel more empowered.

Having worked with thousands of clients, we've seen many people come in because of serious health problems. They've ignored their health for decades, gotten a scary diagnosis, and decided to get healthy. Many people start their weight loss, fitness, and health journeys with personal desires, like finding a new romantic partner after a divorce.

Whatever the reasons you're here, embrace them. However, you can get more power by leveling up your purpose. In his book *Power vs. Force*, Dr. David Hawkins lays out a Map of Consciousness that has several levels. The higher up you go on the map, the more fundamental power you'll have.

Many of us start with low-power purposes, which is fine. It got us into the game. However, to make it all the way, we need more juice. The extra power comes when we shift our purpose to a higher level of consciousness.

We believe that you have arrived once you enter the "love zone." They *love* to work out, and they *love* to eat healthy food. They have fallen in love with the experience of being BIOptimized.

In rarer cases, self-actualization can be the purpose. Being biologically optimized feels awesome! The journey becomes taking your health, performance, and aesthetics to the absolute pinnacle. You're not doing it for others; you're doing it because you're driven to become all that you can be. Inspiring others becomes a cool side effect.

EDGE #26: FLIP THE "GO SWITCH" IN YOUR MIND

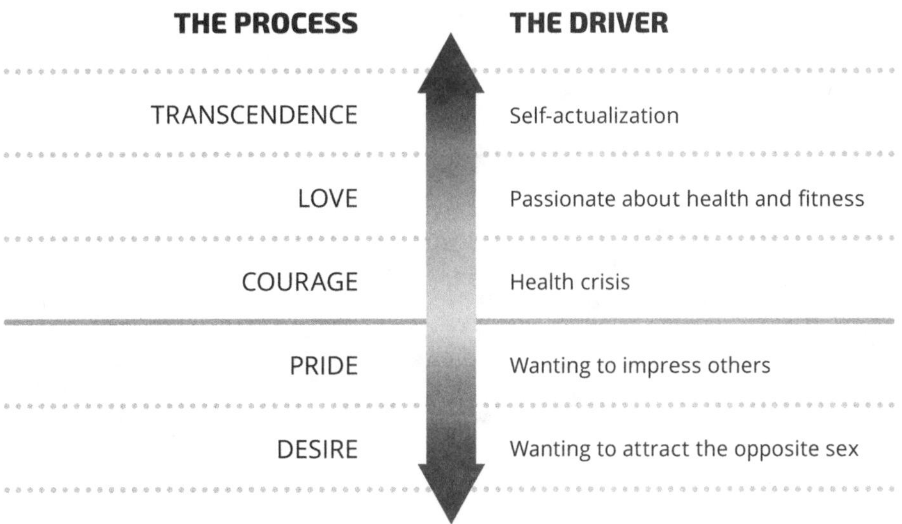

Once you experience the moment of clarity, there's a short window of opportunity that emerges to hit the "go switch." Wade explains, "When I'm ready to go for it and get the results, I turn on a switch in my mind. What happens when I turn on that switch?"

The answer is, these thoughts begin to guide his actions:

- *Food is just fuel.*
- *I'm willing to go to any lengths to get results.*
- *How I feel doesn't matter.*
- *I transcend hunger.*
- *Workouts happen no matter what: if I'm traveling, or it's 4* A.M. *It's the priority.*
- *If I don't have the right foods, I don't eat. I just fast.*

You essentially embrace stoicism. You embrace the obstacles. You're in warrior mode, and the biological impulses for food and inactivity are the enemy.

This is the champion's state of mind that you need to embrace during your final phases. This isn't for everyone. This is a gate that everyone who has chosen to build a world-class level of aesthetics crosses through. Let's flick that GO switch. GO.

EDGE #27: MAKE THE UNBREAKABLE COMMITMENT TO YOUR HEALTH

Commit to becoming the healthiest version of yourself for the rest of your life from this day forward. By doing this, you make an unbreakable commitment that no matter what happens, no matter how many times you fall off your diet or miss a workout . . . you're not stopping.

As Matt's hand-to-hand combat teacher, Christophe Clugston, used to say, "There's no failure, there's only stopping."

Your unbreakable commitment is exponentially more powerful than any short-term goals. This commitment is the missing link for people who come in and out of their weight loss journeys. People who want to get in shape for a wedding or a vacation and don't make this commitment inevitably falter and go back to their old ways.

Humans are like planes. We're off course 90 percent of the time, but we keep adjusting and recalibrating to the destination. We've gone off track more times than we can count. But our unbreakable commitment magnetically draws us back on the path. Nothing will pump wind in your sails like a lifelong commitment to your health.

Here's the great news: once you fall in love with the journey, you've entered the magic zone. Being superhumanly healthy becomes one of life's great joys.

SUMMARY

Achieving long-term success on any diet isn't easy. Maximize your odds of success by stacking every advantage possible.

- Edge #1: Create Your Own Dopamine-Driven Reward Loops
- Edge #2: Layer Your Dopamine Loops
- Edge #3: Always Have the Next Goal
- Edge #4: Take Action Even if You Don't Feel Like It
- Edge #5: Value Long-Term Wins over Short-Term Gratifications
- Edge #6: Success Is a Program of Action
- Edge #7: Find the Gifts in Your Setbacks and Challenges
- Edge #8: Upgrade Your Worst Habits
- Edge #9: Control Your Environment
- Edge #10: Avoid Food Advertising
- Edge #11: The Universal Secret of Physique Champions: Food Prep
- Edge #12: Always Have a Backup Plan
- Edge #13: Hang with the Winners
- Edge #14: Get a Coach
- Edge #15: Get a Personal Trainer
- Edge #16: Build an Emotional Support Team
- Edge #17: Training and Accountability Partners
- Edge #18: Focus on Avoiding the Pain
- Edge #19: Create Reasonable, High-Pressure Deadlines
- Edge #20: Accountability Groups
- Edge #21: Food Journaling
- Edge #22: Tracking Progress
- Edge #23: Choose Self-Acceptance Rather Than Self-Judgment and Shame
- Edge #24: Embrace Extreme Ownership
- Edge #25: Identify Your Why
- Edge #26: Flip the "Go Switch" in Your Mind
- Edge #27: Make the Unbreakable Commitment to Your Health

CHAPTER 6

HOW TO BUILD YOUR ME DIET: THE PYRAMID OF NUTRITIONAL DECISIONS

This chapter provides you with a framework to make smarter nutritional decisions amid all the noise from social media, dietary groups, and influencers.

In this chapter you will learn:

- The hierarchy of nine nutritional factors that help you build the perfect diet for YOU.
- Why spiritual, cultural, emotional, and psychological factors are the baseline keys to keeping you on track with a sustainable diet.
- The five diet optimizers that will take you beyond calorie counting.
- The three fundamentals you must follow after achieving your main goal, and how forgoing them means inevitably sliding back to your old habits.
- You'll have to live with the same exact plan for the rest of your life, right? *Wrong!* Once you've reached your goal, you can lock it in with 20 percent of the effort that it took to get there.

There have been a lot of "nutritional pyramids" built over the years. Most of them attempt to box people into certain diets. In this chapter, we present a new type of pyramid—one that helps you create the best diet for you.

We break down the decision factors in order of importance. We suggest you start at the bottom of the pyramid and move your way up to create your ultimate nutritional game plan.

First, all the factors are important to various levels. Second, know that most nutrition advice you find on social media is one-sided or doesn't take into account all three sides of your BIOptimization Triangle: performance, health, and aesthetics.

More importantly, most dogmatic diet experts rarely take into account your happiness, spiritual beliefs, or lifestyle. This is another reason why 97 percent of people eventually quit and revert to their old habits. We want you to win for life.

There's an order and level of importance for the different decision factors. If you follow our model, you'll be much more likely to be successful and create the perfect sustainable diet for *you*.

Our framework takes into account spiritual, nutritional, emotional, and mental models. It organizes everything in a way that helps you make the right decisions in a personalized way.

We can summarize our Pyramid of Nutritional Decisions™ in four steps:

1. Choose the right approach based on your core values, beliefs, and personality
2. Commit to your goals (this creates direction)
3. Optimize your diet and supplements based on your goals, genetics, food sensitivities, and gut biome
4. Lock in the results for life

Pyramid of Nutritional Decisions
LIFESTYLE
The Final Key to Sustainability
FOOD ALLERGIES AND SENSITIVITIES
SUPPLEMENTS
GUT BIOME
Diet Optimizers
NUTRIGENOMICS
CALORIES AND MACROS
GOALS
Direction
EMOTIONAL AND PSYCHOLOGICAL NEEDS
SPIRITUAL AND CULTURAL COMMITMENTS
Foundational Keys to Sustainability

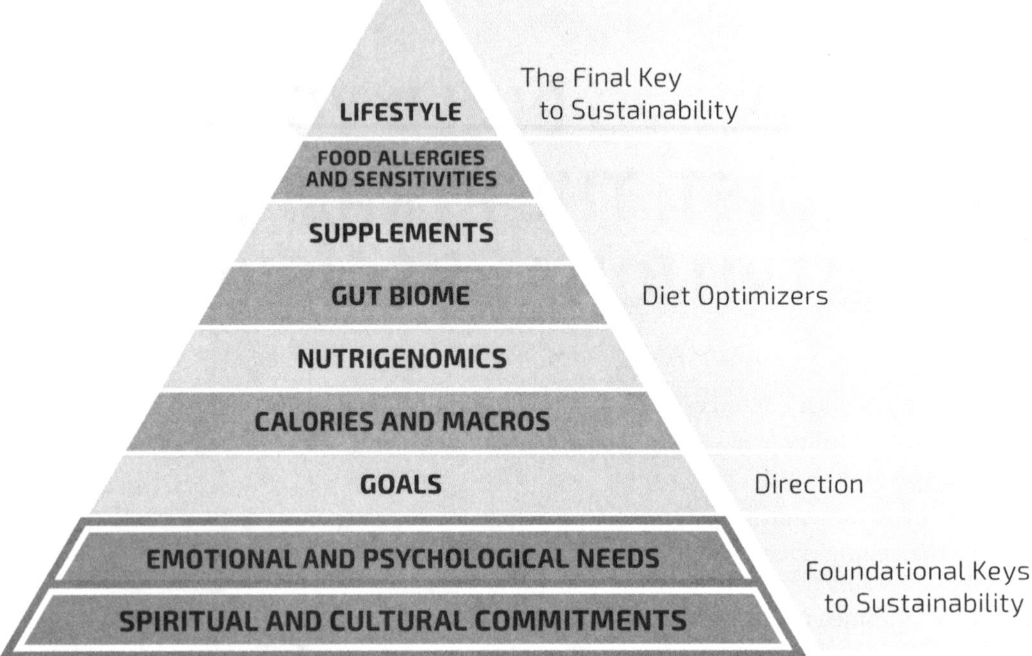

Now let's dive into the Pyramid of Nutritional Decisions model and how to use each layer to help make the right nutritional decisions for you.

NUTRITIONAL DECISION FACTOR #1: SPIRITUAL AND CULTURAL COMMITMENTS

This is about selecting potential diets that are in alignment with your spiritual and cultural core values.

If you have spiritual or cultural beliefs that restrict your dietary choices, we're not here to judge that. Rather, we're here to support you. We can help you thrive on any diet despite the possibility that, physiologically, it might be suboptimal. That way, you can still maximize all three sides of your BIOptimization Triangle.

There are many hacks you can use to counter the potential negative consequences of a diet, especially supplements. We cover those throughout the book.

Why I Became a Vegetarian, by Wade T. Lightheart

Wade was a meat-eating bodybuilder until he read the book *The Holy Science* by Swami Sri Yukteswar, which described how form and function differ between carnivores, omnivores, herbivores, and frugivores (raw fruit eaters).

A few of Yukteswar's key points are:

Carnivores have incisors that can rip flesh, along with shorter intestinal tracts. Plants take a lot more work to digest and extract nutrients from than meat, so herbivores tend to have much longer intestines than carnivores. Our small intestine is about 20 feet long, whereas cat intestines are 3–4.5 feet and dog intestines are 6–16 feet long.[1] So, the undigested meats and animal proteins would deposit in pockets inside the human's longer intestinal tracts.

As Yukteswar wrote in *Holy Science*, abstaining from meat may enhance spiritual practices. Many religions and spiritual traditions use abstinence from meat or animal products as part of theirs.

According to Yukteswar, protein deposits can put pressure on our meridian points and affect our health, as our gut registers every part of the body. Therefore, meat eating could impair meditation. Sensibly, many religious and spiritual traditions throughout the world independently use abstinence from meat and animal products as part of their practice.

So, Wade did a two-week experiment following this philosophy, and he felt really good. He decided to try it for another two weeks, which was followed by another month. The plant-based diet agreed with him so well that he just abandoned all flesh proteins and has been living as a vegetarian for over 20 years.

NUTRITIONAL DECISION FACTOR #2: EMOTIONAL AND PSYCHOLOGICAL NEEDS

We feel it's best to build diet strategies that respect and satisfy your emotional and psychological needs. For most people, psychology is the true make-or-break factor for long-term success beyond a few months. Yet, most diets take zero consideration of your psychology.

NUTRITIONAL DECISION FACTOR #3: YOUR GOALS

Your goals shape your game plan. What do you want to achieve?

The Five Epic Biological Goals

Aesthetics

1. Building lean muscle
2. Burning excess body fat

Performance

3. Maximizing your athletic performance
4. Optimizing your mental performance

Health: Maximizing Your BioSpan

5. Maximizing your life span and health span

This book gives you the best currently known strategies to achieve any goal you desire.

THE FIVE DIET OPTIMIZERS

The next variables are five powerful ways to optimize your diet. We cover each one in depth in this book.

NUTRITIONAL DECISION FACTOR #4: CALORIES AND MACROS

Your goals will be the major determinant of your calories and macros. If you want to lose weight, you need to be in a calorie deficit. If you want to gain weight, you need to be in a surplus. If you're a competitive athlete, then you usually want to keep your calories around maintenance.

No matter what your goals are, protein is the foundational macro. It doesn't matter if your goal is muscle building, fat loss, or athletic performance; you need protein. Then you build the rest of your diet around that. Carbs and fats are adjusted based on genetics, goals, and psychological preferences.

Chapter 7, The Optimized Metabolism System, goes into more details about calories, while Chapter 8 covers how you can cycle calories to both maximize your results and enjoy your favorite foods.

NUTRITIONAL DECISION FACTOR #5: NUTRIGENOMICS

Nutrigenomics refers to the scientific study of the interaction between nutrition and genes. It's a relatively new field, but it's progressing rapidly. Understanding your genetic mutations and optimizing your diet accordingly can help you go to the next level of health and performance.

For example, understanding how your genetic variants influence your nutrient absorption and conversion allows you to overcome gene-based challenges with supplements. It's incredibly valuable information that we believe everyone should have about themselves. To get the test, go to: www.BIOptimizers.com/book/genes.

For decades, people believed that genes were a life sentence. Now we know that what matters more is which genes are expressed. Your genes load the gun, while your environment pulls the trigger. You can have unfavorable genes, but healthy habits can turn on good genes. Conversely, an unhealthy environment and nutrition can turn on bad genes.

While you can inherit both genetics and epigenetics from your parents, your nutrition, fitness, and lifestyle activate your epigenetics.

We've brought in some of the top nutrigenomic experts in the world to help us write Chapter 33, which covers how you can harness the power of nutrigenomics and epigenetics in your nutritional BIOptimization.

NUTRITIONAL DECISION FACTOR #6: GUT BIOME

It's estimated that there are over 1 trillion bacteria in and on your body right now. Your gut microbes are like an ever-evolving back pocket of genes. Your own cells harbor around 22,000 genes, but your microbes have collectively well over 3.3 million.[2]

You have a two-way relationship with your gut microbes. Eating the right foods that are aligned with your gut biome and taking probiotics are effective ways to optimize your intestinal health.

Feeding your body foods that feed the good bacteria in your gut and avoiding foods that aren't ideal for your flora will take your health and performance to new heights.

Chapter 31 covers the latest science on how to live, eat, and supplement in a way that optimizes your gut microbes.

NUTRITIONAL DECISION FACTOR #7: SUPPLEMENTS

If your goal is to achieve optimal nutrient levels to expand all three sides of your BIOptimization Triangle, we believe nutritional supplements are necessary.

Some people want to believe they can get everything their body needs from food. Sadly, modern agricultural practices have greatly depleted the soil of key micronutrients, as well as the microorganisms that help plants assimilate them. As a result, plants and everything up the food chain contain fewer micronutrients than ever before.[3] You just can't trust grocery food to give you the nutrients your body needs. Supplements can give your body the nutrients that are missing from food.

Another critical factor is that most people have genetic mutations that make it hard or almost impossible to metabolize certain foods. Supplements can help counter the negative consequences of this.

Beyond that, for those of us who want to be superhuman versions of ourselves, supplements are some of the most important tools. We can take our health and performance from normal to superhuman with these:

- Bio workers, such as enzymes and probiotics, that can help improve digestion and tens of thousands of metabolic processes in the body
- Optimizers, such as hormone boosters
- Maximizers, such as nootropics
- Activators, which serve to activate mechanisms inside your body, such as the mitochondria, mTOR signaling, or autophagy

To maximize the bang for your buck with supplements, it's important to understand how they work, choose high-quality products, and stack them correctly. More isn't necessarily better; neither do supplements replace an overall healthy diet, sleep, or stress management.

See www.BIOptimizers/book/resources to get our free in-depth supplement guide about how to use them to improve your results.

NUTRITIONAL DECISION FACTOR #8: FOOD ALLERGIES AND SENSITIVITIES

Most people who have food allergies tend to be aware of them because the symptoms are severe, immediate, and potentially life-threatening.

Food sensitivities tend to be more subtle because the reactions are delayed and often milder. In many cases, people may think their inflammatory symptoms are "normal" for years until they eliminate certain foods and discover that they had caused the symptoms. Our brains are constantly normalizing being suboptimal and sick.

Inflammation from food sensitivities affects your entire body, but the symptoms tend to show up first in the weakest link in your body. Therefore, if your goal is to maximize any side of your BIOptimization Triangle, or all three, it's important to identify and avoid foods you are sensitive to.

Because your gut contains 80 percent of your immune system, food allergies and sensitivities are highly linked to your gut barrier integrity, gut flora, and digestive function. In many cases, people can eat the foods again once they fix the gut.

Conversely, factors that cause a leaky gut and dysbiosis can also lead to food allergies or sensitivities, even when you've eaten a food your entire life. To learn more about food sensitivities, refer to Chapter 31.

NUTRITIONAL DECISION FACTOR #9: THE BIOPTIMIZATION LIFESTYLE—HOW TO SUCCEED ON EVERY DIET AND KEEP YOUR RESULTS FOR LIFE

Lifestyle is the final key to lifelong sustainability.

Some hardcore people like David Goggins *love* having a life filled with pain and discipline. However, the rest of us want to be able to enjoy a pizza and ice cream once in a while. We want to enjoy a Christmas dinner with the family without worrying about calories. We want to be able to go on vacation and enjoy the local cuisine.

Here's the great news: once you achieve your final form, you can lock it in with 20 percent of the effort that it took to get there.

Your lifestyle becomes your health style. And, as the great poet James Hetfield said, "My lifestyle determines my death style." If you want to live to be over 100 while rocking and rolling, then implement the advice and Power Moves in this book (and in our other book, *From Sick to Superhuman*).

It's paramount that you always have a goal (even if it's just maintaining your weight), a strategy, and mental vigilance. You need to harness the power of your dopamine loops by constantly setting goals and micro goals. Our most successful clients are the ones who always have constant sequences of goals to keep them motivated and driven.

Once you finish one goal, always have the next one lined up. There is no final destination. Your key to success for becoming a biologically optimized superhuman involves creating endless successions of exciting goals.

SUMMARY

We give you a framework to make the best nutritional decisions and create a personalized diet plan that works for you—one where you'll be able to succeed both short term and long term. This strategy incorporates every model that could be essential to you: spiritual, physical, emotional, and mental.

The Foundational Keys to Sustainability

Spiritual and Cultural Beliefs: Selecting potential diets that are in alignment with your spiritual and cultural core values.

Emotional and Psychological Needs: Building diet strategies that respect and align with your emotional and psychological needs.

The Direction

Goals: What do you want to achieve? The goals shape the game plan.

The Diet Optimizers

Calories and Macros: Your calories and macros are designed around your goal.

Nutrigenomics: These use your genetics to help you pick the right dietary approach and optimize your existing diet.

Gut Biome: These help you optimize your diet further by selecting foods that your gut can easily process and avoiding the ones that are more challenging for your gut biome.

Supplements: These accelerate your results with the right supplement stacks.

Food Allergies and Sensitivities: Knowing these helps you eliminate foods that stress your body.

The Final Key to Sustainability

Lifestyle: Build the diet that you can follow forever while enjoying life and that's still aligned with your goals.

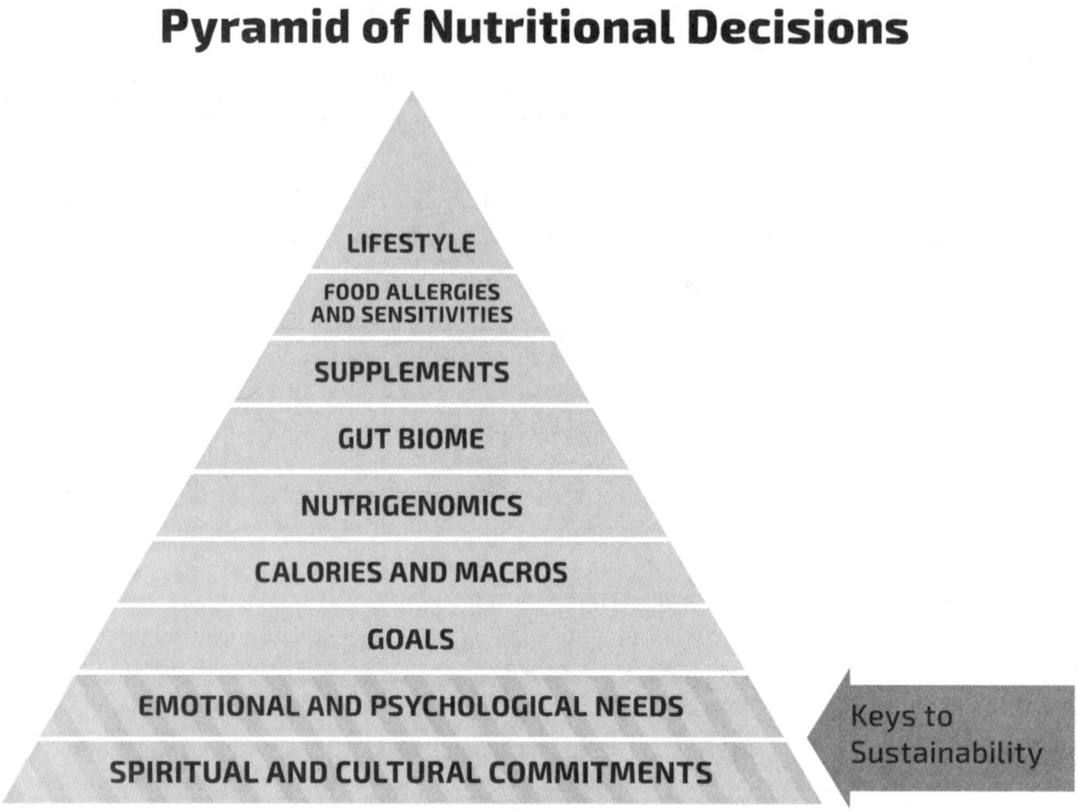

Pyramid of Nutritional Decisions

LIFESTYLE
FOOD ALLERGIES AND SENSITIVITIES
SUPPLEMENTS
GUT BIOME
NUTRIGENOMICS
CALORIES AND MACROS
GOALS
EMOTIONAL AND PSYCHOLOGICAL NEEDS
SPIRITUAL AND CULTURAL COMMITMENTS

Keys to Sustainability

GOAL #1:

YOUR FINAL WEIGHT LOSS JOURNEY

The next eight chapters hold the fundamentals to permanent, healthy weight loss.

CHAPTER 7

THE OPTIMIZED METABOLISM SYSTEM

If your goal is weight loss, this chapter is the most important one in the entire book. This chapter is a major paradigm shift regarding weight loss. Our optimized system keeps your metabolism revving and avoids the pitfalls that may arise from hardcore calorie restriction. This system is the culmination of 50 years of combined real-world experience.

In this chapter you will learn:

- The five optimized strategies to follow to ensure you reach your goals permanently over the long term
- How to turbocharge your metabolism for success without following a model of hard calorie restriction that sacrifices the future for today
- The five main categories of food groups that add up to your calorie intake, and how to understand your total caloric intake
- The 13 practical steps you can start implementing now to maintain muscle mass and healthy BMR, while minimizing metabolic adaptation and the starvation response on a caloric deficit
- Why the diet industry's focus on restricting food intake and burning calories is only effective for a few months, but fails terribly in the long run—and why this is a recipe for a highly restrictive and unenjoyable life
- Why focusing on building and preserving lean muscle mass while revving up the BMR is critical to maintaining your results long term, while still enjoying and living an awesome life to the fullest
- The hierarchy of exercise for fat loss and the benefits of outdoor rather than indoor cardio
- Your three critical tools for slowing down metabolic adaptation—the primary enemy of weight loss
- Why cardio is actually last on the list of the hierarchy of fat loss exercises, and tips to maximize the results of your cardio
- How to optimize calories in vs. calories out
- Five surefire ways to naturally boost your anabolism to maximize weight loss
- The 10 variables for understanding calories out

I think we can declare that fad diets and massive weight loss programs are epic failures. We've already covered the reasons in depth in previous chapters.

Now it's time to give you the solution to the trouble with dieting. The key is to work with your genetics—and your mind.

Focusing on simply cutting calories is the wrong thing to do. Instead, we suggest the eight following strategic items to focus on:

1. Having the right mindset; play the long game and be patient
2. Keeping your metabolism as high as possible during the entire dieting process
3. Maintaining or even building lean muscle
4. Keeping your body feeling safe throughout the journey, which avoids triggering the starvation self-defense systems
5. Rebuilding your metabolism strategically throughout
6. Strategically breaking plateaus when they happen
7. Locking in your final "set point" while living an awesome lifestyle
8. Respecting your limitations and personalizing the system so that it works for *you*

Before we dive into how you can do this, let's examine the classic approach.

WEIGHT LOSS 101: THE CALORIE MODEL

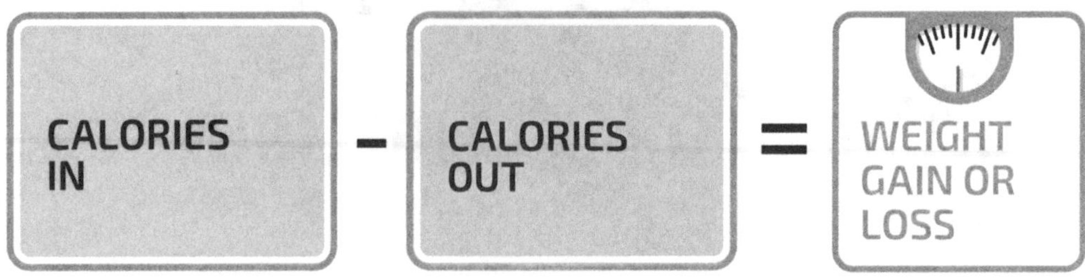

The diagram above sums up the majority of "diet expert" perspectives on weight loss. It is technically accurate. However, it's dangerously incomplete.

The calorie-counting model assumes your body is like a robotic furnace that burns a fixed sum of calories, and the only thing you need to do to lose weight is eat less and exercise more. You just have to create a deficit of 3,500 calories to lose a pound of body fat. Simple, right?

Wouldn't it be awesome if it were that easy? As we explained in previous chapters, our genetic programming has other plans. The body is always adapting. The heart of our strategy is to break homeostasis using a variety of methods vs. constantly lowering calories alone.

THE OPTIMIZED METABOLISM WEIGHT LOSS MODEL

Obviously, for someone to lose weight, "calories out" needs to exceed "calories in" over time. We cannot transcend this law of thermodynamics, despite what some diet experts claim.

Fortunately, science has shown us that it's possible and healthier to leverage other parts of the "calories out" equation and avoid all of its problems. The key to dietary success is not through simple hard calorie restriction that sacrifices the future for today. Instead, this chapter shows you how to turbocharge your metabolism in other ways, which will increase your calories out.

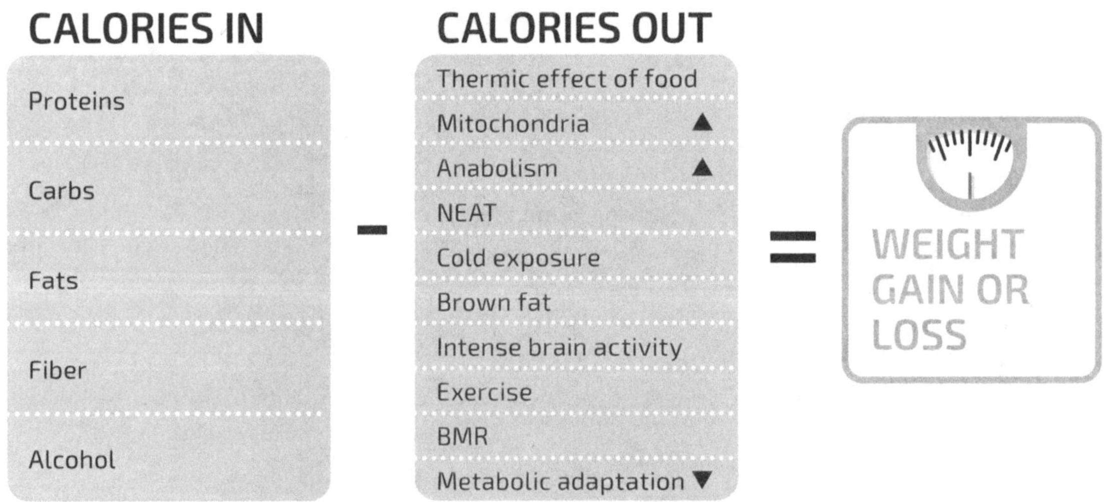

First, let's understand all the pieces of the calorie equation and how we can optimize each one to deliver next-level results.

UNDERSTANDING CALORIES IN

Proteins

Protein is the king macro for weight loss, muscle gain, and athletic performance. One gram of protein contains four calories of energy. This macronutrient is required by your body to carry out essential functions by cells, tissues, and organs. The amino acids from the protein are what repair your muscles, hair, nails, and bones. The three main reasons why protein is so powerful are:

1. The thermic effect of protein, which gives you a 30 percent calorie loss
2. The positive impact on anabolism, which increases metabolism
3. Better satiety, which makes it easier to stay on track and avoid overeating

There's more on this later in the chapter.

Carbs

Carbs are a fuel source in which one gram of carbs has four calories of energy. That's the main function of this macronutrient—to provide your body with energy. It's noteworthy that carbs are a nonessential macro. You can live without carbs. The same cannot be said for protein and fats. That being said, carbs are a superior fuel source for many goals, including athletic performance. And some people (like Wade) thrive on carbs.

Fats

Fats are another essential macronutrient that repairs the body and provides it with potential fuel. One gram of fat contains nine calories of energy. Your body needs fats to build hormones, repair your brain, skin, and hair, and do many other biological functions.

Fiber

Fiber is technically a carbohydrate. One gram of fiber contains around two calories, which makes it a powerful satiety tool for dieting—fiber helps people feel full. The net calories are 50 percent less than in normal carbs. And fiber can help optimize bowel movements.

Alcohol

Alcohol is formed from fermentation with yeast. It is found in wine, beer, and liquors (spirits). One gram of alcohol contains seven calories. Alcohol tends to become belly fat and increases visceral fat.[1]

If this seems too complicated, don't worry. Go to www.BIOptimizers.com/book/dietapp to download our app to make your Me Diet journey simple and easy to follow.

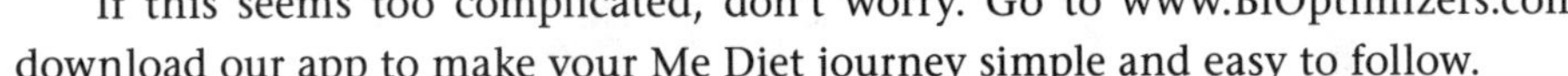

UNDERSTANDING CALORIES OUT

1. Calories Out Variable #1: Increase the Thermic Effect of Food (TEF)

Have you ever experienced the "steak sweats"? You go to a steakhouse and eat a large amount of beef, and your body feels hot for a few hours. That's the thermic effect of protein in action.

The first major key here is that not every macro is created equal. Some macros produce a much higher or lower net amount of "calories in" than others. Your body expends calories to digest and assimilate your food. This is called the thermic effect of food (TEF), which varies based on macronutrients and your meal components:[2]

- Protein has the highest TEF, which is 20 to 30 percent of the four calories per gram that it provides
- Carbohydrate has a 5 to 10 percent TEF of the four calories per gram that it provides
- Fat has a 0 to 5 percent TEF of the nine calories per gram that it provides
- Fiber is great for dieting because 1 gram of fiber is around two calories. Your body absorbs only 50 percent of the four carb calories per gram.

For example, 1,000 calories of protein create 700 "calories in," and 1,000 calories of fiber are around 500 net calories, whereas 1,000 calories of carbs or fats will be much closer to 1,000. These differences can create a huge calorie deficit over time. Because protein and fiber have the highest TEF, and high-protein foods and fiber tend to be satiating, most diets are high in protein and fiber.

Even in overfeeding studies, eating excessive calories of protein resulted in significantly less weight gain than eating the same calories of carbs or fats. Compared to overfeeding with fats, overfeeding protein or a high-protein diet increases daily calorie burn (including during sleep) by about 80 calories per day.[3] Therefore, protein overfeeding may not result in any fat gain.[4]

Proteins also help you build and maintain muscle mass, which people tend to lose when they lose weight. This is why bodybuilders typically rely on high-protein, high-fiber meals to get hyper lean.

Also, high-carbohydrate meals have higher TEF than high-fat meals.[5] However, fat is more satiating than carbohydrates, so choosing your optimal macros requires you to balance hunger management with TEF. See Chapter 29 for more information on macronutrients.

Within the ranges listed above, several factors can affect TEF, including:[6]

- Aging (reduces TEF)
- Obesity (reduces TEF)
- Insulin resistance (reduces TEF)
- Physical activity (increases TEF)[7]
  - This one is why high protein + weight resistance exercise = *big* calories out.
- Meal timing and frequency affects TEF, which is higher earlier in the day. Larger, single meals result in higher per-meal TEF than frequent smaller meals
- Fiber content of the diet and plant-based meals may increase TEF[8]

2. Boost Your Mitochondria

Mitochondria are bacteria in our bodies that produce energy. It makes sense that by increasing the quantity and strength of our mitochondria, we increase our energy output.

Here's what the research says.

In cell-based studies, increasing a protein called PGC-1alpha increases energy expenditure by stimulating the creation of new mitochondria and increasing respiration rates.[9, 10] In muscle cells, increasing PGC-1alpha also increased heat loss through mitochondrial uncoupling.[11]

A high-intensity interval training (HIIT) study had young men performing 10 30-second maximum-effort cycling sprints with 4-minute rest intervals, three days a week. After seven weeks, both fat and carb burning pathways significantly increased in their muscles, suggesting that their muscle metabolism increased.[12]

Another study from McMaster University found that both low-volume HIIT and traditional lower-intensity, steady-state cardio produced similar enzymatic adaptations in the muscles. However, they concluded that HIIT is a more time-efficient way to achieve the same results with your metabolism.[13]

This may explain why HIIT ends up burning more calories than low-intensity, steady state cardio. A HIIT session burns more calories within 24 hours after exercise compared to a low-intensity, steady state cardio exercise session.[14,15] It increases resting energy expenditure.[16]

Power Move

HIIT training increases PGC-1alpha, which stimulates the creation of new mitochondria. It also stimulates anti-aging pathways such as sirtuins and AMPK, which increases fat burning.

Here's the great news: The minimum effective dose for HIIT can be as little as two sessions a week and under 10 minutes. Four 30-second sprints with two minutes in between can yield great results.

A word of caution on HIIT: it's easy to overdo HIIT, cause injuries, and harm your mitochondria. Recent research suggests that doing more is counterproductive. The principle at play is that the optimal dose is best. That's one of the core tenets of Biological Optimization.

In one four-week study, participants increased the number of their HIIT workouts each week. They started with two workouts in week one, then did three in week two and five in week three. They spent week four in some recovery, bumping down the workouts to half in both amount and intensity.

The results? By the end of week two, the participants had improved their blood sugar and boosted their mitochondria. However, in week three, things went bad. Blood sugar spiked and dropped, and mitochondria produced 60 percent of the energy of previous workouts.

The note of caution here is that too many HIIT workouts may suddenly and severely hurt your mitochondria and blood sugar. The metabolic issues seen in the study started to reverse but didn't go away. For those reasons, we suggest starting with once a week, and when you're adapted, go to twice a week. Avoid going beyond twice per week unless you're an athlete working with a professional coach.

3. Activate Anabolism

Bodybuilders and fitness competitors know that focusing on anabolism is the most powerful approach to weight loss for many reasons.

By increasing anabolism, we can boost metabolism 10, 20, or 30 percent (or more). Matt knows of hardcore bodybuilders who did a seven-day experiment wherein they increased their anabolic drive to the max (using a massive stack of anabolic drugs) and doubled their calorie expenditure.

Why? The short answer is that building muscle requires a lot of energy. Based on doing math ourselves and with clients, we estimate that synthesizing one pound of lean muscle burns around 5,000 calories. Yes, the energy cost of building a pound of lean tissue is that high.

Next, muscle increases your BMR, which means you're burning more calories while you watch Netflix. A pound of lean muscle burns on average three times more than a pound of fat. A pound of lean muscle burns around six calories a day, whereas a pound of fat burns around two. A metabolic study found that after nine months of resistance training, resting energy expenditure (REE) went up 5 percent. So, if you add 20 pounds of lean muscle, you're going to burn an extra 120 to 130 calories a day. This adds up over time.

Third, you tend to burn more calories from a weight-lifting workout than you do from cardio. The main calorie-burning difference comes from the post-workout recovery.[17] The calorie difference becomes greater over time because your body adapts far faster to cardio than to resistance training.

Fourth, you will slow down and possibly reverse the typical trend of losing lean muscle while dieting. This means the majority of your weight loss will be fat, which is a key goal.

Five Ways to Naturally Boost Your Anabolism

1. **Optimize Sleep Quality and Quantity**

   Sleep is the most important anabolic thing that people can do. When you sleep well, your leptin and leptin sensitivity normalize, while your growth hormone and testosterone increase. Even one night of sleep deprivation increases muscle catabolism, making you hungrier and more likely to gain fat.[18, 19]

   When Matt had under 15 minutes of deep sleep each night, his body fat got up to 33 percent on the DEXA scan. He also struggled to get his testosterone into healthy levels naturally.

   To maximize your results in any direction, be it toward fat loss, muscle gain, optimized health, or metabolic rehab, you must prioritize and optimize your sleep.

2. **Optimize Your Vitamin D**

   Vitamin D is a master steroid hormone that impacts all the other hormones (including leptin and testosterone), especially in men who are low in both testosterone and vitamin D.[20] It also affects epigenetics, meaning it turns on a lot of healthy genes. It's important for muscle mitochondria function, which helps you burn more calories.[21]

   Vitamin D may also support muscle growth and strength by enhancing the effects of insulin and leucine in mTOR activation.[22, 23]

   Sun exposure can have an energizing effect. When our clients get 15 to 20 minutes of high-intensity sun each week, they lose more body fat and gain more muscle mass.

The sun itself is anabolic beyond just a source of vitamin D, which is triggered by UVB, ultraviolet light in the range that can cause sunburn. The red and infrared spectra of the sun also stimulate your mitochondria, which may increase your metabolism. All of these effects can have an anabolic effect and may burn an extra 10 to 15 percent of calories, in our experience.

If you cannot get all the vitamin D you need from the sun, and you need to supplement, be sure to get tested regularly. To optimize vitamin D metabolism, you'll also want to take Magnesium Breakthrough and vitamin K_2.

3. **Boost Testosterone**

All of your hormones run in symphony with each other.

You can optimize testosterone naturally to a point with diet, exercise, high-quality sleep, and supplements. These should be the first steps to optimizing testosterone levels before you introduce any testosterone boosters or replacement.

Make sure you eat the right foods, manage your stress, and avoid excess sugar. Poor sleep quality and prolonged caloric deficits decrease testosterone.

Unfortunately, most natural testosterone boosters don't increase testosterone as much as can testosterone replacement therapy (TRT). So, if men are at extremely low levels, TRT can benefit them as they get older.

We advise putting off any exogenous hormone intervention as long as you can, because once you get on it, there is almost no way off it. We suggest getting hormone tests every three to six months. If your doctor says your hormones are normal, and they're in the "low normal" zone, take action. You want them to be optimal for your age range. If you do decide to do TRT, make sure you do it intelligently and with a medical professional.

4. **Boost Human Growth Hormone**

Increasing human growth hormone (HGH) is a powerful way to increase metabolic rate.[24,25] Growth hormone typically increases during deep sleep and in response to hormetic stressors like saunas, fasting, HIIT, and high-rep squats. Amino acids, including arginine, methionine, phenylalanine, lysine, and ornithine, can stimulate growth hormone.[26] There are also peptides that boost growth hormone, such as ipamorelin and many others.

Ghrelin increases growth hormone, which is why fasting increases HGH. The increased HGH can help preserve muscle mass.

Using a sauna can be a powerful way to boost HGH by as much as 1,600 percent.

Power Move: The HGH Sauna Protocols

- Two 20-minute sauna sessions at 176°F separated by a 30-minute cooling period elevated growth hormone levels twofold over baseline.
- Two 15-minute sauna sessions at 212°F dry heat separated by a 30-minute cooling period resulted in a fivefold increase in growth hormone.
- A bit extreme: Two one-hour sauna sessions a day at 176°F dry heat for seven days was shown to increase growth hormone by 16-fold on the third day.

5. **Boosting mTOR**

Leucine is one of the most powerful mTOR stimulants. You want to ensure that you have at least 3 to 5 grams of leucine for each protein feeding, which translates to about 6 ounces of meat or 25 grams of whey protein powder. Take MassZymes to maximize your amino acid assimilation.

You can also supplement with 3 to 5 grams of leucine about 15 to 30 minutes before a meal to stimulate mTOR.[27] For maximum anabolism, aim for at least three meals a day. Each meal represents an anabolic opportunity. This is why we believe many people lose lean muscle mass when they overdo intermittent fasting. You can't throw all of your protein into one or two meals and make up for the lack of protein in the rest of the day.

The more of these strategies you combine with weight lifting, the more anabolic you become and the more calories you'll burn.

4. Up Your Non-Exercise Activity Thermogenesis

We mentioned earlier that non-exercise activity thermogenesis (NEAT) is the measurement of calories you burn with random movements, fidgeting, and maintaining your posture. Usually, NEAT accounts for 200 to 300 calories per day, but with a little bit of conscious effort, you can bump this to 400 or 500. People doing hard labor can get up to 2,000 calories a day.

Remember, though, that your body has a mind of its own. When your survival mechanism kicks in, one of the things it does is lower your NEAT. Your body just doesn't want to move unless it has to. You could say it's lazy. As an example, Matt noticed that on his third day of fasting, he'd have to motivate himself to get off the couch.

Once you start to notice this sluggishness and reduced desire to move, it might be time for a refeed, diet break, or try reverse dieting. Nootropics are a powerful way to help find the reduction in NEAT. Check out www.Nootopia.com to learn more

Most NEAT is unconscious. People usually don't notice whether they're moving more or less. However, now that you're aware of your NEAT, you can help consciously override any downregulation of it.

Power Move: Conscious Micromovement

Conscious micromovement means fighting the body's natural drive to move less. Park the car farther from the grocery store. Take the stairs instead of the elevator. Walk to the gym. Get a stand-up desk—or, even better, a treadmill desk. Do push-ups and bodyweight squats once or twice a day. Do abs while you watch Netflix. Start your day with five minutes of yoga.

These can all stack up to burn an extra 200 to 500 calories a day, which is a lot. This will become a big edge once you get deeper into your diet journey. Using nootropics and stimulating your nervous system is another way to help counter any drop in NEAT.

5. Embrace Cold Exposure

Our bodies are always converting food into energy or into heat.

One of the ways you can significantly increase calories out is via heat loss. Submerging your entire body in cold water creates even more heat loss.

Ray Cronise, a former NASA material scientist, attempted to understand how Michael Phelps ate 12,000 calories a day. Phelps was a ripped professional swimmer at his peak. The only way his calories in and out would balance out was when the math took into account heat loss through the water, as Phelps spends many hours a day swimming.

Heat loss increases adiponectin, a hormone released from your fat cells.[28] Adiponectin not only helps with keeping your body warm, but it also increases fat burning and muscle building.[29] The body burns more energy just to reheat your body and keep your core temperature around 98.6°F.

Two vectors can maximize the results of cold exposure:

1. Shivering deeply
2. Maximizing brown fat

Shivering Deeply

In a study among young, lean men, nonshivering cold exposure was shown to increase energy expenditure by 16.7 percent and fat oxidation by 72.6 percent. However, once the cold hit the shivering point, the calorie expenditure increased by 31.7 percent relative to being in a warm room.[30]

Researchers at Harvard University found that thermogenic fat cells accumulate succinate, which is a metabolite of the Krebs cycle, a biochemical pathway in your mitochondria that breaks down carbohydrates and fats into ATP. Succinate also seems to activate calorie burning in brown fat cells, even when they're injected into the blood of mice. They also increase heat loss via mitochondrial uncoupling.[31]

6. Maximizing Your Brown Fat

Optimizing brown fat is another way to get more out of your cold therapy and increase your daily calorie expenditure. It deserves its own place in the "calories out" category.

Brown adipose tissue (BAT), or "brown fat," is the set of heat-producing fat cells that keep you from dying from hypothermia. They have large mitochondria with a lot of uncoupling protein. Typically, your mitochondria produce ATP as an energy currency, but mitochondrial uncoupling generates heat instead.[32]

Cold exposure can convert white fat to brown fat, which increases your overall calorie expenditure through heat loss, even when you're not in ice water.

Power Moves

- Get cold exposure. Take a cold shower, an ice bath, or simply wear less clothing when it's cold out.
- Take Blood Sugar Breakthrough. Many blood-sugar-balancing herbs, such as bitter melon and fucoxanthin, also increase mitochondrial uncoupling.
- Capsaicin seems to be one of the biggest game changers to maximize results from cold exposure. In one experiment, it was found that human BAT can be recruited by chronic cold exposure and capsinoid ingestion, even in individuals who have lost active BAT. So, taking a capsaicin capsule during your cold therapy cycle can produce great results.

If you're going to use cold therapy as a weight loss solution, you must systematize it and commit to it. It can be a powerful way to burn an extra 300 to 1,000-plus calories a day (via heat loss and BAT activation) without doing more exercise or cutting calories.

We suggest programming it in the mid-to-late phases of your weight loss journey. It's a powerful way to break homeostasis. We suggest using it for two or three weeks and then stopping for a week to undo the adaptation. Maximum calorie loss occurs if you shiver. So, if you get used to the cold and stop shivering, it's wise to take a week or two off.

A Word of Caution about Cold Therapy

Hunger can go up significantly when you're using cold therapy.[33] It's a very ravenous, intense hunger. If you're not psychologically ready for its intensity, you're setting yourself up for failure. So, if you do choose to use cold therapy, prepare yourself mentally for the potential hunger spike.

7. Push Your Brain Hard and Deep

Your brain is the most metabolically active organ in the body. Typically, your brain uses up 20 percent of your BMR and 60 percent of your entire body's glucose.[34] So, if you're in a caloric deficit, you'll often find your mental performance declining.

Conversely, if you are intensely pushing your brain, it may burn even more calories. Grandmaster chess players, public speakers, and high performers of all kinds have learned to feed their brains for maximum performance.

Matt finds that he needs to eat 1,500 extra calories a day during his most intense weeks of intensive brain training.

Once, at an A4M conference, Matt unintentionally lost 15 pounds in two days while eating a normal amount of food. He was constantly engaged in challenging intellectual conversations with the doctors who attended the conference. As a result, his brain was burning many more calories than usual from the stress, the environment, the hard questions, and all the talking. Also, constantly moving around meant using more NEAT.

This is something that's hard to program into a workout, but it's useful to understand, especially if you have bouts of intense brain activity. Increasing your calories during important mental activities can be a smart move.

8. Exercise

Exercise is a foundational piece of any healthy weight loss program. What's the best type of exercise for fat loss?

The short answer is the kind of exercise that's on a plan you can commit to and stick with. However, in terms of effectiveness, here's the hierarchy of exercise for fat loss:

- Resistance training
- Walking outdoors
- Rebounding
- Yoga
- Swimming
- HIIT
- Cardio machines

Resistance Training

There's zero doubt that resistance training is the best. Why? Because of the anabolism that we mentioned earlier.

Resistance training protects your lean muscle mass. And if you're really optimized, you'll build lean muscle. This is what we call "The Magic Zone" (which we regularly achieve with our clients). You can *recomp* (as in recomposition) your body, which means that your bodyweight stays the same but you're building lean muscle while losing body fat.

This was Matt's primary strategy for five years before doing the final shredding. Every year, he recomped 3 to 10 pounds (which means he lost 3 to 10 pounds of fat while gaining 3 to 10 pounds of lean muscle).

To get your free training program that we've used with our clients, go to: www.BIOptimizers.com/book/resources.

Walking

Next is walking. Walking is a great form of exercise. Step tracking is readily available via fitness trackers and phones, which makes creating a dopamine loop with walking very easy. Shooting for 10,000 steps a day is a great goal.

Walking has many other benefits beyond just burning calories. Walking is easy on the nervous system, which is important as we ramp up exercise volume. It also synchronizes the right and left hemispheres of the brain.[35] Walking outdoors helps lower cortisol (versus doing indoor cardio).

Shoot for two or three walking sessions a day, ideally after meals. You don't need to walk for hours. A brisk 10-minute walk can lower blood sugar by 20 points. The key is to make walking part of your lifestyle. If possible, walk to work, walk after dinner, walk to the gym, walk the dog, take walks in the park, walk on the beach . . . just walk!

Power Move: Doing Cardio Outdoors (vs. Indoors)

People who exercise outdoors work out on average 30 minutes longer than those who exercise indoors. They also feel that they struggle less to complete their workouts. Another great benefit is the boost to your mood—feeling happier and more satisfied.

Rebounding

We are big fans of rebounding on trampolines. Rebounding is unique among movements because of its powerful lymphatic benefits. This means it can accelerate the body's natural detox processes. Put on some great tunes and start bouncing and dancing for a fun, powerful workout.

One of the reasons we love it is that it's a safe way to do an intense cardio workout. The flexible trampoline material helps protect your joints against wear and tear. Rebounding was developed for astronauts because they lost as much as 15 percent of their bone and muscle mass in a weightless atmosphere in as little as 14 days. Rebounding was the exercise they used to help counter this.

Just make sure you get a high-quality unit. From our research, we feel that David Hall's Cellerciser is the best commercial one.

Yoga

Yoga is powerful and unique due to its parasympathetic activation and its stretching benefits. Yoga is a form of light resistance training for any age or condition and can be made progressively tougher. Plus, yoga routines can always change, which makes adapting to it more difficult than to cardio machines.

One of the most ignored aspects of an extended weight loss journey is managing one's nervous system. This can lead to burnout, which typically means the end of the weight loss program. Make sure to check out Chapter 14, BiOptimizing Your Nervous System, from our book *From Sick to Superhuman* to get more insights on making your CNS as healthy and strong as possible.

Its nervous system regulation makes yoga a great exercise to add on to existing exercise routines while minimizing the overall stress on the body. In fact, it can help reduce overall mental stress as well.[36, 37, 38, 39]

Swimming

Swimming is powerful for two reasons. First, it's great for people with bad joints and injuries. The water protects you against impact. Second, it produces heat loss, which increases your overall burn of calories.

HIIT

We covered some of the benefits of HIIT earlier when discussing the mitochondrial angle. We advise adding this midway through your weight loss journey for another layer of calorie expenditure. Start with once a week, and then add a second HIIT after three or four weeks.

Cardio

When we say "cardio," we're talking about traditional cardio machines and forms of cardio like running and biking. Even though walking, swimming, and rebounding are forms of cardio, their secondary benefits put them in a different class.

Cardio is last on the list for many reasons. First, relying on cardio as your primary exercise is a surefire way to accelerate metabolic adaptation. Second, it accelerates muscle loss. We recommend ramping up as you get into the last phase of your final shredding, if necessary, to break homeostasis (more on this in a moment).

We do recommend doing two hours per week of cardio exercise for overall health benefits, ideally using walking, rebounding, and/or swimming. You can split it however you want.

Here are some tips to maximize the results of your cardio:

- Change up the type of cardio every week or two.
  - Do two weeks of treadmill, then two weeks of elliptical, then two weeks each of rowing, StairMaster, cycling, and so on. This will help minimize the adaptation from the repetitive motions.
- Progressively increase the intensity.
  - The body adapts quickly to cardio. To burn the same number of calories, you must continue making it more difficult. If you're using a treadmill, some of the best ways are to increase the incline and, of course, the speed. Many machines allow you to increase resistance levels as well.

Again, cardio should just be a cherry on top of the metabolic cake (hope we didn't trigger cravings with that analogy).

9. Basal Metabolic Rate

Your basal metabolic rate (BMR), or resting metabolic rate, makes up 60 to 75 percent of your total daily calories burned, making it your biggest category of "calories out."[40] This is how many calories you're burning while doing and eating nothing. Your body burns these calories to sustain life, such as by breathing, pumping blood, and creating new cells. The following factors influence your BMR:

- Muscle mass (increases BMR)
- Aging (tends to decrease BMR)
- Body size (larger people burn more calories)
- Gender (men have higher BMR than women)
- Genetics and epigenetics (see Chapter 34)
- Hormones and neurotransmitters, especially thyroid hormones and orexins
- Drugs and substances such as caffeine, fat burners, and other thermogenic substances (can increase BMR)
- Adaptive thermogenesis, or the generation of heat by the mitochondria when you have extra energy
- Gut microbiota also partly control BMR[41]

When you do most of the strategies we've discussed, your BMR will be much higher.

10. Slow Down Metabolic Adaptation

Metabolic adaptation is the primary enemy of weight loss. We can't stop it completely, but we can slow it down significantly.

We have four primary tools for this:

1. Refeeds and calorie cycling
2. Diet breaks
3. Reverse dieting
4. Changing the adaptive challenges

Refeeds and Calorie Cycling

Bodybuilders have been using calorie cycling for decades. Wade's coach, Scott Abel, is one of the pioneers of this approach and outlined it in his book *The Cycle Diet*. The strategy is to create a calorie deficit for five or six days followed by one or two days of higher calorie intake.

Refeeds are when you increase calories for a short time, usually one to three days. They have several benefits:

- They increase metabolism
- They slow down metabolic adaptation
- They're anabolic and prevent, reverse, or slow down muscle loss
- They provide psychological relief
- They improve lifestyle
- They provide fuel for breakthrough workouts

Refeeds can make it far easier, psychologically, to do diets. It's easier for most people to be extremely disciplined for five or six days when they know they'll have reprieve on a weekly basis.

This might sound counterintuitive, but doing refeeds can help prevent or manage binges in many people.[42] Now, we've seen that with some people who have food addiction problems, it can have the opposite effect and activate binges. So please be true to yourself—do what works for you and avoid what sets you up for sabotage.

Our personal experience, plus that of our clients, has revealed that refeeds can do wonders to prevent loss of lean muscle mass. Research by Bill Campbell and colleagues produced some great data that lines up with our experience. In fact, we believe that if your diet is hyper-optimized and includes refeed days, you can lose body fat and gain lean muscle mass simultaneously on a weekly basis. This is achieved by optimizing the fat loss portion of the week and maximizing the anabolism of the refeed day.

One study showed that this is a superior way to lose weight: 74 patients composed of obese or overweight, nonsmoking women 26 to 50 years old were randomly matched into calorie-shifting and calorie-restricting groups, with under three hours per week of exercise.[43]

Group 1 did the calorie-shifting diet (CSD):

- 11 days of calorie restriction plus 3 days of self-selected diet. Meals were four hours apart.
- The day phases were repeated three times.

Group 2 did plain calorie restriction (CR):

- Six weeks straight of calorie restriction

Both groups lost significant weight by the end of the study; however, the CSD group lost more.

Between-group statistical significance on day 70 was:

- The CSD group lost 5.79 ± 1.17 percent bodyweight, while the CR group lost 3.38 ± 1.4 percent.
- The CSD group lost 12.69 ± 2.72 percent body fat, while the CR group lost 5.18 ± 2.14 percent.

But that's not the end of the story.

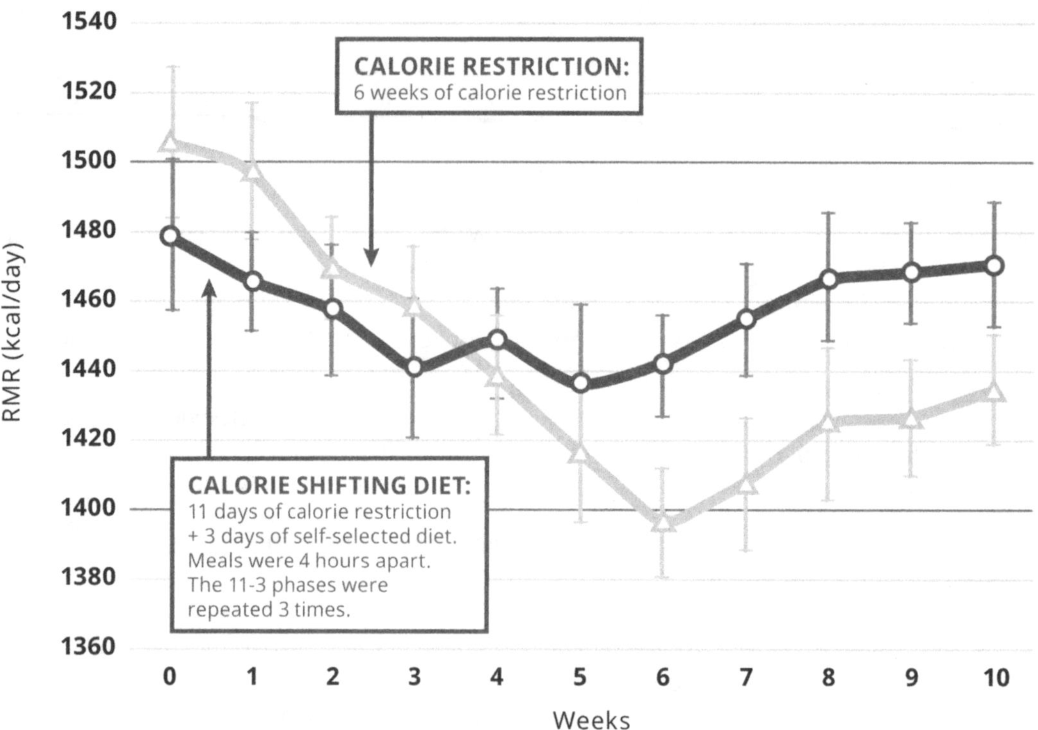

The CR group regained the fat as soon as its members went back to maintenance calories. RMR didn't change significantly in the CSD group, but significantly decreased by about 100 calories in the CR group. This decrease persisted throughout maintenance.

Refeeds tell your mind and body that they're safe. They're not going to starve to death, because there's enough food coming (even if it's just once a week).

Diet Breaks

Diet breaks are one of the best strategies for preventing metabolic adaptation. In an Australian study, 19 obese men went through 16 consecutive weeks of caloric restriction, compared to 17 men who did eight rounds of two calorie-restricted weeks, staggered with seven rounds of maintenance calories. The latter group lost more body fat and had less metabolic adaptation.[44]

Reverse Dieting

Reverse dieting is the final piece of the metabolic puzzle of weight loss. It stops the excessive rebounds that 97 percent of people go through. It's the diet after the diet, and arguably the most important part of the entire journey.

Here's how it works: you slowly increase calories by 100 to 150 per day on a weekly basis until you reach your target calorie maintenance levels. We suggest doing this over 8 to 16 weeks.

This way, we're taking advantage of our body's drive for homeostasis. Increasing calories by 100 to 150 a day is not enough to trigger weight gain. In our experience, it takes 300 to 500 calories a day (surplus or deficit) to break homeostasis. So, when you slowly increase calories, you can ramp up your metabolism back to a healthy level.

If you go from a deep deficit to eating "normally," you will almost certainly regain a lot of fat because your metabolism is lower, even though you're not eating in a calorie surplus.

In cases where someone has lost a tremendous amount of weight and has cut calories down to the bone, reverse dieting is necessary. We can re-boost the BMR by doing a reverse diet over a few weeks and months and prepare the body for the next fat loss cycle.

Our recommended threshold for starting a reverse diet is around 7 calories per pound. We believe that going below that can activate starvation survival effects (we covered those in depth in Chapter 3).

Create New Adaptive Challenges and Strategically Break Homeostasis

Homeostasis is a process in which one self-regulates biological functions by adapting for survival. The body doesn't want change, because change is a threat. The body has one goal: to stay alive. Lose too much body fat, and your body might die. Gain too much fat, and it might die (it's hard to outrun saber-toothed tigers when you're 400 pounds). That's why your body is constantly adapting, striving for homeostasis.

Decrease calories, and your body will adapt by slowing down your metabolism (plus other factors that we discuss in this chapter). Your energy and drive to do things go down the drain. Your physical and mental performance fall off a cliff. Your body starts burning precious lean muscle mass. What truly breaks wills is when progress plateaus despite doing exercises and cutting calories.

Increase your calories, and your body will adapt by increasing its metabolic rate. You may feel warmer and more energized. You may be stronger in the gym and gain muscles more easily. However, you may also store any excess energy as glycogen and fat.

Your metabolism is dynamic. It shifts based on how much you eat, how much you exercise, and your anabolic environment. Your body is always striving for homeostasis. This is why plateaus are normal. We define a plateau as being stuck around the same weight for two weeks.

SMASHING WEIGHT LOSS PLATEAUS

It's impossible to change your body without breaking homeostasis.

One of the best strategies is to introduce new adaptive challenges. The magic zone is where your body is adapting, and the magic stops when you're adapted. This means that when you do something you weren't doing before, your body starts adapting to it. There's a significant increase in calorie expenditure during this adapting phase. Over time, the same activity burns a lot fewer calories because your body becomes adapted.

So, the strategy is to add a new modification when you hit a weight loss plateau. Create a new adaptive challenge. Each modification will break homeostasis (assuming that your diet is on track).

The Key Number: -300

Here's a very key number: -300 calories. In our experience and observation, you need a daily deficit of 300 calories to continue losing weight. If you're under that, the body achieves homeostasis. This means that if you're down only 150 calories, it's not enough to break homeostasis. This is the principle we use to reverse diet (more on that in Chapter 13).

This chapter is loaded with multiple ways to introduce new adaptive challenges and break homeostasis. We recommend that you:

- Upgrade your macros (more protein, more fiber)
- Start lifting weights (if you're not already)
- Change your weight training program
- Increase your weight training frequency each week
- Do an HIIT workout a week
- Progress to two HIIT workouts a week
- Do cold therapy
- Add walking
- Add rebounding
- Add yoga
- Add cardio
- Change the type of cardio
- Increase the intensity of cardio
- Increase anabolism
- Do sauna sessions
- Cut calories

One last key point is to do one modification at a time. Why? Because you want to have more "runway" for later. If you do all your modifications simultaneously, you will get rapid results but eventually adapt and be stuck in homeostasis. You'll run out of runway. Go to www.BIOptimizers.com/book/coaching to have one of our coaches guide you through your journey.

The Tortoise vs. the Hare

Let's compare two potential scenarios with twins who have 60 pounds of fat to lose. We have Carly A, the nonstrategic, impatient "sprinter" versus her twin sister, Carly B, the strategic, patient "marathoner."

Carly A goes from zero to 100—from eating 3,000 calories a day down to 1,500. She goes from not exercising to training six times a week. She's in the magic zone for the first few weeks. She drops three pounds a week the first couple of weeks and then two pounds a week for the following six weeks. Then it goes to one pound per week. Then, she plateaus.

She gets desperate, drops her calories down to 1,200 per day, and adds more cardio. Weight loss resumes for a couple of weeks. Then it grinds to a halt. Carly A has no more runway. She can't do more exercise. She can't drop calories lower. Carly A's metabolism has been run into the ground and activated the starvation self-defense mechanisms. Carly A quits. She regains all of the weight.

Carly B goes from zero to 20. She cuts her calories to 2,200 per day and starts losing one pound per week. Then she adds three workouts a week, and weight loss ramps up to 1.5 pounds per week. After a couple of months, she plateaus. No worries; she does a two-week diet break. Then she resumes her journey and cuts calories to 1,800, dropping one pound per week. She does this for six weeks and then does another two-week diet break. The next week, she comes back and adds a fourth workout. Weight loss continues. She adds one HIIT workout, and a couple of weeks later, she adds a yoga workout per week. Carly B still has many more adjustments she can make, and after a few more months, she reaches her dream weight.

It's the classic tale of the tortoise vs. the hare. When it comes to weight loss, the intelligent, strategic tortoise wins. The hare burns out, activates the starvation effects, and quits. The tortoise keeps chugging along, smelling the roses, and winning huge.

THE ME DIET APP

We know that some of this may be overwhelming for some people. This is why we built a Me Diet app that guides you step by step and makes it easy for you to follow. Go to www.BIOptimizers.com/book/dietapp to download the Me Diet app.

BUILDING YOUR MASTER PLAN OF SUCCESS

We will cover the application of these strategies and tactics and show a real example inside the ultimate fat loss master plan in Chapter 13 and you can download more resources at www.BIOptimizers.com/book/resources.

SUMMARY

- The Optimized Metabolism System is designed to keep your metabolism revving and prevent the pitfalls of hardcore calorie restriction.
- In our opinion, focusing simply on cutting calories is the wrong way to go. Instead, we suggest focusing on the five following strategies.
  1. Keeping your metabolism as high as possible during the entire dieting process
  2. Maintaining or even building lean muscle
  3. Keeping your body feeling safe throughout the journey
  4. Rebuilding your metabolism strategically once goals are achieved
  5. Locking in your final set point while living an awesome lifestyle
- Calories in minus calories out = weight gain or loss.
- For you to lose weight, calories out need to exceed calories in over time.
- It's possible and healthier to leverage other parts of the "calories out" equation and avoid any issues.

- The key to dietary success is not through simple, hard calorie restriction that sacrifices the future for today. Instead, you need to turbocharge your metabolism in other ways that increase your calories out.
  - Mastering calories in:

    Protein: This macronutrient is required by your body to carry out essential functions by cells, tissues, and organs.

    Carbs: The main function of this macronutrient is to provide your body with energy.

    Fats: Your body needs fats to build hormones; to repair your brain, skin, and hair; and for many other core functions.

    Fiber: This helps you feel full and can help optimize bowel movements.

    Alcohol: This tends to become belly fat and increase visceral fat.

  - Mastering calories out:

    Thermic effect of food: Protein gives you a calorie loss of 20 to 30 percent due to its thermic effects because a lot of energy is required to break down and metabolize it.

    Mitochondria: Mitochondria are bacteria in our bodies that produce energy. By increasing their quantity and strength, we increase our energy creation.

    Anabolism: By increasing anabolism, we can boost metabolism 10 to 30 percent—or even more.

    Non-exercise activity thermogenesis: Usually, NEAT accounts for 200 to 300 calories per day, but it can go up to 2,000 in extremely active people.

    Cold exposure: One of the ways you can increase calories out is via heat loss.

    Intense brain activity: If you intensely push your brain, it may burn more calories.

    Exercise: Exercise burns a lot of energy. However, you can never out-exercise a bad diet.

    Basal metabolic rate (BMR): Aka resting metabolic rate, BMR makes up 60 to 75 percent—the biggest category—of your total daily calories burned.

    Metabolic adaptation: This body function is the primary enemy of weight loss. We can't stop it completely, but we can slow it down significantly.

    Brown fat (BAT): Brown adipose tissue, or "brown fat," is a group of heat-producing fat cells that keep you from dying from hypothermia. Optimizing brown fat can increase your daily calorie expenditure.

Pitfalls of Calorie Counting

According to a *New England Journal of Medicine* study, obese people who consider themselves diet-resistant underreported the food they ate by 47 percent and overreported their physical activity by 51 percent, on average. When asked to recall their food intake, they recalled it as 20 percent less than what they ate.[45]

These errors can easily make us feel like we're eating in alignment with our goals when we're really in a calorie surplus (that is, we're gaining fat). Therefore, when you start tracking, it's important to stay aware of this common self-reporting error. Not only that, but we believe that the body can unconsciously sabotage diets by doing this.

Often, weight gain and plateaus happen due to these errors. Fortunately, there are many ways to count calories on autopilot so that it requires less cognitive energy.

Calorie Control the Easy Way

Wade finds that people tend to do best when they eat the exact same thing over and over. Having a rotation of meals with their macros precalculated is a "set it and forget it" version of calorie control without constant counting and measuring. You measure everything the first week, and then you can just repeat without measuring. Just make sure your brain doesn't try to sneak in some stealth calories.

Another approach is to track for one or two weeks before deciding on a plan that will create a deficit. For example, you might want to stop eating when you feel 80 percent full, or remove a portion from your plate to subtract from what you normally eat. Then, keep doing it until the result plateaus off due to metabolic adaptation.

When Calorie Tracking May Be Unnecessary

When starting a new diet, many people see significant results from the initial full feeling. The extra protein combined with the elimination of processed foods can make a big impact. All of these changes are going to help you go from a caloric surplus to a deficit.

When Calorie Tracking Is Absolutely Necessary

Your body will adapt by dialing down your calorie expenditure after a prolonged caloric deficit or significant fat loss, as we've noted. Your metabolism will drop to match your caloric intake, causing a stall in your fat loss progress. At that point, you have to revisit the calorie math and may have to further drop calories to create a deficit, or do a reverse diet if you've gone too low.

If you want to get to elite low levels of body fat, then calorie tracking is absolutely mandatory. You can get very far by progressively improving your diet and metabolism by following the advice in Chapter 7, The Optimized Metabolism System.

However, to lower your body fat below your natural set point, you will have to go to new levels of restrictiveness and accuracy. The leaner you get, the bigger the impact of smaller changes. This is also where world-class coaching becomes vital.

Food Cue #1: Satiety Levels

Notice how hungry you are with:

- Different macronutrient composition (proteins, carbs, and fats) of your meals and overall diet
- Different fiber content in your meals
- Certain food items that make you feel either hungrier or more satiated
- Training intensity and specific exercises
- Quantity and quality of sleep
- Exercise recovery or soreness
- Duration of caloric restriction
- Refeeds

Food Cue #2: Hunger and Cravings

Hunger and cravings play a key role in your long-term success. Noticing which foods leave you satisfied and which leave you hungrier is crucial data to track. Because cravings can crop up for both psychological and physiological reasons, here are some drivers to pay extra attention to during data tracking.

Psychological drivers include:

- Emotional eating
- Anxiety eating
- Habitual patterns, such as eating at the same time every day
- Dehydration, which can also be mistaken for hunger
- Psychological associations, such as sporting events, television, or food commercials
- Gut biome (see Chapter 29)
- Depleted willpower and decision fatigue

Biological drivers include:

- Muscle growth (anabolism), such as in teenage boys
- Sleep deprivation
- Survival mechanisms
- Low or unstable blood sugar
- Nutrient deficiencies
- Hormonal changes
- Heavy cognitive demands

As you diet down, you want to avoid activating your survival mechanisms, which is when your body fights back with a vengeance. Remember how Matt dropped 30 pounds over two years before he aggressively dieted down another 10 to 15 pounds for his wedding. Afterward, he became insatiable for two years and regained most of the weight.

Food Cue #3: Energy Levels

Energy level data helps us understand how our bodies are doing from a high level. As you track your energy, you'll want to note other contributing factors that could be sneaky suspects. Energy drainers include overtraining, undereating, infections, injuries, and poor sleep. Burnout is your biggest enemy.

Low energy can be a signal to lower training volume for a couple of weeks. It's also a potential signal that your body is reducing its NEAT. Remember that this is one of the ways your body increases or decreases its overall calorie expenditure.

CONCLUSION

Most of the diet industry focuses on severely restricting food intake and grueling cardio sessions. This strategy is effective for a few months but fails terribly in the long run.

Keep the body feeling safe and diet more strategically. As Scott Abel says, "Coax the body, don't force it." Minimize the starvation self-defense mechanisms and metabolic destruction.

Focus on anabolism and building lean muscle mass to rev up your basal metabolic rate. And keep your body adapting by strategically introducing new challenges.

CHAPTER 8

ADVANCED CYCLING STRATEGIES

In this chapter, you'll learn:

- What diet cycling is, and why it's so important to implement in order to achieve success in your diet
- How to cycle between muscle building and fat loss like a true bodybuilder
- What a "fat loss sprint" is, and how you can cycle it into your diet
- Various advanced cycling techniques you can use to become biologically optimized
- How you can maximize your body's recomposition (fat loss and muscle gain at the same time)
- The classic cycle diet, which is perfect if you like to enjoy your refeed meals on the weekends
- What the benefits of refeed days are, and why you need to cycle them into your diet
- The ultimate strategy for people who want to add lean muscle mass while minimizing fat gain
- How to cycle between the keto and carnivore diets in the most effective way
- The importance of seasonal food cycling and how to do it
- The story of Wade's 28-day fat loss sprint and how it helped him prepare for a contest he did in 2022
- How to do the inverted muscle-building cycle diet, which is great for people who want to add lean muscle mass while minimizing fat gain

There is a time for everything, and a season for every activity under the heavens:

A time to be born and a time to die, a time to plant and a time to uproot.
A time to kill and a time to heal, a time to tear down and a time to build.

— Ecclesiastes 3:1–11

EVERYTHING CYCLES

Everything in the universe cycles: your heartbeat, circadian rhythms, the seasons, the planet, the sun, and even the universe itself. In this chapter, we share some more advanced calorie-cycling strategies as well as some diet-cycling principles.

Macro Cycling between Muscle Building and Fat Loss

A classic bodybuilding strategy is to cycle between macro muscle-building phases and fat loss phases. To get ready for a competition, a pro bodybuilder usually spends seven to eight months in muscle-building mode and then three to five months in fat loss mode. This was Wade's process for almost two decades.

Your body is a homeostasis machine. Homeostasis means the body is in balance. It wants to be safe and stable, and so extreme changes are seen as a threat. The evolutionary programming dictates that too much weight loss means the body might starve; too much weight gain means predators might get us. Any changes you make cause your body to adjust to reach homeostasis.

This is why people on fat loss programs who are in caloric deficit get lower fat loss results over time, unless they do refeeds or add some reverse dieting.

On the other hand, skinny people attempting to gain muscle also make this mistake—just in the other direction. When you eat more, your body adapts by burning more calories with more body heat and fidgeting. As a result, not taking breaks and pushing through these adaptations means gainers need to gorge even more food to make the same progress with their muscles. Many ectomorphs (people with fast metabolisms) eventually hit the wall; they can't keep up the amount of food they need to eat, and they give up.

Cycling your diet and calories allows you to bypass some of these homeostatic adaptations. You can minimize the activation of your anti-starvation survival response during dieting and minimize fat gain during muscle-building cycles.

A study involved 36 obese men who received either a continuous 16 weeks of 33 percent caloric deficit, or eight 2-week blocks of caloric restriction alternating with eight 2-week blocks of energy balance (30 weeks in total). The 17 men who did diet cycling had more fat-mass loss than the 19 who did continuous caloric restriction.[1]

Lean muscle-mass loss was not significantly different between groups. However, resting energy expenditure decreased significantly more in the continuous diet group. In other words, cycling in maintenance calories reduced the metabolic adaptation and resulted in more fat loss.[2] This is why calorie cycling is vital for extended weight loss journeys.

During extended weight loss cycles, you will lose some lean muscle mass. When you increase calories again, it's normal to quickly regain that lost muscle tissue. We have programmed a variety of advanced cycling strategy in our diet app. Go to www.BIOptimizers.com/book/dietapp to download our app to make your Me Diet journey simple and easy to follow.

Recomposition with Shorter Cycles

In the '80s bodybuilding scene, it was popular to do major bulking cycles. This usually meant extreme overeating for months, and gaining dozens of pounds of bodyweight.

The problem was that sometimes more than half of the weight was fat. Then, bodybuilders would use steroids and other hormones in conjunction with extreme dieting to get to unhealthy levels of low body fat for a competition. And they would rinse and repeat this on a yearly basis. We strongly advise against this strategy.

Instead, we suggest using the same principle but doing shorter cycles. We share a variety of advanced calorie-cycling strategies in this chapter.

Fat Loss Sprints

Layne Norton coined the term fat loss sprints. The idea is short fat loss cycles of two to four weeks with a one to two week diet break (eating at maintenance). This is something Wade has done for many years. Below is an example of a fat loss sprint done by Wade in 2020.

Wade's 28-Day Fat Loss Sprint

On September 8, 2020, I started out at 20.6 percent body fat and 203.8 pounds. I had 41.9 pounds of fat tissue and 153.9 pounds of lean tissue.

I did three weeks of alternate-day fasting, which dropped my body fat to 17.7 percent and weight to 189 pounds. However, my fat dropped to 33.6 pounds. So, I lost almost 8 pounds of fat. My lean mass also went down to 147.9.

Then, one week afterward, I did a refeed when I was 209 pounds at 17.8 percent body fat. So, my body fat only went up 0.1 percent, my fat tissue went up 2.1 pounds, and my lean mass went up to 157.3 pounds. This was essentially almost 10 pounds of muscle gain from the bottom up. It was 3.4 pounds of lean mass gain with 7.7 pounds of fat loss, although I did gain back 1.7. So, net was 6.2 pounds of fat loss and 3.4 pounds of muscle gain.

	Weight (pounds)	Body fat (%)	Fat mass (pounds)	Muscle mass (pounds)
Initial	203.8	20.6	42.0	153.9
After 3 weeks alternate-day fast	189.0	17.7	33.6	147.9
After 1 week refeed	209.0	17.8	35.7	157.3
Net change	+5.0	-2.8	-6.3	+3.4

Wade's diet also didn't put his body into extreme starvation mode, unlike the 11-month insanity diet that he did to prepare for Mr. Universe. After that competition, he developed severe gut, skin, and water retention issues, along with 40 pounds of major rebound weight gain. It took him two years of working with multiple practitioners to get his health and metabolism back.

In hindsight, if Wade could do it all over again, he would have zigzagged in preparation for the show.

ADVANCED CALORIE CYCLING

How to Cycle Your Diet to Maximize Your Recomp

To maximize recomposition (fat loss and muscle gain at the same time), shorter diet cycles work best. In some cases, people with extra body fat may even gain muscle after switching to maintenance calories after a deficit cycle if they're resistance training.

A review of clinical studies compared subjects who used alternate-day fasts with those who had steady daily caloric restrictions. They found that, while both groups lost similar amounts of weight, the weight loss was 90 percent fat and 10 percent lean tissue in the fasted group, and 75 percent fat to 25 percent lean tissue in the steady caloric deficit group.[3]

The Classic Cycle Diet: Staying Lean All Year Long and Enjoying Life

We're big fans of the cycle diet, wherein you get into a caloric deficit for five or six days and alternate that with one or two days of higher-carb eating or caloric surpluses. This tends to work perfectly if you like to enjoy your refeed meals on the weekends.

Here's an example of how this might look:

	MON	TUES	WED	THURS	FRI	SAT	SUN
Energy Balance	-500	-500	-500	-500	-500	-500	+3,000
Effect	fat loss	fat loss	fat loss	fat loss	fat loss	fat loss	muscle building

This is a great strategy for people who want to stay in shape all year long and have a great lifestyle. The extra calorie day on Sunday means you can basically go and eat whatever you want (within calorie range).

The idea is that you're in a calorie deficit for six days and then go into a calorie surplus for one day. If you train properly and minimize catabolism for those six deficit days, you may lose body fat and gain a bit of lean muscle. And the strategy on the calorie surplus day is to maximize anabolism (muscle gain). Go to www.BIOptimizers.com/book/resources to download your free supplement guide that will show which ones can minimize your catabolism and maximize your anabolism.

It's smart to save your biggest workouts of the week (legs and back) for the surplus days. The extra calories will improve your workouts, and thus burn more energy. And the extra calories will help maximize muscle building from those demanding workouts. You will also have a lot of energy on Monday for a tough workout, because your muscles will be loaded with glycogen from the refeed.

We've seen multiple clients, as well as ourselves, use this strategy to recomp 5 to 10 pounds a year. This means you're adding 5 to 10 pounds of lean muscle per year while also losing 5 to 10 pounds of fat.

The Weekly Recomposition Cycle: Fat Loss Focus

This method is ideal for people who are close to their ideal body fat percentage and want to recomp down to their final form.

	MON	TUES	WED	THURS	FRI	SAT	SUN
Energy Balance	-500	-500	-500	-500	-500	-500	+1,000
Effect	fat loss	fat loss	fat loss	fat loss	fat loss	fat loss	muscle building

This is a great strategy for people who want to lose body fat and minimize muscle loss. Using the example above, the net weekly calorie deficit is around 2,000 a week, which produces about a little more than half a pound of body fat loss.

As with the previous method, you're in a calorie deficit for six days and a calorie surplus for one. Training properly and minimizing catabolism on deficit days means you will lose a fair amount of body fat. As before, the strategy on the calorie surplus day is to maximize anabolism (muscle gain).

As we've noted, your biggest workouts of the week (legs and back) are best on the surplus day, where extra calories help improve workouts and help you burn more energy. You'll have extra energy on Monday and Tuesday from stored glycogen, and the refeed calories will help maximize muscle building. The refeed day really helps minimize muscle loss during extended weight loss cycles. And psychologically, many people need the weekly reprieve.

In general, this is ideal for people within 10 to 15 pounds of their ideal shape. If you have more than 15 pounds of body fat to lose, we recommend you start with eight weeks of constant daily deficits before incorporating weekly refeeds. Doing a one- to two-week diet break every six to eight weeks is a great tool for people who are doing extended calorie deficits.

If you're keto adapted and follow a ketogenic diet for fat loss, you can cycle in carbs for those two-day refeeds to replenish your glycogen stores.

The Inverted Muscle-Building Cycle Diet

This is a great strategy for people who want to add lean muscle mass while minimizing fat gain.

The idea is that you're anabolic for five days and go into a calorie deficit for two. If you train properly and maximize anabolism on the surplus days, you will gain lean muscle. And the strategy on the calorie deficit days is to minimize catabolism (muscle loss).

	MON	TUES	WED	THURS	FRI	SAT	SUN
Energy Balance	+500	+500	+500	+500	+500	-1,000	-1,000
Effect	muscle building	muscle building	muscle building	muscle building	muscle building	fat loss	fat loss

The net weekly calorie surplus from this strategy is 500 a week. Theoretically, you would only gain one pound of fat if you did this for seven weeks.

The Inverted Muscle-Building Cycle Diet with Fasting

Many people who have followed the classic bodybuilding advice may believe that their muscles would disappear if they stopped constantly feeding them. However, this isn't true. Fasting is anti-catabolic.

In the times of hunting and gathering, cavemen had muscles because hunting food required strength. So, people would be more likely to survive if their bodies kept their muscles between successful hunts.

Fasting significantly increases your growth hormone and suppresses somatostatin. These changes spare muscles. In a clinical study, a two-day fast increased growth hormone release throughout the day from 2 mg/L to 6.7 mg/L.[4] The liver converts growth hormone into IGF-1, giving you an overall increase.[5]

This is another variation you can do. You go anabolic for six days and fast for one. If you train properly and maximize anabolism on surplus days, you will gain lean muscle, and you'll have little to no muscle loss on the fasting day.

	MON	TUES	WED	THURS	FRI	SAT	SUN
Energy Balance	+500	+500	+500	+500	+500	+500	-2,500
Effect	muscle building	muscle building	muscle building	muscle building	muscle building	muscle building	fat loss

The net weekly calorie surplus from this strategy is 500 a week, which is minimal.

DIET CYCLING

Cycling between Keto/Carnivore and Plant-Based

One of the originators of cyclical ketogenic diets was former Mr. Universe competitor Vince Gironda. He was the first who showed up at Mr. Universe absolutely ripped. In fact, he didn't win because the judges didn't know what to do with a guy that lean.

He would have clients eat a diet of cream and raw eggs while using a lot of glandular supplements and other supplements to maximize anabolism without any carbs. They'd have a serving of carbs every three or four days if their training energy really tanked, but that didn't happen often.

Then, at the end of the 21-day carnivore cycle, he'd switch them to a completely plant-based diet. They'd do cleanses to optimize their digestion and clean out the system. After 10 days, he'd do another cycle of the 21-day carnivore, followed by 10-day plant-based cycles.

It was a radical idea at the time, but he was well known for getting Hollywood elites in shape in record time. This approach was light-years ahead of his time.

Metabolic Flexibility: Cycling from Ketones to Glucose

Metabolic flexibility is the ability to shift your fuel source back and forth between carbs and fats. This means you can go from eating keto to a carb-based diet and back to keto without suffering any negative consequences. It's great for virtually anyone to become fat adapted and reap the benefits of a ketogenic diet (see Chapter 28).

When you get adapted to keto, you build up your lipolytic pathways (fat breakdown into ketones is lipolysis). Once you build this ability, you don't really lose it. The longer you stay on keto or the more times you cycle back and forth, the easier it becomes.

Matt and most of his clients have found that the first time getting into ketosis is the hardest. Then, the second time is a fraction as hard. After that, most people have no trouble getting back to burning fat.

Currently, Matt continues to be in ketosis (over 0.5 mmol) even when he's eating 250 grams of carbs a day. While he has strong ketogenesis genes, he believes that many can achieve the same level of metabolic flexibility once they get sufficiently keto adapted. It probably takes following a ketogenic diet for more than a year to achieve this result.

Matt believes that even for people who want to be keto, it's important to do carb refeeds. Otherwise, the glycolytic pathways (carb-burning capabilities) get very weak. Many people report that their sex-hormone-binding globulins (SHBG) become very elevated during extended keto cycles, which means less free testosterone.

SEASONAL CYCLING

All animals, including humans, have evolved to eat foods that are seasonally available. So, it's natural to eat according to your climate and season.

Winter vs. Summer

Higher-carb foods grow in warmer climates or during the summer in colder climates, so harvest is more available in the summer and fall. Therefore, it's natural to consume more carbs when it's warmer and more fat when it's colder. Also, there isn't one documented culture that thrives year-round in ketosis.

Daylight Length Influences Your Response to Food

Humans are photoperiodic animals. This means the duration of sun exposure, along with UVB light from the sun, affects your epigenetics and circadian rhythms. For example, people who live in temperate zones that have more hours of daylight in the spring experience stimulated fertility.[6]

Many rodent studies have also found that the amount of daylight affects insulin sensitivity and behavior. These studies are almost impossible to do with humans because most of us nowadays are perpetually exposed to light and air conditioning regardless of the season.

A study exposed rats to 6, 12, and 18 hours of light per day. Compared to those with 12 hours of exposure, those with 6-hour light exposure had increased blood glucose, triglycerides, and significantly reduced insulin signaling. In addition, the 18-hour rats developed high blood glucose and some increase in blood lipids, although to a lesser extent than rats with 6 hours of light exposure per day.[7]

Another rat study exposed the animals to 10 hours versus 14 hours of daylight. Obese rats with 14 hours of daylight burned fewer calories. This was measured as reduced thermogenic mitochondria protein for their brown adipose tissues.

However, lean rats didn't have this effect, but they shifted fat storage to inside their bodies. Both obese and lean rats had increased insulin with 14 hours of light exposure. Although their caloric intake didn't increase, obese rats with 14-hour daily light exposure were heavier.[8]

In a mouse model of obesity, long-term UV exposure suppressed weight gain and insulin resistance, even on a high-fat diet. This effect of light exposure was more through nitric oxide rather than through vitamin D.[9]

Vitamin D and UVB Exposure

Vitamin D absolutely affects your metabolism and blood sugar control. And clinical studies show that vitamin D helps with insulin resistance and blood sugar control in vitamin-D-deficient diabetics and in obese people.[10]

Your skin makes vitamin D naturally only with UVB exposure. If you're in a temperate climate—which describes most of the United States and Western Europe—you'll have months with very weak UVB or no UVB at all, even when it's sunny out.

Summer Polyphenols in the Winter Can Throw Off Metabolism

When scientists fed rats that were exposed to shorter daylight hours with dried cherry powder, they had reduced PPAR-alpha function, reducing their ability to produce ketones. The cherry-fed animals also developed more fat cells as well as reduced circadian rhythm and autophagy gene activities.[11] This study suggests that eating summer fruits in the winter can throw off our biology and metabolic rates, making it harder to burn fat.

Shorter exposure to daylight and lower vitamin D levels each make you store more fat and make you less sensitive to insulin. In the summer and fall in temperate climates, your days may be longer than 12 hours and your body may also store more calories to prepare for the colder seasons. Eating summer fruit polyphenols can also put your body in a carb-burning summer mode, which might be detrimental in the winter.

Correspondingly, as you go farther away from the equator, high-carb and sugary foods aren't as available. Fat intake tends to increase, while plant intake goes down. As you get closer to the equator, your daylight length approaches 12 hours, so your fat intake goes down and higher-carb and plant foods become more available.

Therefore, given that nature goes through cycles or seasons, diet cycling is an important strategy that works best with our physiology. You may consider cycling to fewer carbs and fruits during the colder months, and eating a more seasonal variety of foods in the summer and fall.

Humidity vs. Dryness

When Matt moved to Panama, which is a much more humid climate than Canada, he found that certain cravings changed. He used to drink up to a gallon of tea a day, but the craving is now gone. Chinese medicine is highly focused on the effects of environments on the body. It recommends adjusting diets and supplements based on a person's genetics as well.

Athletic Cycles: Off-Seasons and Training Camps

Athletes are masters of cycling both their training and nutrition. As a general rule, they have an off-season cycle and an in-competition cycle. The goal of off-season cycles is generally to build strength, improve technique, and, in some cases, add bodyweight.

In competition, cycles are usually focused on simulating the competition environment and getting bodyweight down to the optimal range.

SUMMARY

This chapter is really about having an experimental mindset. You need to go through the *kaizen* process of experimentation and optimization, and then learn from your cycles. Learn from muscle-building experiments, fat loss experiments, anti-aging experiments, and more. The key is to monitor your biofeedback and keep track of the data (see Chapter 14).

Everyone is different, so to know your individual response, you have to try for yourself. Each time, you'll make adjustments to improve your results.

Along with diet cycling, you'll also have to cycle your training parameters. If your calories and carbs are up, you can train harder and with more volume. You can train with and recover from tougher programs and exercise selections.

If you're dieting, especially for extended periods, you may need to ease up on the training—maybe go to the machines. You want to monitor your muscle mass to prevent any losses there as well as possible.

One of the dangers is that caloric deficits can keep you from recovering well. If that happens to you, it's a sign that you need to stop dieting, especially if your strength starts to drop off a cliff. If you diet for too long and your strength goes down, it's because you're losing muscle mass. Then you need to go the other way.

CHAPTER 9

THE SIMPLEST SECRET OF EVERY SUCCESSFUL DIETER

In this chapter, you'll learn:

- Nutritional strategies to maximize your odds of success on any diet
- How eating a smaller variety of foods can reduce your overall calorie intake and minimize your cravings
- How to leverage structured meal prep so you can achieve your diet results on autopilot
- The most effective secret to a successful diet
- Why the smallest unit of a diet is the meal (and how you will win if every meal you eat is a win)
- The strange phenomenon that happens when you implement the simplest dieting secret
- The six reasons why the simplest dieting secret actually works
- How structure gives you higher odds of success
- How to build structure within your diet that guarantees success every time
- How to eliminate reactive diet destruction so your diet never fails again
- How pro athletes and bodybuilders achieve and maintain world-class physiques
- How to plan meals with ease and remove the dread of deciding what to eat every day

WHAT IS THE SIMPLEST DIET SECRET EVER?

If you look at the diets of pro athletes, bodybuilders, and physique competitors, you'll see one common thread: they eat the same meals over and over and over again.

Now, before you jump to the next chapter and dismiss this strategy because it sounds boring, stay with us. There's game-changing gold in this chapter.

The wider the variety of foods you eat, the more cravings you will have—and thus your odds of success drop significantly.[1] The world's elite physique competitors know this and eat a handful of perfectly calibrated meals. Almost every meal has the ideal amount of calories and macros. Most competitors use meal prep and often eat the same meals for months or years. Wade lived this lifestyle too. Why? Because it works.

All You Need Are 12 Winning Meals

The strategy is to choose or create about a dozen winning meals.

What is a winning meal?

- It has flavors you enjoy
- It satiates you
- Its calories are in the right range
- Its macros are in line with your diet goals

That's it. You don't need to figure out 100 meals, 50 meals, or even 20 meals. You just need 12 (or fewer).

The smallest unit of a diet is the meal. Ultimately, if every meal you eat is a win, you win the day. If each day is a win, you win the week. If you win enough weeks, you achieve your goals. The key is simply to create 12 winning meals. Twelve isn't a magic number. But from our experience, that's all people need, and many people succeed with even fewer.

To boil it down, select or create optimized meals that sound delicious, and eat the right amount of them. That's it.

THE CHAMPION'S MINDSET

Many professional athletes and physique champions adopt the mindset strategy of thinking of food only as fuel—nothing more, nothing less. They cut off all the emotional and psychological baggage that they may have associated with food.

These people need a strong emotional reason to do this without feeling like they're losing out on pleasure. They have their weekly meal plans and get their foods ready, and they eat those meals. There's no thinking. The thinking was done when the game plan was created.

High-performance athletes like Shannon Sharpe have had the same breakfast for over 30 years, and he's a physical specimen in his 50s. He removes the thinking from it and just does it—it becomes effortless.

A Paradox of Choice

One of the reasons that the population as a whole is gaining weight is our environment—we have so many more choices and flavors available to us 24/7. Food companies are constantly creating new products that taste better and are more addictive. So, a simple way to cut calories is to limit the variety of foods that you typically eat.

The larger the variety of foods you eat, the more cravings you create. There's little to no structure, and no structure means low odds of success.

The smaller the variety of food you eat, the more successful you will be, because following your plan will be far easier. Portions will be incredibly easy to manage. You will actually start craving and enjoying just the food you eat.

Structure gives you the best chance of success. The more structured your diet is, the less thinking you need to do, and the more successful you're going to be. This is true for both your diet and your training program.

The Novelty Seeker's Antidote

There's a part of your brain that seeks novelty. Some people who really love novelty (like Matt) tend to break mentally when they don't get something new for an extended time. Here are two strategies that solve this problem.

Update Your Winning Meals

Your 12 winning meals aren't a prison sentence. When you get bored of a meal, change it. It's that simple. Swap out the meals you don't enjoy as much for something new. Ideally, you're not doing an entire diet overhaul unless the entire diet isn't working for you. If that's the case, then you're probably not following the right type of diet to start with.

Every few weeks or months, feel free to rotate in a few new winning meals. Keeping your mind satisfied is vital for long-term success.

Some people who get bored easily simply have more winning meals in their rotation. One of our clients had 80 different winning meals and a private chef to help prepare them. Interestingly, though, this client eventually simplified everything and went to the "12 winning meals" strategy.

Create a "Window of Freedom" Every Week or within Your Meals

This second strategy is great for people who do weekly refeeds. Matt's strategy is to add some new restaurants or meals on refeed days (while staying on track with his calorie targets, of course).

YOU'RE PROBABLY ALREADY USING THE SIMPLEST SECRET

Most people aren't conscious of it, but they do tend to eat the same meals over and over again on rotation. Maybe it's 12 meals, 15 meals, or 20, sprinkled with a new restaurant once in a while. The difference is, you may not have used this winning strategy when building your Me Diet.

As Matt and Wade grew up, their parents had about 15 meals on rotation. It's a natural pattern.

SIX REASONS WHY YOU SHOULD USE THE SIMPLEST SECRET

1. It's Easy to Prepare Your Winning Meals and Have Them Ready

It's exponentially easier to do meal prep when things are simpler and you've done it before. You know what to buy at the grocery store, and how much. You know how to prepare the meals. Once you've calculated portions and made a meal, it's a lot easier the second and third time, and so on.

2. It's Easier to Eat Less at Each Meal

This is perhaps the biggest reason to use our strategy. Studies have shown that if you eat fewer things with less variety, you will end up eating less.[2] The more food and flavor variety you have, the more your cravings go up and your odds of success drop.

Some fascinating experiments have been done on this topic:

- In two separate studies, sandwiches with different fillings instead of just one kind prompted an increase in meal size.[3, 4, 5]
- When three different pasta shapes were served compared to a single favorite, study subjects ate 14 percent more.[6]
- In another study, yogurts differing in flavor, appearance, and texture led to a 12.6 percent boost in intake compared to a single preferred style.
- A four-course lunch of different foods presented with more variety compared to a plain meal with the same foods raised energy intake by 60 percent, mostly at the third and fourth courses.[7]
- Subjects ate more ice cream when they were offered three different kinds than when offered only one.[8]

3. It's Easier to Reduce Portions

This is the next biggest reason to use our strategy. When you eat the same meals, it's super simple to adjust portion size down. Some examples:

- If you eat six eggs for lunch every day, just cut out two of them, and you've lowered your weekly calories by 1,260.
- Let's say you have 1.5 cups of rice with dinner. It's easy to cut that by a half cup (-600 calories for the week). Then cut another half cup later (another -600 calories per week).

If you're looking to build lean muscle and want to increase calories while minimizing fat gain, it's very easy to incrementally add to your portions to reach your target goal.

4. It Reduces Decision-Making

You want to eliminate making unnecessary new decisions. Why? Because there is always a potential "F-it" moment when we get tired and hungry. If you have to decide what to eat and use willpower multiple times a week, the odds of you blowing your diet and giving in to temptations go up big time!

If you know what you're eating for every meal of the week, you eliminate dozens of decisions. You only need to think about your dozen winning meals *once,* and that's it.

By removing the thinking and decision-making on what to eat every day, you'll minimize decision fatigue and maximize your odds of success. If you have all your meals planned and figured out, then it's just a logistics game. Just follow the plan, and success will come much more easily. This cannot be overemphasized.

Matt shares his experience of when he made the shift:

> When I just planned what I was going to eat and had my chef prepare it without having to change anything, it lowered my mental RAM significantly. I didn't realize how much time and energy I was wasting thinking about what I was going to eat every day.

Lowering your mental RAM being spent on useless things is one of the biggest wins in life. It opens up creative space in your mind to focus on other high-value activities.

5. You Have Reduced Cravings

We believe that your gut biome is one of the biggest drivers of specific food cravings. Matt has done "before and after" gut health tests going from keto to plant-based. His gut bacteria changed. Bacteria have about a 48-hour life cycle. This means that specific types of bacteria that thrive on certain foods die if you don't feed them. Conversely, you create new colonies of bacteria when you start eating new foods.

Eating a greater variety of foods feeds a bigger variety of bacteria strains, which drives more cravings. However, once you stick to a set menu for a few weeks, your palate and microbiome will adapt to these foods, and you'll grow to like them.[9]

You Start Craving What You Eat

Story time: A couple of decades ago, Matt was a hardcore keto zealot. He was open to trying something new, so he asked Wade to design him a meal plan. One of the core elements was a "big-ass salad." Matt had never faced a salad like this before. The surprising thing was that after a week, Matt found himself *craving* the big-ass salad. This shocked him. He didn't understand how this was possible.

This strange phenomenon happens every time you stick with a new meal plan long enough. After a few days, you start craving what you eat!

6. It Eliminates Reactive Diet Destruction

Proactively plan and implement your strategy so that you have food ready when you need it. That way, you don't raid the fridge or cupboard. Also, you should never go to a restaurant or supermarket when you're hungry.

When you make a meal plan, always have a few extra meals each week to bring with you in case you get stuck in traffic or something else happens. You should have emergency protein bars, shakes, nuts, or anything else that's compliant with your plan everywhere to make it easier to stick to. These on-the-road snacks are part of your winning meals. Protein bars that are in line with your macro and calorie parameters are a great solution.

SUMMARY

The simplest secret of every successful dieter is to eat the same things over and over again. Create a set of winning meals that are compliant with your diet plan to prep ahead and have on rotation. This allows you to eat on autopilot.

The more structured your diet is, the less thinking you need to do and the more successful you're going to be. Not thinking about your meals or training program is vital.

All you need is a set of 12 winning meals that:

- Have flavors you enjoy
- Satiate you
- Have calories in the right range
- Have macros that are in line with your diet type

The 12 winning meals aren't permanent; if you get bored of a meal, change it!

There are six main reasons why the simplest secret works:

1. It's easy to prepare your winning meals and have them ready.
2. It's easier to eat less at each meal.
3. It's easier to reduce portions.
4. It reduces decision-making.
5. It reduces cravings.
6. It eliminates reactive diet destruction.

The smaller the variety of food you eat, the more successful you will be, because following a plan is far easier. Portions are incredibly easy to manage, and you'll actually crave and enjoy the food you eat. It's the champion's secret.

CHAPTER 10

CONQUERING HUNGER

The irrefutable fact about any extended weight loss program is that you will face hunger. What are the best strategies and tactics to manage hunger? This chapter gives you the answers.

In this chapter you will learn:

- How to manage your hunger so that as you lose weight, you won't develop a ravenous appetite and destroy your progress by relapsing into binge eating
- Four intra-day optimization strategies to manage cravings and stay on track with your goals despite experiencing hunger
- Two simple pre-meal optimization tactics to help lower your potential hunger
- Seven psychological and spiritual hunger management strategies, including how to make hunger feel like winning instead of suffering
- The ways in which low blood sugar levels will make you hangry, and what that means for your weight loss goals and the types of foods you might crave as a result
- The importance of filling your diet with high-satiety foods and how to compare the least satisfying to the most satisfying
- How to use visual hacks to reduce the amount you eat and listen to your body's signals more effectively

It's crucial for anyone doing an extended weight loss cycle to master hunger and cravings. As a general rule, if your hunger increases during a weight loss program, you're most likely burning body fat. As usual, stacking strategies and tactics will give you the best possible results.

UNDERSTANDING CRAVINGS, HUNGER, AND EMOTIONAL EATING

If you're in a caloric deficit and your body is burning fat, you're going to feel hungry sometimes. It's inevitable, but it doesn't have to become a nightmare. The first step is to reframe being hungry as a good thing—because it means you're burning fat. Create a dopamine loop with feeling hungry because you know you're in a calorie deficit.

UNDERSTANDING THE FOUR TYPES OF HUNGER

Many people nowadays are completely disconnected from their bodies. They inhale their meals. The first step to managing hunger is to relearn what it feels like.

There are four different types of hunger with different physiologic root causes:[1]

1. **Physical hunger** is real hunger—it's when your body wants calories.
2. **Nutritional hunger** is when your body is hungry for specific nutrients, which may manifest as cravings for specific foods.
3. **Emotional hunger** is when you feel an impulse to eat something to soothe an emotion or increase certain neurochemicals. You may not even be truly hungry.
4. **Programmed hunger** is when you get hungry in response to a cue. For example, your body increases ghrelin about an hour prior to your regular mealtimes.

UNDERSTANDING CRAVINGS

Cravings can fall into two different categories: physical and psychological.

Physical Cravings

Physical cravings may indicate that your body needs certain nutritional or energetic nourishment from foods with those properties. Cravings for energetic nourishment may include those for tea, soups, and stews during cold seasons, and salads or more cooling foods in the summer.

Salt cravings could mean that you're low in salt or certain other minerals. Instead of gorging on chips, try having more unrefined salt—such as Himalayan pink salt or other sea salt—in your food. Don't be afraid of salt.

If you're on a ketogenic diet or lose a lot of salt through sweat, you have to consume more salt in general.

Some people are low in other minerals, such as magnesium and zinc. Many minerals require healthy stomach acidity to absorb, and you can be low in minerals just because you're not absorbing them. If you test low for many key minerals, be sure to use HCL Breakthrough with your meals.

Sugar cravings may include those for any high-carb or sweet items such as bread, pizza, pasta, pastries, candy, ice cream, and more. These can come from a blood sugar crash after a meal that spikes your blood sugar (reactive hypoglycemia).

Insulin resistance and blood sugar roller coasters are extremely bad for your health. The blood sugar issues can manifest as mood issues and irritability. These can go hand in hand and create a truly vicious cycle.

Psychological Cravings

Psychological cravings mean you're using foods to get a certain type of neurochemical hit in your brain or to change your emotional state.

Gorging on your favorite sugary, hyper-palatable foods will spike both dopamine and serotonin. This is a powerful, addictive neurochemical stack.

Associative cravings are a type of psychological craving triggered by memory, sight, smell, or sound cues.

Most associative cravings appear when you attend an event that triggers certain fond memories and behaviors. Craving popcorn at the movie theater, eating chips during the football game with the boys, and your mom's fresh bread when you visit her are classic examples of this.

Marketing-Driven Cravings

Food marketers are masters at activating associative cravings. Before his first bodybuilding contest, Wade had never eaten a Snickers bar or had any desire for one. During his prep for the competition, though, he saw a Snickers bar ad with caramel rivers and nuts falling off chocolate mountains on his friend's TV. Suddenly, he had a desire for a Snickers bar. He realized that the advertising had anchored him. Now, we face this even more as restaurant and food companies advertise on social media. The best strategy is to avoid food advertisements.

Emotional Eating

Emotional eating is when people use food as a psychological escape, just like a drug. We discussed emotional eating earlier, but with that being said, we aren't psychologists. If you're suffering from any type of eating disorder, we strongly suggest working with a trained professional.

RIDING THE HUNGER SPECTRUM

The diagram below puts hunger on a scale of 1 to 10. If you hit a 9 or a 10, you're famished. This is usually when diets go out the window and people do the "see food" diet—they see food and they eat it.

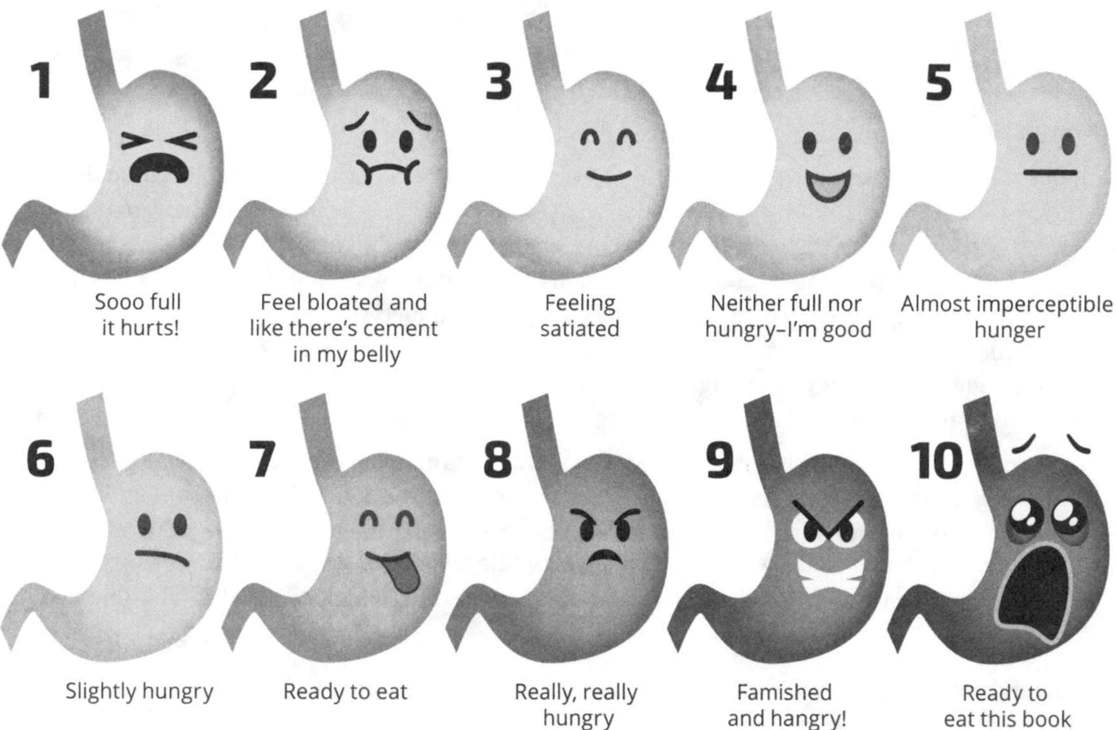

There are plenty of tactics in this chapter, and they all help. However, there is one core strategy: Embrace hunger as part of the process—because it is. The goal is to stay between 3 and 6 on the hunger scale. This is manageable psychologically.

Increase Your Self-Awareness

First, become highly tuned to the sensations in your body when hunger comes on. Be present with yourself, take a deep breath, and scan your body for all the sensations:

- Is your stomach growling?
- Are you getting hunger pangs?
- Do you feel cold, lightheaded, tired, or grouchy?
- What emotions are you feeling along with hunger?
- Are specific food items calling your name?
- Have your senses of taste and smell become more acute?
- Do the sensations go away when you drink water or go for a walk?
- Is what you thought was hunger only frustration or an urge to procrastinate on something else?
- Where is the hunger coming from? Is it just an associative craving?
- Do you feel anxiety or anger because you're hungry?

Becoming contemplative and understanding yourself will help you troubleshoot problems in the future. The more you understand the source of your hunger and how your brain and body work, the better you'll become at giving them what they want and need. We go deeper into the very effective "no-resistance technique" later in the chapter.

As with all other strategies and tactics, the more of these you stack together, the more successful you'll be.

INTRA-DAY HUNGER OPTIMIZATION STRATEGIES

1. Get Enough Sleep

A good night's rest sets up your entire day for either success or struggle. If you get enough high-quality sleep, your food cravings will be far lower than if you have poor sleep. Here's what the research has discovered:

A two-week experiment was done on 10 overweight adults.[2] Those who got 5.5 hours of sleep per night lost 55 percent less fat and 60 percent more muscle than those with 8.5 hours of sleep per night. Beyond this, the group getting 5.5 hours of sleep also reported greater cravings. Cravings kill diets.

If you can't manage hunger and cravings, your odds of success with any diet are close to zero. Sleep deprivation can easily lead to out-of-control food cravings.

The problems don't end there. Here are some other eye-opening data points around sleep deprivation:

- It's been shown to increase levels of ghrelin (the hunger hormone) by 28 percent.[3]
- Short-term sleep deprivation increases energy intake and can lead to a net weight gain in women.[4]
- It has a harmful impact on carbohydrate metabolism and endocrine function, with effects similar to those in normal aging (and therefore it may increase the severity of age-related chronic disorders).[5]
- It takes more food to make someone feel satiated after breakfast, which can lead to snacking and eating, according to research.[6]

For a comprehensive guide to maximizing the quality of your sleep, check out Chapter 11, Sleep Deep and Dominate, in our book *From Sick to Superhuman*.

2. Drink Coffee (Preferably Decaf)

Another adrenaline activator is coffee, which can lower appetite. However, there's another pathway on which coffee works. Research shows that it increases the release of peptide PYY,[7] which helps create a feeling of fullness and may have metabolism-boosting benefits.[8]

One of the most interesting findings was that decaffeinated coffee may produce the biggest reduction in hunger—appetite suppression can last up to three hours after consumption. So, as an appetite-suppression strategy, drink decaf coffee throughout the day (especially if you're genetically slow at metabolizing caffeine).

3. Maté's Magnificent Properties

There's a popular South American tea called yerba maté that can help reduce appetite.[9] Yerba maté may stimulate the body's production of GLP-1 and leptin levels. Wade personally loves drinking yerba maté instead of coffee. The L-theanine in it helps create a much smoother caffeine experience.

4. Stabilize Your Blood Sugar and Avoid Hangry Foods

Low blood sugar can make you hangry—irritable, tired, brain-fogged, and starving—leading you to make worse food choices overall. Any blood sugar roller coaster is a recipe for hedonic hunger—when pizza, donuts, and pastries call your name.[10]

Blood sugar roller coasters can happen after meals that spike your blood sugar and/or insulin. High blood sugar triggers big insulin releases so your cells quickly remove the glucose from your blood about two to four hours after you eat. That blood sugar dip can put your body in red-alert mode, making you hungry and craving anything that will get your blood sugar back up.

So, one of the most important keys to managing your hunger is to find a diet that keeps your blood sugar even-keeled (see Chapter 15). That includes focusing on low-glycemic-impact foods and picking a macronutrient split that keeps you satiated with enough proteins and fats.

Recent research has found that blood sugar responses to each high-glycemic-impact food differ widely from person to person, depending on their gut bacteria.[11] Wade finds that potatoes make him feel very even-keeled, but they can cause major blood sugar roller coasters for other people. Matt, for example, finds it easier to manage hunger on keto.

The key is to observe your own response to different foods, both in terms of post-meal hunger and blood sugar. Then, if you do eat carbs, stick mostly to the ones that don't throw you off. It doesn't matter how healthy the carb appears. If the carbs make your blood sugar crash, they're bad for you.

Now, some protein foods can trigger huge spikes of insulin, and thus hunger. Dairy proteins, especially whey, are very insulinogenic. If you get hungrier consuming these, you may want to replace them with another protein source that makes you more satiated.

If you struggle with blood sugar crashes and cravings, Blood Sugar Breakthrough can help you improve your overall blood sugar control. Many of its ingredients also help manage appetite. If you know certain foods make you ravenous, Blood Sugar Breakthrough is your friend on the occasion that you decide to eat them.

PRE-MEAL HUNGER OPTIMIZATION TACTICS

These tactics are simple things you can do *before* a meal to lower your potential hunger.

5. Exercise before a Meal

Higher levels of adrenaline have an appetite-lowering effect. High-intensity workouts are another healthy and effective appetite suppressant. A review based on 20 different studies[12] found that the appetite-suppressing hormones PPY and GLP-1 are released immediately after a tough, high-intensity workout. The review also found that HIIT helped lower ghrelin (the hunger molecule).

6. Pound Fluids before Every Meal

Pounding a large glass of water before eating has been found[13] to make a person feel more satiated *after* the meal.

A study tracked the appetite of 50 overweight women who drank 1.5 liters of water a day for eight weeks.[14] They found that it lowered appetite and weight, and also led to better fat loss results.

There may be wisdom in the tradition of starting your meal with a soup. Some research has shown that people report feeling more satiated after the meal when they do.[15]

MEAL HUNGER OPTIMIZATION TACTICS

Here are things you can do *during* a meal to lower your potential hunger.

7. Fill Your Diet with High-Satiety Foods

This is a powerful strategy for anyone who eats carbs. Keto followers can move on to the next tip.

In 1995, a study done by Holt et al. studied the satiety levels of various foods.[16] The higher their score, the more satiated you will feel, while lower scores mean feeling hungrier faster. On this scale, "100%" represents the satiety level of white bread.

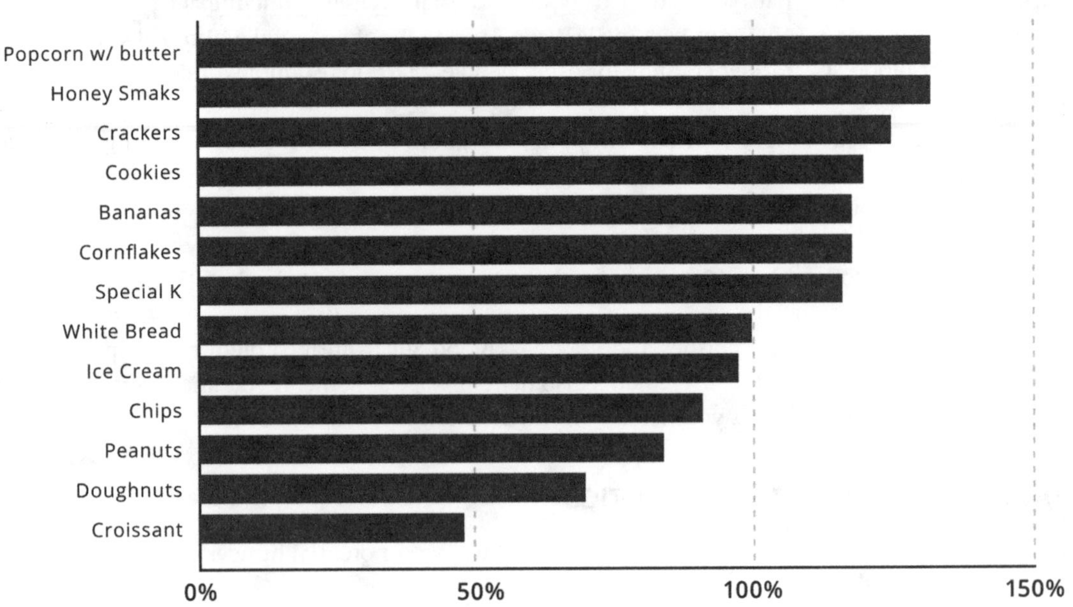

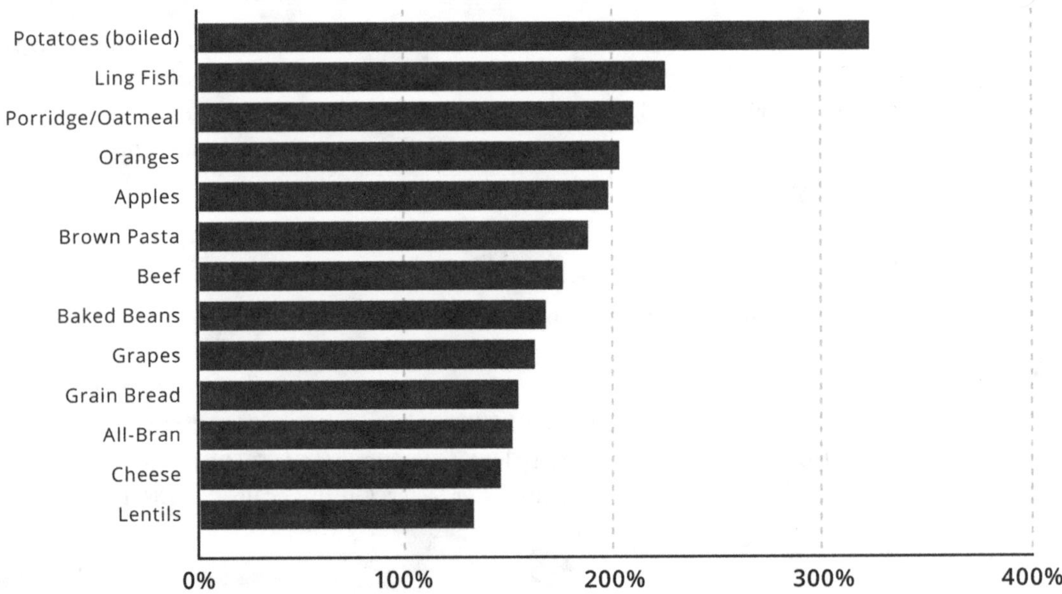

Source: https://www.researchgate.net/publication/15701207_A_Satiety_Index_of_common_foods

The data is clear. If you eat sugary, baked, and fried foods, you will be hungrier sooner. If you eat complex carbs and protein, you will feel fuller longer.

8. Eat Protein and Healthy Fats with Every Meal

Protein, fiber, and fats are the most satiating macros. Making sure that you've got enough protein and/or fats in each meal is important. Most of us have had the experience of having a high-carb takeout meal and feeling hungry 90 minutes later.

Some proteins satiate more than others. Dairy proteins like whey and casein are good options. When Matt is dieting and he's hungry, he likes eating high-protein, low-sugar cereals (like Magic Spoon) because he finds the protein in the milk satiating.

Bonus Tip: *Start* your meal with fats, fiber, and protein. This will slow down your absorption of carbs. If you want to see awesome examples of real world experiments, follow The Glucose Goddess on Instagram.

9. Eat More High-Fiber Foods

As we've said in previous chapters, fiber is a powerful dieting tool. In Wade's recent final shredding as of this writing, maximizing fiber was one of his main strategies. Fiber slows down digestion and helps you feel full throughout the day, and it can help suppress appetite.[17] Data shows that people who eat high-fiber diets tend to have lower obesity rates, although this might simply be because people who eat fiber tend to eat more vegetables and thus fewer calories.

10. Switch to Dark Chocolate

If you've got a sweet tooth like Matt, then chocolate is probably part of your diet. No shame in that. The key is to enjoy dark chocolate versus sugar-loaded milk chocolates. Dark chocolate has been shown to suppress appetite in comparison.[18]

If you're used to eating normal milk chocolate, then we suggest you progressively increase the cacao level. Go from regular chocolate to 45 percent cacao and then keep raising the level by another 5 percent. Many keto followers even find themselves enjoying 100 percent pure cacao. The interesting thing with cacao is that it has many different notes—like wine. Some kinds are naturally sweeter, and some are more bitter. If you go down this road, you'll eventually become a cacao connoisseur and join the endless hunt for the world's best.

11. Eat Some Ginger

Ginger is an absolute powerhouse spice. You should use as much ginger as you can possibly handle. If you can do 5 grams a day, then great. In one study, consuming 1 to 3 grams a day helped improve CRP and lipid profiles. In another study, it boosted men's testosterone by 17 percent. In another study, ginger helped increase the thermic effect of food (see FREE supplement guide www.BIOptimizers.com/book/resources) and helped lower appetite.[19] We could fill an entire chapter with ginger research. The data is clear: you should find a way to incorporate ginger into your life (preferably fresh). You can buy ginger powder or grind it fresh in a healthy shake.

12. Pick Solids over Liquids

It's classic dieting advice: *eat*—don't drink—your food. This is a good rule. One review found that people who ate a solid versus a liquid snack were 38 percent less likely to overeat at their next meal.[20] Another study confirmed that liquid calories have a low satiety level. One of the reasons for this is that solids require more chewing, which slows down your calorie consumption speed and gives more time for the fullness signal to reach the brain.[21]

We formulated Protein Breakthrough to be a satiating meal. The combination of protein, fiber, and fats will leave you feeling satisfied for a few hours.

~~13. Drink Carbonated Water~~

Note the strikethrough on this one. Many people who diet resort to drinking copious amounts of carbonated water because the gas makes them feel fuller. However, this may be a bad idea. In both rats and humans, it seems that carbon dioxide gas increases ghrelin release and hunger response.[22]

14. Eat Omega-3 Fats

Omega-3 fats, like those found in fish and algae oils, can raise levels of the hormone leptin, which helps you feel full.[23] Leptin is a key hormone in metabolism. When calories are restricted for weight loss, a diet high in omega-3 fats may help promote satisfaction after meals.[24] Note, though, that these impacts have only been seen in overweight and obese people so far. More research is needed to establish whether it's true for lean individuals.

One of the greatest trainers of all time, Charles Poliquin, had a protocol for weight loss: 1 gram of fish oil for each percentage of body fat. That means someone with 20 percent body fat would consume 20 grams a day. It's a very high dose, but based on the data we just mentioned, he was probably on to something.

PSYCHOLOGICAL AND SPIRITUAL HUNGER MANAGEMENT STRATEGIES

15. Wire Your Brain so That Hunger Equals Winning

The difference between starving and fasting is simply a conscious decision. When you're starving, you want food, but you can't have it for some reason, and it creates psychological suffering. When you're fasting, you make the conscious decision that you're not going to eat. People who fast feel that they're winning.

This idea goes back to Chapter 5: whatever you label as a win will help create a dopamine loop.

Hunger is similar. If you decide that you're winning when you're hungry, you'll release more dopamine, and it will help lower your noradrenaline. American neuroscientist and tenured associate professor in the Department of Neurobiology at Stanford University School of Medicine, Dr. Andrew Huberman, says that when noradrenaline gets too elevated, that's when people quit.

When we flip the mental switch to weight loss mode, it helps us embrace hunger. We know it's coming. We don't fear it. We just embrace it as part of the journey.

16. Stress Less

Stress eating is a real thing. More than 43 percent of people report using food to manage stress.[25] Stress-driven eating is not the same as real hunger. It's usually activated by stressful events, anger, fear, or sadness. The serotonin and dopamine from food are like drugs that help numb the pain. Stress has been associated with binge eating, non-nutritious food consumption, and an increased desire to eat.

Finding healthier ways to manage painful emotions is the way. The Emotional Freedom Techniques (EFT—more on this in a moment), meditation, and neurofeedback are all great tools that are proven to help. Getting high-quality sleep, a good circle of loving friends, and taking time to relax can all assist to reduce stress. Mindful eating is another part of the solution.

17. Mindful Eating

Mindful eating, according to one study, can help people prevent stress-related binge eating and comfort eating.

Your visual system plays a key role in determining what and how much to eat. When you concentrate on your food rather than watching TV during a meal, you're more likely to consume less. The journal *Appetite* did research wherein people ate supper in the dark, and they consumed 36 percent more.[26] During meals, paying attention to food can help you avoid overeating.

Wade likes to give people the following challenge: Order a large movie theater popcorn and take it home. Then sit at the table without any TV and try eating it all. It's hard. Most people can't finish it. Without the adrenaline and dopamine from the movie, the popcorn isn't that appealing.

Eat slowly and mindfully, and watch out for the fullness signal.

Be present with your meals and chew your foods thoroughly, almost to a meditative level. Between each bite, take a deep breath and scan your body.

- Do you feel stomach distention?
- Do you feel satisfied? Physically and emotionally?
- Do you notice hunger sensations going away?
- Are you energized, or stuffed and sleepy?

Stop eating when you feel about 80 percent full, not when you feel stuffed and need a nap. Then put the food away. Some people, like Wade, have a gene variant that makes the message from their belly to their brains slower. That's one of the reasons Wade can eat too much if he turns off his mental vigilance. And that's why the big-ass salad is a winning strategy for him.

18. Eat on Smaller Plates

This is another visual hack: shrink your dinnerware. It's a good way to trick the brain and help reduce your meal size without even realizing it. There's a reason why all-you-can-eat buffets give you small to medium plates. Chinese buffet diners with large plates piled on 52 percent more, ate 45 percent more, and wasted 135 percent more food than those with smaller plates.[27]

Matt once sat down next to a man on a plane ride who explained how he had lost 150 pounds. Interestingly, he shared this hack (as well as the "no carbonated drinks" tactic).

Surprisingly, even nutrition experts aren't immune to the big-plate phenomenon. For example, when given larger bowls of ice cream, even they unconsciously served themselves 31 percent more ice cream, according to research.[28]

So, there you have it. Research shows that when you have more food on your plate, you're more likely to eat more without even realizing it.[29] The takeaway is simply to shrink your plate sizes and put less food on your plate.

19. Emotional Freedom Techniques (Tapping)

Emotional Freedom Techniques (EFT), also known as "tapping," is one of Matt's favorite emotional health tools. Matt is a certified EFT practitioner and believes that it's one of the simplest, most powerful tools anyone can use. EFT tapping lowers cortisol, a stress hormone, by shifting your nervous system into a parasympathetic (rest and digest) state. EFT can lower and even completely eliminate stress and anxiety in minutes. In Matt's experience, the more you do it, the faster the results.

There's some evidence that tapping can help you lose weight, according to certain studies, and it's an amazing tool for managing cravings, especially emotionally driven ones.

Additionally, over an eight-week period, acupressure administered to pressure points on the ear successfully helped reduce body mass index (BMI) in 84 obese volunteers between the ages of 18 and 20.[30] What's great about acupressure is how fast it works. The sessions were just 10 minutes long.

In a 2019 study, acupressure was demonstrated to lower BMI in 59 people when done twice a week for eight weeks.[31] The participants who used an app to track their progress had superior results.

Weight gain and binge-eating behaviors are linked to elevated cortisol levels. So, if EFT tapping helps you stabilize your cortisol, it could help you lose weight.[32] EFT researcher (and dear friend) Dawson Church did a weight loss study using EFT.[33] Weight decreased an average of one pound per week during the course and two pounds per month between pretest and a one-year follow-up. The results show how EFT can address the emotional influence of food in the external environment, assist weight loss, and promote beneficial long-term change.

20. The No-Resistance Technique

Dr. David Hawkins teaches a technique of identifying bodily sensations once you feel hunger or a craving coming on. First, don't label it as hunger or cravings; just sit and be one with the feeling. Don't intellectualize it. Instead, focus on the *sensation*.

In the moment, what he suggests is actually to lie down without identifying the sensation and simply focusing on it until it passes. When you first start this technique, you'll probably have to do it two or three times the first day, a couple times the second day, maybe once or twice the third day, and then usually the sensations will pass. Your body will become faster at processing the sensations the more you practice.

Intermittent fasting is a good practice because you'll put yourself through the four types of hunger and feel their differences. It also tends to eliminate the ghrelin bursts that come one hour before your mealtimes, so you can eat less frequently and eat only when you're hungry.

It's common to fear that hunger will amplify itself exponentially during your fast. However, the truth is that hunger comes in waves and goes away even when you're fasting. So, it's a way to condition your mind that hunger isn't torturous or catastrophic. By fasting, you learn the powerful lesson, "I can survive without food."

Intermittent fasting may or may not be part of your caloric deficit strategy, but you should try it at least once to learn about your own hunger sensations, as long as you don't have contraindications (see Chapter 30).

Dr. Hawkins has a simple strategy for managing hunger: eliminate all resistance. Here's an excerpt from his *Healing and Recovery* book.

When the feeling we call hunger arises, we simply do this:

1. Sit or lie down someplace quiet, and fix our attention on the feeling
2. Stay with it without trying to resist it or do anything about it
3. Stop giving it labels; we simply focus on the sensations in the body.
   E.g., a diffuse sensation of discomfort around the belly instead of calling it "hunger"
4. Next, we let go of trying to change the sensations
5. We stop visualizing it, we remove all images from the mind
6. We open the gates to the sensation, "I want more of whatever that is"
7. When allowed to come up unresisted, the sensation runs itself out
8. If we resist it or try to change the sensation, it persists and grows

Our final note on this is that we both believe that Dr. Hawkins has created one of the greatest bodies of spiritual work ever. If you have the spiritual drive to grow and improve your level of consciousness, we strongly recommend reading all of his books. You can learn more about Dr. Hawkins' books and see his video lectures at www.veritaspub.com.

A Japanese Hunger-Management Prayer

Prayer is another powerful tool. By asking your higher power to give you the strength and the wisdom to do the next right thing, miraculous changes can happen in your psyche.

There's a Confucian teaching that instructs, "*Hara hachi bun me.*" Roughly, this translates to "Eat until your belly is 80 percent full."

When you find yourself struggling with your diet and your psychological shortcomings, we suggest using the powerful Seventh Step Prayer from 12-step programs:

> My Creator, I am now willing that you should have all of me, good and bad. I pray that you now remove from me every single defect of character which stands in the way of my usefulness to you and my fellows. Grant me strength, as I go out from here, to do your bidding. Amen.
>
> — Anonymous

Miraculous things can happen when you surrender.

SUMMARY

It's a well-known fact that any long-term weight loss regimen will result in hunger. So, what are the best strategies and tactics to manage it?

Among the numerous strategies that will assist you, one key is to embrace hunger as part of the process, because it is.

Some basic strategies for reducing hunger include:

- Get enough sleep. If you get enough high-quality sleep, your food cravings will be far lower than if you have poor sleep.
- Drink coffee (preferably decaf). Coffee can lower appetite, and decaffeinated coffee appears to be better for that.
- Worship the gourd. There's a popular South American tea called yerba maté that can help reduce appetite.
- Stabilize your blood sugar and avoid hangry foods. Stick to carbs, macros, and foods that make it easier for you to maintain your blood sugar.
- Exercise before a meal. Increased adrenaline levels suppress hunger.

- Pound fluids before every meal. A large glass of water before a meal lets you feel more satiated after the meal.
- Focus on high-satiety foods. Anyone who eats carbs should use this method.
- Eat protein and healthful fats with every meal. The most satiating macronutrients are proteins and fats.
- Eat more high-fiber foods. Fiber aids digestion, keeps you full throughout the day, and can help suppress appetite.
- Switch to dark chocolate. Compared to milk chocolate, dark chocolate suppresses hunger better.
- Eat some ginger. Ginger is an absolute powerhouse spice. Use as much as you possibly can.
- Pick solids over liquids. *Eat* your food, don't drink it.
- ~~Drink carbonated water~~. Carbon dioxide gas increases ghrelin release and the hunger response.
- Eat omega-3 fats. Omega-3 fats can raise leptin levels, which helps you feel full.
- Stress less. Stress eating is a real thing.
- Eat mindfully. Mindful eating can help prevent stress-related binge eating.
- Eat on smaller plates. Shrinking your dinnerware is a good way to trick the brain and reduce your meal size without even realizing it.
- Use EFT tapping. Matt, as a certified EFT practitioner, believes that EFT is one of the most powerful tools for managing weight.
- Stop the resistance. Use Dr. David Hawkins's simple strategy for managing hunger: eliminate all resistance.
- Prayer. Asking your Higher Power to give you the strength and the wisdom to do the next right thing can cause incredible changes in your psyche that can ultimately lead to hunger control and achieving your goals.

This chapter would be remiss if we didn't mention the new breakthrough GLP-1 weight loss drugs. GLP-1 agonist drugs are a type of medication used to treat type-2 diabetes. These drugs work by mimicking the effects of the natural hormone GLP-1, which is produced in the gut and helps regulate blood sugar levels. GLP-1 agonists stimulate the pancreas to release insulin in response to rising blood sugar levels and slow down the absorption of glucose from the gut. Additionally, they can reduce appetite and promote weight loss.

Their impact on ghrelin diminishes appetite and makes it much easier for people to eat less food. In our opinion, the success of these drugs proves our point concerning the starvation self-defense mechanisms. By diminishing the intensity of those mechanisms, weight loss becomes much easier.

CHAPTER 11

CLEARING THE EMOTIONAL BLOCKS TO VICTORY

There's a classic saying in health. "The mind shapes the body, and the body shapes the mind."

We've experienced the truth of this countless ways, and so have our clients. Your mind creates your reality, including your body. And, as you transform your body, your mind evolves. The two are constantly transforming together.

This chapter is critical for everyone who wants to become emotionally healthy, which, in our opinion, is as important as a healthy body. And for people who have food issues or food addictions, this chapter is one of the most important. It gives you the tools to quickly remove any emotional obstacle.

In this chapter you will learn:

- The four potential causes of "small-T" traumas and how they can impact your ability to lose weight and keep it off
- Two powerful ways to clean your limbic system (aka your "emotional brain")
- The nine steps for clearing negative emotion, including resentment
- How to become aware of *how* your brain works and *what* drives you or keeps you motivated so you can design a diet that satisfies your psychological needs
- Which of the four discipline styles is yours and how to leverage it to craft the best dietary plan for you
- A powerful four-letter acronym for food addiction struggles that you can use to manage yourself and your triggers
- The three major psychological keys to long-term diet results and how to implement them
- The incredibly effective nine-step forgiveness process that will help you overcome emotional traumas
- The importance of knowing yourself so that you can leverage and manage your tendency for success
- What a "dietary cyborg" is—and how you can become one
- Why it's so important to surround yourself with people who already are what you strive to become
- The reality of emotional eating and an addictive personality

The psychology of your diet strategy can be boiled down to two categories of action:

1. Eliminating the negatives
2. Building a diet that's aligned with your core psychological nature

The most successful people in life are extremely self-aware. To achieve long-term results, you have to be aware of your personal drives and what your psychological and emotional needs are around food. You must be self-aware about your traumas and resentments, and what your brain needs to be driven, satisfied, and motivated. This chapter gives you both.

MAJOR PSYCHOLOGICAL KEY #1: FOR LONG-TERM RESULTS, GET EMOTIONALLY HEALTHY

The scientific consensus is clear that adverse childhood experiences predict a struggle with being overweight or obese, vulnerability to all kinds of diseases, and a shorter life span.[1]

If you have the novelty-seeking genes and an addictive personality, like Matt, your tendencies can increase your risk of food addiction and emotional eating. In this case, it's even more important to develop self-awareness and handle your traumas accordingly. Matt works with addicts in his personal life, and he's found that the behavior of most addicts is driven by past traumas.

Cleaning House and Eliminating Traumas

According to EFT experts Craig Weiner and Alina Frank, the average person has anywhere from 300 to 500 small-T traumas stored in their nervous systems (*average* here means not coming from an abusive upbringing).

What classifies an experience as a small-T trauma?

1. It's emotionally painful
2. It's unexpected
3. The person experiencing it isn't resourced to process it (they don't have the emotional toolbox)
4. The person feels alone

In our professional opinion, trauma is one of the biggest reasons that health industries fail to help most people to get healthy, and why 97 percent of those who lose weight gain it back.

If you don't clean house emotionally, the odds of long-term success with your diets are close to zero because you'll continue to use food as a coping mechanism to deal with emotional pain.

We believe that addressing traumas and learning healthy ways to cope with stress are critical to achieving any health and nutrition goals. The traumas themselves also keep your body in an unhealthy, defensive state that you can't train, diet, or supplement your way out of.

Studies have shown that traumatic memories are stored in your nervous system and throughout your body, rather than in your conscious thought.[2] In fact, many traumatized people aren't even aware of the exact events that traumatized them. So, you can't rationalize or think your way out of traumas; you need to clear them by working with your limbic system.

Reactive rage and anger often arise when events remind us of unresolved, painful events from our past. These are fight-flight-freeze responses created by our nervous systems. Our brains see current situations as threats and then react.

It's pretty rare in today's world to be chased by sharks, knives, or tigers. So why does the body have these stress responses? It's because your brain doesn't differentiate between a physical threat and an emotional threat. The biological response is the same to both.

When someone loses their job, their mind can start racing and projecting the worst-case scenario. Feelings of financial insecurity and fear take hold. Questions like, "What if I can't pay my rent?" or "What if I can't buy food for my family?" and so on start running through the mind.

When someone leaves a relationship, it's common for the other person to feel insecure. "What if I'm not good enough? What if I can't attract someone else? What if I'm alone the rest of my life?"

The root of these modern stress responses is unprocessed trauma.

When we experience a painful event, unless we process it and heal from it, it gets stored in the limbic system as a way to protect us in the future. This is how post-traumatic stress disorder (PTSD) develops. The key word in that phrase is *traumatic*.

When trauma happens to them, people usually resort to emotional repression and suppression to cope with it. This buries the trauma in the emotional limbic system.

Then, the amygdala—the security guard of the brain—scans for threats. Any time it sees anything remotely close in nature to those old traumas, it reacts. The nervous system goes straight to fight, flight, or freeze.

We all know people who have been bitten by a dog and are scared of dogs for their entire life. They may be 40, 50, or 60 years old and still feel scared of a chihuahua, even if it's friendly. If a dog comes into the elevator with them, their adrenal glands get activated. There's sweat, tension rises, and the heart rate speeds up.

Fortunately, there are many effective tools for clearing traumas. A couple of the best are EFT and forgiveness work.

Potent Emotional Healers

The limbic system is one of the components of your nervous system. It's considered your "emotional brain." Some of the most powerful techniques for cleaning the limbic system include:

1. EFT

We mentioned EFT in the previous chapter. It's one of our favorite tools for clearing traumas that lead to emotional eating. EFT is safe, inexpensive, and now proven to have lasting results.

In a clinical study from Bond University in Australia, 49 overweight and obese adults who received four-week EFT treatments were compared with 47 who were placed in a waitlist group. A year after the study, the EFT group had experienced significant weight loss, fewer food cravings, better craving restraint, and psychological coping.[3]

A randomized, controlled trial examined portion control combined with online EFT treatments as compared to portion control and treatment as usual. At six months, the portion-control-and-EFT group experienced the greatest improvement in emotional eating, uncontrolled eating, and self-esteem.[4]

The Naturally Thin You study evaluated 76 participants who enrolled in an online EFT group program. At a 12-month follow-up, participants lost a significant amount of bodyweight. On average, each lost almost 8 pounds over the 6 weeks, and 16.9 pounds during the 12-month follow-up. Also, depression symptoms, low restraint, and subjective power of food scores significantly decreased.[5]

In healthcare workers who were under a lot of stress, EFT reduced addictive food cravings, along with distress, pain, and psychological symptom severity.[6]

A randomized controlled trial found that EFT significantly reduced salivary cortisol immediately and 30 minutes after a single session. This effect was comparable to that of talk therapy or rest.[7] Measures of brain electrical activity found that EFT reduces anxiety brain waves.[8]

2. Effective Forgiveness

Traumas usually create resentments that cause emotional suffering and can drive self-destructive behaviors. The word *resentment* comes from the French word *resentir*, which means to "re-feel." If you think about past events that happened to you with *any* negative emotions, that qualifies as resentment. Harboring resentment, as some have said, is like drinking poison and thinking it's going to hurt the other person.

The question is, how can you clear these negative emotions? Here's the incredibly effective process that we learned by working with experts in this field.

1. Write a list of every fear, resentment, and other negative emotion you have.
2. Get into a relaxed, meditative state.
3. Choose one negative experience you would like to clear.
4. Replay the event and feel the emotional pain and sensation in your body.
5. Go through this forgiveness process:
   - Gratitude: Ask yourself, "What's the gift in healing from this experience?"
   - Responsibility: While you may not be responsible for the actions of others, take ownership of your healing.
   - Understanding: Put yourself in the other person's shoes and aim to understand why they did what they did.
   - Empathy: Feel compassion for their shortcomings.
   - Unconditional Love: Aim to let go and give as much love as possible to the other person.

Having both done hundreds of emotional cleanings, we can attest it's one of the most powerful things anyone can do to improve their quality of life. Our emotional reactivity has been reduced by 99 percent. A serene state of mind is the baseline. Our emotional intelligence has significantly improved. The best way to do this is through neurofeedback, specifically targeting alpha brain waves. When you effectively forgive, your alpha brain waves will increase significantly. The synergy between the neurofeedback and the forgiveness process is profound.

If you do the work, you will become a better version of yourself, *guaranteed*.

Some people with serious food issues should find trained experts that specialize in those areas, whether it's bulimia, food addiction, or anorexia.

Many people find success by using the 12 steps of Overeaters Anonymous (OA). Going through a proven 12-step process will make most into better humans.

MAJOR PSYCHOLOGICAL KEY #2:"TO THINE OWN SELF BE TRUE"

People fall into different psychological profiles. Becoming aware of how your brain works and discovering what drives you is vital to designing the Me Diet that satisfies your needs.

Here are a few examples of emotional and psychological factors you need to take into account when making nutritional decisions:

What's Your Discipline Style?

There are a few different archetypes with respect to discipline. It is important to know yourself so that you can leverage and manage your tendency for success.

1. Dietary Cyborgs

Cyborgs are people who are naturally hardwired for discipline. They're willing to do whatever it takes to achieve a goal, including eating the same thing every day, giving up pleasures from food, and paying the full social cost of sticking to a diet. They have Terminator-like programming and won't waver, no matter what.

Many of the most successful athletes are this way. We learned from having coached, met, and spoken to a lot of people that only a very small percentage of the population has this mentality. Very few are naturally this disciplined. Neither Wade nor Matt is a naturally hardwired dietary cyborg, according to our personality tests.

That being said, discipline is a muscle. Everyone can put in an effort to improve it. However, if it's not natural to you, you need to follow step #2.

Strategies for Natural Cyborgs

- Find other cyborgs to train with and hang with. They will strengthen your programming and help you cement your hyper discipline.

2. Obsessed with a Purpose

Some people, like Wade, develop their cyborg mentality when they have a purpose. They build a heart-based connection to an outcome and use that to overcome any challenges. When Wade doesn't have a committed goal that he deeply cares about, he's not naturally disciplined.

Now, thanks to our understanding of dopamine's attenuation effect on noradrenaline, we have a neurochemical explanation of this process. Both of us are focusing on our purpose and mission to educate the world about health and nutrition as our driving force.

Despite being an exercise physiologist and nutrition expert, Matt found it challenging to stay on hyper-restrictive diets, even for a month. He could stick to them for maybe five or six days because he knew a reprieve was coming. This is the psychological reason why Matt loves refeed strategies. It allows him to have one day of freedom.

However, after five years of this, he flipped the switch and made the choice to push himself to final form. Why? Because of this book. Matt made the decision to be a walking example for the rest of his life that this book is the way. Matt found the purpose he needed to go to the world-class zone.

However, during those five years of 80 percent effort, he achieved very good results. He was able to recomp by over 20 pounds. (As we've explained, this means he built over 20 pounds of lean muscle and lost 20 pounds of body fat while his weight remained the same.) His tools include refeeds, coaching, training partners, systematization, diet breaks, and scheduling, which we talk about throughout this book.

Strategies for Purpose-Driven People:

- Find ways of deepening your commitment to your purpose. Meditate about it. Focus on the massive positive impact it's going to have on others. Visualize that impact.

- Create ways of constantly reminding yourself of your purpose. Share it with your friends, family, and teams.
- Find your tribe of purpose-driven people. They will keep your soul charged.

3. Nurture

Some people become their best when they're working with others. The power of groups has been demonstrated by the success of 12-step programs and other group-driven organizations. "Together, we can do what we can't do alone," is a saying that sums this up.

The people around you inspire or drain you. This is why it's so important to spend time with people who have become what you want to be.

Strategies for People Who Need Nurture:

- Hire experts like coaches, trainers, dietitians, etc.
- Join a gym or health club. You'll be surrounded by people of various levels working toward the same goal you are.
- Build your workout squad. Get two more people, commit to a new training program together, and rock it.

Power Move: Build Your Me Diet Family

We strongly suggest that you build your "Me Diet Family." Be the leader who initiates the action. Join the gym. Design the diet that works for you. Find at least two more people who are willing to follow along and support you. Choose your crew carefully. The most important qualities you want them to have are willingness and open-mindedness. To join our Me Diet community, go to www.BIOptimizers.com/book/dietapp to download our app.

4. Necessity

Sometimes people need life-and-death situations to wake up and become self-aware. Dire medical diagnoses are often the catalyst for many people to start on their health journey.

Another form of necessity is often the loss of a romantic partner. We've had countless clients hire us after a divorce. They want to maximize their attractiveness so they can find another mate.

Strategies for People Who Are Driven by Necessity

- Find other forms of drive because, more often than not, when the necessity is gone, people slip back into their old ways. Why? Because they didn't find a stronger source of drive.

5. Are You a Moderator or an Abstainer?

In her book *The Happiness Project*, Gretchen Rubin explains two ways in which people deal with their vices. People can either be a moderator or an abstainer.

Wade is an abstainer, or "all or nothing" person. Once he's on a diet, if he slips, there is no going back. He enters an out-of-body dissociative state where he can't control himself. For Wade, it's safer and healthier for him to mostly abstain from treats or hyper-palatable foods. It takes more energy for him to stop mid-binge than to never start bingeing in the first place. Abstainers aren't easily tempted by things that they've made off-limits. The thought of giving up a food item doesn't bother them.

However, Matt is the opposite—he's a moderator. He enjoys regular treats and can moderate himself. For Matt, having to abstain from treats and new foods makes him feel restricted and dissatisfied. For moderators like Matt, being able to indulge once in a while strengthens his resolve to stay on his nutrition plan the rest of the time.

Moderators find that occasional controlled indulgences are pleasurable and strengthen their resolve. On the other hand, the idea of never enjoying a food item again can cause them to panic.

Your nutritional decisions and strategies need to take your own tendencies into account. For example, Matt builds in regular refeed meals and refeed weekends and has learned to use these to support his overall goals. Wade, though, rarely ever has cheat meals. On the rare occasion that Wade does enjoy treats, he has the exact strategies and tools he needs to get out of nonstop eating.

Understanding whether you're a moderator or an abstainer will help you better design sustainable dietary compliance strategies.

Fasting and Feasting vs. Regular Feeding

Do you enjoy fasting and feasting? Matt does. He has good genetics for fasting. It shows up in his nutrigenomics and also in his biofeedback (his HRV goes up and HR goes down). He gets a massive dopamine rush from feasting. Matt has used this approach for years because it satisfies his psychological desires and preferences.

Do you enjoy a more predictable feeding schedule or more frequent feedings? This is more Wade's style.

Some people enjoy eating big meals and fasting in between, while others prefer small and more frequent meals. If you participate in many social events that involve feasting, then fasting *and* feasting, or calorie cycling, may work better for you. If you feel good and experience better performance while fasting, it might be something you want to build into your lifestyle.

Novelty vs. Familiarity

How much novelty does your brain crave? Do you prefer the same meals all the time?

Regions in the brain called the substantia nigra (SN) and ventral tegmental (VT) areas have recently been studied; they're full of dopaminergic neurons. About 25 percent of them fire when you're exposed to unfamiliar things.[9,10] They may influence your tendency to be a novelty explorer versus a familiarity seeker.

The intensity of the dopamine release in the SN/VTA area predicts your tendency to be a novelty seeker. By definition, novelty seekers find new stimuli (such as new foods) exciting even when they're not otherwise rewarding (delicious).[11]

Your upbringing and genetics may have to do with these personality traits. For example, if your parents raised you to explore many new experiences, you may be more exploratory than if your parents hadn't encouraged new experiences. Also, human geneticists have found that genetic variants that affect dopamine and serotonin function predict novelty seeking.[12] You can learn more about some of your genetically driven personality traits by going to: www.BIOptimizers.com/book/genes.

It's typically easier to stick to a nutrition plan if you always eat the same rotation of foods. However, if you're a foodie and love having food experiences, it's important to find a way to make a plan work for the long term. Matt is this way. Fortunately, with the right nutritional strategies, you can build a good plan into your lifestyle.

We've discussed Matt's strategy before: five to six days of eating the same things, and then one day of total variance. That one day satisfies Matt's desire to eat something different, allowing him to be okay with having the same things for most of the week.

Strategies for Abstainers

- Go for longer diet cycles of 8 to 12 weeks.
- Avoid refeeds until you reach your final form. Instead, do strict diet breaks.
- Avoid buffets and other places that make it easy to binge.
- Use the "simplest diet secret" in this book.

Strategies for Moderators

- Consider following an IIFYM dieting approach.
- Consider programming refeeds. Make sure to read Chapter 8 about this before you do.

Wade's Donut Story

Over 15 years ago, while on a restrictive diet, I was attending an event where I was first introduced to Krispy Kreme by a friend. The first bite literally blew my brain. Research shows that sugar creates a heroin-like response. So, I had one donut . . . and then another.

The next day, I saw the donut place again. I felt like I needed more. So, I did the same thing.

And the next day, I gorged on donuts again.

I woke up the next morning craving one of those donuts. Immediately, I recognized that I was having an addictive response and knew I needed to reroute my nervous system's conditioning surrounding the donuts. I decided I was going to turn this "positive" psychological experience into a negative one.

I went down to the donut store in the hotel lobby and bought two full boxes. I sat there and ate donut after donut until I felt sick. I kept eating more so that the negative feelings would overcome the euphoria the donuts had initially created. That was how I fixed my Krispy Kreme donut addiction.

Thankfully, I was conscious of this phenomenon and had the tools from my earlier experience to overcome it.

6. How Do You Comply with Expectations?

Rubin has also categorized people according to their tendencies to follow internal (their own) and external expectations:

1. Upholders are people who have no trouble complying with their own and other people's expectations, sometimes to a fault.
2. Questioners question all expectations. They only comply with expectations if they understand the reasons why, so they're more likely to succeed when given the right information. This is how Matt is wired.
3. Obligers struggle with following through with their own expectations of themselves, but have no problem following through with other people's expectations. Therefore, they're more likely to succeed with external accountability. We also call obligers "oxytocin type."
4. Rebels defy both their own and other people's expectations, so they are more likely to succeed when no expectations are placed upon them. Rebels are more likely to succeed if they focus on the why, change their identity, and do things that set them apart from other people. This is how Wade is wired. How are YOU wired?

Obligers are the most common type, followed by questioners, upholders, and rebels. Some people do have mixed tendencies. You can take a personality-type questionnaire to determine which one you are and share with your coach so they can adapt your communication for your success.

Strategies for Upholders

- Find a great coach you believe in and follow the plan.

Strategies for Questioners

- Find a science-driven coach who's really knowledgeable. You need someone who lets you ask all your questions and gives you satisfactory answers.
- Try developing a little bit of faith in the process of meeting your expectations.

Strategies for Obligers

- Stack the odds by surrounding yourself with accountability
- Consider joining Overeaters Anonymous with a 12-step program
- Hire a trainer or coach
- Train with friends
- Create weekly sporting events with friends

Strategies for Rebels

- Focus on learning the core principles in this book.
- Create your own program with all the variance that fits your personality.
- Come up with challenging goals for yourself, ideally that are unusual.

7. Emotional Eating and Addictive Personality

Food has druglike effects. That's why it's so often used as a coping mechanism. For people who do this, comfort eating is their drug and escape from emotional pain and anxiety. Carbs release serotonin,[13] and the neurochemical combination of that and dopamine strengthens addiction even more.

This type of engineered food response is a key strategy of almost every food company. If you're susceptible to it, you'd better be conscious of that and have a strategy to deal with it. Otherwise, it can keep you fat and unhealthy for the rest of your life.

Strategies for Emotional Eaters

- Consider joining Overeaters Anonymous.
- Find healthier ways of getting dopamine and serotonin, like going out in the sun and exercising.
- Avoid hyper-palatable foods, which can kickstart massive binge cycles.
- Focus on eating unprocessed fruits, vegetables, nuts, meat, and seafood. Learn how to make them tasty while hitting your calorie and macro targets.

8. Which Neurotransmitter Type Are You?

One of the biggest drivers of human behavior is neurochemicals. For example, addictive behaviors can be explained with dopamine.

Dopamine

Dopamine is the reward neurotransmitter. It spikes when you're moving toward something you want, such as anticipating your favorite food or going for your goals.

Dopamine-type people are very strong-willed, dominant, confident, and rational, and they make up 17 percent of the population. They're also more comfortable with logic and facts than emotions. They have a lot of energy and may need less sleep. These people do well with strength, such as powerlifting, strongman, CrossFit, and high-intensity interval training.

Low dopamine can appear in dopamine types and other types. This deficiency can result in weight gain, hypertension, depression, carbohydrate craving, and metabolic issues. Supplement solutions we recommend for low dopamine include Nectar X, Apex, and Ultimate Focus by Nootopia.

Acetylcholine

Acetylcholine is important for learning and memory, and the parasympathetic nervous system. Acetylcholine types, which account for another 17 percent of the population, are highly creative, charismatic, and open to new ideas. They may also enjoy the world through different senses. They're quick thinkers, spontaneous, and exploratory. Because acetylcholine is also important for language and comprehension, acetylcholine-type people may be very social and choose careers that involve interacting with others. This type tends to do well with speed, such as in Olympic lifting and sprinting.

An acetylcholine deficiency can result in reduced sensations and enthusiasm, and in forgetfulness. People with low acetylcholine may also suffer from attention issues, isolation, and disorganization. Weight gain, fatigue, joint aches, low mood, and cravings for ice cream and fried foods are symptoms of acetylcholine deficiency. Many components of Cognibiotics support acetylcholine levels. In addition, egg yolks and liver are high in choline, as are many high-fat foods. Mental Reboot AM is a great way to quickly boost your acetylcholine.

GABA

GABA is a calming neurotransmitter that is important for sleep and relaxation. It counteracts stimulating brain signals in your nervous system.

GABA-type people are about 50 percent of the world's population. They are consistent, social, and nurturing. They make others comfortable. They can also be very laid-back and calm, reliable, and level-headed. GABA-type people have to be careful with very stimulating fitness programs and should focus instead on activities like team sports, rock climbing, and yoga.

A GABA deficiency can make you anxious, nervous, and irritable. Other symptoms include headache, burping, disturbed sleep, dizzy spells, and clammy hands. GABA levels can be restored with high-GABA foods and supplements such as GABAlicious from Nootopia.

Serotonin

Serotonin is your happy neurotransmitter. Psychiatry believes that a serotonin deficiency can be responsible for depression.

Serotonin types make up 17 percent of the population. When balanced, these people are playful and social, yet serene. They thrive on change and novelty. These people are sensitive to different senses, in touch with both their minds and bodies; they're practical and often physically coordinated. They may be the life of the party and not easily discouraged by setbacks. Like GABA types, serotonin types have to be careful with very stimulating fitness programs and should also focus on activities like team sports, rock climbing, and yoga.

Overexertion, or not allowing time for their brains to recover, can cause serotonin deficiency, even in serotonin-type people. Symptoms include lack of confidence and desire for social interaction, emotional eating, carb cravings, poor sleep, reduced productivity, insomnia, and sexual dysfunction. You can support your serotonin levels with high-serotonin foods and supplements such as Upbeat from Nootopia.

Oxytocin

If you don't have the dopamine drive but you're more of a connection-based GABA or serotonin type, you might be an oxytocin person. Connection means more to you than outcome. While you won't show up for your own goals, you'll show up when you're a part of a team, group, or membership. Also, group leaders are often dopamine or acetylcholine types.

If you go to www.nootopia.com/quiz, you can take a neurochemical assessment. The test categorizes people based on neurotransmitter dominances and deficiencies, which is a great starting point.

9. What Foods Do You Like?

One last psychological factor for choosing what type of diet to follow is determining the foods that you love. This can only be accurately assessed once you move past any hyper-palatable addiction response. Are you a meat lover? Veggie lover?

Many factors govern your food and diet preferences, such as your:

- Genetics and heritage (for example, you may crave more fish if you don't make omega-3 well)
- Epigenetics
- Upbringing or associative memory surrounding a food
- Gut microbes
- Nutritional needs at any given time (certain nutrient deficiencies are linked to food cravings and preferences)

Pay attention to the somatic experience that you feel when you eat your favorite foods or diet. They should make you feel good.

However, there are a few exceptions to this:

1. Food sensitivities and allergies can make you feel good initially, because inflammation from food can increase cortisol.[14] In the short term, cortisol can feel energizing and anti-inflammatory. But once the response subsides, you start to feel the inflammatory symptoms, such as joint pain or skin breakouts.

2. Dietary transitions typically require a period of adjustment while your epigenetics and gut microbes adapt to the new diet.

We've seen with both ourselves and our clients that everyone experiences some degree of craving and irritability when they switch to a new diet. You may need to use willpower to get through a few days of this. Know that the symptoms will subside and you'll start to like the new foods you eat regularly.

MAJOR PSYCHOLOGICAL KEY #3: MENTAL VIGILANCE

Developing and maintaining mental vigilance is the key psychological program for lifelong success. If you're only motivated by a short-term goal and don't make that lifelong, unbreakable commitment to be healthy, at some point you will fail.

Mental vigilance is like a security system in your brain. It monitors activity, and if you program it correctly, it will keep you focused and on track.

For example, create a 10-pound alarm in your brain. This means if your weight goes up more than 10 pounds, it's unacceptable and you will instantly take action to lose the 10 pounds. Or, if your body fat goes up 3 percent, it triggers the alarm. Create the right alarms for your brain that keep you on track over the long haul.

Protect Yourself at All Times: Managing Environmental Threats and Triggers

It's important (especially early on in your journey) to remove all of the potential triggers from your environment. Avoiding potentially dangerous people, places, and things is Recovery 101.

Dangerous People: Those Who Want You to Suffer with Them

If you're currently hanging out with people who don't want to change when you decide to do your metamorphosis, protect yourself. Don't expect support from them. In fact, expect the opposite: envy, jealousy, and sabotage.

The grand majority of people will feel envy when they see you take action and transform. They may even try to convince you that it's a bad idea, you're fine as you are, and other dangerous rationalizations. Protect your mind. Build a shield there that doesn't let those poisonous thoughts enter.

Spend less time with those people and see them less often. Make new friends who want to see you grow into the healthiest version of yourself. And, even better, become friends with people who are what you want to become.

Dangerous Places: TV, Sporting Events, Mindless Eating Occasions, Buffets, and Free Food

Wade notices that when he's watching television, attending a sporting event, or around certain friends, the food frenzy guy in his brain comes alive.

Some people will go off the rails at a buffet or when they're around free food, because they feel the need to get their money's worth.

Power Move: Eating a Great High-Protein Meal before Dangerous Events

A critical power move is: don't go hungry. If certain situations could trigger your food-munching gene and cause you to overeat, it's a great idea to fill up on a high-protein meal before going.

Protein helps you feel full and satisfied. This will massively lower your impulse to eat foods that aren't part of your plan.

Another variation of this is to bring protein to the party. Bring protein powder or bars, a meat snack, or some form of protein that you can enjoy while you're having fun with your loved ones.

Dangerous Things: Hedonic Foods

Hedonic foods, such as engineered foods that are saturated with hyper-intense flavorings, salt, sugar, and fat, can cause you to eat more even after you're full. Some people also have favorite foods that give them a hedonic response. They're irresistible beyond hunger and negative consequences.[15] Wade knows that once he goes off his diet, it's hard to stop.

If there are hedonic food triggers that tend to cause you to overeat, plan out the amount you will eat, and don't eat from large containers of them. Most importantly, make sure you're not constantly surrounded by easily accessible hedonic foods. Remove foods that trigger binging from your house and life.

COMING BACK FROM MOMENTARY LAPSES OF REASON

Some situations can cause you to overeat or put you in a hypnotic state that causes you to lose control.

First, it's important not to beat yourself up when you lose it. Nothing productive comes from that. The guilt and shame that comes from self-flagellation is extremely destructive and often leads to a bad case of the F-its. That's usually when the diet comes to an end. "Oh, F-it! I went off the rails yesterday, I might as well eat whatever I want today," or "I already gained five pounds, might as well keep going." This is a self-destructive thought pattern that must be deleted from your mind *today.*

Here are the ways to get back on track:

- Make your next meal a winner.
- Go work out or walk.
- Call your trainer or coach and tell them what happened. The coach can help you do a postmortem and turn the mistake into a learning opportunity.
- Journal about it.
- Attend a 12-step OA meeting.

Remember, food acts as a drug on your brain. In drug and alcohol recovery, there's a powerful four-letter acronym that you can use to manage yourself and your craving triggers: HALT. It stands for "hungry, angry, lonely, or tired."

These are dangerous states in which willpower drops down and the chance of catching the "F-its" goes up massively. Why? Because food gives a temporary reprieve from those painful emotions (just like drugs). Let's dive a bit deeper into each one:

Hungry

Hunger is a part of weight loss; there's no escaping it. However, hunger should be manageable. When it starts dominating your thoughts virtually every waking hour, you're in trouble. First of all, you're either following a bad diet (for your body), or you've activated the starvation survival mechanisms. Either way, you need to change your game plan immediately.

There are many strategies to manage hunger, which we cover in Chapter 10.

Angry

Anger is another dangerous state where the ability to think clearly can go out the window. The odds of saying, "F-it!" go up exponentially.

Tapping is incredibly effective against anger. You can reduce it within minutes.

For a more permanent solution, we've both found that nothing beats clearing out resentments. The processes we outlined earlier have changed our lives.

Lonely

Loneliness kills. Humans are social creatures that need interaction to be fulfilled. According to some recent research, it's believed that loneliness is a bigger threat than even obesity.[16]

On the flip side, a 75-year study from Harvard showed that close relationships, more than money or fame, are what keep people happy throughout their lives.

Nothing feels emotionally fulfilling like being a part of a family, of brotherhoods and sisterhoods, of fellowships and groups.

When you have a close group of friends and allies, the quality of your life goes up exponentially. And remember the classic cliché "you become the average of the five people you spend the most time with." As far as your health journey goes, make friends with people who have achieved what you're striving for. Build your own crew of people working toward the same vision. And later on, help others who are inspired by your own story.

When you feel lonely, food can feel like your only friend. It's dependable. It gives you a temporary reprieve from sadness. However, it doesn't solve the problem, and it doesn't fill the emotional void. For many people, only a relationship with a Higher Power can fill that "God-shaped hole."

Tired

Matt's hand-to-hand combat teacher, Christophe Clugston, used to say, "The root of all evil is sleep deprivation."

If you were to ask Matt, "What's the number one thing I can do to improve all three sides of the BIOptimization Triangle?" his answer would be, "High-quality sleep."

Here's what Matt says, in his own words: *I realized that improving the quality of my sleep was the number one thing I could do to improve every aspect of my life. By dramatically improving my sleep, I would improve my appearance, improve my brain, improve my productivity, improve my sex life, and improve my health. I realized that it was the best investment I could make in myself by a long shot.*

We could fill an entire book with research showing the negative effects of sleep deprivation. However, that's not very helpful, so let's switch gears and get into the solution. Make sure to read Chapter 11 in our book *From Sick to Superhuman*, Sleep Deep and Dominate.

SUMMARY

There is an undeniable link between mind and body. Therefore, to be successful in both the short term and long term, you must address your two core psychological needs around food:

1. Address Traumas and Get Rid of Resentments

- Small-T traumas can be created by anything that is emotionally painful, unexpected, something you lack resources to handle, or feel alone about.
- If you don't address emotional traumas, you can fall back on using food to dull the pain and be unsuccessful at managing your body in the long term.
- To clear emotional traumas, you can use EFT (tapping), effective forgiveness, and the 12 steps of Overeaters Anonymous or some other modality that resonates with you.

2. Create a Diet Around Your Psychological Nature—What Drives, Satisfies, and Motivates You

Incorporate a nutritional strategy based on your discipline style:

- If you're a dietary cyborg (super disciplined), then you'll do whatever it takes to achieve and maintain your goal.
- If you're obsessed with purpose, then build an outcome that's close to your heart to keep you emotionally motivated.
- If you're more of a "nature, nurture, or necessity" type, then discipline for long periods of time is more difficult. Incorporate refeeds or diet break to compensate for the restrictiveness and have something to look forward to.

- If you're an abstainer, it can be difficult to get back on track when you slip, so the best thing to do is to stay moderate with—or better yet, abstain from—treats that will derail you.
- If you're a moderator, you feel restricted and unhappy if you have to abstain from treats, so you want to be able to indulge from time to time (diet breaks and refeeds are great).
- If you enjoy feasting or big meals, then fasting is a great strategy for you.
- If you prefer frequent meals, then small and regular feedings are best for you.
- If you like novelty, you can incorporate one day to have something completely different and satisfy this need.
- If you prefer familiarity, it's easier to stick to a diet plan, and you can eat close to the same thing every day.
- It's important to note that more food variety creates more cravings, which makes it more difficult to succeed. So, we suggest paring down the number of your "winning meals" as much as possible. It's a key that virtually every professional bodybuilder uses.
- If you're an emotional eater or have an addictive personality, hyper-palatable foods have a druglike effect and can endanger your goal. These foods include anything salty, sugary, fatty, crunchy, or carby. You should be careful with these and have a strategy for how to deal with them.
- The mind shapes the body, and the body shapes the mind.

CHAPTER 12

POST-DIET SUCCESS

In this chapter, you will learn:

- The three core reasons why more than 97 percent of people fail in their diet journeys
- The two post-diet psychological strategies that can help you remain successful
- What is reverse dieting? And the importance of implementing it into your plan
- The 12-week reverse dieting strategy we highly recommend for post-diet success
- The 9-week reverse exercising strategy we highly recommend to remain successful post diet
- The perfect exercise maintenance plan for a healthy, strong body
- The three psychological strategies for lifelong weight loss success
- The three vital groups of people who should definitely reverse diet
- Wade's words of wisdom for achieving diet maintenance
- How to achieve lifelong weight loss success and fall in love with health
- Which key tactic will protect you more against relapse like nothing else
- Why once you accomplish one goal, it's important to find a new one—and that there's so much more for you to discover and experience

In many ways, this is the most important chapter in the book if your goal is to achieve lifelong weight loss success. How many people do you know who have successfully lost the weight only to regain most of it? We've already mentioned that 97 percent of people fall into this category. If dieters implemented our simple strategies, their success rates would be far greater.

Why?

There are three core reasons:

1. Dieters don't understand the starvation survival mechanisms or how to create a winning strategy.
2. They don't understand how the brain's dopamine system works.
3. When people hit their weight loss goal, they think, "that's it!" Yet they're only about a third of the way to the REAL goal.

The solutions are twofold:

1. Post-diet physiological strategies. Rebuild your metabolism and lock in the results.
2. Post-diet psychological strategies. Create a new series of goals.

THE PHYSIOLOGICAL STRATEGIES FOR LIFELONG WEIGHT LOSS SUCCESS

Once you achieve your final form, your next goal is to slowly rebuild your metabolism. How? The reverse diet is the answer.

Carrie's Predicament

One of Matt's most frustrating experiences as a trainer was working with Carrie. And it wasn't her fault. Matt had always gotten great results with every client, until he met Carrie 20 years ago.

Carrie had done the Bernstein diet, which is a harmful low-calorie diet. She had wrecked her metabolism by eating 800 calories a day and overdoing cardio for an extended period. Matt didn't have the reverse dieting strategy back then. And even though he helped Carrie build lean muscle and get stronger, he failed to help her with her weight loss goals.

Today we know better. The first thing for someone like Carrie to do is to reverse diet slowly for three to four months. The second most important thing is to reduce cardio and increase weight training.

So, if you've done a diet where you went under 1,200 calories and did a ton of cardio, you've probably done a lot of metabolic damage. In that case, the first phase of your weight loss journey should be a reverse diet.

What's a Reverse Diet?

A reverse diet is your final dieting phase. The process includes slowly increasing calories until your metabolism builds back to "normal." Each week, you increase your calories by about 5 to 10 percent, or 100 to 150 calories a day. You're taking advantage of the body's drive for homeostasis. It has a small buffer zone when it comes to variance in calories. This means that if you increase or decrease calories a little bit, your body just maintains homeostasis and you won't gain or lose weight.

One of Matt's coaches, a physique champion, recommends reverse dieting for as long as you've already dieted. We suggest reverse dieting for at least 12 weeks and until your caloric intake is close to 14 to 16 calories per pound. If you've been dieting for more than a year, we suggest reversing for 18 weeks.

There is variance per person depending on how active someone is. For example, for someone who's 150 pounds, target maintenance calories might be 2,250 per day (150 pounds x 15). Below are two examples, using two different final form bodyweights.

Final Form Bodyweight	120 pounds	180 pounds
Reverse Diet Strategy	**Daily Calories**	**Daily Calories**
Week 1	960	1,440
Week 2	1,060	1,590
Week 3	1,160	1,740
Week 4	1,260	1,890
Week 5	1,360	2,040
Week 6	1,460	2,190
Week 7	1,560	2,340
Week 8	1,660	2,490
Week 9	1,760	2,640
Week 10	1,860	2,790
Week 11	1,960	2,940
Week 12	2,060	3,090

When reverse dieting is done properly, there's very little fat gain. You might gain a couple of pounds of fat over the whole process.

Whom Is a Reverse Diet For?

So, whom would a reverse diet be good for? Let's talk about three key groups:

Group #1: Final Form Fat Loss Goal Achieved, and Calories Are Too Low

Let's say someone achieves their goal; however, their calories are down to around seven calories per pound. This is too low. At that point or beyond, energy and brain function become compromised.

Group #2: Physique or Bodybuilding Competitors

Calorie deficits are almost always pushed to extremely low levels during contest prep. It's critical to slowly add calories back in over time to prevent "ballooning." This is one of the reasons why Wade gained 42 pounds after his Mr. Universe contest. He didn't add calories back in slowly enough.

Group #3: Final Form Goal Not Achieved, and Calories Are Too Low

As stated above, when calories reach around 7 per pound, it's time to consider reverse dieting. Can you push calories down further? Yes, but at what cost? The harder you push your body, the harder it will fight back with its starvation survival mechanisms. It's not a fight you want to take on.

So, obese people who are doing long, extended weight loss journeys usually have to do at least one reverse dieting phase if they want to truly achieve world-class form—and sometimes two.

For example, if someone has 200 pounds of body fat to lose, they will usually lose the first 100 to 150 pounds relatively easily. However, at that point, their body is probably highly adapted to exercise and their calories might be down to 7 per pound or less. To lose the final 50 pounds, they need to rebuild their metabolism.

It's wise to proactively schedule and program in reverse diets for long dieting journeys. For a multiyear weight loss quest, it can make sense to do an 8- to 12-week reverse diet every 6 to 9 months.

Now, let's get back to more post-diet success strategies.

Decreasing Exercise Load

As someone follows their weight loss journey, their usual process is to decrease calories and increase exercise. For people who want to reach elite body fat levels, it's not unusual to reach two to three hours of exercise a day at peak.

However, just like in the reverse dieting strategy, you want to reverse your exercise load, especially cardio. For optimal health, two hours of zone 2 cardio a week is the maximum. There is no need to do more. So, if you're beyond two hours a week of cardio, slowly ramp down your cardio volume by five minutes per workout until you reach your target volume.

Final Form Bodyweight	120 pounds	180 pounds
Reverse Diet Strategy	**Daily Cardio Volume**	**Weekly Cardio Volume (6x/week)**
Week 1	60 min	360 min
Week 2	55 min	330 min
Week 3	50 min	300 min
Week 4	45 min	270 min
Week 5	40 min	240 min
Week 6	35 min	210 min
Week 7	30 min	180 min
Week 8	25 min	150 min
Week 9	20 min	120 min

Power Move

Increase your intensity as you lower your volume. Try to push yourself a little harder and beat your speed or power records as you ramp down. It's a good way to create a new wave of adaptation while letting your body heal and recover.

THE PERFECT EXERCISE MAINTENANCE PLAN

This is the minimum effective dose you want to ramp down to for a healthy, strong body:

1. Three full-body weight lifting workouts per week
2. 120 minutes of zone 2 cardio

Your cardio can be done whatever way suits you: 3 x 40-minute workouts or 20 minutes a day. It's up to you. Of course, you can do more, but this will be enough to lock in your gains once you reach final form.

Wade's Words of Wisdom on Maintenance: Create Alarms

I always strove to be in good shape even in the off-season. Here are a few key strategies I use.

There's a simple rule for weight management that is really critical. Every time I've made a mistake on this, I've paid the price. You want to create a mental body fat alarm.

And, if you don't have a DEXA scanner handy, create a mental bodyweight alarm.

Your body fat percentage alarm should be 3 percent. This means, if you're at 12 percent body fat at your best and you find yourself at 15 after hitting the Las Vegas buffets a little too hard for a week, it's time to do another fat loss cycle.

And for bodyweight, I recommend an alarm at eight pounds. Whatever your target bodyweight is, if you go above eight pounds from that, it's time to focus and get it back down.

THE PSYCHOLOGICAL STRATEGIES FOR LIFELONG WEIGHT LOSS SUCCESS

The Power of Love

The ultimate power is love. People who achieve lifelong weight loss success fall in love with health. They fall in love with exercise, enjoy healthy eating, and experience joy when they improve. They love every minute of the journey. We've rarely seen people fall off the wagon once they achieve this level of consciousness with their health. It becomes too good to even think about giving up.

Share the Message

In the recovery community, there's a saying: "Nothing will protect you against relapse more than helping someone else." In our experience, this is 100 percent true. If you choose to become a health professional and help others go through their journeys, you also experience tremendous benefits. It forces you to learn more and go deeper. You get tremendous satisfaction seeing others change. When Matt helped his best friend lose 191 pounds in 18 months, it changed both their lives. Helping others can change yours too.

Goals and Your New Quest

Once you select your direction, it's time to create goals to get you there. The true power of any goal is the dopamine loops it creates. And the first thing we love to do with our clients after they reach a goal is set them up on new quests. There's so much more for you to discover and experience!

See Chapter 12 to discover how to stack the odds of winning in your favor and to learn about all the exciting quests you can take with your body.

SUMMARY

This is the most crucial chapter in the book if your goal is to achieve lifelong weight loss success.

Most people who diet end up gaining their weight back. There are three core reasons:

1. No knowledge about starving survival mechanisms or how to devise a successful approach
2. No idea how the dopamine pathway in the brain operates
3. Going too quickly from "deep" dieting back to "normal" without reverse dieting into it

The solutions are:

1. Post-diet physiological strategies to rebuild your metabolism and lock in the results
2. Post-diet psychological strategies for a new series of goals

Reverse dieting is good for those who:

- Have achieved their "final form" fat loss goal and whose calories are too low.
- Are physique competitors or bodybuilders.
- Have not achieved their final form and their calories are too low.

It's wise to proactively schedule and program in reverse diets for long dieting journeys.

The psychological strategies for lifelong weight loss success include:

- Goals and Your New Quest. The true power of a goal is the dopamine loops it creates. We love setting our clients up on a new quest, because there's so much to discover and experience.
- The Power of Love: People who achieve lifelong weight loss success fall in love with health. They love every minute of the journey.
- Share the Message. "Nothing will protect you against relapse more than helping someone else." Teaching others forces you to learn more and go deeper.

CHAPTER 13

THE ULTIMATE FAT LOSS MASTER PLAN: HOW TO LOSE THE WEIGHT AND KEEP IT OFF FOREVER

It's time to get practical.

In this chapter, you will learn the following:

- An in-depth example of what an ultimate fat loss master plan looks like
- Many strategies and tactics you can use to apply the fat loss master plan to your own life
- How to transition out of the realm of research, theory, and science and into the real-world application of fat loss strategies
- The difference between yo-yo dieting and reverse dieting
- The 16 mini-weight-loss phases that will help you succeed psychologically by constantly setting up motivating dopamine loops
- The 14 key principles, strategies, and tactics that will help you apply a fat loss master plan to your life
- Identifying your fat loss goals and the importance of sticking to them throughout your master plan
- How to take notes for each phase of your fat loss master plan
- How to reach the two-year maintenance phase of your fat loss journey so that you can keep the weight off
- The importance of diet breaks and how to implement them into your fat loss master plan to ensure success

The Master Plan sections are about getting out of the realm of research, theory, and science and showing you a real-world implementation.

To demonstrate, we show you some of our previous clients and walk you through what we did step-by-step.

Please note that these are examples, and your situation will most likely be different. It's impossible to cover every possible variation. The key is to focus on the similarities. The principles that we use are universal, and you can tweak them to fit your life.

Of course, we take out all of the guessing and use our formulas to design your personalized journey designed with the Me Diet app. Go to www.BIOptimizers.com/book/dietapp to download our app to make your Me Diet journey simple and easy to follow.

Our first Ultimate Fat Loss Master Plan is for Frank.

Frank weighs 350 pounds.

- His body fat percentage is 50 percent.
- His lean body mass is 175 pounds.
- His fat mass is 175 pounds.

Goal: Get his body fat to 20 percent or lower.
Target fat loss: 105 pounds
Target timeline: 24 months
Average target weight loss per week: 1 pound per week
Notes: Frank is currently not lifting weights. So, it's possible for him to build some lean body mass for the first 6 to 12 months due to the "beginner's adaptive response" to weights. There's a magic zone of adaptation for the first year when people start to lift.

However, he will probably start losing some lean muscle later in the weight loss phases. For the purpose of this chapter, we're going to keep Frank's lean body mass the same throughout. If, for example, he loses 15 pounds of lean muscle mass (which is expected), then he would have to lose more than 120 pounds of bodyweight to hit his goal. However, we're going to keep it simple for the purpose of illustration.

For the first few months, Frank will lose two to five pounds a week. That will slow down the longer he goes. Frank will also take several diet breaks, which extends the total time.

Frank likes to eat meat and the idea of eating carbs on the weekend, so we chose a cyclical ketogenic diet for him. This means he will be following a ketogenic diet during the week and do a carb refeed on the weekends.

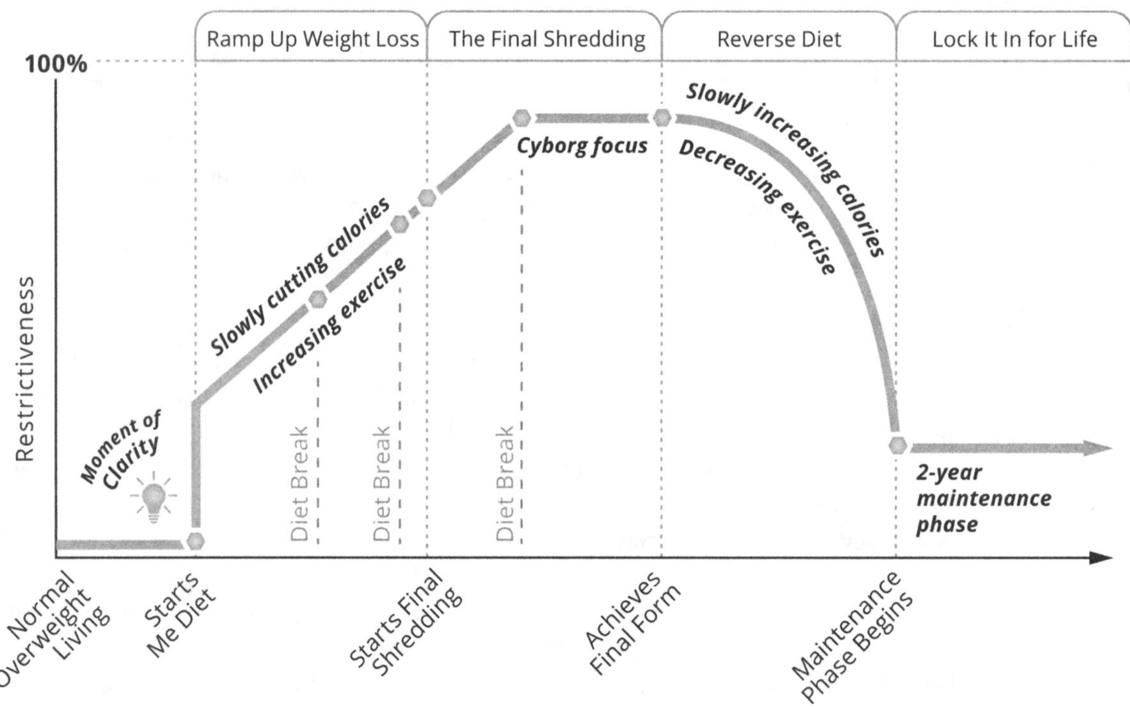

This framework is key. We're going to break up Frank's weight loss journey into 16 mini-weight-loss phases. This will help him psychologically by constantly setting up motivating dopamine loops (see Chapter 16 for more insights). There will be a lot of diet breaks, which will allow him to stay focused throughout.

Here's how we break up the journey:

Weight Loss Phase 1: 11 weeks

Week 1 to Week 10

Target weight loss: 30 pounds (3 pounds per week)

Week 11: Diet break

Notes: Rapid weight loss is normal in the beginning for people who are obese. We estimate Frank's calorie burn to be around 4,500 a day. He was eating around 5,000 calories a day prior to starting this process. We are starting Frank off slowly with three weight training workouts a week. He's doing 7 exercises (one exercise per body part) x 3 sets. Plus, he's walking for 20 minutes between weight-training workouts.

	MON	TUES	WED	THURS	FRI	SAT	SUN
Calories Burned	4,500	4,500	4,500	4,500	4,500	4,500	4,500
Calories Consumed	3,000	3,000	3,000	3,000	3,000	3,000	3,000
Energy Balance	-1,500	-1,500	-1,500	-1,500	-1,500	-1,500	-1,500
Nutritional Strategy	Keto	Keto	Keto	Keto	Keto	Carb refeed	Carb refeed
Exercise	Weights full body 21 sets	20 min walk	Weights full body 21 sets	20 min walk	20 min walk	Weights full body 21 sets	20 min walk

Weight Loss Phase 2: 10 weeks

Week 12 to Week 20 (9 weeks)

Target weight loss: 20 pounds (2.5 pounds per week)

Total weight loss: 50 pounds

Week 21: Diet break

Notes: We are expecting weight loss to slow down a bit. Frank's BMR (basal metabolic rate) is lowering as he's losing bodyweight. Also, he's adapting to the exercises. This is why we're increasing his weight training volume from 21 sets per workout to 28 sets (4 sets per exercise x 7 body parts). And we're increasing his walking time to 25 minutes.

	MON	TUES	WED	THURS	FRI	SAT	SUN
Calories Burned	4,250	4,250	4,250	4,250	4,250	4,250	4,250
Calories Consumed	3,000	3,000	3,000	3,000	3,000	3,000	3,000
Energy Balance	-1,250	-1,250	-1,250	-1,250	-1,250	-1,250	-1,250
Nutritional Strategy	Keto	Keto	Keto	Keto	Keto	Carb refeed	Carb refeed
Exercise	Weights full body 28 sets	25 min walk	Weights full body 28 sets	25 min walk	25 min walk	Weights full body 28 sets	25 min walk

Weight Loss Phase 3: 10 weeks

Week 22 to Week 30 (9 weeks)

Target weight loss: 16 pounds (2 pounds per week)

Total weight loss: 66 pounds

Week 31: Diet break

Notes: We are expecting weight loss to continue slowing down (from 2.5 pounds to 2 pounds per week). A lot of people have unrealistic expectations about continual rapid weight loss, and it sets them up for disappointment. Frank's BMR (basal metabolic rate) continues to go down as he's losing bodyweight. He's also adapting to the exercises.

This is why we changed his workout routine up with completely new exercises (4 sets per exercise x 7 body parts). And we're increasing his walking time to 30 minutes.

	MON	TUES	WED	THURS	FRI	SAT	SUN
Calories Burned	4,000	4,000	4,000	4,000	4,000	4,000	4,000
Calories Consumed	3,000	3,000	3,000	3,000	3,000	3,000	3,000
Energy Balance	-1,000	-1,000	-1,000	-1,000	-1,000	-1,000	-1,000
Nutritional Strategy	Keto	Keto	Keto	Keto	Keto	Carb refeed	Carb refeed
Exercise	Weights full body 28 sets	30 min walk	Weights full body 28 sets	30 min walk	30 min walk	Weights full body 28 sets	30 min walk

Weight Loss Phase 4: 9 weeks

Week 32 to Week 39 (8 weeks)
Target weight loss: 10.5 pounds (1.5 pounds per week)
Total weight loss: 77.5 pounds
Week 40: Diet break

Notes: We're expecting weight loss to continue slowing down (from 2 to 1.5 pounds per week). We're also slowly starting to shorten the windows between diet breaks (going from 10 to 9 weeks). We do this to slow down metabolic adaptation. Frank's BMR (basal metabolic rate) continues to go down as he's losing bodyweight. He's also adapting to the exercises.

This is why we changed his weight training routine again, and why we changed his cardio from walking to biking. It's very easy for the body to adapt to any form of continuous cardio. When you change the form, it creates a new wave of adaptation, which usually helps break homeostasis.

	MON	TUES	WED	THURS	FRI	SAT	SUN
Calories Burned	3,700	3,700	3,700	3,700	3,700	3,700	3,700
Calories Consumed	2,800	2,800	2,800	2,800	2,800	3,200	3,200
Energy Balance	-900	-900	-900	-900	-900	-500	-500
Nutritional Strategy	Keto	Keto	Keto	Keto	Keto	Carb refeed	Carb refeed
Exercise	Weights full body 28 sets	30 min bike	Weights full body 28 sets	30 min bike	30 min bike	Weights full body 28 sets	Day off

Weight Loss Phase 5: 8 weeks

Week 40 to Week 46 (7 weeks)

Target weight loss: 6 pounds (1 pound per week)

Total weight loss: 83.5 pounds

Week 47: Diet break

Notes: We are expecting weight loss to continue slowing down (from 1.5 to 1 pound per week). We also continue to shorten the windows between diet breaks (going from 9 to 8 weeks) to slow down the metabolic adaptation.

We changed Frank's weight training program again. Every time we do this, we create a fresh wave of adaptation. There's an extra level of calorie burning that occurs when your body is in adaptation mode. We also changed his cardio to an elliptical machine.

	MON	TUES	WED	THURS	FRI	SAT	SUN
Calories Burned	3,400	3,400	3,400	3,400	3,400	3,400	3,400
Calories Consumed	2,800	2,800	2,800	2,800	2,800	3,200	3,200
Energy Balance	-600	-600	-600	-600	-600	-200	-200
Nutritional Strategy	Keto	Keto	Keto	Keto	Keto	Carb refeed	Carb refeed
Exercise	Weights full body 28 sets	30 min elliptical machine	Weights full body 28 sets	30 min elliptical machine	30 min elliptical machine	Weights full body 28 sets	Day off

Weight Loss Phase 6: 6 weeks

Week 47 to Week 50

Target weight loss: 4 pounds (1 pound per week)

Total weight loss: 87.5 pounds

Weeks 51 to 52: 2-week diet break

Notes: We dramatically shortened the window between diet breaks (going from 6 to 4 weeks) to slow down the metabolic adaptation. Metabolism continues to slow down a bit. For that reason, we also took out one day of carb refeed. Going from two days of carb refeed to one day can make it easier for some people to lower their overall weekly calories.

We're also changing the structure of his weight training program. We're going from three days of weight lifting to four days and doing a full-body split (half the body divided into two workouts). And we're changing his cardio to yoga. Yoga is harder to adapt to. Movement wise, it's not as repetitive as walking, biking, or using an elliptical. It's also great for flexibility, and the difficulty level can be adjusted as needed. And yoga allows us to increase overall exercise volume without taxing the nervous system.

	MON	TUES	WED	THURS	FRI	SAT	SUN
Calories Burned	3,200	3,200	3,200	3,200	3,200	3,200	3,200
Calories Consumed	2,600	2,600	2,600	2,600	2,600	2,600	3,200
Energy Balance	-600	-600	-600	-600	-600	-600	0
Nutritional Strategy	Keto	Keto	Keto	Keto	Keto	Keto	Carb refeed
Exercise	Weights half day split 1 28 sets	Weights half day split 2 28 sets	1 hour of yoga	Weights half day split 3 28 sets	Weights half day split 4 28 sets	1 hour of yoga	Day off

Weight Loss Phase 7: 6 weeks

Week 53 to Week 57 (5 weeks)
Target weight loss: 3 pounds (0.75 pounds per week)
Total weight loss: 90.5 pounds
Week 57: 1 week weight training break
Week 58: 1 week diet break

Notes: We are expecting weight loss to continue slowing down (from 1 to 0.75 pounds per week). We also continue with a diet break every four weeks to slow down the metabolic adaptation.

On week 57, we have Frank take an entire week off from weight training. Why? We want to detrain his body a little bit and give his nervous system a break. When Frank comes back from this, he'll be more responsive to the weight training. But, for that week, he's going to walk every day for an hour to remain active.

	MON	TUES	WED	THURS	FRI	SAT	SUN
Calories Burned	3,000	3,000	3,000	3,000	3,000	3,000	3,000
Calories Consumed	2,400	2,400	2,400	2,400	2,400	2,400	3,000
Energy Balance	-600	-600	-600	-600	-600	-600	0
Nutritional Strategy	Keto	Keto	Keto	Keto	Keto	Keto	Carb refeed
Exercise	Weights half day split 1 35 sets	Weights half day split 2 35 sets	1 hour of yoga	Weights half day split 3 35 sets	Weights half day split 4 35 sets	1 hour of yoga	Day off

Weight Loss Phase 8: 5 weeks

Week 58 to Week 62 (5 weeks)

Target weight loss: 3 pounds (0.75 pounds per week)

Total weight loss: 93.5 pounds

Week 63: 1 week diet break

Notes: There are no changes in expectations or diet break timing. However, we're going to change Frank's weight training program to five days a week, followed by 20 minutes of high-incline walking on the treadmill. He will keep one yoga workout a week.

	MON	TUES	WED	THURS	FRI	SAT	SUN
Calories Burned	2,800	2,800	2,800	2,800	2,800	2,800	2,800
Calories Consumed	2,400	2,400	2,400	2,400	2,400	2,400	3,000
Energy Balance	-400	-400	-400	-400	-400	-400	0
Nutritional Strategy	Keto	Keto	Keto	Keto	Keto	Keto	Carb refeed
Exercise	Weights Day 1 + 20 min walking	Weights Day 2 + 20 min walking	Weights Day 3 + 20 min walking	Yoga	Weights Day 4 + 20 min walking	Weights Day 5 + 20 min walking	Day off

Weight Loss Phase 9: 5 weeks

Week 64 to Week 67 (4 weeks)

Target weight loss: 1.5 pounds (0.5 pounds per week)

Total weight loss: 93.5 pounds

Week 68: 1-week diet break

Notes: We are expecting weight loss to continue slowing down (from 0.75 to 0.5 pounds per week). We continue with diet breaks every 3 weeks to slow down metabolic adaptation. We are going to maintain this structure of the rest of Frank's weight loss journey.

Losing 0.5 pounds a week is a good target for those who have more than 15 pounds of body fat to lose, or those that have been dieting for more than a year. We did a slight reduction in calories consumed (100 fewer per day).

We're keeping Frank's weight training to five days a week. And we're switching his cardio to stair-climbing (which is one of the hardest forms of cardio).

	MON	TUES	WED	THURS	FRI	SAT	SUN
Calories Burned	2,600	2,600	2,600	2,600	2,600	2,600	2,600
Calories Consumed	2,300	2,300	2,300	2,300	2,300	2,300	2,600
Energy Balance	-300	-300	-300	-300	-300	-300	0
Nutritional Strategy	Keto	Keto	Keto	Keto	Keto	Keto	Carb refeed
Exercise	Weights Day 1 + 30 min stair climber	Weights Day 2 + 30 min stair climber	Weights Day 3 + 30 min stair climber	Yoga	Weights Day 4 + 30 min stair climber	Weights Day 5 + 30 min stair climber	Day off

Weight Loss Phase 10: 5 weeks

Week 68 to Week 71 (4 weeks)

Target weight loss: 1.5 pounds (0.5 pounds per week)

Total weight loss: 95 pounds

Week 72: 1-week diet break

Notes: We're sticking with the same structure as in the previous phase, except we're changing stair-climbing to jumping rope—a great form of cardio that can be done virtually anywhere. We reduced calories slightly (100 fewer per day).

	MON	TUES	WED	THURS	FRI	SAT	SUN
Calories Burned	2,500	2,500	2,500	2,500	2,500	2,500	2,500
Calories Consumed	2,200	2,200	2,200	2,200	2,200	2,200	2,500
Energy Balance	-300	-300	-300	-300	-300	-300	0
Nutritional Strategy	Keto	Keto	Keto	Keto	Keto	Keto	Carb refeed
Exercise	Weights Day 1 + 30 min jumping rope	Weights Day 2 + 30 min jumping rope	Weights Day 3 + 30 min jumping rope	Yoga	Weights Day 4 + 30 min jumping rope	Weights Day 5 + 30 min jumping rope	Day off

Weight Loss Phase 11: 5 weeks

Week 73 to Week 76 (4 weeks)

Target weight loss: 1.5 pounds (0.5 pounds per week)

Total weight loss: 96.5 pounds

Week 77: 1 week diet break

Notes*:* We made *major* changes this week. First, we're going to have Frank walk in the morning for 30 minutes. That little bit of movement gives him a bit of metabolic boost for the first part of the day, helping to increase his overall calorie burn. We did a slight reduction in calories consumed (100 per day). We're also going to assign six days of weight lifting per week.

	MON	TUES	WED	THURS	FRI	SAT	SUN
Calories Burned	2,400	2,400	2,400	2,400	2,400	2,400	2,400
Calories Consumed	2,100	2,100	2,100	2,100	2,100	2,100	2,400
Energy Balance	-300	-300	-300	-300	-300	-300	0
Nutritional Strategy	Keto	Keto	Keto	Keto	Keto	Keto	Carb refeed
Workout 1 (A.M.)	30 min walk	30 min walk	30 min walk	30 min walk	30 min walk	30 min walk	Day off
Workout 2 (P.M.)	Weights Day 1	Weights Day 2	Weights Day 3	Weights Day 4	Weights Day 5	Weights Day 6	Day off

Weight Loss Phase 12: 5 weeks

Week 77 to Week 80 (4 weeks)

Target weight loss: 1.5 pounds (0.5 pounds per week)

Total weight loss: 98 pounds

Week 81: 1-week diet break

Notes: We changed the exercises in Frank's weight training program. This should help increase his overall calorie burn. We did a slight reduction in calories (100 fewer per a day). And we changed walking to biking.

	MON	TUES	WED	THURS	FRI	SAT	SUN
Calories Burned	2,300	2,300	2,300	2,300	2,300	2,300	2,300
Calories Consumed	2,000	2,000	2,000	2,000	2,000	2,000	2,300
Energy Balance	-300	-300	-300	-300	-300	-300	0
Nutritional Strategy	Keto	Keto	Keto	Keto	Keto	Keto	Carb refeed
Workout 1 (A.M.)	30 min biking	30 min biking	30 min biking	30 min biking	30 min biking	30 min biking	Day off
Workout 2 (P.M.)	Weights Day 1	Weights Day 2	Weights Day 3	Weights Day 4	Weights Day 5	Weights Day 6	Day off

Weight Loss Phase 13: 5 weeks

Week 82 to Week 85 (4 weeks)
Target weight loss: 1.5 pounds (0.5 pounds per week)
Total weight loss: 99.5 pounds
Week 86: 1-week diet break

Notes: We changed up the weight training exercises again and reduced calories by 100 per day. And we changed walking to yoga.

	MON	TUES	WED	THURS	FRI	SAT	SUN
Calories Burned	2,200	2,200	2,200	2,200	2,200	2,200	2,200
Calories Consumed	1,900	1,900	1,900	1,900	1,900	1,900	2,200
Energy Balance	-300	-300	-300	-300	-300	-300	0
Nutritional Strategy	Keto	Keto	Keto	Keto	Keto	Keto	Carb refeed
Workout 1 (A.M.)	30 min yoga	30 min yoga	30 min yoga	30 min yoga	30 min yoga	30 min yoga	Day off
Workout 2 (P.M.)	Weights Day 1	Weights Day 2	Weights Day 3	Weights Day 4	Weights Day 5	Weights Day 6	Day off

Weight Loss Phase 14: 5 weeks

Week 87 to Week 90 (4 weeks)
Target weight loss: 1.5 pounds (0.5 pounds per week)
Total weight loss: 101 pounds
Week 91: 1-week diet break

Notes: We changed the weight exercises. We also added three sprint workouts per week for 3 weeks. He'll stop the sprinting on his diet break week. We reduced calories by 100 per day.

	MON	TUES	WED	THURS	FRI	SAT	SUN
Calories Burned	2,100	2,100	2,100	2,100	2,100	2,100	2,100
Calories Consumed	1,800	1,800	1,800	1,800	1,800	1,800	2,100
Energy Balance	-300	-300	-300	-300	-300	-300	0
Nutritional Strategy	Keto	Keto	Keto	Keto	Keto	Keto	Carb refeed
Workout 1 (A.M.)	15 min sprints	30 min yoga	15 min sprints	30 min yoga	15 min sprints	30 min yoga	Day off
Workout 2 (P.M.)	Weights Day 1	Weights Day 2	Weights Day 3	Weights Day 4	Weights Day 5	Weights Day 6	Day off

Weight Loss Phase 15: 5 weeks

Week 91 to Week 94 (4 weeks)
Target weight loss: 1.5 pounds (0.5 pounds per week)
Total weight loss: 102.5 pounds
Week 95: 1-week diet break

Notes: We changed the weight exercises and ramped up the yoga to six days a week (45 minutes per workout). We reduced calories by 100 per day, getting close to the limit of calorie reduction. Fortunately, we only have two more phases to go.

	MON	TUES	WED	THURS	FRI	SAT	SUN
Calories Burned	2,000	2,000	2,000	2,000	2,000	2,000	2,000
Calories Consumed	1,700	1,700	1,700	1,700	1,700	1,700	2,000
Energy Balance	-300	-300	-300	-300	-300	-300	0
Nutritional Strategy	Keto	Keto	Keto	Keto	Keto	Keto	Carb refeed
Workout 1 (A.M.)	45 min yoga	45 min yoga	45 min yoga	45 min yoga	45 min yoga	45 min yoga	Day off
Workout 2 (P.M.)	Weights Day 1	Weights Day 2	Weights Day 3	Weights Day 4	Weights Day 5	Weights Day 6	Day off

Weight Loss Phase 16: 5 weeks

Week 96 to Week 99 (4 weeks)

Target weight loss: 1.5 pounds (0.5 pounds per week)

Total weight loss: 104 pounds

Week 100: 1-week diet break

Notes: We changed the exercises as usual, but he'll maintain the yoga since it's not very demanding on the nervous system. We reduced calories again with only one more phase to go.

	MON	TUE	WED	THURS	FRI	SAT	SUN
Calories Burned	1,900	1,900	1,900	1,900	1,900	1,900	1,900
Calories Consumed	1,600	1,600	1,600	1,600	1,600	1,600	1,900
Energy Balance	-300	-300	-300	-300	-300	-300	0
Nutritional Strategy	Keto	Keto	Keto	Keto	Keto	Keto	Carb refeed
Workout 1 (A.M.)	45 min yoga	45 min yoga	45 min yoga	45 min yoga	45 min yoga	45 min yoga	Day off
Workout 2 (P.M.)	Weights Day 1	Weights Day 2	Weights Day 3	Weights Day 4	Weights Day 5	Weights Day 6	Day off

Weight Loss Phase 17: 2 weeks

Week 101 to Week 102 (2 weeks)
Target weight loss: 1 pound (0.5 pounds per week)
Total weight loss: 105 pounds
First major goal has been achieved!
Notes: We changed the exercises and reduced calories for the last time. Yoga continues.

	MON	TUES	WED	THURS	FRI	SAT	SUN
Calories Burned	1,800	1,800	1,800	1,800	1,800	1,800	1,800
Calories Consumed	1,500	1,500	1,500	1,500	1,500	1,500	1,800
Energy Balance	-300	-300	-300	-300	-300	-300	0
Nutritional Strategy	Keto	Keto	Keto	Keto	Keto	Keto	Carb refeed
Workout 1 (A.M.)	45 min yoga	45 min yoga	45 min yoga	45 min yoga	45 min yoga	45 min yoga	Day off
Workout 2 (P.M.)	Weights Day 1	Weights Day 2	Weights Day 3	Weights Day 4	Weights Day 5	Weights Day 6	Day off

Frank's journey isn't over. Far from it. Now it's time to lock in the results for life. So, we begin a two-year weight loss maintenance goal, which is for Frank to stay within 10 pounds of his new bodyweight. If he goes over the 10 pounds, he'll start a new weight loss phase to get back to his target bodyweight of 245 pounds.

To keep Frank motivated from here, we've set some athletic goals. Frank wants to compete in CrossFit. Remember that continually creating new goals is *vital* to staying on the path. As soon as you have no goal, your motivation disappears.

We're also going to do a reverse diet for 13 weeks while reducing Frank's training volume over the next few months. He'll go back to one workout a day and increase his calories by 100 per week to help rebuild his metabolism.

Frank's Reverse Diet

Weekly Calorie Targets

Week 1	1,600
Week 2	1,700
Week 3	1,800
Week 4	1,900
Week 5	2,000
Week 6	2,100
Week 7	2,200
Week 8	2,300
Week 9	2,400
Week 10	2,500
Week 11	2,600
Week 12	2,700
Week 13	2,800

Now, if Frank wanted to, he could start another weight loss phase to go from 20 percent body fat down to 15 percent or lower. Or he can just choose to maintain at 20 percent and focus on other goals. The choice is up to him.

We can create the ultimate personalized fat loss plan for you. Go to www.BIOptimizers.com/book/coaching to have one of our coaches guide you through your journey.

HOW TO APPLY THIS CHAPTER IN YOUR LIFE

You can apply many strategies and tactics, but we wanted to use a more extreme case to illustrate what a long-term weight loss master plan looks like.

- If you have 100 pounds to lose, aim to achieve that in two years.
- If you have 50 pounds to lose, aim for a timeline of one year.
- If you have 30 pounds to lose, give yourself 6 to 8 months.
- If you have 20 pounds to lose, give yourself 4 to 6 months.
- If you have 10 pounds to lose, give yourself 8 to 10 weeks.

Here's a summary of key principles, strategies, and tactics:

- Figure out your daily calorie burn. A good starting point is 10 per pound. So, if you weigh 200 pounds, start with a total of 2,000 calories in per day.
- In the beginning, you can aim for a maximum of 1,000 calorie deficit per day. This means 500 cut from food and 500 burned with exercise, for a total of about two pounds lost per week.
- As you progress with your weight loss journey, slowly lower calories by 700 per week (that is, reduce total calories per day by 100, and stay there all week). If you're stuck for more than two weeks, lower by 300 calories, or add a bit more activity.
- Weight training is the base of your weight loss program for all the reasons we outlined earlier in the book.
- Start with three days of weight lifting per week.
- Change your weight training program at least every eight weeks.
- Every couple of months, add an extra day of weight lifting. Start at three days per week and go up to six days per week total. For extreme cases (to get to superhuman levels of muscularity and conditioning), lifting can go up to 12 times a week.
- Progressively increase the intensity and difficulty of your weight training. This means adding more weights and pushing yourself more. Always train safely.
- On non-weight-lifting days, do cardio. Walking 20 minutes a day is a good start. Slowly add more cardio time. Adding five minutes per workout per week is a good way to do it. However, don't go beyond 60 minutes of cardio per workout unless you're training for a marathon.
- Change the form of your cardio every few weeks. Go from walking to biking to stair-climbing to rope-jumping and back to walking. We're trying to slow down adaptation to the exercise.
- Do refeeds every week. Start with two days a week, and then as you go deeper, lower it to one day a week. You must still be mindful of calories on refeed days. This isn't an all-you-can-eat refeed day.
- Do a diet break every four to eight weeks. In the beginning, go eight weeks straight. Then, as you progress, up the frequency to once every seven weeks, every six weeks, every five weeks, and every four weeks. Some people like going two weeks in calorie deficit and taking a one-week diet break. Do what psychologically works best for you.
- If your calories go below 7 per pound of bodyweight, consider doing a reverse diet. So, if you weigh 150 pounds, the lowest you want to go is 1,050 calories per day.
- Once you've reached your goal, do a slow reverse diet. Slowly add 100 calories per week until you reach about 12 calories per pound of bodyweight or until you start regaining body fat.

CYCLING AND REFEEDS FOR OPTIMAL LONG-TERM FAT LOSS

One of the most important keys to keeping your body safe is to take diet breaks or refeeds. Numerous clinical studies have shown that it helps maintain the metabolic rate and reduce metabolic adaptation in the long term.

In a fasting and refeeding study, leptin was shown to decrease from 12 hours into fasting and bottoms out at about 36 hours in. Once the subjects returned to eating like normal, their leptin levels return to baseline within 24 hours. Therefore, we recommend at least one or two days of refeeding to reset your leptin.[1]

Zigzagging in Two-Week Breaks

If you start off with extra body fat, it's beneficial to take two weeks of maintenance diet breaks for every 5 to 10 pounds that you lose. A clinical study showed that two-week breaks reduce the impact of fat loss on long-term metabolic adaptation.[2]

Some obese people have leptin resistance, and overeating tends to make it worse.[3] So, if you're still in the obese-to-overweight range, taking diet breaks at maintenance with healthy foods is more beneficial than overeating for refeeding.

11 Days On, 3 Days Off

A study compared 74 overweight men who went through four solid weeks of caloric restriction against those who went through 11 days of a controlled diet followed by 3 days of a self-selecting diet.

The basal metabolic rate of the 11 days on, 3 days off group dropped during each day of the diet and increased slightly during their diet breaks. On the other hand, the calorie-restricted group's basal metabolic rate stayed low and continued to decrease.

During the four-week follow-up period, the calorie-cycling group regained 2 pounds, while the calorie-restricted group regained 5 pounds out of around 12 pounds lost in total.[4]

Reverse Dieting to Maximize Your Maintenance Calories and Prevent Fat Rebound

Your metabolism works like a slingshot. It adjusts, to an extent, to your day-to-day fluctuations in caloric intake. This is why most non-dieting people stay at a steady weight even though their food intake fluctuates. Now, a mistake that most dieters make is to go right back to eating whatever they want to their (now-increased) appetite.

Yo-Yo Dieting vs. Reverse Dieting

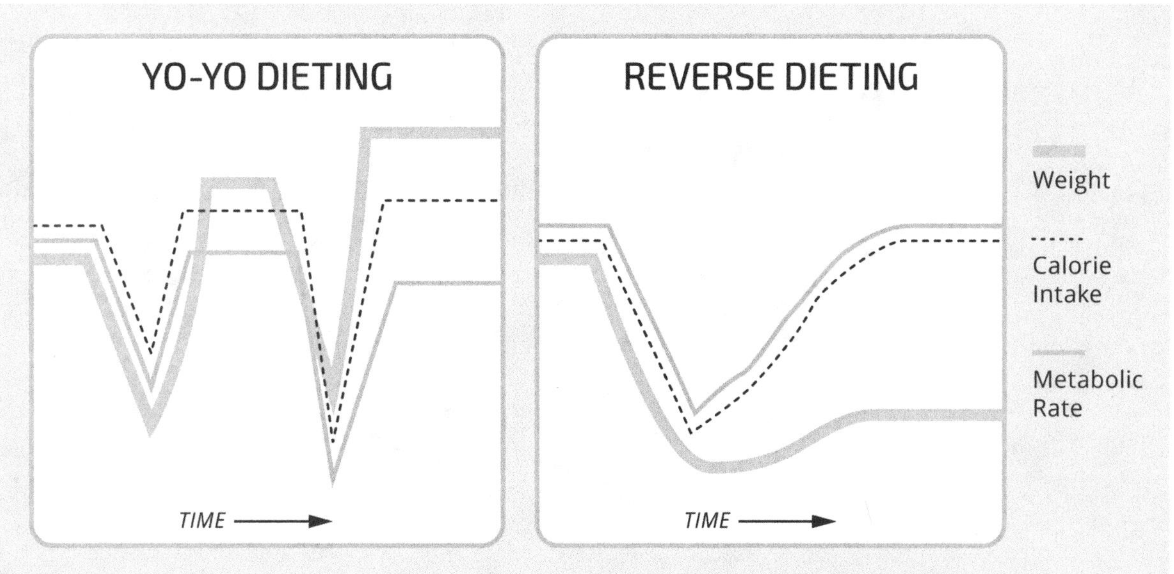

With every successive cycle of yo-yo dieting, weight rises, while metabolic rate drops.

Reverse dieting helps to maintain weight loss and metabolic rate over time.

These graphs represent general trends. Real life data may vary, as weight loss/gain is not usually linear.

The leaner you are away from your original body fat set point, the harder your body wants to fight back to regain the fat. Going right back to eating whatever you want right away is a recipe for disaster: you'll most likely overshoot the metabolic slingshot and regain the fat, undoing your hard work.

The good news is that you don't have to be stuck dieting with lower calories forever. The solution is to reverse diet out of your caloric deficits. You'll slowly increase calories within the range that won't overshoot your metabolic slingshot. This would be 50 to 100 calories per week above your starting calories until you reach your target intake.

By reverse dieting, you slowly stretch your metabolic slingshot to a new set point of maintenance calories. At this new set point, your body learns to expend more energy rather than store everything as fat. So, you'll feel more energized, perhaps have a higher sex drive, and perform better both physically and mentally.

It's possible to gain some body fat as you reverse diet, so it's important to monitor your body composition and adjust. Sometimes you need to slow down the calorie increase or take a break too.

Keep in mind that reverse dieting can take a lot of discipline to stick to, as it can take months to reach your prediet maintenance calories. You have to be able to stick to your calorie count perfectly for it to work, but the effort you put in will be worth it in the long run.

CHAPTER 14

CREATING THE ULTIMATE HEALTHY LIFESTYLE

Do you have a cyborg-like focus and discipline?

Would you challenge Jocko and David Goggins to a battle of wills?

Can you ignore the food you love for decades to come?

If you answered no to any of these questions, then this chapter is for you.

The fact is that very few people would answer yes. Only a select few choose and develop the love of a disciplined life. For this elite group, the more spartan their lives are, the more dopamine they get. This chapter is for those of us who are not naturally wired this way.

Don't get us wrong; we can all benefit from having more discipline. It's your last line of defense when you're fighting your mind's desire to do (or not to do) something. Discipline can be the process you use to propel you into action when you're fighting procrastination.

However, we believe that for you to achieve lifelong dietary success, the strategies that work are the ones that you stick with. Therefore, an enjoyable lifestyle must be one of the top factors of your nutritional pyramid. This chapter focuses on integrating your dietary strategies with your dream lifestyle.

In this chapter, you will learn:

- How to strategically ramp up your discipline to a peak and then lower it for maintenance
- Why dietary "cyborgs" tend to lose friends and alienate people—and that you don't need to be one to get the results you want (we aren't either)
- Strategies to build in dietary flexibility so you can achieve your nutrition goals (while enjoying your life)
- Why people who use dietary flexibility tend to be more successful
- How to use holidays, family gatherings, vacations, and social events to your advantage
- How to literally have your cake and eat it too
- How you can achieve better results by being less disciplined
- How Wade's personal experience as a bodybuilder teaches us that extreme practices can cost you relationships and opportunities
- What questions you need to consider when you navigate what's most important to you
- Why your total potential results are determined by the quality of your overall BIOptimized health strategy
- The role neurochemical imbalances play in food addiction and disordered eating
- Why you need a "suffering is winning" mindset instead of using willpower and self-control to resist temptations
- Why daily calorie counting is a mistake, and how to leverage your fasting, cycling, and refeeds with weekly calorie math
- 10 tactics you can use to enjoy dinners and parties without getting off track from your weekly calorie goal
- 12 strategies to keep your diet on track while enjoying vacations and holidays
- The importance of HIIT workouts, short bursts of exercise, and daily walking
- How to reach your "magical promised land" using temporary, progressive restriction combined with nutrition and lifestyle

Wade tells this story of one of his clients, Dale, and his journey to falling in love with exercise:

Dale's Story

"I hate exercising . . . that's why I hired you."

This confession came to me from a wildly avant-garde hairstylist almost two years after I first began coaching him.

I ran a juice bar next to a gym where I coached clients. As I got to know Dale, I realized he was one of the most balanced people I had ever met, despite his outwardly radical appearance. We got him in fantastic shape in short order, as he was also one of the most dedicated people I've ever trained.

It came as a shock two years into working with him when he commented offhandedly that he had hated working out, even though he never missed an early-morning appointment.

When pressed, he said, "I hired you because it literally was a struggle to go to the gym, and I knew that if I didn't have skin in the game as leverage on myself, I would never go on my own." He then said almost sheepishly, "I didn't have the heart to tell you, but I can now—because after two years, my back doesn't hurt anymore, I can run circles around my peers, and I actually enjoy coming to the gym."

Dale fell in love with exercise!

That's the ultimate goal. Once you fall in love with exercise and eating healthy, they become effortless.

Now in his 70s, Dale continues to work in the salon at a reduced load, maintains his garden at the cottage, and still has a zest for life. With Dale, we never tried to build a life of restriction; rather, we gave him a consistent training program with a sensible diet. We created winning strategies that allowed him to enjoy life, be healthy, and look great.

Dale is enjoying lifelong benefits due to his dedication to living the principles of biological optimization.

Here's the good news: like Dale, you don't need to have cyborg-like discipline to be in fantastic shape and enjoy a great lifestyle. You *do* need to be restrictive, committed, and focused for a small portion of your life. And yes, you do need to maintain mental vigilance for the rest of your life. But this doesn't mean you can't enjoy food *and* maintain a healthy, fit, lean body.

How long does the restrictive period last? That depends on how much physical change you're trying to create. If it's 20 pounds, then maybe it's three or four months. If you have 200 pounds of fat to lose, it might take a couple of years. If you're trying to become Mr. or Mrs. Olympia, it could be 20 years.

Let's break down the diagram of restrictiveness over time on page 155.

The average overweight person has close to a zero level of restrictiveness. They eat and drink whatever they want, whenever they want. Then they experience a moment of clarity when they realize they're heading in the wrong direction and choose to change. So, they start their Me Diet.

A lot of people want to go from zero to 100 on restrictiveness. As we covered in previous chapters, that's a physiological mistake. It's much better to ramp up exercise—the right kinds—and slowly ramp down calories. In our app, we have made this complex system super simple. You just have to follow the plan. Go to www.BIOptimizers.com/book/dietapp to download our app.

However, as your body adapts, you need to keep ramping up activity and lowering calories even more. For those of you who want to achieve elite body fat percentages, you will have to push it to another level. As you enter the "final form" phase (your last phase of weight loss), you may need to go to 100 percent restrictiveness. How long does that last? Usually a few months.

Once you reach your final form goal, you need two more phases: the reverse diet and the lock-in phase. The reverse diet usually lasts a couple of months. The lock-in phase is when you maintain your bodyweight within eight pounds for two years. If you just go back to your old ways without these pieces, you're going to lose all your gains. It will all be for nothing.

We've got another word for the lock-in phase: the lifestyle phase. This is where you can maintain your health and aesthetics while enjoying your favorite foods, and even go on epic culinary adventures.

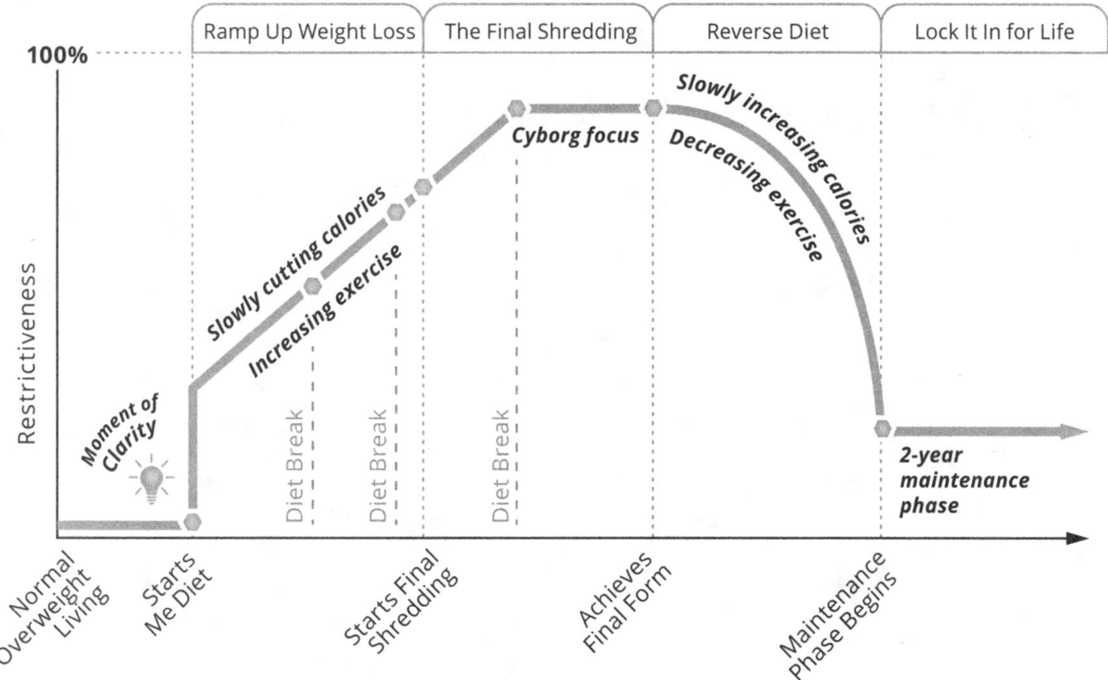

For people who decide to pursue bodybuilding or other aesthetic careers, there is no final form. They're on a multi-decade pursuit of a dream vision, continuing to improve their form year after year. This decision certainly isn't for everyone. Here's a cautionary tale about the price of world-class aesthetic success.

Wade's Story: How to Lose Friends and Alienate People with Super-Restrictive Lifestyles

For 15 years, I competed in professional bodybuilding, one of the most restrictive lifestyle sports in the world. It requires achieving super-low body fat levels and high levels of muscle mass, which go against our evolutionary survival programming. I literally trained, ate, and slept bodybuilding. There was no room for anything else.

Over that time, I never had butter or dessert, because my goal was to become the best bodybuilder I could. The goal superseded everything else, and I was going to make sure I gave it my best effort.

My only way around natural tendencies was to maintain cyborg-like rigidity. There was no deviation from the diet. There was no flexibility at any social occasion. There was just Terminator-like focus, because I knew that if I slipped, I would go off track.

When I got to very low body fat during long periods of dieting, I would constantly think of food. I'd have to count out mini rice cakes; I allotted myself 20 to 25 of them, in bowls of five at a time. If I did it any other way, my brain would skip the count, causing me to want to cheat and eat more rice cakes. I couldn't keep the count down. My brain was trying to fool me into eating more. It was a constant battle against my starvation self-defense mechanisms.

I could date only people with the same mentality: bodybuilders and fitness competitors. It was very difficult for a "normal" woman to tolerate my restrictive ways.

I would either skip social occasions or bring my own food to them. If challenged, I would leave the occasion or fight back against anybody who suggested that I deviate from my diet, regardless of whatever rationalization they had.

I would not get invited to certain events and things just because I was the weirdest guy they knew. As an outgoing person, this was a major sacrifice for me.

Wade's story serves as a cautionary tale of what it might take to transcend your natural lack of discipline, although some might find it inspirational. If you want to go extreme with your physique, you need to engage in extreme practices that can cost you relationships and opportunities.

Here's a diagram to help illustrate the throughput of effort compared to results.

Speed of Results Based on Commitment
Full Commitment
EFFORT
THE BEST STRATEGY
THE BEST EXECUTION
THE BIOPTIMIZED LIFESTYLE
RESULTS
Half-ass Commitment
EFFORT
BAD STRATEGY
POOR EXECUTION
UNOPTIMIZED LIFESTYLE
RESULTS

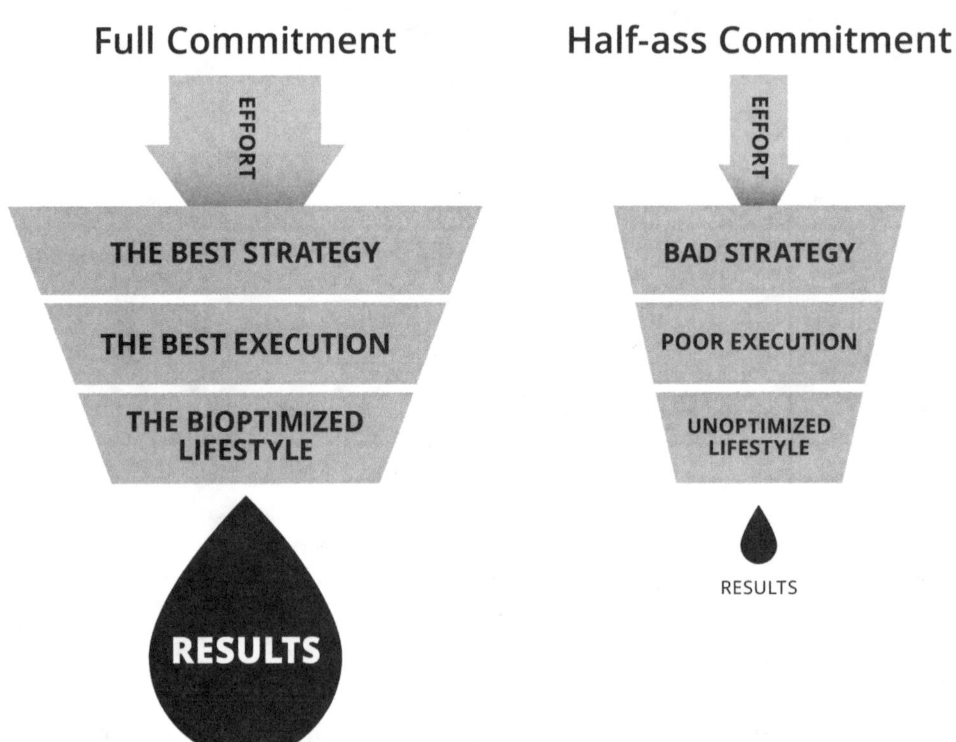

Effort flows into the pipe. Your total potential results are determined by the quality of your overall strategy. The better the strategy, the better the potential results. Don't worry, this book has every top strategy you need to succeed.

Then comes execution. How effectively are you executing your strategy? If you're at 80 percent or above, you'll get good results. If you want great results, you need to go to 90 percent or higher. If you want to go to the world-class zone, you're living at close to 100 percent. This is why lifestyle is the final piece of the pipe. The closer you get to total throughput, the more restrictive your lifestyle is.

There's another way to use this framework. If you want to reach your final form as fast as intelligently possible, then this is highly relevant. In other words, you could go to 95 or 100 percent restrictiveness for a few months and then strategically and slowly shift down into an awesome lifestyle.

BUILDING IN DIETARY FLEXIBILITY

Food Is One of the Pleasures of Life

When you eat, your body creates neurochemical rewards in the form of dopamine, opioids, cannabinoids, and serotonin. By hitting your body with this intense pleasure response, eating enhances your chance of survival. The responses become hedonic with meals that are rich in fat, sugar, and salt, which can promote eating even when you're not hungry.[1]

In other words, food provides us with such a strong neurochemical hit that many people would find it hard to go for a long time without their favorite foods. Foods can act like drugs on your brain.[2]

If you have a strong dopamine system genetically (another important aspect of nutrigenomics), you will have a much stronger response to hyper-palatable foods. There is a spectrum of how strong the response is.[3, 4] Matt's is probably a 7 out of 10, whereas food addicts or disordered eaters might score at 9 or 10.

Food addiction and disordered eating are often symptoms of neurochemical imbalances. They're forms of substance abuse in the guise of food and exercise.[5] Such problems are also common among people with preexisting mental health issues.[6] If you have these tendencies, work with a mental health professional and be mindful about your neurochemistry, with regard to both your diet and lifestyle.

The Mental and Emotional Cost of Deprivation

Beyond the social cost, there is a mental and emotional cost to the feeling of deprivation. Unless you've hardwired your mind to believe that suffering is winning, you will have to use willpower and self-control to resist temptations.

Research has shown that willpower is a limited resource,[7] so food restrictions can have mental and emotional costs. The more willpower you expend, the closer you get to a breaking point.

Long-term diet studies also show that people with more dietary flexibility and the ability to personalize their diets to their preferences have more diet sustainability and better long-term results.[8] This is what we mean when we say you'll be more successful with structured windows of food freedom.

EFFECTIVE NUTRITIONAL LIFESTYLE STRATEGIES

Now, let's get into nutritional lifestyle strategies and tactics that you can apply to enjoy life and stay on track with your goals.

Almost Every Successful Diet Has Refeeds

Many of the most successful diets, including Body for Life, 4-Hour Body, and the Anabolic Diet, have excellent long-term outcomes because they employ refeeds as a strategy. On these plans, you can have five or six days of highly structured eating and one or two days of diet breaks.

Refeed Day vs. Cheating

There's a key mindset difference here. We don't like to use the terms *cheat meals* or *cheat days*, because the word *cheat* implies something is not part of the plan. There is no cheating here; these days are planned. However, you still need to be mindful of calories.

If you're not mindful, you can easily wipe out your entire week of effort in a day or even one meal. One 12-inch pizza is around 3,000 calories. Add an appetizer, a Coke, and a dessert, and you're at 4,500 for a single meal. For some people who are deep in a diet deficit, that's almost three days' worth of calories.

Instead, we use refeeds, which is a planned dietary strategy to refill your glycogen store, refeed your muscles, and stoke your metabolism a bit. You'll also get muscle-sparing and leptin benefits.

The goal here is to maintain the flexibility to enjoy life as much as possible and not become a dieting recluse. At the same time, you'll be able to stick to the diet and not go too far off track.

Dinners and Parties

The core strategy at social occasions is to align your refeeds with parties and events. If you're having a birthday party on Friday, then that's your refeed day.

Many people make the mistake of looking at their calories from a daily perspective. If you're fasting, calorie cycling, and doing refeeds, it's better to do the calorie math on a weekly basis. What matters at the end of the week is if you are in a deficit or a surplus.

10 Tactics You Can Use to Enjoy Dinners and Parties without Getting off Track

1. **Save your calories for one meal.**

   Look at calories like a budget. If your budget is 2,500 calories a day, you can save them all up for the party or dinner. In other words, fast for the entire day and enjoy one big meal. Matt loves doing this for dinners and parties.

2. **Fast the day before.**

   Using the same budget analogy, you get a certain amount per week. Say your budget is 12,600 calories a week (1,800 per day). If you skip one day of eating, you can overeat the following day. Theoretically, you can eat 3,600 calories and achieve the same results if you fast one day.

3. **Fast the day after.**

   You can also fast the day after you enjoy your feasts and parties.

4. **Train legs hard and heavy before the feast.**

   By activating the anabolic response (especially from a demanding leg workout), you can put those excess calories to good use and build muscle. Remember, anabolism is a great way to increase calories out. Nothing burns calories and activates anabolism like squats and deadlifts.

5. **Optimize your blood sugar response.**

   We suggest taking two capsules of Blood Sugar Breakthrough before every high-carb meal. This will optimize your body's ability to use those carbs.

6. **Optimize your digestive system.**

   We suggest increasing your digestive aids and taking Gluten Guardian (digestive enzymes that break down gluten and milk proteins), MassZymes (the strongest proteolytic enzyme formula), P3-OM (probiotic blend), and HCL Breakthrough.

7. **Maintain a minimum level of mental vigilance.**

   It is possible to blow your week's progress with one or two days of refeeding, especially if you've got a big appetite. Many people can eat 7,000 to 8,000 calories in a day when they activate feasting mode, which can easily wipe out five or six days of dieting results.

8. **Focus on protein and fiber first.**

   When you eat protein, fat, and fiber before carbs, you blunt the blood sugar response. This can help prevent a blood sugar roller coaster that makes you overeat. They increase satiety and lower the odds of overeating. So, we suggest you focus on those first and add tasty carbs last.

9. **Watch the alcohol.**

   Alcohol is seven calories per gram, and many alcohols have a lot of sugar and other carbs. The best options are wine, light beer, hard liquor with low-calorie mixers, and champagne. Worse options are sugary cocktails (some are more than 500 calories), frozen beach drinks, and craft beer.

10. **Drink lots of water.**

    Instead of alcohol, why not drink water or carbonated water? Throw in a lime or a spritz of juice, and you've got a great-tasting, low-calorie mocktail.

Offsetting Jet-Setting

We both love to travel and see the world, but let's face the facts. Very few things stress your body more than flying and traveling.

First, you're exposed to high levels of radiation as you soar 35,000 feet above the planet.

Planes have poor air quality, you stay seated for long hours, and the food isn't very good whether you're in economy, business, or first class.

On top of that, the change in time zones disrupts your circadian rhythms. Also, when you're traveling, getting workouts in and maintaining your healthy diet can be a struggle most of the time.

It took us years to figure out how to minimize the damage and optimize travel through a variety of tricks we've learned over the decades. Even then, it takes an extra amount of focus and attention to ensure you get the most out of your travel while optimizing your health.

We recommend the following flying habits:

- Bring your own food
- Fast on the plane, rather than eat
- Exercise as soon as you can once you land, even if you're tired (half of your normal workout is fine)
- Hydrate, hydrate, hydrate. The humidity level in most planes is lower than that of a desert—between 5 and 20 percent. (A desert is between 10 and 30 percent.) Flight attendants don't offer enough water, so on short flights, buy one liter; for long-haul flights, buy two.
- Before you go to sleep, block out as much light as possible, including lights on clocks, TVs, and wall sockets (add blue-light blocking glasses before sleep if you're flying at night)
- Pick hotels that have good-quality exercise equipment
- Before you land, have healthy meal places already dialed in (pin them in Google Maps to get there easily once you're there)
- After you land, get some time in the sun with your bare feet on the ground as soon as possible, if you can
- After you land, go floating in a sensory deprivation tank, if you have the chance, to help your nervous system recover

When you fly over more than three time zones, make a decision around resetting your circadian rhythms. If your trip is only a couple of days long, we suggest keeping the same schedule as you do back home. However, if it's more than three days *and* more than three time zones away, here are the top ways to reset your circadian rhythms:

On the plane

- Use an optimal dose of melatonin at the time you want to sleep at your destination. We suggest using 4 to 6 sprays of Dream Optimizer, which allows you to control your dose. Combine that with Sleep Breakthrough for the best plane sleep ever. For example, if you're flying from Los Angeles to Paris and want to sleep at 11 P.M. Paris time, take your melatonin at 2 P.M. PST.

When you wake up in your new time zone, do the following for the first three days:

- Go outside and expose your eyes to direct sunlight for at least 15 minutes
- Do a workout
- Eat a big, high-protein breakfast
- Take a 20-minute nap in the afternoon if needed

At night

- Go to bed at the same time every night
- Use a micro amount of melatonin for two nights, taken at the same time each night. We suggest using the Dream Optimizer from BIOptimizers.

Vacations and Holidays: 12 Strategies and Tactics

1. **Align time off with your diet breaks.**

   Remember, diet breaks are a bit of a misnomer. You're still on a structured diet; however, you're not shooting for a calorie deficit on breaks but eating at maintenance—usually for one to three weeks. Your goal is to give your brain a break and rebuild your metabolism a bit.

2. **Focus on anabolism.**

   The best strategy to minimize fat gain during vacation is to focus on building lean muscle. If you can, train hard every day with a tough weight lifting routine. Your body can use the extra calories in combination with weight lifting to build lean muscle. Then the calorie expenditure from muscle building helps offset fat gain. If you stop weight lifting and go off your diet, it can be a recipe for body fat disaster.

3. **Still (kind of) track your calories.**

   Do you need to weigh everything you eat? Count calories? No, not unless you're trying to become a bodybuilding or fitness champion. That being said, keep a rough tally of your daily calories. Remember that your goal is to stay at maintenance. Not gaining weight is a win.

4. **Weigh yourself daily.**

   Weighing yourself daily helps keep you aware during vacation. However, point #5 is critical . . .

5. **Don't freak out!**

   If your weight goes up by three or five pounds, don't freak out. You're retaining water and glycogen. You've got more intestinal bulk (aka poop) in your body. All of those together can easily create a five-pound weight swing with just one epic feast.

6. **Create a ceiling.**

   You should set a maximum weight gain limit of five to seven pounds. If you go past that, you're probably overeating. If you do cross the threshold, do a day of fasting.

7. **Use all ten of the "dinners and parties" tactics above.**

   The tips we gave are all highly applicable, especially on holidays. For example, it's normal to eat 4,000 to 6,000 calories on Christmas Day. Use all of the tactics to mitigate consequences. During a vacation, you might have a couple of days where the feasts are epic and the booze flows deep. Optimize around those party days to slow down the damage.

8. **Forgive yourself.**

   As we've already said, avoid beating yourself up. If you do end up going over the top, don't worry. You're in this for the long haul.

9. **Have fun.**

   Enjoy the holidays. *Enjoy* your vacation. *Enjoy* the feasts. *Enjoy* your family. These are special moments.

10. **Do a three-day fast before.**

    One thing Matt's a fan of is three-day fasts at the end of a diet phase for the final extra fat burn—up to an extra percent of body fat lost. However, it also depletes your body of glycogen, so be cautious of overeating after the fast. Your hunger can be ravenous. Read about how to end a fast in Chapter 30.

11. **Do a three-day fast after.**

    Similarly, you can lose some fat after the vacation and also get rid of excess water, sodium, and glycogen. Always remember that when you get the "10 pounds in a week" effect on vacation, 8 or 9 pounds of it are water, glycogen, sodium (salt), and intestinal bulk. A three-day fast will usually get you back to where you were before the vacation.

12. **Have a comeback plan and date.**

    You must plan your comeback before you go. Make sure you set a time limit for how long your less restrictive period is. Some people struggle to return to a diet once they go off their original structured lifestyle. If you typically struggle to return, you need a well-structured plan in place to follow next. Otherwise, you risk going back to your old habits and regaining a lot of body fat.

LIFESTYLE AND EXERCISE

We've covered lifestyle and nutrition. What about lifestyle and exercise? How devoted to exercise do you need to be?

Here's the great news: maintaining takes only 33 percent of the effort to build. A recent study proved that this amount of resistance training maintains strength, myofiber size, and muscle mass gains.

This two-phase exercise trial studied 72 adults divided into young (20 to 35 years) and old (60 to 75 years) groups. For phase one, they did resistance training three days per week for 16 weeks. Phase two was maintenance, consisting of 32 weeks with random assignments of reduced doses to either one-third or one-ninth of phase one.

The results for the younger group concluded that both maintenance prescriptions (one-third and one-ninth) preserved the gains, and the one-third dose actually led to additional myofiber hypertrophy.

For the older group, strength was retained during the maintenance phase and was at even higher levels than the younger group. However, they required a higher dose of weekly loading to retain their myofiber hypertrophy gains.[9] For both groups, myofiber-type shift was maintained better with the one-third dose.

Our suggestion for minimum effective dose is three hyper-efficient, full-body resistance workouts per week. They can be done in as little as 20 minutes (but more realistically in 30). This is enough to maintain your lean muscle and bone density.

Add one eight-minute HIIT workout per week. Warm up for one minute; do a 30-second burst at 90 percent effort. Rest for one minute. Repeat the work and rest two more times, and cool down for one minute. This will help maximize your VO_2 max.

And then move daily. Aim to walk two times a day; 10-minute walks are enough. Wake and walk for 10 minutes in the sun, and walk for 10 minutes after each meal. Walk the dog. Walk to the gym. Walk to work. Just move. Movement is life: 20 minutes of walking divided into two 10-minute sessions can do wonders.

If you combine all of these recommendations before adding walking, you can stay very fit and healthy with as little as 70 minutes of exercise per week. And if you add walking, it's only an extra 20 minutes a day.

SUMMARY

To enjoy lifelong physical success, you need dietary strategies and a lifestyle that you enjoy. You can create your dream lifestyle by integrating dietary strategies. You begin by being restrictive, committed, and focused for only a short period of your life—just until you reach your goal.

- You'll start the Me Diet. The strategy here is to slowly lower your calorie intake and ramp up exercise. Once your body adapts, you lower calories even further and increase your workouts even more. You don't go from 0 to 100 at the beginning.
- Then you enter the "final form" phase, in which you go to 100 percent restrictiveness for a couple of months.
- Once you achieve your goal, you go on to the "reverse diet" phase for two months.
- Finally, you get into the "lock-in" phase for two years (aka your lifestyle). The goal is to stay at the current weight for two to five years. You can maintain your aesthetics, your health, and your performance while enjoying your favorite foods and even taking full advantage of your vacations.
- You still need to maintain mental vigilance to protect your gains and stay on track for life.
- Some strategies to maintain your goal and enjoy dinners, parties, and vacations are:
  - Refeeds (diet breaks): You can align your parties, short vacations, and holidays with your refeed days.
  - Save your calories for the *big* meal. Eat light or fast the whole day before the feast.
  - Alternatively, you can fast the day before the feast, or the day after.
  - Have an intense leg workout before the big meal.
  - Optimize your blood sugar. Take Blood Sugar Breakthrough 20 minutes prior to every high-carb meal.
  - Optimize your digestive system with enzymes, probiotics, and HCL to help break down food and make the best use of nutrients.
  - Consume more protein and fiber. They have fewer calories and make you feel full faster.
  - Go slow on the alcohol. The best options are wine, light beer, hard liquor with low-calorie mixers, and champagne.
  - Drink a lot of water. If you're not a fan of plain water, drink carbonated water or add a lime or a spritz of juice.
  - Maintain vigilance. Count your calories (a rough tally will do), weigh yourself daily, and have a maximum weight gain limit of five to seven pounds.
  - Have a comeback plan and date. Plan how long you'll be off for, when you'll return, and how you plan to go forward (meal plan, workouts, timeframe, etc.).

CONCLUSION

Lifestyle is the peak of the pyramid of your nutritional decisions. It's the final piece that makes health and fitness a joy instead of a sacrifice. Yes, you can have cake and abs too. Yes, you can be fit without training every day.

Be aware that you need to pay the price to get to this magical promised land. The price is temporary, progressive restrictiveness with nutrition and lifestyle, plus progressively more time and effort on the exercise side. Once you achieve your final form, your goal becomes to lock it in for life.

GOAL #2:

YOUR LEAN MUSCLE JOURNEY

The next two chapters reveal the fundamentals to permanent, healthy lean muscle mass.

CHAPTER 15

HOW TO SUCCEED WITH A MUSCLE-BUILDING DIET

This chapter gives you the best possible muscle-building nutrition advice. It's simple, straightforward, and highly effective. Just follow the steps along with a good weight lifting program, and you will gain muscle.

In this chapter, you'll learn:

- How optimal levels of muscle mass expand all three sides of the BIOptimization Triangle: aesthetics, health, and performance
- Cautionary tales against muscle mass maximization: what you don't see when you look at legendary bodybuilders
- How to maximize your mTOR and insulin functions for muscle anabolism while minimizing fat gain
- Why calories are often the most important limiting factor in muscle gain for dedicated bodybuilders, but not without monitoring key biofeedback data
- How to maximize your nutrification and minimize gut discomfort to assimilate the extra calories needed for muscle gain
- Why "bulking up" could be a bad idea for most people, and what to do instead
- Matt's and Wade's own muscle-building journeys
- The importance of balancing anabolism and catabolism
- About massive differences between optimal calories for bodybuilding, depending on genetics
- The seven most basic tenets of bodybuilding nutrition
- The simple process of monitoring the scale and body fat to make the proper adjustments to your muscle-building journey
- How to prevent gaining fat during your muscle-building journey

You can gain muscle on almost any diet, provided that it has enough protein and calories. That being said, many things can be optimized to maximize your results. You can turn virtually every diet into a muscle builder, including a keto diet (Matt did this), a vegan or vegetarian diet (Wade did this), paleo, and If It Fits Your Macros (IIFYM).

Both of us have bad genetics for bodybuilding. We're both ectomorphic, which forced us to truly figure out what works for us. Over multiple years of experimenting with thousands of different clients all over the world and getting their feedback, we created a powerful system for natural trainees to maximize muscle gains in a healthy way.

Wade's Muscle-Building Journey

At age 15, five feet six inches tall, and a skinny 130 pounds, I started training in my barn and got myself up to 176 pounds over four years by the time I left for college. Then, I started on the quest of getting as big as possible, following Arnold Schwarzenegger's *Encyclopedia of Bodybuilding* and training nine times a week.

I was very athletic and worked a manual-labor job, so I'd have to eat a total of 5,000 to 6,000 calories, broken into six meals a day. These included force-feedings at night where I would blend my shake at 2 A.M. (I still feel bad for waking up my roommate all these times). I ate every three to four hours to get above the 200-pound mark without drugs.

Eventually, I got up to 190 pounds on Dorian Yates's training, looking good without drugs. Then I started on anabolic drugs, which got me up to 230 pounds and looking like a Marvel superhero. Then I dieted down for the '98 Nationals to about 4 percent body fat at 196 pounds. You could see striations in my jawline when I ate.

Six weeks later, I was 230 pounds with veins in my abs. According to my coach, my liver enzymes and everything else were fine. He wanted me to take it to the next level and add GH and other stronger anabolics.

However, I had developed sleep apnea, edema, and skin breakouts, and was wondering, "Where is this all going?" I knew I didn't have the genetics to beat freaks like Ronnie Coleman and Dorian Yates, the world's best bodybuilders at the time.

So, I left. I stopped anabolic drugs in 1998 and never did them again. I decided to focus on natural bodybuilding. I stepped on stage at 176 and 183 pounds, and at single-digit body fat. I might not have been as ripped or full as I was before, but I also didn't sacrifice my life span and put up with the health consequences of drug-driven bodybuilding.

Matt's Story

I was 147 pounds and 16 years old, feeling small and weak when I saw a couple of bodybuilders at the beach (fortunately, they didn't kick sand in my face). I decided I wanted to look like they did and got bitten by the bodybuilding bug. I became totally obsessed and trained twice a day for three years. Every dollar I made went into bodybuilding magazines and supplements.

The first year, I was able to go from 147 to 175 pounds, most of it lean tissue, on a standard bodybuilding diet.

Then, I discovered the Anabolic Diet by Dr. Mauro DiPasquale, which took me from 175 to 235 pounds. I made a ton of mistakes on the way.

In the last six years, my goal has been to recomp. I now believe this is the best way to improve body composition. I've stayed at about the same weight over that time, losing three to eight pounds of body fat and gaining the same amount of weight in muscle, according to DEXA scans.

BENEFITS OF MUSCLE MASS

Lean muscle mass isn't just about looking good. It extends both your life span and health span.

Professor Claudio Gil Araújo followed the health of 3,878 people for 6.5 years. The participants in the weakest quartile had a risk of dying that was 10 to 13 times higher than that of those in the top third or fourth quartile. As you get older, the quality of your life becomes highly correlated with your lean muscle mass and strength.[1]

- Leg strength is what determines whether you avoid falling down easily, cross the street quickly, or go up and down stairs with ease
- Arm strength affects how you carry your groceries

Now let's discuss the impact of muscle mass on health span. At a certain point, people can become too weak to maintain good balance. Their bone density becomes compromised, which makes their bones prone to break.

As Matt witnessed firsthand, this can then be the beginning of the end. As he was growing up, Matt's grandfather, who lived with the family, got hit by a car. A couple of years later, he fell down and broke his hip. Once his mobility went downhill, so did his health. The last few years of his life were spent in agonizing pain. He was literally praying for death. It was very sad and traumatizing to witness this experience. If Matt's grandfather had lifted weights, he could have rebuilt his strength and possibly gained an extra decade of quality living.

The point is to recognize that lifting weights is a requirement for a superhuman health span.

Muscle is alive. It's metabolically active and burns energy. It also stabilizes your balance and helps you move in the world. It stores glucose, keeping your metabolism healthy by preventing blood-sugar-related problems. Here's what Dr. Gabrielle Lyons, who calls muscle "the organ of longevity," has to say about this:[2, 3]

> Muscle plays a central role in whole-body protein metabolism by serving as the principal reservoir for amino acids to maintain protein synthesis in vital tissues and organs in the absence of amino acid absorption from the gut and by providing hepatic gluconeogenic precursors. Furthermore, altered muscle metabolism plays a key role in the genesis, and therefore the prevention, of many common pathologic conditions and chronic diseases.

Your organs need amino acids for repair. It can get them from your muscle mass. There are massive blood sugar management benefits of lean muscle mass.

We could write an entire book on the health benefits of lean muscle mass. Hopefully, this short discussion was enough to sell you on it. For most people, it's not about bodybuilding. Not everyone wants to look like a superhero. Most people don't. However, virtually everyone looks better when they add 10 to 20 pounds of muscle. The Adonis ratios get amplified, and we're hardwired to find that more attractive.

The great news is that it doesn't matter how old you are; whether you're a man or woman, you can build muscle mass. Tons of research has been done with elderly people, and they can build muscle too—and gain strength.

The solution is simple. Resistance training combined with proper nutrition (which we cover in this chapter) will add decades to your health span and most likely improve your life span. Not to mention, muscle mass supports good posture and makes you look more athletic, younger, and more attractive.

The sweet spot for how much muscle mass is best for your life span and health span depends on your goals and genetics. To learn about your genetics, go to: www.BIOptimizers.com/book/genes.

While many nutritional strategies in this chapter apply to muscle maximization and the sport of bodybuilding, we are not advocating putting on as much muscle mass as humanly possible. You can likely maximize your muscle mass, but pushing past the optimal zone takes major trade-offs in time, effort, and health.

Most men benefit from gaining 20 to 40 pounds of muscle, whereas for women, it'd be 10 to 20 pounds. This is achievable in 12 to 24 months, depending on the level of your dedication and effort. These targets are achievable for someone untrained, and without using drugs.

METABOLIC BENEFITS OF MUSCLE

The metabolic benefits of muscle mass are huge. One is glucose disposal. Your muscles act like sponges for glucose. This means the more you build lean muscle, the more carbs your muscles can absorb. So, instead of turning the glucose into fat through gluconeogenesis, you can absorb a lot more of it. Extra lean muscle mass has a real anti-diabetic benefit.

Of course, as we outlined in Chapter 7, The Optimized Metabolism System, lean muscle mass is essential to healthy, lifelong weight loss. The caloric burn from your extra muscle tissue is one of the keys.

Activating Anabolism

To build muscle, your body must be anabolic. This means it's in a state of growth and repair. The enemy of anabolism is catabolism. Catabolism is when your body is in a state of breakdown. There's a constant balancing act between anabolism and catabolism. To activate muscle growth, we must tip the scales in favor of anabolism.

Here are some frameworks to help illustrate this:

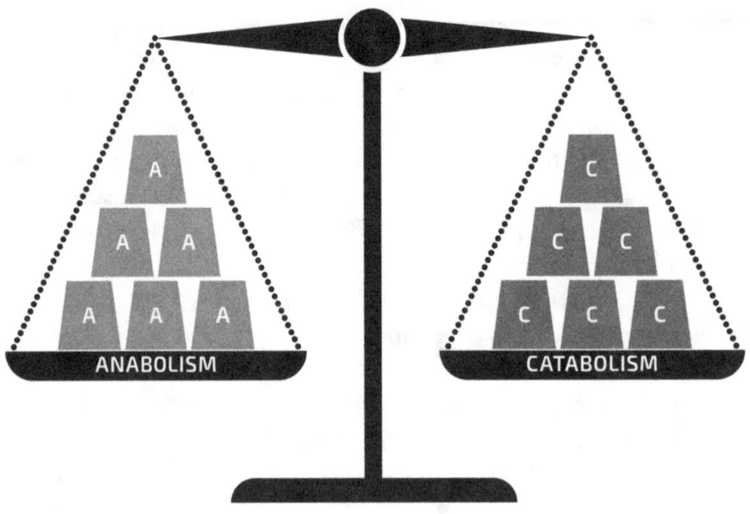

The first diagram illustrates homeostasis. This means your body is in balance; it's not anabolic or catabolic. The key point is that your body is always striving for homeostasis. It's the safest state to be in for survival.

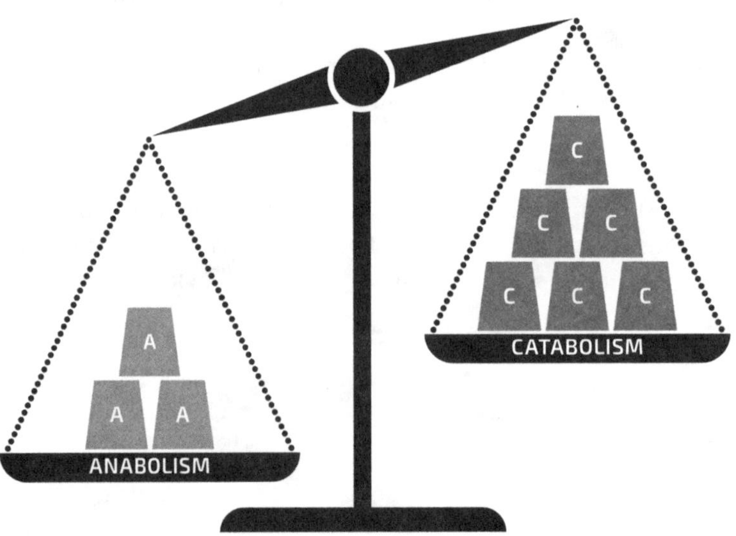

The second diagram is what catabolism looks like. There's an overload of catabolic activity, and it creates a breakdown of muscle. Some people are more genetically prone to be catabolic. Usually, they produce too much cortisol, which destroys muscles when it's elevated chronically.

The next diagram is the goal for muscle building. We want to maximize the anabolic factors and break homeostasis.

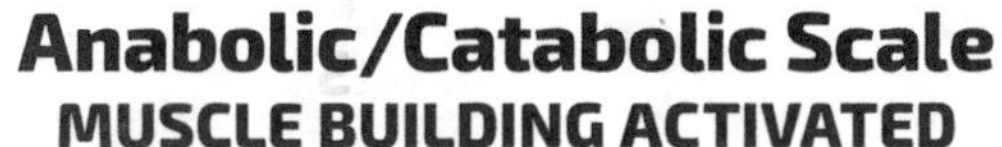

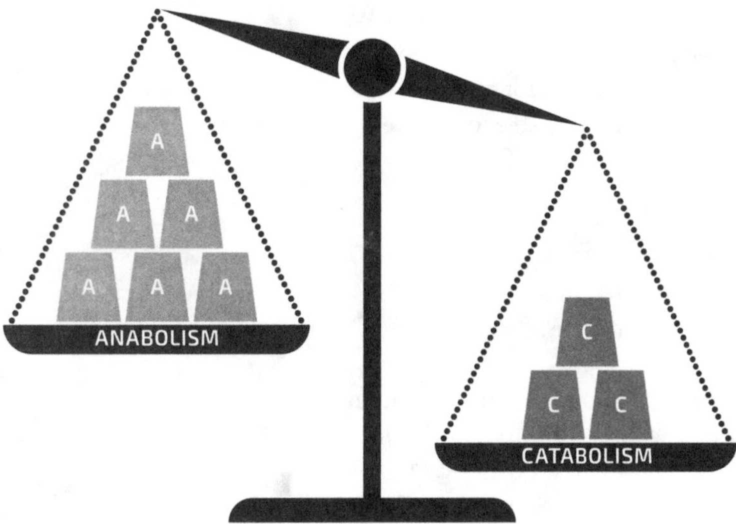

How do we tip the scales in our favor? The next diagram shows all of the major anabolic and catabolic components. The goal is to maximize the ones on the anabolic side and minimize the ones on the catabolic side. Make sure to check out the Supplements Guide www.BIOptimizers.com/book/resources to see all of the different ways you can give yourself the anabolic edge.

Anabolic/Catabolic Balance
COMPONENTS

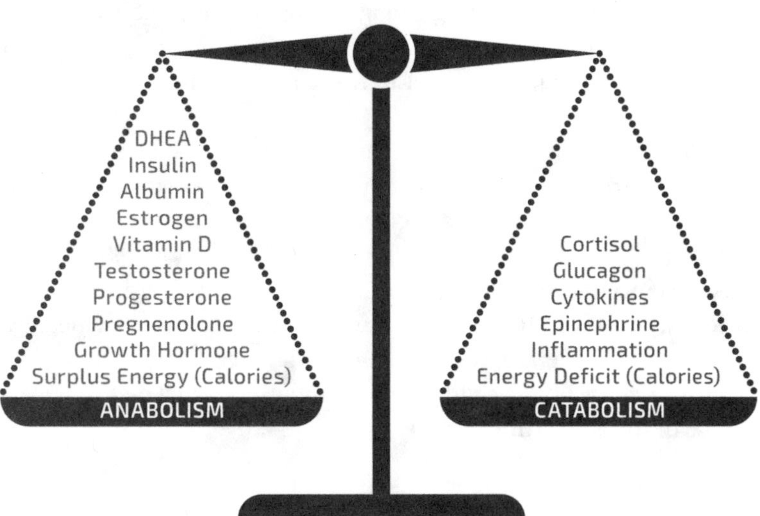

THE SEVEN BASIC TENETS OF BODYBUILDING NUTRITION

To best fuel yourself for building muscle, aim to optimize your:

1. Calorie levels: Over time, you must be in a slight calorie surplus.
2. Protein levels: Your protein dosage per day should be 1.6 to 2.2 g/kg (or 0.7 to 1 per pound) of bodyweight.
3. mTOR response: Consume 3 to 5 grams of leucine with each meal.
4. Meal frequency: Consume three to six meals a day.
5. Carb macros: This is for energy and calories.
6. Fat macros: This is for health and for calories.
7. Digestive system: You want to be able to handle your food intake.

Now let's dive into each one.

The Optimal Calorie Level for Muscle Building

There are massive differences in what number of calories is optimal for each of us. It depends on personal genetics. Here are some general starting guidelines:

1. Ectomorphs (naturally skinny people): 20 times bodyweight in pounds. For example, a 125-pound ectomorph might need 2,500 calories to be in a surplus.
2. Mesomorphs (people who easily gain muscle): 18 times bodyweight in pounds. For example, a 180-pound mesomorph would start with 3,600 calories.
3. Endomorphs (people who easily gain fat): 16 times bodyweight in pounds. A 200-pound endomorph would eat 3,600 calories.

Again, these are just starting points. You'll have to monitor the scale and body fat to make the proper adjustments.

The process is simple. If you're not gaining weight, you need to eat more calories. If you're gaining too much body fat, you need to lower your calories.

Muscle anabolism and protein takeover are metabolically expensive—building muscle requires a lot of calories. By some estimates, it takes 5,000 calories to synthesize a new pound of lean tissue.

The minimum effective calorie surplus seems to be about 300 to 500 calories a day. There's a key point that relates to reverse dieting as well. If people go above or below 150 to 200 calories, it doesn't break homeostasis. It's not enough to shift the body into muscle growth mode. We can use that to our advantage, or it can be a disadvantage. Remember, this is a moving target, though. As you gain muscle and bodyweight, your BMR will increase.

Some people (especially ectomorphs) have a metabolism that ramps up quickly with the increased calories and added lean muscle mass. So, the math changes. One client with whom Matt worked was a hardcore ectomorph.

The biggest challenge for an ectomorph is eating enough food. This client added 10 pounds of lean muscle mass quickly. However, he was eating 4,000 calories a day, and if he missed one meal, he would go catabolic and start losing lean muscle. If you're an ectomorph, the answer to this challenge is to maximize your digestive capabilities. We cover that later in the chapter.

If you're a mesomorph or endomorph, you must be very mindful of too many excess calories. There's no sense in mega-bulk cycles in which 50 percent of the weight gained is body fat. We made these mistakes so that you don't have to. Based on our personal results and those of our clients, we know now that it's completely unnecessary unless you want to be a sumo wrestler.

One study using elite resistance-training athletes examined the effects of different calorie surplus levels. The first group, with an average bodyweight of 165 pounds, ate energy ad libitum—this means they ate as much as they wanted without counting calories. On average, they ate 2,964 calories each day (which was a very small surplus).

The second group, with an average bodyweight of 156 pounds, received a diet in which participants consumed 600 more calories than those in the ad libitum group.[4]

Both groups did the same resistance training program over a period of 8 to 12 weeks. The researchers hypothesized that the 600 excess calorie group would have greater gains in bodyweight and lean body mass (LBM). Although the excess-calorie group achieved slightly better increases in LBM compared to those eating ad libitum, the difference failed to reach statistical significance (1.7 kg vs. 1.2 kg, respectively).

Here's the key difference. The excess-calorie group gained a lot more body fat than the other group, increasing their fat mass by 1.1 kg vs. 0.2 kg.[5] So, in our opinion, it's better to cut your fat gains by 80 percent even if it means you make slightly lower muscle gains. At the end of the chapter, we share a variety of strategies to help minimize fat gain while you're building lean muscle mass.

Optimize Protein for Muscle Building

Let's start with the bottom line, which is that you need protein for building muscle. Simply eat enough protein with every meal. As we've previously discussed, protein is the king macro.

As long as you're consuming around 0.7 grams per pound per day, you should be okay. If you're training hard five or six days a week, then you may have to increase it to 1 gram per pound per day.

Should you take a protein supplement? The answer is that you probably should. For most people, it's not easy to eat enough protein to hit their protein macros goals. This is where having a protein shake or two each day can easily solve the problem. That's why we built Protein Breakthrough. We have both plant-based and keto versions.

Is there a superior form of protein for building lean muscle? According to research, whey is the most anabolic. Why? Because it contains a high percentage of leucine. However, many people don't digest whey well, and if you're one of them, then taking a leucine supplement with your protein is an effective hack. For plant-based diets, pea protein has almost the same percentage of leucine as whey.

The BIOptimized Intra-Workout Amino Acid Shake

A high concentration of amino acids in the bloodstream during exercise significantly increases exercise-induced protein synthesis. Blood flow from the workout increases amino acid delivery to the muscles by 650 percent. The key is to predigest your protein. One of the best ways to do this is with the following mix:

- 1 scoop of your favorite protein (we recommend Protein Breakthrough)
- 1 cup of fruit or 1 banana
- ½ tsp of Himalayan salt
- 2 capsules of MassZymes
- 2 capsules of P3-OM

MassZymes and P3-OM break down protein into amino acids. The carbs help fuel your energy. The salt gives you electrolytes. This BIOptimized Intra-Workout Shake will help maximize your workout performance and your lean muscle gains. Take 1 to 2 grams of leucine before your workout to kick it up another level.

Optimize mTOR Response for Muscle Building

The amino acid leucine is a potent stimulator of mTORC1. Leucine has about a 10-fold greater impact on protein synthesis than any other amino acid. Mammalian target of rapamycin (mTOR) is the nutrient-sensing pathway that turns on anabolism with enough leucine and insulin signaling. Therefore, mTOR is one of the biggest anabolic levers.

You need to eat enough protein to have enough leucine. Because there is a threshold to activate mTOR (above 25 grams per meal for older adults), it's better to split your protein consumption into multiple meals rather than just consume it all in one big meal.[6] Overall, you want to get three to seven grams of leucine per meal so you stimulate muscle protein synthesis multiple times a day.

Nutrition expert and powerlifting champion Layne Norton gives a good analogy for how leucine works:

> Imagine a contractor building a new skyscraper. The contracting company is mTOR, the skyscraper is the protein you are trying to synthesize, the machines (bulldozers, cranes, etc.) you use to make the building are the protein synthesis pathway components, and leucine is the cash needed to make the project work.
>
> When enough cash is available (increasing leucine concentrations), not only can the contracting company start building the skyscraper (synthesizing muscle protein), it can also purchase more machines (increased synthetic components) to increase the capacity and speed at which it constructs the skyscraper (the muscle protein being synthesized).[7]

According to Dr. Donald K. Layman, formerly a protein researcher in the Department of Food Science and Human Nutrition at the University of Illinois, it takes about 2.5 grams of leucine to initiate protein synthesis. On the whole, this isn't much at all.[8]

Power Move: Eat Leucine-Rich Foods and Proteins (or Supplement It)

If your goal is to maximize muscle growth, then you should target at least 3 grams of leucine per meal. This is hard to achieve with natural foods. Protein powders make it easier. And leucine is an inexpensive supplement that can make hitting your targets very easy.

Food Leucine per 100 Grams

Food	Leucine	Food	Leucine
Whey protein	10 g	Pork chop	2.2 g
Pea protein	9 g	Chicken leg	2 g
Casein protein	8 g	Sesame seeds	1.3 g
Soy protein	8 g	Cottage cheese	1.27 g
Hemp protein	6.8 g	Canned navy beans	0.7 g
Pumpkin seed protein	6.3 g	Milk	0.3 g
Tuna	2.4 g		

Optimize Meal Frequency for Muscle Building

The bottom line is to do what works for you. There's no magic meal frequency, despite some of the old bodybuilding gospel.

That being said, to gain maximum muscle mass, more protein feedings per day are better than fewer.[9] In other words, three protein-based meals per day is better than two, four is better than three, and so on. Why? Because there's a limit to how much protein you can absorb from each meal. You just can't eat all your proteins in two meals and get the same effect as in six meals a day.

Should you eat six meals a day? We don't think it's necessary, unless you're trying to become a pro bodybuilder. Is there a big difference between four and six meals? It seems to be incremental. So, for lifestyle reasons, we usually recommend four meals a day if you're bodybuilding seriously.

Here's an excerpt from a research summary paper from Helms, Aragon, and Fitschen:

> Bodybuilders typically employ a higher meal frequency in an attempt to optimize fat loss and muscle preservation. However, the majority of chronic experimental studies have failed to show that different meal frequencies have different influences on bodyweight or body composition.[10]

Lifestyle and digestive speed are probably the biggest considerations with this variable. Some people prefer eating moderately sized meals five or six times a day, whereas others prefer three bigger meals. Some people don't have time to eat six times a day due to their hectic schedules.

Our opinion is that four times a day is probably the sweet spot for most people. It's an achievable, sustainable target. You get four opportunities for protein feeding and mTOR activation. If time is a challenge, use protein shakes. They take just a couple of minutes to make.

How fast you digest your food is another variable. Some digest faster and find themselves hungry soon after a meal. They can handle eating more frequently. Digestive enhancers like MassZymes, P3-OM, and HCL Breakthrough can make a big difference in optimizing your digestive speed (more on this in a minute).

Optimize Carbs for Muscle Building

In muscle building, carbs have three purposes:

1. Fueling tough workouts
2. Helping you achieve a calorie surplus
3. Supporting post-training recovery and anabolism

Looking at the research comparing keto vs. carbs, neither appears to have a significant advantage for building muscle. You can build muscle both ways. High-intensity sports is a different story. There is no denying that some people have much better high-intensity workouts on a carb-based diet (see more in Chapter 17). Wade is one of these. When he experimented with a ketogenic diet, his workout performance plummeted.

If you can burn fat and ketones, turning them into cellular energy (ATP), you'll produce a lot of ATP. However, this entire process is slow compared to burning glucose to get ATP. So, if you need a lot of ATP very fast, you'll need carbs.

This is why carbs are *king* for high-intensity performance.[11] Resistance training at 6 to 20 repetitions max takes carbs either from the bloodstream or from your liver and muscle glycogen stores.

As glycogen stores go down after an hour of intense training, your performance starts to drop. Correspondingly, you'll also enter a catabolic state just by running out of glycogen stores.[12] So, carbs are important for training performance, training adaptation, and recovery.

If you can train hard on low-carb diets, like Matt can, it's because your body has learned to produce glucose anew from fats, ketones, or amino acids to replenish your glycogen stores. Keep in mind that Matt still finds his workouts to be significantly better after carb-load days.

Carbs also increase insulin, which will help you get into the anabolic state, especially post workout.[13] By increasing your blood sugar, you'll stimulate insulin release. Generally, combining carbs with protein post workout at a two-to-one ratio triggers the most insulin release.[14] The post-workout carbs and proteins will help bring glucose and amino acids into your muscles.

What are the best sources of carbs for muscle building?

If you're looking to maximize calories, you'll want to consume faster-digesting carbs. White rice is probably the best source for doing this while minimizing digestive distress.

This is why bodybuilding legend Stan Efferding, who is known as the "World's Strongest Bodybuilder," chose it as the foundational carb source for his Vertical Diet plans. The Vertical Diet is an intelligently designed system that optimizes digestive health so people can maximize their calorie intake.

If you're looking for more of a moderate carb increase, then some of the best sources are complex carbs such as:

- Sweet potatoes
- Yams
- Oats
- Quinoa
- Potatoes

Optimize Fats for Muscle Building

The type of fats you eat can make an impact on your muscle-building results.

Supporting Testosterone Production

Studies show that diets low in saturated fats and high in polyunsaturated and monounsaturated fats lead to lower testosterone.[15] This is possibly because such diets reduce blood cholesterol, which provides a backbone for testosterone. The Leydig cells in men's testicles take cholesterol in your blood and turn it into testosterone.

In a study of 49 older men, higher dietary and serum cholesterol are associated with better responses to resistance training.[16]

If you're plant-based, you need to ensure that you're consuming enough saturated fat to support your testosterone levels. Wade finds that he needs some coconut oil to maintain his testosterone levels, even when he's dieting for a show.

Your muscle-building results will be enhanced when you increase your testosterone, insulin, growth hormone, and IGF-1. The free-testosterone-to-cortisol ratio is an indicator of physical strain, which can result from insufficient recovery.[17] Factors that may influence this number include:

- A diet too low in carbs or calories to fuel your workout, which can reduce testosterone relative to cortisol
- Your age, which also determines your capacity to recover from training
- Your sleep quality and quantity, which also determines your growth hormone levels

If you're doing everything right but don't seem to be getting the muscle gain results you want, it's a good idea to test these hormones and work to optimize them.

Supporting Training-Induced Inflammation and Exercise Response

Muscle building requires creating inflammation during your training and healing from it. The inflammation process requires a long-chain omega-6 fat called arachidonic acid, while the healing and anti-inflammatory process requires omega-3.[18, 19] Sensibly, omega-3 supplementation helps with soreness.[20]

A study was conducted on 31 resistance-trained men in which half were given arachidonic acid and the other half were given a placebo over a four-day resistance training regimen.

The study concluded that arachidonic acid supplementation during a resistance training regimen can enhance aerobic capacity and decrease inflammatory response. However, arachidonic acid didn't provide significantly larger gains in muscle mass or strength, or influence muscle hypertrophy. A good target dose is 1,500 mg taken 30 minutes before your workout.

High-cholesterol foods also tend to contain a lot of arachidonic acid, which may explain why eating a lot of cholesterol helps with muscle building.

How Much Fat to Eat on a Muscle-Building Diet

Our general approach is to rely on your biofeedback. Too little fat, and you may start to feel your testosterone, and hence your mood, motivation, and energy nosediving. Too much fat, and your workout quality may drop or you may start to gain some fat.

Start with a reasonable amount of fat—between 0.22 to 0.68 grams per pound of bodyweight per day.[21] For a 200-pound guy, that's between 44 and 136 grams.

In elderly men, at least 2 grams of omega-3 intake helps with muscle building and maintenance.[22] For younger adults, taking omega-3 improves strength and exercise recovery, and it reduces fat tissues more than directly increasing muscle mass.[23]

Fatty Foods to Eat on a Muscle-Building Diet

These animal fats are great sources of omega-3, dietary cholesterol, and arachidonic acid:

- Wild-caught salmon and other fatty fish (make sure they're not farmed and corn-fed)
- Fatty cuts of grass-fed steak
- Pasture-raised pork and their products
- Poultry
- Eggs
- Dairy (if tolerated), ideally pasture raised

Plant-based fats:

- Avocados
- Coconut and coconut products
- Nuts
- Olive oil
- Algae oil for DHA (crucial for vegans/vegetarians)

Fats to avoid on a bodybuilding diet:

- Trans fat
- Hydrogenated fats, including margarine and shortening
- Vegetable seed oils

Optimize Digestion for Muscle Building

Ben Pakulski shared with Matt once that the hardest part of high-level bodybuilding is eating all of this food. We've talked about ghrelin before in this book. When you start consuming massive amounts of food, your ghrelin levels become very low. You're not hungry. However, you must eat. This is harder than it sounds. You're essentially force-feeding yourself.

The first key is to eat foods that are easy on your gut. That's why we support Stan Efferding's Vertical Diet approach, where you identify a few healthy foods that you can digest easily.

Avoid high-FODMAP (fermentable oligosaccharides, disaccharides, monosaccharides, and polyols) foods and any that can cause bloating, gas, or digestive discomfort (such as broccoli, onions, and garlic). If you develop gas or digestive troubles from eating legumes or certain grains, then avoid these foods as well.

Another powerful tool is the BIOptimized Gut Health Test, which helps you identify foods that your gut biome digests easily and others that it struggles with based on your bacteria. Go to www.BIOptimizers.com/book/guthealth to do a gut health test, this will help you choose better foods for YOUR gut biome.

However, there is a solution if you have digestive trouble: massive amounts of MassZymes. We have a special protocol for hardcore bodybuilders and aspiring athletes who want to maximize recovery and gains.

MassZymes was designed to help optimize high-protein diets. Our advanced MassZymes protocol for maximum digestion is one capsule for every 100 to 200 calories. We've had clients on 10,000-calorie diets eat 100 capsules a day and see incredible results, including close to zero digestive distress.

To optimize your digestive powers even more, add P3-OM with each meal. P3-OM is a proteolytic probiotic that will help further break down protein into usable amino acids. We suggest three capsules with each meal, along with the MassZymes. The final piece of the ultimate digestive trio is HCL Breakthrough. We suggest using one to two capsules of that with each meal as well.

These three solutions combined are an absolute game changer for people trying to eat more food and maximize the value they get from it. In our opinion, you triple the value you get from your food with enough MassZymes. You can eliminate digestive discomfort and increase your digestive speed. This allows you to eat more throughout the day.

PREVENTING FAT GAIN DURING MUSCLE-BUILDING JOURNEYS

Back when we started bodybuilding, the approach was to do six-to-nine-month "mass building cycles" and gain a lot of body fat along with the muscle. Next, we would diet for three months. And then we'd repeat the process. We do not advise this. There is a better way.

Fat Gain Minimization Key #1: Go for the Minimum Effective Calorie Surplus

As a general rule, 300 to 500 calories above maintenance are a good starting point. If you just increase by 100 or 200 calories, your body can quickly achieve homeostasis, and you won't gain weight (you've already seen that this is how we reverse diet). Taking in those 500 calories seems to be enough to kick anabolism into gear.

The key is in the adjustments. Every day, weigh yourself first thing in the morning. Each week, if your weight hasn't increased by more than 0.5 pounds, then increase calories by 300 per day the following week.

Fat Gain Minimization Key #2: Reverse Calorie Cycling

This is kind of a reverse calorie-cycling strategy. When we're dieting, we can increase calories for one or two days to refeed the muscles and help slow down metabolic downregulation. Now, we're doing the reverse.

You're in a calorie surplus for five to six days a week. You will be gaining lean muscle during that time (assuming you're training correctly and following most of our suggestions).

A one- to two-day micro diet isn't going to kill your gains. We suggest going for a 500-to-1,500 calorie deficit on those days. This will help minimize fat gain. Your net weekly calorie surplus will be lower. You can do this on your off days if you wish. We cover these strategies in greater depth in Chapter 8, Advanced Cycling Strategies.

Our favorite way to implement this type of calorie cycling is to add fasting.

Incorporate Fasting

If you're an endomorph or mesomorph, we suggest adding one day of fasting (which ends up being around 30 to 36 hours) per week during your muscle-building phases. There are many advantages to building in these micro cycles instead of being in the same or increasing caloric surplus throughout your muscle gain program.

- Slow down your metabolism a notch

  When you're on a constant caloric surplus, your body adapts by wasting more energy as heat. It increases NEAT, exercise energy expenditure, and diet-induced thermogenesis. As a result, you'll need to eat even more to have the same number of calories available for muscle gain. This is especially true for skinny men and women who have high metabolism to begin with.

  Fasting can help counter this. When you fast, you dial down your metabolism a little bit. This makes it easier to get into a calorie surplus long term.

- Maximize fat loss during those days

  You'll get a tremendous bang for your buck in terms of calorie deficit during these one-day fasts because your metabolism is revved to the max from your high-calorie dieting and muscle building. These are massive calorie-loss days compared to those for someone who's been dieting for 12 weeks and whose body is adapted.

  The fasting also helps reset insulin and leptin sensitivity, making it easier for nutrients to get into your muscles.

- Reprieve from gorging and pushing through your hunger hormones

  Many bulking bodybuilders enjoy the temporary psychological reprieve from gorging as they go on diet breaks or even fasting days. Building up a bit of hunger again through fasting can be helpful.

- Enjoy the longevity benefits

  Although muscle mass is a determinant of longevity, most professional bodybuilders are neither healthy nor long-lived. We believe that anabolism should be cycled on and off for the best longevity results.

  Constantly pushing anabolism comes with health downsides because your biology is built to cycle between anabolic (mTOR and IGF) and autophagy pathways (sirtuins and AMPK).

  Too much anabolism can contribute to cellular aging, which makes your mitochondria less efficient. That can significantly increase oxidative stress, age-related inflammation, and cancer risk. To counteract the problem, you need to cycle in periods of autophagic pathway upregulations, such as with some caloric deficits and fasting.

  By upregulating your sirtuins, the number one anti-aging gene, you reduce your cellular age and age-related inflammation. You strengthen your mitochondria, boost cellular repair, and increase your exercise endurance.

Fat Gain Minimization Key #3: Ben Pakulski's "Two-Inch Rule"

Our friend and bodybuilding legend Ben Pakulski had a simple set of rules to prevent excess fat gain. Measure your waist, and when you've gained two inches, start dieting. Once you've lost the two inches, refocus on weight gain.

Depending on how well you execute everything, you may find yourself on a weight-gaining cycle for six to eight weeks and then dieting for two to four weeks. This will help keep you in good shape while you make progress.

The best way to monitor body fat is to use a DEXA scanner if you have one available in your area. As you track your results along with your macros and calories over time, you'll know exactly how to tweak your diet to maximize your muscle gains and minimize the fat gains. You become a master of your biology. You have control over your body's aesthetics. It's an incredibly powerful place to be.

Fat Gain Minimization Key #4: Maximize Your Anabolism

We aren't talking about using anabolic steroids. There are many things you can do as a natural trainee to maximize anabolism. This is truly the ultimate strategy. If you increase your anabolism enough, you can lose body fat and gain muscle simultaneously. We've experienced this and seen it many times with our clients.

Some of the best ways to maximize anabolism naturally are:

- Getting high-quality sleep, especially deep sleep
- Maximizing mTOR response to every meal with leucine
- Optimizing hormones

Power Move: Maximize Anabolism with the Sun

We've already noted that vitamin D is a prohormone produced phytochemically in the skin, and unlike traditional vitamins, vitamin D has its own hormone receptor (VDR).

We recommend you go outside for 15 to 20 minutes of sunscreen-free sun exposure three to four times a week.

Studies have found:

- The addition of vitamin D to insulin and leucine significantly enhances the activity of the mTOR pathway and protein synthesis.
- Vitamin D has the potential to directly alter protein synthesis in muscle cells. Additionally, several studies have found that low vitamin D is associated with low testosterone levels.
- Men with sufficient vitamin D levels have significantly higher testosterone levels and a lower sex hormone-binding globulin (SHBG) count than men with insufficient amounts of the vitamin (or hormone) in their blood serum.
- When healthy male participants take 3,332 IUs of vitamin D daily for a year, they end up having 25.2 percent more testosterone on average when compared to placebo.

Getting out in the sun may be more than just relaxing; it is anabolic for anyone who wants to build muscle. In our opinion, three to four sunbathing sessions a week activate a new level of anabolism for most people.

Fat Gain Minimization Key #5: Optimize Your Blood Sugar

Fasting blood glucose is an easy way to measure insulin sensitivity. We suggest tracking this daily to monitor your metabolic health. To keep track of it on a regular basis, you can use a simple glucometer or a continuous glucose-monitoring device. If your fasting blood glucose is creeping up, it's often a sign that you need to stop the muscle gain cycle and start fixing your insulin resistance first.

A good goal is to stay below 90. If your fasting blood glucose creeps above 100, we suggest taking measures. Options are:

- Incorporate Blood Sugar Breakthrough (two caps, 20 minutes before each meal with carbs)
- Walk 10 minutes after every meal
- Consider doing a two to three-week mini-diet

Blood Sugar Breakthrough makes a *big* difference in minimizing fat gains in a calorie surplus.

BODYBUILDING PITFALLS: HOW NOT TO BUILD YOUR MUSCLES

Every year, millions of men partake in the endeavor to look like Greek gods. Sadly, 90 percent of them stop going to the gym within three months.[24] Of the ones that remain, 97 percent of them fall back into their old habits and patterns, losing their results in under three years. Here are the most common mistakes we see.

1. Following Generic Internet Bodybuilding Advice or Programs for Pro Bodybuilders

Generic Internet bodybuilding advice—or, as seen in the '90s, books like Arnold Schwarzenegger's *Encyclopedia of Modern Bodybuilding*—is typically based on programs for ectomorph physique competitors. Such men may also have hours to train and can take the rest of their time to recover. This is their job. They're typically not the average guy with a family and a day job.

You should follow training programs that are tailored to your:

- Genetics
- Goals
- Training level
- Lifestyle

Some key suggestions are to:

- Change your workout every 12 weeks
- Add progressive challenges to every new workout plan
- Cycle your training volume

We're big fans of cycling from three sets per exercise to four and five sets, then cycling back down and repeating the process.

We suggest changing programs every three months, and they should get progressively harder with increases in training volume, exercises, and intensity. We offer highly effective training programs for free in our BIOptimized app.

2. Not Using Data as Feedback

Muscle building happens when all parameters are dialed in, so not tracking your results is a guaranteed way to fail. These parameters include nutrition, sleep, hormones, training, and more. It is, therefore, critical to track all of these, along with your progress in terms of muscle and fat gain (see Chapter 32, Data Shapes Destinies).

With our coaching clients, we help them monitor and adjust based on all of these metrics. We also teach them to listen to their bodies and speak up if something feels off.

Monitoring Results

We believe that DEXA, pictures, scale, and tape measurements are the best tools for progress monitoring. See our recommendations below.

- In general, the gold standard for body fat measurements is the DEXA.
- However, your muscles may improve in quality (shape and form), but the DEXA won't reveal that. That's why pictures are important. Fluctuations in hydration create big changes in lean body mass measured on the DEXA scan. This is why we suggest doing all scans at the same time of the day.
- On the other hand, the downside of pictures is that you may look worse from one week to another. Fluctuations in water retention or how "full" your muscles are with glycogen can make you look worse in a picture.
- If your weight is staying the same but the tape measurements of your waist and hips are changing, then you're probably recomping (losing body fat and gaining muscle).
- Weigh yourself daily, but have close to zero emotional attachment to the number. It's normal to fluctuate three to five pounds (sometimes more) based on water retention and intestinal bulk.

For optimal progress tracking:

- Get a DEXA scan monthly
- Take pictures monthly
- Take tape measurements weekly
- Weigh yourself daily

3. Not Accounting for Metabolic Adaptations

Weight gain and loss are all about calories in and calories out. While you have full control of calories in, calories out can be a moving target. So, you may have to increase calories over time to continue gaining lean muscle mass.

4. Not Optimizing Gut Health

If you start off with suboptimal gut health in the first place, it can be a major bottleneck for your bodybuilding efforts. Most people's biggest challenge is eating enough food to activate muscle growth.

In Chapter 31, we discuss food sensitivities and allergies, which can worsen your gut health and cause other symptoms. In addition, we also recommend digestive and gut biome support, including MassZymes, HCL, and P3-OM, to maximize your muscle gain results. Go to www.BIOptimizers.com /book/guthealth to do a gut health test. This will help you choose better foods for YOUR gut biome.

5. Not Training Hard Enough

If your nutrition is on point, your sleep is good, and you're not making steady gains, then the training is probably the problem.

Here are some simple training guidelines for maximizing muscle gains:

- Your first goal is to master exercise performance. The key is to connect your mind with your muscle in every exercise. Use 80 percent of the weight that you can lift, but make it harder by going slower. This will help you learn optimal form. You can maximize the weights once you've achieved a strong mind-to-muscle connection.
- Emphasize the negative portion of the rep (the eccentric phase). This means that you slow down the negative. It should take two to three seconds.
- Every set should be close to failure. This means that the last couple of reps should require significant strain. The last rep should be slow despite the fact that you're going as fast as you can. As you age, training to absolute failure is counterproductive. It's best to end the set when you're one or two reps away from failure.

Muscle-Building Supplements

- MassZymes can maximize protein digestion and help break down gut irritants.
- Gluten Guardian contains enzymes that can digest gluten and casein.
- HCL Breakthrough supports healthy HCl levels, which is important for protein digestion and healthy gut movement.
- P3-OM contains *Lactobacillus plantarum OM*, which produces proteolytic enzymes that can help you digest and better assimilate proteins.
- Protein Breakthrough is our great-tasting plant-based protein powder that can supplement your protein intake without the side effects of dairy proteins.
- Blood Sugar Breakthrough can help maintain insulin sensitivity, so you put more carbs and amino acids into your muscle cells.

SUMMARY

You can gain muscle on almost any diet, provided that you get enough protein and calories. You can turn virtually every diet into a muscle-builder.

Power Moves

Restorative sleep is one of the biggest ingredients of a successful muscle-building program. The best way to maximize your growth hormone, which is also important for your testosterone levels, is to optimize your sleep quality by doing the following:

- Block out blue light a few hours before bed with blue-light-blocking glasses.
- Sleep in total darkness by creating a pitch-black room. Use two layers of blackout curtains on your windows and cover all lights emitted from electronics in your rooms with black tape.
- Ensure that your sleep environment is cool, with air conditioning and a cooling pad on your bed.
- Use an organic memory-foam mattress that doesn't create pressure points.
- Sleep consistently and early.

We suggest using Sleep Breakthrough and Dream Optimizer to help you maximize the quality of your sleep which will help you maximize your muscle gains.

This chapter provides the best possible muscle-building nutrition advice. It's simple, straightforward, and highly effective. Just follow a good weight-lifting program along with the steps outlined below, and you will gain muscle.

Master the Keys to Minimize Fat Gain:

- Go for the minimum effective calorie surplus
- Reverse calorie cycling one to two days a week
- Follow Ben Pakulski's "two-inch rule"
- Maximize your anabolism
- Optimize your blood sugar
- Incorporate fasting
- Make sure you have four to six servings of protein a day (30 to 50 grams per meal)
- Use muscle optimization supplements
- Aim for a 300- to 500-calorie surplus
- Watch your body fat. Go for a calorie deficit one to two days a week. Do mini-diet cycles every few weeks.
- Try to do four to six resistance workouts a week
- Change your program every 12 weeks

CHAPTER 16

THE ULTIMATE MUSCLE-BUILDING MASTER PLAN

In this chapter, you will learn:

- The common differences in aesthetics that men want to achieve vs. what women want to achieve, and how much muscle to build based on each
- The importance of selecting a fitness role model
- How long it should take you to achieve your muscle-building goals based on your achievable and best possible gains
- The three main categories your aesthetics can be broken down into and what determines each
- Aesthetic ranges for men vs. women
- How much you need to train based on the goal you want to achieve
- The seven different phases you'll go through over the course of your muscle-building master plan
- The seven most important muscle-building nutrition tips
- What your future could look like after you complete your muscle-building master plan
- How to calculate a fat-free mass index and why it's important
- The various muscle mastery training systems you will use throughout each phase of your muscle-building master plan

This is another hyper-practical chapter. However, before we begin, we want to emphasize more vital facts about the value of lean muscle.

HOW MUCH MUSCLE SHOULD I BUILD?

If we had a Bitcoin for every time someone said, "I'm worried about weight lifting. What if I get too big?" we would be billionaires. The short answer is that you won't. Very few people have the genetics to get "too big." Researchers have found there are about 13 genes (and probably many more undiscovered ones) that affect how people respond to exercise.[1]

We estimate that around 1 to 2 percent of the population can easily build muscle mass. As we noted before, they are called mesomorphs. About 5 to 10 percent struggle to build muscle; they're ectomorphs. The majority are somewhere in the middle. Something else worth noting is that you can epigenetically push your body toward one or another body type with exercise and proper nutrition.

The other reason you don't need to worry about getting too big is that you can easily stop building muscle and simply maintain where you are. Just lower your calories a little bit to maintenance, and do three moderate weight-lifting workouts a week. You can maintain your gains without adding more lean muscle mass.

Aesthetics are a personal thing. Some people want to look like Brad Pitt in *Fight Club*. Some want to look like Chris Hemsworth in *Thor*. And some just want to look fit.

Regardless of whether they're women or men, or how old they are, virtually everyone would benefit from adding 10 to 15 pounds of lean muscle mass.

For men:

- If you want to look fit, then you should aim for 15 to 25 pounds of lean muscle.
- If you want to look muscular, then 25 to 40 pounds or more will usually get you there.
- If you want to look like a bodybuilder, you usually need an extra 40 pounds or more.
- These numbers will fluctuate based on your starting point.

For women:

- If you want to look fit, then you should aim for 10 to 15 pounds of lean muscle.
- If you want to look muscular, then 15 to 25 pounds will usually get you there.
- If you want to look like a bodybuilder, you usually need around 25 pounds or more.
- These numbers will fluctuate based on your starting point.

SELECT YOUR ROLE MODEL

If you're struggling with motivation to lift weights, we suggest finding an inspiring role model. When Wade was a hardcore bodybuilder, Arnold was his role model. Now that he's a bit older, Wade looks up to legends like Bill Pearl. Matt loved Tom Platz's freaky legs when he started. Now he loves physiques like Greg Plitt's in his prime (RIP, brother).

Find inspiring figures in your age category that you can relate to and aspire to look like. Challenge what you think is possible to achieve. Put your favorite picture of them on your walls and fridge. The constant reminder of your ultimate ideal will inspire you to stay on track. It's a powerful technique that keeps you focused.

HOW LONG WILL IT TAKE TO ACHIEVE MY MUSCLE-BUILDING GOALS?

The short answer is that it depends on your commitment level. If you do the majority of things correctly, you can achieve your goals relatively quickly.

Here's a table that can help you choose some achievable targets:

	Achievable Gains	Best Possible Gains
Year 1	10–15 pounds	25–50 pounds
Year 2	5–10 pounds	10–20 pounds
Year 3 and beyond	3–5 pounds	6–12 pounds

What makes the difference between "achievable gains" and "best possible gains" are your:

- Genetics
- Commitment level with exercise; are you training three times a week, or six?
- Commitment level with nutrition; are you eating enough to be anabolic?
- Age; people in their teens and twenties tend to respond better due to hormone levels.
- Anabolic environment; sleep quality, sun, and supplementation are the big difference-makers. See the complimentary Ultimate Supplement Guide for more insights: www.BIOptimizers.com/book/resources.

WHAT DETERMINES MY AESTHETICS?

Let's discuss the art of bodybuilding. Back in the 1980s, Vince Gironda calculated the body part and weight-to-height ratios for every single Mr. America and Mr. Universe winner in the world. What he found is that the development of their muscle tissues worked off the Adonis ratio, which was also used in Greek statues. It seems to be hardwired into our minds: the majority of the world is unconsciously attracted to those proportions.

For men, it's a 1.68 to 1 shoulder-to-waist ratio. This means the shoulders are 1.68 times wider than the waist. This is the primary measurement for the Adonis ratio, but it includes many other body-part calculations.

For women, it's primarily about waist-to-hip ratio. The great news is, by adding lean muscle mass, you can certainly dramatically improve yours. To do this, follow training programs with a lot of deadlifts, squats, lunges, and other glute and leg exercises.

What affects your look can be broken down into the following factors:

1. Bone structure
   a. Some men have wide shoulders
   b. Some women have wide hips
   c. Some people have bigger or smaller bones
2. Muscles
   a. How much muscle do you have?
   b. How is the muscle mass dispersed?
   c. Where are your muscle insertions?
3. Body fat level
   a. The leaner you are, the more muscle definition you have.

Fat-Free Mass Index (FFMI)

Here are the various health ranges for body fat and FFMI. To calculate it, take your fat-free lean body mass and divide by your height in inches.

Aesthetic Ranges for Men

Range	Body Fat Levels	Fat-Free Mass Index
Unhealthy Danger Zone	35%+	Below 14
Unhealthy	25–34%	15–17
Average/Healthy	18–25%	18–19
Optimal/Athletic	8–18%	20–27
Maximization Zone (Danger)	7% or less	Over 28

Some notes on this chart:

- Past a FFMI of 27, you're entering the maximization zone, and it will almost certainly require steroids, testosterone, and other enhancers.2
- Body fat percentage-wise, less is better up to a point. Below 8 percent, the body will go into starvation self-defense mode unless you're a genetic freak.
- Every person has an optimal body fat range depending on their genetics and life history. The body has a set point. When you try to push the body past that point, expect the body to start fighting back. This can create severe metabolic damage and other health problems. For some men that will be 18 percent and for others it will be 9 percent.

Aesthetic Ranges for Women

Women Range	Body Fat Levels	Fat-Free Mass Index
Unhealthy Danger Zone	40%+	Below 11
Unhealthy	30–39%	12–14
Average/Healthy	23–29%	15–17
Optimal/Athletic	11–22%	18–22
Maximization Zone (Danger)	10% or less	Over 23

Some key points on this chart:

- This chart was created by examining the stats of fitness competitors as well as female pro bodybuilders.
- Past 23 FFMI, you're entering the Maximization Zone and it will almost certainly require steroids, testosterone, and other enhancers.
- Just like men, women have an optimal body fat range depending on their genetics and life history. For some women, that will be 11 percent and for others it will be 22 percent.
- Body fat percentage wise, less is better up to a point. Women need a higher percentage of body fat than men. For most women, body fat levels below 10 percent can lead to health problems unless they're genetic freaks. This can lead to a host of serious health issues including hormonal problems and metabolic damage.

HOW MUCH DO I NEED TO TRAIN?

If the goal is just health, longevity, and BioSpan, the minimum effective dose is three 20-minute workouts a week (assuming they're effective). A challenging 20 minutes of weight lifting is going to produce significant results, especially starting from zero.

If your goal is to build significant lean muscle, then between four and five times a week is optimal. If somebody is driven to build as much muscle mass as possible, then 6 to 12 times a week might be needed to maximize their potential.

Matt trained 12 times a week for three years and made incredible progress. He went from 147 to 235 pounds without any drugs or steroids. But to do this, your lifestyle becomes bodybuilding. You're waking up early in the morning. You train, shower, eat, work. Train again in the evening. Shower, eat, and sleep. It's a major commitment, and this is what most professional athletes do.

Important caveat: the more you train, the smarter you have to be about recovery and workout programming. You can definitely overtrain at 12 times a week. So be mindful of that.

TONY'S MASTER PLAN

For our Master Plan example, we're going to use Tony, who wants to build 20 pounds of muscle in the next year and get his body fat below 12 percent. Again, if your goal is only to build 10 pounds of muscle, then it will take you less time. If you want to build more than 20 pounds, it will take you more time.

Tony's Starting Stats:

Weight: 160 pounds
Body Fat: 15 percent
Lean Body Mass (LBM): 136 pounds
Fat Mass: 24 pounds

Tony should be able to add about 20 pounds of LBM the first year. His best gains will come in the first six months due to the intense adaptation response his body will have.

Tony's Diet Strategy

Our goal is to have around a 300- to 400-calorie surplus six days per week, and then one day of calorie deficit. This should keep Tony's body fat percentage in check while he adds lean muscle mass.

MON	TUES	WED	THURS	FRI	SAT	SUN
+400 surplus	+400 surplus	+400 surplus	+400 surplus	+400 surplus	+400 surplus	-1,500 deficit
Muscle building	Muscle building	Muscle building	Muscle building	Muscle building	Muscle building	Fat loss

We'll use an IIFYM strategy and aim for about 35 percent carbs, 40 percent protein, and 25 percent fat. For meal frequency, we're shooting for four feedings a day: three meals and one protein shake.

Phase 1: 8 Weeks

Goal: Gain 5 pounds of muscle
Fat Mass Gained: 1 pound
Weight: 166 pounds
Body Fat: 15 percent
LBM: 141 pounds
Fat Mass: 25 pounds
Notes: Tony is going to make his best gains in the first few months. He's going to do two different workouts and repeat them twice a week, for a total of four. He'll do three sets per exercise. His target rep range is 8 to 12 per set.

We're estimating Tony's caloric maintenance levels with exercise at around 2,500 a day. We'll target 2,900 calories a day for six days a week, with one at a 1,500-calorie deficit. The net weekly calorie surplus from this strategy is 900 a week, which is minimal. Tony might gain an extra pound of fat each month. We'll do a four-week dieting phase every six months to reduce that. By using these calorie-cycling strategies, Tony can reach his muscle goals with minimal body fat gains.

Visit www.BIOptimizers.com/book/resources to get our $300 Muscle Mastery Training System for FREE.

	MON	TUES	WED	THURS	FRI	SAT	SUN
Calories Burned	2,500	2,500	2,500	2,500	2,500	2,500	2,500
Calories Consumed	2,900	2,900	2,900	2,900	2,900	2,900	1,000
Energy Balance	+400	+400	+400	+400	+400	+400	-1,500
Exercise	1A workout	1B workout	30 min walk	1A workout	1B workout	30 min walk	Day off

Muscle Mastery Training

This book isn't really a training book; however, no muscle-building master plan would be complete without a proper exercise routine. We've included routines from our natural bodybuilding system called Muscle Mastery. It was a $300 system that yielded mind-blowing results for anyone who followed it.

Muscle Mastery Training System 1A: Chest, Shoulders, Back, and Abs

Day 1: Reps 10–12
Day 4: Reps 10–12
Sets: 3

	Set 1	Set 2	Set 3
Exercise	**Reps**	**Reps**	**Reps**
Incline Barbell Press			
Seated Side Laterals			
Flat Bench Press			
Bent Over Laterals			
Dumbbell Flyes			
Bent Over Db Rows			
Upright Row			
Pulldown to Front			
Standing Shoulder Press			
Abdominal Exercise 1			
Abdominal Exercise 2			
Abdominal Exercise 3			
Hyper Extensions			
Seated Calf Raise			

Muscle Mastery Training System 1B: Legs and Arms

Day 2: Reps 10–12
Day 5: Reps 10–12
Sets: 3

	Set 1	Set 2	Set 3
Exercise	**Reps**	**Reps**	**Reps**
Leg Extensions			
Lying Leg Curls			
Leg Press			
Toe Press			
Triceps Pressdowns			
Seated Incline Db curls			
Lying Triceps Extensions			
Close Grip E-Z Bar Curls			
Dips			
Hammer Curls			
Wrist Curls			
Reverse Wrist Curls			

Phase 2: 8 Weeks (weeks 9 to 16)

Goal: Gain 4 pounds of muscle this phase
Total LBM gained: 9 pounds
Fat mass (FM) gained this phase: 1 pound
Total FM gained: 2 pounds
Weight: 171 pounds
Body fat: 15.2 percent
LBM: 145 pounds
Fat mass: 26 pounds

Notes: Tony will continue making rapid gains. One important note is that his metabolism will increase for two reasons. First, he's eating a surplus of calories. Second, he's gaining muscle. We'll change the routine and increase his sets to four per exercise.

	MON	TUES	WED	THURS	FRI	SAT	SUN
Calories Burned	2,600	2,600	2,600	2,600	2,600	2,600	2,600
Calories Consumed	3,000	3,000	3,000	3,000	3,000	3,000	1,000
Energy Balance	+400	+400	+400	+400	+400	+400	-1,600
Exercise	2A workout	2B workout	30 min walk	2A workout	2B workout	30 min walk	Day off

Muscle Mastery Training System 2A: Chest, Shoulders, Back, and Abs

Day 1: Reps 8–10
Day 4: Reps 8–10
Sets: 4

	Set 1	Set 2	Set 3	Set 4
Exercise	**Reps**	**Reps**	**Reps**	**Reps**
Flat Bench Press				
Rear Deltoid Machine				
Incline Db Press				
Wide Grip Upright Rows				
Dips				
Pulldown to Front				
One Arm Cable Side Laterals				
Bent Over Barbell Rows				
Alternate Db Front Raise				
Behind the Head Pulldowns				
Abdominals Exercise 1				
Abdominals Exercise 2				
Abdominals Exercise 3				
Hyperextensions				

Muscle Mastery Training System 2B: Legs and Arms

Day 2: Reps 8–10
Day 5: Reps 8–10
Sets: 4

	Set 1	Set 2	Set 3	Set 4
Exercise	**Reps**	**Reps**	**Reps**	**Reps**
Front Squats				
Seated Leg Curls				
Lunges				
Standing Calf Raises				
Incline Triceps Extensions				
Incline Alternate Db Curls				
Lying Triceps Extensions				
E-Z Bar or Barbell Curls				
Triceps Machine Extensions				
Preacher Curls with Barbell or DB				
Low Bar Triceps Dips				
Cable Curls				
Wrist Curls on Bench				
Reverse Wrist Curls on Bench				

Phase 3: 9 Weeks (weeks 17 to 26)

Goal: Gain 3 pounds of muscle this phase
Total LBM gained: 15 pounds
FM gained this phase: 1 pound
Total FM gained: 3 pounds
Weight: 175 pounds
Body fat: 15.4 percent
LBM: 148 pounds
Fat mass: 27 pounds

Notes: We continue to slowly increase Tony's calories to keep up with his increasing metabolism. And with this training cycle, we'll do one of our favorite strategies: ramping up training volume and then taking it down again. When you ramp up volume, each additional set creates additional stress and thus adaptation. Then you ramp down to give the body a rest and start over. We repeat this process three times.

We'll also change the rep ranges more—to alternate higher and lower rep ranges with each workout. We believe this also creates new stresses and adaptations. We also increase the number of exercises per workout. It's important to keep adding the appropriate amount of stress as time goes on.

	MON	TUES	WED	THURS	FRI	SAT	SUN
Calories Burned	2,700	2,700	2,700	2,700	2,700	2,700	2,700
Calories Consumed	3,100	3,100	3,100	3,100	3,100	3,100	1,000
Energy Balance	+400	+400	+400	+400	+400	+400	-1,600
Exercise	3A workout	3B workout	30 min walk	3A workout	3B workout	30 min walk	Day off
Rep Range	13–15	13–15		6–8	6–8		

Training Volume:

Week 1: 3 sets
Week 2: 4 sets
Week 3: 5 sets
Week 4: 3 sets
Week 5: 4 sets
Week 6: 5 sets
Week 7: 3 sets
Week 8: 4 sets
Week 9: 5 sets

Muscle Mastery Training System 3A: Chest, Shoulders, Back, and Abs

Day 1: Reps 13–15
Day 4: Reps 6–8
Sets: 3–5

	Set 1	Set 2	Set 3	Set 4	Set 5
Exercise	Reps	Reps	Reps	Reps	Reps
DB Incline Press					
One Arm Side Lateral Cable					
DB Flyes					
Bent Over Barbell Rows					
Dips or Decline Bench Press					
Wide Grip Upright Row					
Alternate Db Press (standing)					
Close Grip Pulldown to Front					
Side Laterals (machine or DB)					
One Arm DB Rows					
Abdominals Exercise 1					
Abdominals Exercise 2					
Abdominals Exercise 3					
Hyperextensions					

Muscle Mastery Training System 3B: Shoulders and Arms

Day 1: Reps 13–15
Day 4: Reps 6–8
Sets: 3–5

	Set 1	Set 2	Set 3	Set 4	Set 5
Exercise	**Reps**	**Reps**	**Reps**	**Reps**	**Reps**
Leg Press					
Lying Leg Curls					
Squats (Smith Machine)					
Leg Curls					
Triceps Pressdowns					
Standing Alternate Db Curls					
Incline Tricep Extensions					
One Arm Preacher Curls					
Overhead Rope Extensions					
Machine Preacher Curls					
Dips (Bench or Regular)					
Cable Curls					
Wrist Curls					
Standing One Legged Calf Raise					

Phase 4: 4 Weeks (weeks 27 to 30)

Goal: Lose 4 pounds of fat this phase and 1 of lean muscle
Total LBM gained: 14 pounds
FM gained this phase: -4 pounds
Total FM gained: -1 pounds
Weight: 170 pounds
Body fat: 13.5 percent
LBM: 147 pounds
Fat mass: 23 pounds

Notes: There's a major shift happening this phase. We're doing a fat loss cycle to help lower Tony's body fat. He'll have an aggressive calorie deficit for four weeks with the intent of losing five pounds total. Tony will lose a little bit of muscle, but as long as it's 25 percent or less of the total weight, it's acceptable.

Not only will we eliminate all the extra fat he gained, but he'll go below what he started with in terms of total fat mass. He'll be leaner than when he started, with an extra 11 pounds of muscle. One key point: Going from 15 to 13.5 percent is a significant shift in visual aesthetics. When you get below 15, every percentage point makes a big impact on "the look."

Our goal is to keep lowering Tony's body fat level as he adds lean muscle mass. We can do that with cycling strategies such as these, where we:

- Increase Tony's reps on the early workouts to 15 to 20. Higher rep ranges like these are superior for improving mitochondria, which is one of the ways we can increase overall calorie burn.
- We also ramp up his cardio to 60 minutes on non-weight-lifting days.
- We're ramping up volume to five sets per exercise. This will be a challenging phase for Tony, but he's ready.

	MON	TUES	WED	THURS	FRI	SAT	SUN
Calories Burned	2,800	2,800	2,800	2,800	2,800	2,800	2,700
Calories Consumed	2000	2000	2000	2000	2000	2000	3,100
Energy Balance	-800	-800	-800	-800	-800	-800	+400
Exercise	4A workout	4B workout	60 min walk	4A workout	4B workout	60 min walk	Day off
Rep Range	15–20	15–20		8–10	8–10		

Muscle Mastery Training System 4A: Chest, Shoulders, Back, and Abs

Day 1: Reps 15–20
Day 4: Reps 8–10
Sets: 5

	Set 1	Set 2	Set 3	Set 4	Set 5
Exercise	**Reps**	**Reps**	**Reps**	**Reps**	**Reps**
Db Flat Bench Press					
Seated Side Lateral Machine					
Incline Db Flyes					
Supported Bent Over Rows					
Decline Bench Press or Flyes					
Wide Grip Upright Row					
Front Cable Raise, 2 Arms					
Reverse Grip Pulldowns to Front					
One Arm Bent Over Cable Lateral					
T-Bar Rows					
Abdominals Exercise 1					
Abdominals Exercise 2					
Abdominals Exercise 3					
Reverse Hyperextensions					

Muscle Mastery Training System 4B: Legs and Arms

Day 2: Reps 15–20
Day 5: Reps 8–10
Sets: 5

	Set 1	Set 2	Set 3	Set 4	Set 5
Exercise	Reps	Reps	Reps	Reps	Reps
Hack Squats					
Single Leg Curls					
Leg Extensions					
Seated Leg Curls					
Decline Triceps Extensions					
Standing Alternate Db Curls					
Incline Triceps Extensions					
Concentration Curls Db					
Low Bar Triceps Dips					
Cable Curls					
One Arm Triceps Pressdown					
Alternate Hammer Curls					
Reverse Wrist Curls					
Donkey Calf Raises					

Phase 5: 12 Weeks (weeks 31 to 42)

Goal: Gain 3 pounds of lean muscle
Total LBM gained: 17 pounds
FM gained this phase: +1 pound
Total FM gained: 0 pounds
Weight: 174 pounds
Body fat: 13.7 percent
LBM: 150 pounds
Fat mass: 24 pounds

Notes: Metabolism will be a little bit down after that aggressive mini weight loss cut. The big changes this phase are as follows:

- Increasing from four workouts a week to five
- 12-week vs. an 8-week phase (or less)

Both of our coaches, Scott Abel and Kevin Weiss, are big advocates of 12- to 16-week workouts. Doing the same program for 12 to 16 weeks can really create great gains. We have noticed that as well in our own routines.

	MON	TUES	WED	THURS	FRI	SAT	SUN
Calories Burned	2,700	2,700	2,700	2,700	2,700	2,700	2,700
Calories Consumed	3,100	3,100	3,100	3,100	3,100	3,100	1,000
Energy Balance	+400	+400	+400	+400	+400	+400	-1,600
Exercise	5A workout	5B workout	30 min walk	5A workout	5B workout	5C workout	Day off
Rep Range	13–15	13–15		8–10	8–10	6–8	

Training Volume:

Week 1: 3 sets
Week 2: 4 sets
Week 3: 5 sets
Week 4: 3 sets
Week 5: 4 sets
Week 6: 5 sets
Week 7: 3 sets
Week 8: 4 sets
Week 9: 5 sets
Week 10: 3 sets
Week 11: 4 sets
Week 12: 5 sets

Muscle Mastery Training System 5A: Chest, Shoulders, Back, and Abs

Day 1: Reps 13–15
Day 4: Reps 8–10
Sets: 3–5

	Set 1	Set 2	Set 3	Set 4	Set 5
Exercise	Reps	Reps	Reps	Reps	Reps
Incline Barbell Press					
Seated Side Laterals					
Decline Db Presses or Flyes					
Rear Deltoid Machine					
Pec Deck Flyes					
Close Grip Pulldowns					
Upright Row					
Straight Arm Pulldown					
Standing Calf Raise					
Hyperextensions					
Abdominal Exercise 1					
Abdominal Exercise 2					
Abdominal Exercise 3					

Muscle Mastery Training System 5B: Legs and Arms

Day 2: Reps 13–15
Day 5: Reps 8–10
Sets: 3–5

	Set 1	Set 2	Set 3	Set 4	Set 5
Exercise	**Reps**	**Reps**	**Reps**	**Reps**	**Reps**
Triceps Pressdown					
Standing Db Curls					
Incline Triceps Extensions					
Incline Db Curls					
Overhead Triceps (elbows on bench)					
E-Z Bar or Barbell Curls					
Leg Extensions					
Jump Squats					
Lying Leg Curls					
Db Stiff Legged Deadlifts on Bench					

Muscle Mastery Training System 5C: Legs and Arms

Day 6
Sets: 3–5
Reps: 6–8

	Set 1	Set 2	Set 3	Set 4	Set 5
Exercise	Reps	Reps	Reps	Reps	Reps
Clean and Press					
Seated Calf Raise					
Power Deadlift					
Pec Deck Flyes or Db Flyes					
Leg Extensions					
Barbell Curls					
Lying Leg Curls					
Dips					

Phase 6: 12 Weeks (weeks 43 to 54)

Goal: Gain 3 pounds of lean muscle
Total LBM gained: 20 pounds
FM gained this phase: +1 pound
Total FM gained: 1 pound
Weight: 178 pounds
Body fat: 14 percent
LBM: 153 pounds
Fat mass: 25 pounds
Notes: The big changes this phase are the following:

- We're continuing with a structure similar to the last program.
- This is Tony's *last* muscle-building phase to achieve his goal.

	MON	TUES	WED	THURS	FRI	SAT	SUN
Calories Burned	2,800	2,800	2,800	2,800	2,800	2,800	2,800
Calories Consumed	3,200	3,200	3,200	3,200	3,200	3,200	1,000
Energy Balance	+400	+400	+400	+400	+400	+400	-1,600
Exercise	6A workout	6B workout	30 min walk	6A workout	6B workout	6C workout	Day off
Rep Range	13-15	13-15		8-10	8-10	6-8	

Training Volume:

Week 1: 3 sets
Week 2: 4 sets
Week 3: 5 sets
Week 4: 3 sets
Week 5: 4 sets
Week 6: 5 sets
Week 7: 3 sets
Week 8: 4 sets
Week 9: 5 sets
Week 10: 3 sets
Week 11: 4 sets
Week 12: 5 sets

Muscle Mastery Training System 6A: Chest, Shoulders, Back, and Abs

Day 1: Reps 13–15
Day 4: Reps 10–12
Sets: 3–5

	Set 1	Set 2	Set 3	Set 4	Set 5
Exercise	**Reps**	**Reps**	**Reps**	**Reps**	**Reps**
Incline Db Press					
One Arm Db Side Lateral Standing					
Flat Bench Flyes					
Reverse Cable Crossover					
Seated Machine Bench Press					
Reverse Grip Pulldowns					
Alternate Standing Db Press					
Seated Cable Rows					
Seated Calf Raise					
Reverse Hyperextensions					
Abdominal Exercise 1					
Abdominal Exercise 2					
Abdominal Exercise 3					

Muscle Mastery Training System 6B: Legs and Arms

Day 1: Reps 13–15
Day 4: Reps 10–12
Sets: 3–5

	Set 1	Set 2	Set 3	Set 4	Set 5
Exercise	**Reps**	**Reps**	**Reps**	**Reps**	**Reps**
Lying Db Extensions					
Seated Db Curls					
Low Pulley Triceps Extensions					
Db Preacher Curls					
Triceps Pressdowns					
Alternate Hammer Curls					
Leg Press					
Frog Jumps					
Seated Leg Curls					
Db Lunges					

Muscle Mastery Training System 6C: Legs and Arms

Day 6: Reps 6–8
Sets: 3–5

	Set 1	Set 2	Set 3	Set 4	Set 5
Exercise	**Reps**	**Reps**	**Reps**	**Reps**	**Reps**
Db Clean and Press					
Donkey Calf Raises					
Deadlift or Power Deadlift					
Db Pullovers					
Jump Squats					
Standing Hammer curls					
Seated Leg Curls					
Dips					

Phase 7 (Fat Loss): 6 Weeks (weeks 55 to 60)

Goal: Lose 6 pounds of body fat + 1 pound of muscle
Total LBM gained: 19 pounds
FM gained this phase: -6 pounds
Total FM gained: -5 pounds
Weight: 171 pounds
Body fat: 11.1 percent
LBM: 152 pounds
Fat mass: 19 pounds

Notes: This is the final fat loss cycle for Tony. He'll be below 12 percent body fat and look like a totally different guy. The visual difference between 14 and 11.1 percent is night and day. After this, he'll shift to a maintenance program, which we discuss in a minute.

- Five weight-lifting workouts a week
- Two 60-minute walks a week
- We'll alternate between four-set and five-set weeks

	MON	TUES	WED	THURS	FRI	SAT	SUN
Calories Burned	2,800	2,800	2,800	2,800	2,800	2,800	2,700
Calories Consumed	2,000	2,000	2,000	2,000	2,000	2,000	3,100
Energy Balance	-800	-800	-800	-800	-800	-800	+400
Exercise	7A workout	7B workout	60 min walk	7A workout	7B workout	7C workout	60 min walk
Rep Range	15–20	15–20		8–10	8–10	6–8	

Training Volume:

Week 1: 4 sets
Week 2: 5 sets
Week 3: 4 sets
Week 4: 5 sets
Week 5: 4 sets
Week 6: 5 sets

Muscle Mastery Training System 7A: Chest, Shoulders, Back, and Abs

Day 1: Reps 15–20
Day 4: Reps 8–10
Sets: 4–5

	Set 1	Set 2	Set 3	Set 4	Set 5
Exercise	Reps	Reps	Reps	Reps	Reps
Db Flat Bench Press					
Bent Over 1 Arm Cable Raise					
Incline Bench Press					
Two Arm Cable Front Raise					
Decline Bench Press or Flyes					
Bent Over Barbell Rows					
Machine Side Laterals					
Pulldowns to the Front					
Standing Single Leg Calf Raise					
Machine Pullovers					
Abdominal Exercise 1					
Abdominal Exercise 2					
Abdominal Exercise 3					

Muscle Mastery Training System 7B: Legs and Arms

Day 2: Reps 15–20
Day 5: Reps 8–10
Sets: 4–5

	Set 1	Set 2	Set 3	Set 4	Set 5
Exercise	**Reps**	**Reps**	**Reps**	**Reps**	**Reps**
Decline Triceps Extensions					
Incline Db Curls					
Bent Over Cable Triceps Extensions					
Barbell Preacher Curls					
Low Bar Overhead Triceps Dips					
Db Concentration Curls					
Jump Squats					
Leg Extensions					
Lying Leg curls					
Db Lunges					

Muscle Mastery Training System: Power, Size, Endurance 7C: Legs and Arms

Day 6: Reps 6–8
Sets: 4–5

	Set 1	Set 2	Set 3	Set 4	Set 5
Exercise	**Reps**	**Reps**	**Reps**	**Reps**	**Reps**
Jump Squats					
Db Pullovers					
Dips					
Chins					
E-Z Bar Curls or Barbell Curls					
Incline Triceps Extensions					
Push Ups on Swiss Ball					
Reverse Chops with Medicine Ball					

Tony's Future

Now that Tony has achieved his muscle-building and body fat goals, his body composition will be far easier to maintain.

For maintenance and a great lifestyle, all he needs is:

- Three weight-lifting workouts a week. He can use any of the routines and rotate every 8 to 12 weeks.
- Two hours of zone 2 cardio a week
- To follow the cycle diet calorie strategies from our previous chapter

As we've said, it's critical to have new goals constantly. Tony's is to become the best pickleball player on the planet and crush his friend Todd on his home court.

SUMMARY

Lean muscle mass isn't just about looking good. It's a crucial part of maximizing your bio span and aging gracefully. The main point is that lifting weights is a requirement for superhuman health. Muscle mass has enormous metabolic benefits. This means that the more lean muscle you have, the more carbs your body can absorb.

So, how long should it take to achieve your muscle-building goals?

The quick answer is that it depends on your level of dedication. You can reach your objectives relatively quickly if you do things correctly.

For you, the difference between "achievable gains" and "best possible gains" is in your:

- Genetics
- Commitment level with exercise
- Commitment level with nutrition
- Age
- Anabolic environment

Your "look" can be broken down into the following factors:

- Bone structure
- Muscles
- Body fat level

Activating anabolism

Your body must be anabolic to create muscle. Anabolism is the state in which your body undergoes growth and repair. Catabolism is anabolism's enemy. It's your body's state of breakdown.

So, how much do you need to train?

- If your goal is health, longevity, and greater bio span, the minimum effective dose is three 20-minute workouts a week.
- If your goal is to build significant lean muscle, then between four and five times a week is optimal.
- If you're obsessed with building as much muscle mass as possible, then 6 to 12 times a week might be needed.

Muscle-Building Nutrition Tips:

- The minimum effective calorie surplus seems to be about 300 to 500 calories a day
- To gain maximum muscle mass, more protein feedings per day are better than fewer
- Eliminate all FODMAP foods to minimize digestive distress
- Calorie quality matters
- Make sure to choose protein sources your body digests the best
- Monitor results with DEXA, pictures, scale, and tape measurements
- Keep your posture optimized

SPECIAL THANKS TO OUR MENTORS

The results, programs, and strategies we outlined have worked for thousands of our clients both in person and online. We'd like to give special thanks to all of our mentors who taught us the way: Scott Abel, Kevin Weiss, Tom Platz, Leo Costa Jr., Arnold Schwarzenegger, Ben Pakulski, Bill Pearl, Vince Gironda, and many, many more.

GOAL #3:

ACHIEVING ATHLETIC DOMINANCE

The next chapter will show you how you can maximize your training and game-day performances.

CHAPTER 17

ASSEMBLING THE ULTIMATE ATHLETIC PERFORMANCE MASTER PLAN

In this chapter, you will learn:

- The nine performance considerations you should include if you want to optimize all facets of athletic nutrition
- The three categories of optimizing athletic performance
- The five categories of bodyweight and body composition required for success in different sports
- The four-stage process for achieving your final athletic form
- A chart of 22 sports showing the ideal body fat percentage for your specific sport (whether you're male or female)
- How to balance power and performance needs when figuring out your ideal bodyweight, and which is the biggest advantage for reaching your goals
- How bodyweight fluctuation can negatively influence your athletic performance
- An estimate of how much protein you should have in grams and which supplements you can take to maximize the value of the protein you eat
- The difference between "maximum absolute strength and power" vs. "maximum relative strength and power," and how you as an athlete can optimize performance for each type
- The truth about carbs and the best kinds for athletes
- The axiom of the body is how your body becomes its function

On game day, the goal is simple: get into a peak physiological and psychological state. We cover both sides at the end of this chapter.

All of the principles, strategies, and tactics we've laid out in the book are vital for athletic performance, including:

- Optimizing your diet based on your genetics
- Optimizing your supplements based on your goals, bloodwork, and genetics
- Optimizing your foods based on your gut health test results

Optimizing all facets of athletic nutrition can make a massive impact on performance. Athletic nutrition has unique considerations, because the desired key attributes can vary radically from sport to sport. Athletic performance considerations include:

1. Maximum relative power output
2. Maximum absolute power output
3. Body fat optimization
4. Bodyweight optimization
5. Optimal nutrition for off-season goals
6. Optimal nutrition for training camps
7. Optimal nutrition for peak workouts
8. Optimal nutrition for post-workout recovery
9. Optimal nutrition for game-day performance

This chapter gives you some key points to help you with all nine of these factors.

OPTIMAL BODYWEIGHT AND BODY FAT LEVELS

The primary objective for most athletes in the majority of sports is maximizing relative power. Because they're competing at a certain weight limit, they want to gain a relative power advantage over other competitors in the same weight class. Their goal is to maximize their strength/power-to-bodyweight ratio, which is called "relative strength" or "relative power output." Achieving this requires an extremely high level of nutritional accuracy.

There are a few sports like football, sumo wrestling, and others where athletes try to get as big and strong as possible. If you're competing in one of those sports, then we suggest following our protocols from the muscle-building chapters. The process is pretty simple: do the right training and keep eating in a calorie surplus.

Athletes aren't rewarded for being lean and ripped like in bodybuilding. In other words, they seldom need to push themselves to sub-5-percent body fat, unless they're a horse jockey. The first key is to figure out what the ideal body fat range is for your sport. There is a body fat sweet spot for each athlete where they perform their best. This is usually a range, and athletes should track their body fat percentages and correlate the data to their athletic performances. This is a great process for figuring out your optimal body fat zone.

Different sports have different requirements in terms of bodyweight and body composition. You can divide sports into five groups in which different athletes excel:

1. Athletic gravitational sports: These are where the body moves athletically against gravity. An athlete's key attributes here are high relative power and high levels of athleticism. Examples include skateboarding, mountain biking, ski jumping, and jumping field sports. Explosive power, lighter bodyweights, and lower body fat percentages are ideal.
2. Endurance sports: The body moves against gravity here too, but the key athletic attribute is very different: it's maximum power over time (aka endurance). Examples include: long-distance running, cross-country skiing, cycling, and long-distance swimming. Lower levels of muscularity and low body fat are optimal.
3. Power sports, including combat sports: In most of these, the key athletic attribute is maximum relative strength and power. Examples include mixed martial arts (MMA), wrestling, judo, boxing, tae kwon do, rowing, and weight lifting. In some sports, such as MMA and wrestling, athletes seek a bodyweight advantage as well. They achieve this by cutting weight aggressively and rehydrating for events (more on this later in the chapter). These athletes should pursue higher levels of muscle and power and lower levels of body fat.
4. Athletic aesthetic sports: The two key attributes here are ideal aesthetics and high levels of coordination and agility. Examples include rhythmic and artistic gymnastics, figure skating, diving, and synchronized swimming.[1, 2] Unlike bodybuilding, the aesthetics here are based on impressive movements. Moderately low bodyweight with lower body fat are desirable.
5. Maximum strength and power sports: The key attribute is maximum power and strength regardless of bodyweight. Examples include open-weight sports such as strongman contests, sumo wrestling, superheavy combat divisions, and certain National Football League (NFL) positions. Maximum weight, power, and strength are the goals. Body fat is almost irrelevant.

Most popular sports such as basketball, MMA, soccer, hockey, and others are hybrids of the above types. This means they require a mixture of endurance, power, and athleticism.

THE PROCESS OF ACHIEVING YOUR FINAL ATHLETIC FORM

- Figure out the ideal body fat and bodyweight for your sport.
- Gain or lose the ideal amount of weight you need for your sport. If you need to gain weight, your goal should be that 75 percent of your weight gain is lean muscle mass. If your goal is to lose weight, then 75 percent of your weight loss should be body fat (instead of lean muscle).
- Once you're within striking distance of your final athletic weight and form, shift your strategy to recompositioning (maintaining your bodyweight while slowly losing body fat and gaining lean muscle mass). This makes sense for men when they're around 15 percent body fat or lower and for women around 20 percent. Slowly recomp to your ideal body fat percentage.
- Maintain your ideal weight and focus on improving your power, strength, and athletic performance.

Your chosen process may take a few years to achieve.

The Ideal Body Fat Percentage for Your Sport

There's no absolute best body fat percentage for each sport. However, there are researched ideal ranges. The best body fat for each individual can differ based on genetics. Some people can easily lower body fat and maintain performance. Others lose too much strength and power when they push their bodies too low.

Being absolutely shredded like a competitive bodybuilder leads to a massive drop-off in athletic performance. It usually begins to rapidly decline below 8 percent body fat, although there are some genetic exceptions.

In football, they optimize the body fat percentages based on each position's purpose. Receivers have extremely low body fat because they want to maximize athletic speed. Running backs have a higher body fat percentage because they're taking hits. Linemen are around 20 percent body fat because they need maximum force.

Perhaps the most extreme examples of low body fat are seen in horse jockeys. They aim to be as light as humanly possible. Body fat percentages as low as 2.5 percent have been reported. However, a recent review of nutritional practices showed that most jockeys lack major key nutrients.

Average body fat percentages found in research into different sports are shown below.[3]

Sport	Male	Female	Sport	Male	Female
Baseball	12–15%	12–18%	**Rowing**	6–14%	12–18%
Basketball	6–12%	20–27%	**Shot put**	16–20%	20–28%
Bodybuilding	5–8%	10–15%	**Skiing (cross-country)**	7–12%	16–22%
Cycling	5–15%	15–20%	**Sprinting**	8–10%	12–20%
American Football (Backs)	9–12%	No data	**Soccer**	6–18%	13–18%
American Football (Linemen)	15–19%	No data	**Swimming**	9–12%	14–24%
Gymnastics	5–12%	10–16%	**Tennis**	8–18%	16–24%
High/long Jumping	7–12%	10–18%	**Triathlon**	5–12%	10–15%
Ice/field hockey	8–15%	12–18%	**Volleyball**	11–14%	16–25%
Marathon running	5–11%	10–15%	**Weight lifting**	9–16%	No data
Racquetball	8–13%	15–22%	**Wrestling**	5–16%	No data

FIGURING OUT YOUR IDEAL BODYWEIGHT: THE BATTLE BETWEEN POWER AND PERFORMANCE

For athletes competing in weight classes, the key questions about your advantages are:

- Do you have a bigger edge trying to cut weight?
- Do you compete closer to your natural weight?
- Do you focus on getting bigger and stronger?

No matter what you decide, if you're an athlete in this group, you need to be far more precise with your nutrition, because your goals include:

1. Increasing lean body mass slightly
2. Decreasing body fat slightly
3. Increasing strength and power dramatically
4. (In some cases) gaining a bodyweight advantage

Avoiding Extreme Weight Cuts

In some sports, like wrestling or MMA, bodyweight plays a big role. As Matt's former fighting teacher used to say, "Bodyweight . . . you've got to deal with it." Some competitors resort to extreme water cutting to gain an advantage the day of a fight.

They usually cut 10 or 20 pounds of water weight 24 to 72 hours before the weigh in, and then focus on rehydrating before the event.

It sounds good on paper to gain a weight advantage over your opponent. However, doing it this way can severely compromise performance. Dehydration from weight cutting is one of the most brutal things anyone can do for athletic performance.

We've seen many fighters in the Ultimate Fighting Championship (UFC) fight in multiple weight classes. Finding themselves too drained from weight cuts, many decided to move up to a higher weight class, and their performance improved. Others struggled to stay competitive when they moved up in weight. There are no objective rules. Experiment and see where you perform your best.

Fluctuating Bodyweight Impacts Performance

One of the most important points is that when you move either up or down in weight, your athletic performance will be compromised for a while. When you change weight classes, there's a learning curve of moving your new bodyweight in a new way. When you move up, you typically gain power but lose athleticism. When you go down in weight, you can lose power and strength; however, you may be able to pull off techniques you couldn't before.

These differences are apparent when you watch the UFC and mixed martial arts. You see the lighter weight classes fight totally differently than the heavyweights, especially in grappling exchanges.

Our point is, it's usually best to choose a weight class and focus on improving at that one. Your training and performance will be maximized when your bodyweight is at maintenance.

ATHLETES WHO MAXIMIZE BOTH STRENGTH AND POWER

This group divides into two subcategories:

1. Maximum *absolute* strength and power
2. Maximum *relative* strength and power

Maximum Absolute Strength and Power

Athletes focused on maximum absolute strength and power have no weight class limitations. The World's Strongest Man contest and sumo wrestling are good examples of this. These athletes' goal is to continue gaining as much weight, strength, and power as possible. Yes, they want muscle more than fat, but they will accept an increase in body fat as long as their strength and power are maximized. Most of the world's strongest men weigh between 350 and 400 pounds at their peak.

Moving Up Weight Classes

In some cases, athletes want to be as big as possible, so they want to move up in weight and power. A good goal in those situations is to target adding around 15 pounds a year. If training and nutrition are optimized, 8 to 10 pounds of that can be lean muscle mass. In some cases, younger athletes may gain even more lean muscle mass than that. When gaining weight, aim for around 75 percent of it to be lean muscle mass.

It's better to go slower and gain more muscle mass than to go up in weight quickly and gain a lot of body fat. Excess body fat can become another challenge that you end up fighting your entire sports career.

We've seen a lot of mixed martial arts athletes go up in a weight class and do a lot better. It's not always the case, but oftentimes it is. This is because they were previously compromising their performance with aggressive weight cuts. There is an ideal weight for you to compete at, and finding that is key.

Off-Season: The Time for Muscle, Strength, and Power

One of the classic bodybuilding calorie-cycling strategies is a meso-cycling approach: increase calories and bodyweight off season, cut calories and body fat during training camp. As long as the bodyweight swings aren't too extreme, the off-season is a good time to focus on building muscle, strength, and power. Good targets are staying within 15 or 20 pounds of your competition weight, and aiming for 5 to 10 pounds of your competition weight before weight cutting.

Avoiding Massive Off-Season Bodyweight Swings

One of the biggest mistakes any athlete can make is to have huge bodyweight and body fat swings off season.

Some undisciplined athletes balloon up 30 to 50 pounds off season and then get into an aggressive body fat cutting cycle and, in some cases, aggressive water cutting before they compete. These athletes' strength, power, endurance, and performance become severely compromised compared to when they're in homeostasis. We strongly suggest avoiding this process. It's bad for performance and for health.

Maximum Relative Strength and Power Athletes

Most athletes fall into this category: focusing on maximum relative strength and power. We'll outline some key strategies to help you achieve this athletic goal in the healthiest way possible.

If you gain too much lean body mass, it can become extremely difficult to make your target weight. The key is in managing calories and anabolism.

Process: Slowly Recomp Your Body to Its Final Form

One of the key strategies is to slowly recomp (your bodyweight stays around the same, while you lose body fat and gain lean muscle). This means your overall caloric balance is to achieve maintenance. However, there's constant cycling between anabolism and fat loss. We're big fans of shorter calorie cycling for recomping.

Your teenage years and early 20s are a great time to shift your body composition to your final form. The process is to keep bodyweight around the same while slowly increasing your lean body mass and decreasing your body fat. Ideally, take a year or two to do a healthy body recomp. The best nutritional strategy to accomplish this is strategic calorie cycling. Read Chapter 8, Advanced Cycling Strategies, for the best strategies.

As an example, when Matt was preparing for a mixed martial arts fight, his coach had him lower his bodyweight while getting stronger. The goal was to eat just enough food and to get stronger from the workouts while slowly losing body fat with a target of 175 pounds. The goal with his calories was to be in a slight deficit, but not so much as to get drained. Matt changed his training style and his relative strength was about 30 percent stronger than now.

Once you achieve final form, focus on maintaining it while improving your athletic performance. Maintenance is easier and will allow you to focus on maximizing your athletic abilities.

Extreme Endurance Training Means Extreme Calorie Needs

Athletes who do 10 to 20 hours of endurance training a week need a high level of calories to recover and maintain their bodyweight. The primary goal of people in this group is to prevent muscle loss and lower body fat. In other words, they focus on being anti-catabolic. Catabolism is very bad for performance, including endurance sports.

Michael Phelps, the world-renowned Olympic swimming champion, is one of the most famous examples. He ate between 10,000 and 12,000 calories a day due to heat loss from being in the pool and his hours of swimming.

In these situations, we strongly recommend increasing enzyme and probiotic dosage to maximize your digestive capability. Many of our high-calorie athletes take between 30 and 75 capsules of MassZymes a day, and it allows them to eat as much as they need without suffering digestive issues.

Moving Down Weight Classes

Sometimes, some athletes want to move down in weight to try to gain an advantage. It's very common in combat sports, especially wrestling and mixed martial arts. The best strategy is to minimize aggressive weight cutting.

To move down in class, you may have to lower your overall body fat. The best approach is to follow a plan like the ones we outlined in the previous chapter. Avoid fast, aggressive weight cuts and instead use the principles in this book for healthy, permanent results.

One note is that some athletes have too much muscle, and the only way they can move down a weight class is to lose some of it. This requires going through a catabolic phase and breaking down excess muscle mass. Of course, being in a calorie deficit is the main key; however, sometimes drastic changes in training are required. Doing less weight training and increasing aerobic endurance work is usually needed in those situations.

How Much Protein Do You Need?

As a rule of thumb, shoot for 0.5 grams to 1 gram of protein per pound of bodyweight. If your goal is to maintain your weight, then move toward 0.5 grams. If your goal is to gain lean muscle and weight, move toward 1 gram per pound. Also, you may need to increase your protein intake if your training volume increases past a certain threshold.

As a competitive bodybuilder, Wade's average protein intake per day would range between 80 and 120 grams per day, with gusts up to 150. He was able to maintain a muscular 200-pound physique.

Also maximize the *value* from the protein that you're eating instead of just eating more protein. The best way to do that is to use proteolytic enzymes. With each meal, we suggest using:

- Five MassZymes capsules
- Three P3-OM capsules
- One to two HCL Breakthrough capsules

If you want to increase calories, it's better to increase protein instead of just carbs and fats. You'll gain less body fat and maximize anabolism. Studies suggest that a higher-protein diet leads to improvements in body composition (vs. more carbs and more fats).

Best Carbs for Athletes

As an athlete, your goal with carbs is to fuel your energy, your workouts, and your competitions. The best thing is to have stable blood sugar. Slower-digesting carbs are superior for stabilizing blood sugar. They tend to also have a higher satiety factor.

Faster-digesting carbs can be useful during workouts or training events. To keep their energy reserves high, many athletes drink glucose while they're competing.

Use a CGM to Optimize to the Next Level

Every serious athlete should spend a month or two monitoring their blood sugar response to various foods. Pay attention to which carbs make you feel best and give you a more stable blood sugar curve. People's responses differ according to their genetics and gut biomes, and that's why you can't just go off those glycemic index and glycemic load charts.

Here's the million-dollar question: What's the best type of diet for sports—keto, or one with carbs? There is *zero* doubt which one is superior for strength and power sports. Carbs rule.

THE TRUTH ABOUT CARBS

For power performance athletes, the proof is undeniable that carbs are a superior source of energy. You'll be able to generate high levels of power. When you're pushing your body to the max and cortisol gets excreted, blood sugar utilization ramps up. So, when you're pushing yourself, glucose is definitely superior.

Blood Sugar Breakthrough will improve athletic performance if you're eating carbs. Even if you have great carbohydrate metabolism, you will go to another level.

- Your glycolytic pathways will be stronger
- You'll be able to break down carbs easier and faster
- You'll produce more ATP

It's a great tool for workouts and for athletic performance.

LONG-DISTANCE NUTRITION STRATEGIES

Dual Fuel

Some long-distance runners are experimenting with going dual fuel, which means carbs and ketones. Some pro racers consume 25 to 50 grams of ketone esters, along with glucose, amino acids, and other nutrients. We actually use this protocol during our intensive MetaMorphosis brain trainings.

It is possible that for long-distance endurance events, ketones are better. During long-distance races, the body uses both glucose and ketones for energy. For that reason, it makes sense for most long-distance racers to become fat adapted.

In our opinion, it takes around 12 months to become fully fat adapted, so we suggest following a ketogenic diet for that long. The good news is, once you achieve it, you'll be set for life for fat adaptation. Read Chapter 20's section on ketogenic diets for more insights.

Another underrated benefit of ketosis for long-distance athletes is anti-catabolism. You want to minimize muscle loss (unless that's one of your bodyweight goals). Being in a catabolic state impacts athletic performance massively. The key for this is to drink sufficient fast-digesting amino acids during the race. For more information, read the Ultimate Supplement Guide at www.BIOptimizers.com/book/resources.

YOUR BODY BECOMES ITS FUNCTION

Throughout this chapter, we talk about key attributes like athleticism, power, strength, and agility. Those are byproducts of the training. The stimulus comes from the training (and we're not going to get into that in this book, because that would double its size).

The axiom of the body is: your body becomes its function. This means your body changes and adapts based on what you do. If you do long-distance running, your body will adapt for long-distance running. If you sprint, your body will adapt to sprinting. If you lift weights, it will get bigger and stronger.

The basic formula for adaptation = stimuli x recovery.

The majority of your recovery comes from food and sleep. Seek out the best coaches in your field to give you the best protocols for stimuli. Training mastery is necessary to becoming a master athlete.

Training Camp Strategies

Training camp is the transition phase between the off-season and in-competition, where you fine-tune the body in preparation for the competitive season. It's the right time to lose any excess body fat from the off-season. If you need to do that, target about one pound per week of weight loss, and give yourself ample time. When the season starts, you don't want to be cutting or gaining weight.

Sport-specific training volume begins to ramp up. When you ramp up your training volume, you need to ramp up your nutrients. Many athletes have suboptimal levels of key minerals and other vital nutrients.

Treat Workouts Like Game Day

Your workouts should be ramping up in intensity as well. Aim to simulate the actual event as much as possible during training. Remember: your body becomes its function.

The axiom of the mind is: "what fires together, wires together." This is vital to understanding state-dependent training. Aim to make your training almost as intense as game day. You want to re-create its stress and intensity during training—this will help you perform better when the big day comes.

Winning Game Days

On game day, the goal is simple: get into a peak physiological and psychological state. We're going to cover both sides.

Optimize Your Hydration

One ounce of water per pound of bodyweight is a good target for hydration. It curbs appetite and accelerates the clearing of metabolic waste products. It enhances the overall fat loss on a diet, partly because it suppresses hunger (and most people mistake dehydration for hunger).

- If you're 200 pounds, drink about 200 ounces per day (which is about 1.5 gallons).
- If you're 120 pounds, drink 120 ounces (which is a little less than a gallon).

Most people are dehydrated, and they do things that dehydrate them more. Being hydrated is anti-catabolic. In one experiment, weightlifters did squats while dehydrated. A massive cortisol spike occurred, which will break down muscle. So, water is anabolic. Every athlete should be obsessed with staying hydrated and mineralized.

Optimizing Electrolytes

One key consideration for anyone training is to replenish not just water, but electrolytes. As we mentioned earlier, even a 1 percent dehydration level impacts performance.

When people train hard, they sweat more, and they lose more minerals. A high-volume athlete could sweat out three to six liters of minerals and water a day with long workouts in a warm environment.

Most serious athletes should consume:

- 5 to 10 grams of sodium a day
- 3 to 7 grams of potassium a day
- 1 to 2 grams of magnesium (we recommend Magnesium Breakthrough)

Most people have too much sodium and not enough potassium, which affects their performance. Read Chapter 27 on micronutrients. Should you worry about being overmineralized? It's hard to do. The body has many mechanisms for excreting mineral excess—like aldosterone, which binds to excess sodium. So, in our opinion, it's a bigger concern to be undermineralized. Of course, monitor your blood pressure.

We're also big believers in trace minerals. We believe they are co-factors in hundreds of biological pathways and bioconversions.

THE ULTIMATE PEAK-PERFORMANCE STATE HACK: OPTIMIZE YOUR NEUROCHEMICALS

Perhaps the most underrated game changer is optimizing your neurochemicals (molecules that are part of neural activity). They can shift your entire sense of being. The right stack of neurochemicals is vital to becoming a champion.

Charles Poliquin is arguably one of the greatest strength and conditioning coaches of all time. He's best known for working with more than 800 Olympic athletes and trained medalists in 24 different sports.

Before working with any athlete, he would have them do the Braverman test, which helps to assess neurotransmitter dominance and deficiencies. He wouldn't even work with athletes who weren't dopamine and acetylcholine dominant. He felt they just wouldn't be able to compete with those who were.

Incredibly successful people are usually dopamine driven. They're naturally good at building dopamine loops in their minds (see Chapter 18 to learn how to do this). This allows them to train harder and longer, because the dopamine attenuates noradrenaline—the neurochemical that makes people and animals quit. If you want to be the best in your sport, it's important to have the capacity to go really deep in the pain zone.

Next is acetylcholine, the focus molecule. To perform at your best physically, you need world-class focus. Every rep of every set needs focus. Even something as simple as a bicep curl can be enhanced with better focus. Former Mr. Olympia contender Ben Pakulski went to the University of Tampa's muscle research facility, where they ran tests and found that higher levels of mental focus increased his muscle activation.

Think about athletic performance in a game. That laser-beam focus to stay on task and hyper-aware of every moment can be the difference between winning and losing.

As soon as you're deficient in acetylcholine, your ability to focus drops. Focusing becomes a struggle.

Here's the great news: you can hack your focus with nootropics. You can easily increase acetylcholine using a stack of choline donors. You can also increase dopamine with certain nootropics. We go deep into brain optimization nutrition and supplementation throughout this book.

On the choline side, eggs are the most abundant natural source you can get. That's one of the reasons why eggs are more than just protein and fat—the choline in them is really powerful for focus.

GAME TIME: NEUROCHEMISTRY AND HORMONE OPTIMIZATION

The right levels of dopamine, acetylcholine, adrenaline, and noradrenaline are vital for peak performance. The best strategy is to have your neurochemicals and hormones peak during your game and workouts. Time your nootropics and supplements for that. We've worked with many athletes to help them beat their best performances.

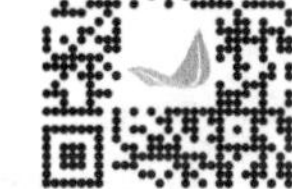

The epic news is, Nootopia can give you a *massive* edge over your competitors by helping you optimize your neurochemistry. Visit www.nootopia.com for more info.

Game-Time Nutrition

Perhaps the most underrated aspect of nutrition timing is game-time nutrition. Let's talk about the ultimate intra-workout shake (or "game-time drink"). Its purpose is to:

- Replace lost water
- Replenish lost minerals and vitamins
- Feed the body glucose for fuel
- Feed the body amino acids for recovery

Matt was working on an optimal intra-workout formula when Wade visited him in Panama. One day, we decided to see how many sets we could do with our friend Sherman.

The 300-Set Experiment

We wanted to see if we could do 300 sets of weight lifting in less than three hours. We ended up doing well over 300. A few notes on the workout:

- We did triplexes for everything. This means we grouped three different body parts and did one exercise for each (for example: chest, calves, and abs). We did more than 60 exercises for around five sets per exercise.
- We had close to zero rest between sets. We took between 5 and 15 seconds between each exercise in the triplexes.
- We didn't go to failure. We went until there were 1 or 2 reps left and stopped. Rep range was 8 to 10 on most sets.

The Result?

All three of us were shocked at how good we felt during and after this mega-volume workout. We felt great. We had no doubt that if we hadn't fueled and replenished our bodies, we would have crashed at around 100 to 150 sets. This was a powerful experiential lesson for us in intra-workout drink design.

Each of us drank the following three drinks, which totaled about one gallon of optimized fluids each:

Drink #1: BIOptimized Electrolyte Water

Purpose: to hydrate the brain and body with water and electrolytes

- 2 liters of water
- trace minerals
- ½ teaspoon of Himalayan salt (for sodium and trace minerals)
- ¼ teaspoon of cream of tartar (for potassium)

Drink #2: The Ultimate Intra-Workout Shake

Purpose: energy and recovery

- ½ cup of strawberries (for fructose/glucose)
- ½ frozen banana (for fructose/glucose)
- 2 scoops of Protein Breakthrough Berry Bliss (for amino acids)
- 3 MassZymes capsules (caps are opened, and powder is blended in shake)
- 3 P3-OM capsules (caps are opened, and powder is blended in shake)
- 1½ cup of coconut water

Mix the ingredients together about 30 minutes before your workout begins, and leave at room temperature for at least 20 minutes before drinking. Sip throughout the workout, starting at the beginning and aiming to finish by the end. You'll be rocking your workouts hard, fast, and deep.

Note: The enzymes and probiotics are the game changers of this recipe. They break down any protein into usable amino acids and also help break down the carbs. This means you're drinking easily digestible aminos and carbs. Because they're easy to absorb, the shake won't disturb your digestive system and affect your workout or performance.

This is crucial. Make sure that your intra-workout drinks have zero impact on your digestive system. If they do, it will impact your performance.

Amino Acids are the Real Kings

We've said multiple times in this book that protein is the king macro. However, the real truth is that amino acids are the apex molecules. The real goal is to feed your body enough amino acids so it can quickly recover from workouts and competitions.

Protein + Proteolytic Enzymes = Amino Acid Heaven

The key to getting amino acids in your system is proteolytic enzymes. They're the ones that do all the bio-work and break down big proteins into usable amino acids. However, during training or sporting events, you don't want protein sloshing in your stomach. It weighs you down and impacts performance. That's why you want to mix MassZymes with P3-OM and protein, and drink this while you're training.

There's research to validate the use of predigested amino acids during training.

The protocol is simple: Mix your favorite protein with three to five capsules of MassZymes plus two capsules of P3-OM. Open the capsules and blend it all up. The longer you wait before drinking, the more protein will convert into amino acids. You want amino acids in your body while you're training, because as soon as you stress a muscle, it begins adapting immediately. Yes, there's a cycle of recovery that lasts 48 to 72 hours. However, the body starts adapting immediately after a set.

Drink #3: Matt's Zamner Coffee

Purpose: to boost adrenaline, ketones, and nootropic absorption

This is Matt's tweak on the classic Dave Asprey buttered coffee recipe, and it's designed to be taken along with nootropics.

- 2 cups of organic coffee (any level of decaf works too)
- 1 teaspoon of grass-fed butter
- 1 teaspoon of MCT oil
- Trace minerals
- 30 to 60 milligrams of CBD oil
- 1 tablespoon of organic raw cacao powder (you get a much stronger nootropic effect from raw cacao)
- 3 kApex capsules (to assist in breaking down the fats)

Make your coffee of choice and then blend all ingredients. Sip over a one-to-three-hour period. We sipped it throughout our three-hour workout.

We love stacking this recipe with Nootopia Breakthrough Brain Stacks. This will enhance the absorption of your fat-soluble nootropics.

Note: Watch how much MCT oil you put in, because it gives a lot of people digestive discomfort. That's why we advise using just 1 teaspoon. And if that still gives you problems, replace it with another source of fat.

Warning: Adjust the caffeine levels of the coffee based on your stimulant tolerance. If you're a fast caffeine metabolizer, then you can go full caffeine. If you're hypersensitive to caffeine, use decaf or half-caf.

Optimal timing: You don't want fats in your stomach while you're training or competing, so the best timing for this drink is to finish it about 45 to 60 minutes before your workout or event, which is also when the fat-soluble Nootopia capsules will hit you.

Power Move for Keto Followers: Microdose Carbs

Even keto followers can microdose carbs to boost performance when training. Highly respected scientific researcher and keto advocate Dr. Dom D'Agostino talked about it on a podcast we did together.

Take 40 to 80 grams of carbs during a workout, adjusting the amount based on difficulty. If it's a lighter workout, like arms, then 40 grams is enough. If you're training legs or back or just training really hard, then do 80 grams. Don't worry, there's no change in ketosis. So, you can basically stay in ketosis while just using the glycogen in real time to get that boost in performance.

Post-Game Recovery

Post-workout nutrition is important. You usually want a large meal after a workout or a competition. Your body is depleted, and a good meal is how you ensure anabolism. Eating enough calories and protein is vital. Of course, all of our advice on the best types of foods is important. Read previous chapters to learn more.

Optimizing Recovery

Last but certainly not least is recovery. Optimizing recovery doesn't just come from food. There are many modalities you can stack together to maximize recovery, whose other key drivers are:

- Supplements
- Sleep
- Nervous system optimization (learn more on this in our book *From Sick to Superhuman*)

The first thing is to shift to a parasympathetic state as soon as your workout or game is done. The more you train and compete, the more crucial this is. If an athlete trains two or three times and is always sympathetically activated (in fight-flight-freeze) during the day, they easily become overtrained, and their nervous system gets fried. This is when performance goes off a cliff.

Taking naps, chilling out, floating, getting gentle bodywork, taking sufficient magnesium, or listening to classical music will all help shift the nervous system over and allow the body to recover. Matt believes that nothing beats floating for nervous system recovery. He's seen it with the athletes he coaches.

You can use music to enhance the nervous system shift. Music is an activator and enhancer of neurochemistry. Go from Metallica during your workout to Mozart after.

SLEEP DEEP AND DOMINATE

The most important thing for recovery is sleep. Total sleep time depends on your training volume. The more you train, the more sleep you need. Also, the harder you train, the more sleep you need. If you're squatting and deadlifting a couple of times a week, you'll notice a greater need for sleep.

High-quality sleep is everything. The formula for athletes is 8 hours + 1 hour for every hour that you train. So, for now if I just train 2-3 hours a day, it should be 10-11 hours of sleep. Total sleep time can include naps and meditation. So, it's not necessarily just sleeping 10 or 11 hours straight at night.

For an in-depth sleep optimization guide, read our chapter on this topic in our book *From Sick to Superhuman*.

THE WOLVERINE INJURY PROTOCOL

Injuries are a part of competitive sports. Hopefully, you haven't had any major ones. However, it's critical to maximize your recovery if it does happen. In our experience, you can speed up your recovery time like the Wolverine and cut it from 30 to 50 percent using the following protocol.

Matt recently tore his Achilles tendon and got reconstructive surgery. Using the process we outline, he cut his healing time by almost half.

Phase 1: Optimize autophagy and repair

Phase 2: Optimize anabolism

1: The Autophagy and Repair Phase

Focus on maximizing autophagy through fasting and proteolytic enzymes.

Fasting Speeds Up Healing

One research group found that fasting twice a week for 24 hours helped speed up wound healing.[4] Another group found that fasting accelerated healing of spinal injuries in mice.[5]

For the first 30 days:

- Fast twice a week
    - We suggest not eating for two days per week for the first few weeks.
- 60 MassZymes capsules per day
    - Load the body with proteolytic enzymes (we'll share some mind-blowing research with you in a moment)

        25 in the morning on an empty stomach
        25 in the afternoon on an empty stomach
        Plus 3 to 4 with each meal
- Healing peptide stack: BPC 157 + TB 500
    - Matt used several vials of each during the first month.
    - Consult with your doctor for dosage.

Proteolytic Enzymes Speed Up Healing

During the first few weeks after an injury or surgery, your body is focused on autophagy and inflammation. Proteolytic enzymes help speed up this process. Here are some epic findings on using high doses of proteolytic enzymes to heal athletes faster.

- Dr. Fulgrave believes that with enzymes, recovery from sprains and strains can go from eight weeks of inactivity to two.[6]
- J. M. Zuschlag's "Double-Blind Clinical Study Using Certain Proteolytic Enzymes Mixtures in Karate Fighters" study showed mind-blowing reductions in healing times for:[7]
    - Hematoma: 15.6 days to 6.6 days
    - Swelling: 10 days to 4 days
    - Restricted movement: 12.6 days to 5 days
    - Inflammation: 10.5 days to 3.8 days
    - Being unfit for training: 10.2 days to 4.2 days
- Dr. Baumuller used enzymes in a double-blind study for ankle-related injuries and found people would recover up to 50 percent faster.[8]
- Dr. Lichtman treated boxers and found that he could drop black eyes from 10 to 14 days of recovery to 1 to 3.[9]

When Matt tore his Achilles and got reconstructive surgery, he was taking 60 MassZymes a day on an empty stomach. It works.

2: The Anabolism Phase

After a few weeks of autophagy and reduction in inflammation, it's time to focus on anabolism. You want to strengthen your muscles, ligaments, and tendons. You also want to activate your nervous system and start rebuilding neural pathways between your brain and your body. Of course, work with a highly skilled physical therapy (PT) expert during this time.

Increase Calories and Protein

It's time to increase overall anabolism, and this requires a calorie surplus. A good target is around 500 a day. Keep in mind that you can still fast one or two days a week to get rid of calorie excess. Also be mindful that your overall calorie expenditure is lower now than normal, because you're probably not as active and are training a fraction of what you were. It's time to slowly increase the intensity of your resistance training and get stronger.

Amino acids are still key to everything on the recovery side. To maximize anabolism, continue optimizing your digestion with proteolytic enzymes, proteolytic probiotics, and HCL.

SUMMARY

Optimizing all aspects of athletic nutrition can have a huge impact on performance.

Optimal Bodyweight and Body Fat Levels

The first step is to determine the appropriate body fat range for your particular sport.

Sports can be divided into five categories:

- Athletic gravitational
- Endurance
- Power
- Athletic aesthetic
- Maximum strength and power

The process of achieving your final athletic form is as follows:

- Figure out the ideal body fat and bodyweight for your sport
- Gain or lose the ideal amount of weight
- Recomp to your ideal body fat percentage
- Maintain your ideal weight and focus on maximizing your power, strength, and performance

Maximizing Strength and Power

There are two types of goals for maximizing strength and power:

Maximum absolute strength and power. The goal of these athletes is to gain as much weight, strength, and power as possible.

Maximum relative strength and power. The key for these athletes is to manage calories and anabolism.

Your Body Becomes Its Function

Your body changes and adapts based on what you do. If you do long-distance running, your body will adapt for long-distance running. It will get bigger and stronger if you lift weights.

The basic formula for adaptation = stimuli x recovery.

Winning Game Days

Optimize your:

- Hydration
- Electrolytes
- Neurochemicals
- Hormones
- Recovery
    - Supplements
    - Sleep
    - Nervous system optimization

Injury Protocol

The autophagy and repair phase. Maximize autophagy through fasting and proteolytic enzymes.

After a few weeks of autophagy and reduction in inflammation, it's time to focus on anabolism.

The anabolism phase. Strengthen your muscles, ligaments, and tendons. Activate your nervous system and rebuild neural pathways between your brain and your body.

GOAL #4:

MAXIMIZING YOUR BRAIN POWER

The next chapter will show you how you can maximize your cognitive performance in the short term and long term.

CHAPTER 18

ASSEMBLING THE PEAK MENTAL PERFORMANCE MASTER PLAN

This chapter is for people who really want to push their brains. That's highly driven entrepreneurs, high performers, business executives, and creatives. If you need your brain to be at its peak, this chapter is for you.

In this chapter, you will learn:

- What the "perfect brain day" is and how you can achieve it
- How to honor your chronotype to determine when you should be waking up each day
- Six great rituals you can implement in the first 30 to 60 minutes of your morning to take some time for yourself
- Three examples of the ultimate morning ritual stacks
- How to stack biohacking processes for peak mental performance
- Seven benefits that adding nootropics to your daily routine will have on your mental performance
- A few examples of nootropic Power Moves to get the most out of your Nootopia formulas
- Key evening rituals for nightly downshifting to optimize sleep and maximize your next day's mental performance
- How to cycle between intensity and recovery to become a high performer (and stay one for the rest of your life)
- The ultimate brain optimization program
- The three levels of recovery for peak mental performance so you can manage your energy like an athlete

It's important to realize that we're all fighting aging, including brain aging. Some people have genetic tendencies for Alzheimer's disease and dementia, and if they don't proactively optimize their brains, they could lose a decade or more of quality life as they get older.

The great news is, there are many things you can do to optimize your brain and live in a peak mental state for the rest of your life. Actively optimizing your brain can lift your daily performance to a new level as well as add years and decades to your career.

The difference between a normal-functioning brain and dementia is 100 milliseconds, according to Dr. Braverman.[1]

In this chapter, we cover the "perfect brain day" as well as create a yearly master brain optimization plan.

The Perfect Brain Day

The perfect brain day is a 24-hour view of all of the activities, foods, and supplements you can take to be in a peak state all day.

The perfect brain day starts when you go to sleep the night before. Sleep is essential for peak performance. We could write an entire chapter on sleep . . . actually, we did, and that chapter is Chapter 11 in *From Sick to Superhuman.*

WHEN SHOULD YOU WAKE UP? HONOR YOUR CHRONOTYPE

Next, it's important to align your day with your chronotype. *The Power of When* is the best book we've seen on this topic. It breaks people down into four chronotypes:

- Lions: morning people
- Wolves: night people
- Bears: people in the middle
- Dolphins: light sleepers who struggle to get a good night's sleep

The main point is, if possible, don't try to force your brain to be at its peak when it's not aligned with your circadian rhythms. Lions can wake up very early and get great deep work done. Wolves are more productive in the evening.

No one type is better than another. Just be true to yourself and rock your work when your body is rocking. Matt has tried waking up before 6 A.M., and all he felt was pain. Of course, it is possible to shift your circadian rhythms if you wish.

It's worth noting that you can use light to retrain your circadian clock. By waking up at your target time and shining sunlight into your eyes as soon as possible, you can reset your clock within a few days.

Waking Up

The goal is to go from sleepy to optimized within 15 minutes of waking up.

The Power Move is to have water next to your bed when you go to sleep. As soon as you wake up, drink 500 ml of mineralized room-temperature water—the entire thing. Your body is definitely dehydrated from the night before. It's not unusual to lose one to four pounds of water while sleeping. Even minor levels of dehydration hurt mental performance.

Of course, go take care of business in the bathroom. And we suggest weighing yourself every morning to keep your weight in check.

Sunlight in Your Eyes

Kudos to Dr. Andrew Huberman for explaining the power and importance of this Power Move in Episode 28 of the *Huberman Lab* podcast:

> Getting sunlight in your eyes first thing in the morning is absolutely vital to mental and physical health. It is perhaps the most important thing that any and all of us can and should do in order to promote metabolic well-being, promote the positive functioning of your hormone system, and get your mental health steering in the right direction.
>
> The protocol is to get outdoors, ideally with no sunglasses . . . Even if there's cloud cover, more photons, light information are coming through that cloud cover than would be coming from a very bright indoor bulb. How long should you do this? It depends on the brightness of the environment. Two minutes would be a minimum and 10 minutes would be even better. And if you can, 30 minutes would be fantastic.[2]

So, go outside (no windows or sunglasses) and aim to get 10 to 30 minutes of sunlight (even if it's overcast) in your eyes. This is the ultimate biological cue to kickstart your circadian clock. There's also a boost in dopamine and serotonin that comes from sunlight, which will help you maximize your performance.

Your Morning Rituals

Morning rituals can become life-changing habits if they are well designed and adhered to long enough. They will become a part of your life, and the benefits will compound over time. We will cover a few examples, but just use them as inspiration. Create the ultimate morning ritual that works for you.

Stacking Contemplation + Biohacking

The Power of Contemplation, Prayer, and Meditation

Your first 30 to 60 minutes upon awakening are a great time to take for yourself. Aim to not use your phone the first 30 minutes. Some great morning rituals include:

- Meditation
- Breathing practice
- Journaling
- Prayer
- Walking outside (with sun in the eyes)
- High-impact learning
- Playing with your kids and pets

All of these rituals help get your brain waves into a calm, optimized state. Playing with your kids and pets helps boost your oxytocin. This sets the tone for a beautiful day.

Some people do just one of these, some do a combination, and some even do all of them.

Stacking Biohacking Technologies and Processes

One of the great things about biohacking is, you can stack processes (combine several at the same time). This creates hyper efficiency.

- Photobiomodulation, also known as red light therapy, offers a host of great benefits. Here are a few options that you can run:
  - Low-level laser therapy (LLLT) panels for the body, which can help with pain and inflammation
  - LLLT for the face for anti-aging benefits
  - LLLT for the brain (such as Vielight). Five to 10 minutes of gamma pulsing or alpha pulsing can get your brain into an optimized state quickly.
- Pulsed electromagnetic field therapy (PEMF) is a set of technologies that use waves and frequencies to positively affect your body and your brain.
  - Visit www.BIOptimizers.com/book/resources for which technologies we recommend. Our opinions on which ones are the best change with time.
- Cyclic Variations in Adaptive Conditioning (CVAC) is an atmospheric trainer that simulates massive fluctuations in atmospheric pressure. It seems to enhance gamma and delta brainwaves as well as blood flow.
- Neurofeedback is probably the ultimate way to start your day. Doing 15 minutes of alpha training or theta training with 5 to 10 minutes of gamma will get you into a peak performance zone. (There's a new, affordable groundbreaking technology that you can use at home. Go to www.BIOptimizers.com/book/neurofeedback for more information.)
- Grounding. Just put your bare feet on the grass or dirt for 30 minutes. This reduces your body's inflammation. So, by simply walking outside on the grass, you're getting a three-fer: movement, sunlight, and grounding.

Morning Ritual Stacks

The ultimate stacks combine journaling, meditation, and contemplation with biohacking. Here are a few examples:

Stack 1: The Outdoor Primer Ritual

- Go outside (to get the sunlight in your eyes)
- Ground (put your feet on the earth)
- Do neurofeedback, meditation, or journaling for 20 minutes

Stack 2: The Ultimate Photobiomodulation Meditation Ritual

- Put on a photobiomodulation mask
- Use a photobiomodulation panel on your body
- Use the Vielight on your brain
- Meditate or do a breathing process

Stack 3: The Walk, Light, Learn Ritual

- Walk outdoors for 10 to 30 minutes while getting sun in the eyes
- Listen to a high-quality audiobook

Experiment with what works for you. The right rituals will prime your brain and body for the perfect brain day.

OPTIMIZING YOUR NEUROCHEMISTRY

In many ways, neurochemicals are the strongest driver of human behavior. They completely change your experience of reality. By learning how to optimize your neurochemistry, you'll be able to experience perfect brain days regularly.

It's important to note that having a great night's sleep is critical for the production of multiple neurochemicals. There are seven key players in your brain's chemical makeup.

1. Dopamine: The Molecule of Drive and Motivation

If you've been feeling overwhelmed and burnt out, with zero energy to get through your day, there could be another mischievous, lurking reason as to *why* that is.

It all has to do with your neurochemicals—most notably, dopamine. When your levels of dopamine are rocking and rolling, life is pretty great. This is because dopamine is responsible for your body's reward system, which helps you feel motivated.

So, when you've got great levels of dopamine, you feel awesome as you work step-by-step toward your goals. It will reinforce behavior and make you feel good, like that giddy feeling you get when you're looking forward to something exciting.

This in turn helps you get into good habits and avoid the low-energy or burnout feeling. For example, say you know you've got to get in a morning run. When you have good dopamine levels, you'll think about something fun in that run that will get you moving and grooving and ready to crush your routine. Dopamine even reinforces memories. Having good levels of dopamine is critical to success.

Here are some natural ways to boost your dopamine:

- Sunlight: Sunlight in the eyes boosts dopamine and serotonin—another reason to lock in that morning sunlight ritual
- Cold therapy: Exposure to cold has been shown to boost dopamine by 250 percent (an incredible gain)
- Nootropics: Nootropics are brain-enhancing supplements that can directly level up your neurochemicals, including dopamine

We created a company that produces the most powerful and personalized nootropic stacks on the market. We have several formulas that increase dopamine, including Powerful Solution, Apex, Dopa Drops, and Ultimate Focus.

2. Acetylcholine: The Molecule of Focus

On a day-to-day basis, you have to rely on your brain to maximize on all the necessary steps that will get you to your end goal. This is true whether you want to triple your revenue growth, overcome your strongest competitor, or anything else.

That's why investing in your brain is one of the most critical things you can do for your career long term. With all of this in mind, it's important to answer three questions. How long does it usually take you to do the following:

1. Think up new project ideas
2. Recall information
3. Learn something new

Imagine for a moment what your day would look like if you increased your ability to do all of those things at lightning speed. You'd be able to:

- Come up with creative new project proposals faster, see results faster, and grow your business faster.
- Boost your memory and attention span to accomplish double the work you usually do in a day.
- Learn more at faster speeds to reach your goals and rise above the competition.

The key to making this a reality is acetylcholine. Your thinking, memory, focus, and attention all rely on it.

Eggs are the best source of choline, which your body converts into acetylcholine.

Nootopia has several formulas that boost your acetylcholine on demand, including Apex, Mental Reboot AM, and Nectar X.

3. Oxytocin: The Bonding Molecule

Oxytocin is one of the most important molecules for great health. Men thrive on testosterone, and women thrive with oxytocin.

The best part of oxytocin is that it's free! You can get a significant boost by simply hugging someone for at least 22 seconds.

Kids and pets are powerful oxytocin generators. Just playing with them will give you a potent boost for a very positive impact on your health and mental perspective.

4. GABA: The Molecule of Chill

Do you find yourself getting easily irritated by the following daily frustrations?

- Traffic
- Nowhere to park
- Coffee getting cold
- Dying phone battery

Do you feel like your brain is going a mile a minute with jittery nervousness, and you're unable to get calm for big meetings or social interactions?

Would you like to tap into a state of mind where you feel groovy, ready to rock and roll, and able to maintain a positive attitude through anything your day throws at you?

If you answered yes, odds are, you're low or deficient in the neurochemical gamma-aminobutyric acid (GABA). GABA is the anti-stress "molecule of chill." It's a critical neurochemical not only for keeping stress levels low and "chillaxed" levels high, but it also plays a major role in keeping all of your other neurochemicals balanced.

GABA is flexible. You can control your dopamine, serotonin, and acetylcholine levels with GABA to make them each act more effectively, or reduce it to avoid jitters.

In other words, GABA is key for connectedness. When your GABA levels are optimal, everything works in harmony to bring you groovy vibes.

The great news is that if your levels are currently low, you can get GABA flowing in just two minutes.

Nootopia has two powerful GABA-boosting formulas: Zamner Juice and GABAlicious.

5. Serotonin: The Molecule of Stability

If you're low in serotonin, a few things start to happen . . .

- You always feel blue and struggle to get into a good mood
- You lose the drive to do things you have to do
- Your brain becomes foggy 24/7
- You no longer take pleasure in what you used to enjoy

Low levels of serotonin are linked to depression, anxiety, and poor sleep—all of which keeps these four main negative impacts going in a vicious cycle. That doesn't sound like a very good way to enjoy life to the absolute fullest. So, if you've started to notice some of these traits in your own daily life, try the following:

- Getting sunlight
- Eating carbohydrates (although this is one reason why sugar and carbs can be addictive)
- Nootopia blends, including Upbeat, Zamner Juice, and Nectar X

6. Noradrenaline: The Molecule of Initiation

Do you ever realize partway through a conversation that you're not really "there" with the other person? That you feel a bit disconnected, or not very present? Have you ever found yourself in the middle of a task when you realize you're not very focused on what you're actually doing?

Would you like to increase your wakefulness to boost your presence, reduce distractions, and pump out hard work effortlessly?

If you answered yes to any of these questions, a key neurochemical is at play: noradrenaline. Not to be confused with adrenaline, *noradrenaline* is responsible for arousal and wakefulness. We're not talking about sexual arousal, but rather alertness and presence.

When your levels of noradrenaline are low, you feel:

- A lack of energy
- An inability to concentrate
- Unfocused
- Disconnected

All of this adds up to an unproductive day, with your task list piling up. You'll have trouble communicating and connecting with others and difficulty keeping your projects and deadlines straight.

This is not a great way to get to the next level of your career or increase your business growth.

The good news is, your noradrenaline levels don't have to stay low. You can boost them to optimal levels. However, it's a tricky neurochemical. Get too much, and you'll feel wired and burn out fast. You want to find that zone of magic, the sweet spot, without overkill. That's when you unlock a gentle extension of focused attention that lights up your brain, with the ability to control your focus throughout the day.

The best two Nootopia formulas for noradrenaline are Nectar X and Ultimate Focus.

7. Adrenaline: The Molecule of Aggression

When you hear the word *adrenaline*, what do you think of? Maybe it's one or more of the following:

- Stress
- Fear
- Your heart racing
- Feeling your heartbeat throbbing in your temples
- Rapid breathing

Yes, adrenaline is an important neurochemical for keeping us safe in dangerous moments where we need heightened senses or a flood of energy. But many people don't know how adrenaline can be used for success. The optimal levels of adrenaline can fuel your performance for athletic endeavors, workouts, and other situations that require intensity and aggression.

It's possible to access adrenaline without tipping over into fear or the physical signs of stress. When you're in control of your adrenaline levels, some pretty incredible things happen:

- You're able to push through barriers.
- You rise to the next level of focus to push your projects forward.
- You surge with intensity and drive, which is key for any physical task.
- Your mental drive gets combined with your physical capacity to do something.

Listening to aggressive music is one of the best free ways to activate adrenaline. What type of music is best for adrenaline differs from person to person. For some it's rock and metal; for others it's EDM and gangster rap.

Many people, including fighters, soldiers, and athletes, can generate adrenaline on demand. They've learned how to activate it by switching into an aggressive, high-performance state.

Nootopia has created effective stacks that will boost your adrenaline, including Power Solution and Ultimate Focus.

OPTIMIZING MENTAL PERFORMANCE WITH COGNITIVE SUPPLEMENTS

We could write an entire book on supplements that boost your cognitive performance. Here's a review of some of our favorite nootropics. With Nootopia, we create personalized blends of these ingredients.

Celastrus paniculatus

In one study, two different doses of *Celastrus paniculatus* extract were administered to rats (350 and 1,050 milligrams per kilogram) and to mice (500 and 1,500 milligrams per kilogram). In an elevated plus maze and sodium-nitrite–induced amnesia model, *Celastrus paniculatus* extract significantly improved memory process compared to a control group.[3]

Lion's Mane

This is the rock star of brain fungus. The brain-derived neurotrophic factor (BDNF) boost is off the charts.

One study examined the effects of lion's mane on amyloid β(25-35) peptide-induced learning and memory deficits in mice. Amyloid *β*(25-35) peptide plays a role in diseases like Alzheimer's.

The peptide was injected into mice on days 7 and 14 of the study, and over the course of the 23-day experiment, they were fed a diet containing lion's mane. The findings revealed that the fungus reduced amyloid-peptide–induced short-term and visual-recognition memory loss.[4]

For people, 500 to 1,000 mg is recommended one to three times per day.[5] Our favorite way to get lion's mane is to drink CollaGenius in the morning.

Pregnenolone (Especially When Optimally Paired with DHEA)

Add 15 to 50 mg of pregnenolone (natural, not an acetate of it). You'll help activate the cholesterol hormone cascade and light up neurogenesis in profound ways.

One study examined the effect of pregnenolone on depressive symptoms in bipolar disorder (BPD). For 12 weeks, adults with BPD who experienced depressed mood states were randomized to pregnenolone (500 mg per day) or a placebo group. The results suggest that pregnenolone may improve depressive symptoms.[6] Check out DH-HE-A and DH-SHE-A from Nootopia.

Centrophenoxine

The big brother of dimethylethanolamine (DMAE), centrophenoxine is both a self-regulating choline donor *and* a critical molecule in removing "lipofuscin"—the detritus that builds within the brain, leading to poor mental function. It's even used to slow senile dementia and Alzheimer's disease.

One study analyzed six chronic alcoholics with marked memory disturbances. For 12 days, they were each given three doses of 250 mg of centrophenoxine, which was shown to significantly improve the subjects' learning processes and short-term memories.[7]

You can take one to six 250 mg doses of centrophenoxine daily.[8]

Phosphatidylcholine

Wrap choline in a phospholipid (the outer shell of most cells in your body), and you have an incredibly effective acetylcholine precursor. You also improve cellular integrity, a serious bonus.

In a 1995 study on mice with dementia, 100 mg of either phosphatidylcholine or water (in the control group) were administered for 45 days. The control mice with dementia had poorer memory and lower acetylcholine.[9]

The recommended daily dose of phosphatidylcholine is 1.5 to 5 grams.[10]

Huperzine A

Acetylcholinesterase is the fancy name for the enzyme that breaks down acetylcholine in the brain. Huperzine A reduces that pesky enzyme. It keeps more choline available in the synapse, improving mental capacity and reducing "focus fade." Supplementation tends to range from 50 to 200 mcg daily.[11]

One double-blind clinical study found that 200 mcg taken twice daily measurably improved memory, cognitive function, and behavioral factors in 58 percent of Alzheimer's patients compared to 36 percent in the placebo group.[12]

Aniracetam

Aniracetam is one of the most popular and effective "racetams" in existence. Most users find aniracetam, which is derived from the amino acid GABA, gives a gentle, positive boost in mental energy while also increasing serotonin levels.

This often results in a positive, uplifting feeling without any grittiness or anxiety. Because it's oil soluble, aniracetam cleaves to any oils taken concurrently, extending its half-life considerably.

In one mouse study, researchers dosed 50 mg/kg of oral aniracetam each day.[13] Another trial employed 1,500 mg per day in people with Alzheimer's disease, with good tolerance levels found.[14]

Oxiracetam

Oxiracetam is currently the most popular "racetam." It's fast acting and water soluble. Gently stimulating (it modulates AMPA receptors and stimulates the release of glutamate).

It's also experiential, in that you can feel the results within 20 to 40 minutes. The gentle mental lift and cognitive performance increase make it a favorite of biohackers and students. Daily dose ranges from 1,200 to 2,400 mg in two or three evenly spread periods.[15]

In one study on senior people with organic cognitive decline, 400 mg of oxiracetam (built up over six weeks to 2,400 mg daily, then administered for another six weeks) was able to minimize symptoms of cognitive decline both subjectively and empirically while boosting memory formation.[16]

Nefiracetam

One of the most overlooked "racetams," "nef" is a powerhouse when stacked correctly. It opens the calcium channel, supporting cognitive enhancement and memory. And it activates receptors similar to those motivated by nicotine (another popular nootropic compound). It's great for chill clarity with an edge. The daily dose ranges from 150 to 450 mg.[17]

According to an animal study, 1 to 10 mg of nefiracetam improved learning and memory deficits in amyloid-β-(1–42)-infused rats. And 3 mg increased the activity of choline acetyltransferase in the hippocampus.[18]

Phenylpiracetam

If you want the benefits of piracetam with a fraction of the dose and an additional lift in energy, this is your pick. In certain trials, 200 mg of phenylpiracetam has been shown to reduce symptoms associated with cognitive decline.[19] Daily dosages of this supplement range from 200 to 600 mg.[20]

Noopept

Science says Noopept is a thousand times more powerful than its big brother piracetam. With an increase in nerve growth factor (NGF) and a sensitizing effect on acetylcholine receptors, Noopept is a workhorse in helping improve memory formation. It's recommended that you take 10 to 30 mg once daily.[21]

In one study, taking 10 mg twice daily appeared to be more effective in aiding in recovery of brain damage from vascular damage than 12 grams of piracetam.[22]

Sunifram

A solid AMPAkine—any of a class of synthetic compounds that facilitate transmission of nerve impulses in the brain and appear to improve memory and learning capacity—sunifram works a lot like nefiracetam but at a fraction of the dose (5 to 10 mg). A derivative of piracetam (the mother of all racetams), it has shown measurable results in animals with impaired mental performance. Both glutamine and choline levels are enhanced.

CDP-Choline

CDP-choline, aka citicoline, is the gold standard in choline donors. Its low-dose, fast-acting, long-lasting benefits make it a nootropic as well as a powerful choline donor for racetams and the like. You'll get a slight boost in mental capacity and endurance with a dose as low as 100 to 200 mg.

One study showed memory performance in recall tests (immediate and delayed object recall, word recall, etc.) significantly improved with supplementation of CDP-choline at 500 to 1,000 mg daily in older people with memory deficits.[23]

Phosphatidylserine

Take 300 to 600 mg a day (in divided doses of 100 or 200 mg) and watch your cortisol-induced anxiety plummet while your mental and physical endurance climbs noticeably. Also neuroprotective, phosphatidylserine can help attention-deficit/hyperactivity disorder (ADHD) sufferers stay on task. Also, it's effective for reducing the refractory period in men.

One study showed that symptoms of cognitive decline and dementia were improved with phosphatidylserine supplementation in elderly people with 300 mg over six months.[24]

Acetyl-L-tyrosine

Acetyl-L-tyrosine increases noradrenaline and dopamine in a noninvasive way, helping improve focus and follow-through. But it's such a good precursor to both, it helps keep adrenal fatigue from rearing its ugly head during high-stress events.

Acetyl-L-tyrosine can preserve mental performance during physically strenuous situations or instances of sleep deprivation when taken in doses ranging from 45 to 68 mg per pound.[25]

Schizandrol A

This berry extract is a powerhouse when it comes to both dopamine stimulation and cardiovascular enhancement. Used correctly, it seems to quickly promote focus and optimism. The peripheral benefits are so exhaustive that some consider it a superfruit. Daily dose ranges from 100 to 400 mg three times a day, but you can also take a dose as low as 50 mg.[26]

Caffeine

Caffeine is the most popular nootropic in the world (especially as found in coffee beans, green coffee bean fruit, and guarana). Adding it to just about any nootropic stack can increase stack performance. Aside from increasing vigilance and touching just about every key neurotransmitter, caffeine has a semisecret purpose with nootropics.

While the brain is processing certain nootropics (converting to or optimizing the key neurotransmitters for mental performance), you can experience a slight brain performance downshift. Caffeine can "upregulate" receptors to overcome that lag, so when the nootropics hit, you're primed for performance. Coffee fruit extract also increases BDNF by as much as 140 percent (a significant rise).

While the consumption of caffeine is correlated with a higher risk of cardiovascular diseases, including elevated blood pressure and plasma homocysteine, consuming moderate amounts of caffeine (300 to 400 mg per day) has little-to-no health risks and some evidence of health benefits.[27]

Theanine

Though caffeine can speed things up, it's also a great way to put you on a roller coaster of performance peaks and valleys. To smooth things out, theanine—a compound most commonly extracted from green tea—acts on GABA and glutamate receptors, balancing calmness with gentle wakefulness (at low dosage, about 200 mg).

Higenamine

This is a very cool stimulant, especially paired with gingerol (shogaöl), that is unique in that it has shown to both burn fat and improve breathing potential. For nootropics, it can provide a unique rise in cognition without increasing dopamine levels. Combined with 6-8-10 gingerol (and their resulting shogaols), the heart-protective and fat-burning benefits measurably increase. Doses range from 20 to 30 mg taken two to three times daily.[28]

Uridine Monophosphate

Uridine mono is a fantastic solution to increasing dendrites and raising phosphatidylcholine levels at the synapse.

Giving rodents a single dose of the uridine source uridine monophosphate increases their brain levels of CDP-choline by 50 percent.[29] The recommended dose is 150 to 250 mg per day.[30]

Triacetyluridine

This is uridine mono's big sister (at five times more potent), with the additional ability to radically improve mood and help remove detritus from overactive glutamate receptor activity. A small dose (25 to 50 mg) at night can prime the brain for a clear morning.

N-acetyl-L-cysteine

Currently under fire by the FDA, n-acetyl-L-cysteine (NAC) is a precursor to glutathione, the body's most powerful antioxidant. Research also indicates it can quiet the overactive mind, and it's finding many uses in psychology and psychiatry.

Five studies provided data on 574 participants, showing that n-acetyl-L-cysteine treatment alleviated depressed symptoms more than placebo treatment.[31]

Daily dose ranges from 500 to 3,000 mg.[32]

Vitamin D_3 Cholecalciferol

Modern medicine is just now realizing that a large swath of the world is potentially deficient in vitamin D_3 (as it's made primarily from UVB rays on the skin).

A good 5,000 IU of D will help upregulate many critical brain functions and may also alleviate some symptoms of depression. People ages 18 and older can take as little as 4,000 IU per day.[33]

Omega-3 Oils (Fish, Krill, or Algae)

Everything in the brain works better with DHA and omega-3 (anti-inflammatory) oils. In fact, coupling these natural oils with nootropics is all but guaranteed to multiply your results. We've found that taking 3,000 to 6,000 mg of a good DHA or EPA source can support the benefits of nootropic stacks by 150 to 500 percent in terms of duration and experiential performance.

Researchers believe that long-chain omega-3s safeguard cognitive function by assisting in the maintenance of neuronal activity and cell membrane integrity in the brain.[34] In support of this hypothesis, certain case-control studies show that patients with Alzheimer's disease have lower DHA levels in their blood than cognitively healthy people.[35, 36]

The recommended daily doses of these key nootropics ranges so widely because optimal amounts vary from person to person. That's why personalized products are so imperative for maximizing mental performance. Nootopia has done all of the hard work of combining these ingredients (and more) into powerful stacks and then personalizing them for you.

NOOTROPIC POWER MOVES

There are key things you want to do (and don't want to do) to get the most out of your nootropics.

Nootropic Power Move #1: Stack Your Fats

Many nootropics are fat soluble—they look for a source of fat to bond to, which helps the nootropics cross through the blood-brain barrier (BBB). It also helps modulate the effective release of the nootropic's key neurotransmitters for a longer half-life and a more measured uptake. This helps eliminate peaks and valleys, providing you with more effective, longer-term benefits.

Stacking all your fat-soluble supplements with fats with creates a major breakthrough in nutrient absorption. For example, research has shown you can boost CBD absorption in the bloodstream 800 percent by taking it with a high-fat meal. You can get similar absorption gains with many other key nutrients.

We suggest taking 5 to 10 grams of high-quality fats, fat-soluble nootropics, and fat-soluble supplements in one shot. These might include:

- Fish or krill oil
- Algae oil
- Buttered coffee with MCT oil or butter (See Matt's Zamner Zone coffee recipe on page 223)
- Other high-quality fats: olive oil, macadamia nuts, Brazil nuts, pecans
- Vitamins A, D, K, and E
- Nootopia caps (Brain Flow, Upbeat, Focused Savagery, and Apex)
- CBD, CBG, or CBN oil

Nootropic Power Move #2: Movement Is Life

Many people take supplements and immediately become sedentary. They sit in one place and expect the supplement to do their heavy lifting. That's not how it works.

With nootropics, first, you're in a race to get the active ingredients (the "stack") into the bloodstream and then through the BBB. It takes blood flow to make that happen. Passivity is the enemy of blood flow. Sitting sucks for optimizing brain performance.

The ideal would be a 5-to-15-minute moderate cardio workout: biking, walking, yoga, swimming, and so on.

For peak mental performance throughout the day, you must move—ideally every 30 to 60 minutes. Your body starts downshifting health wise and energy wise if you don't move after an hour.

Pressed for time? Don't worry, because you don't need to do a full workout to activate your nootropics and reenergize your body. Every hour, just 60 seconds of movement will make a massive difference in your energy and brain performance. The key is to make it a habit. Put an alarm or notification on your phone "to move." Micro bouts of movement are all that's needed.

Here are a few simple Power Moves you can do:

- Walk around the block
- A set of air squats
- A set of push-ups
- A few yoga poses
- Dance!

Whatever you can do to accelerate blood flow will dramatically aid the performance of your nootropic stacks.

Avoid Protein with Nootropics

Protein is the seed of life, but it blunts the effects of nootropics. Many nootropics are created from amino acids (pyroglutamic acid, glutamate, GABA, and tryptophan are typical precursors). So, protein, an amalgam of 20 amino acids, competes with the more fragile nature of nootropics.

Taking your Nootopia stacks "away from" protein is how you best experience the nootropic benefits. We suggest taking them 60 minutes before, or 45 or more minutes after, a high-protein meal. That will help you maximize your nootropic absorption.

Timing Your Nootropics: Peaking around Key Events

The goal with your nootropic planning is to focus it around the most important thing in your day—a key event. It could be a presentation, a sales pitch, a deep work session, a team meeting, a creative work session, and so on. That's when you want to peak.

For example, if you have a presentation at 2 P.M., then taking your Apex 90 minutes before will help you be in a peak state for your talk.

Other Helpful Brain Supplements

Here are a few key supplements that can really help you get the most out of your day:

- kApex: take three to five capsules on an empty stomach. This will give you 6 to 10 hours of enhanced energy without using any stimulants.
- Cognibiotics: the combination of mood-enhancing herbs and brain-enhancing probiotics will help boost your dopamine, serotonin, and BDNF.
- Magnesium Breakthrough: take one to two capsules to give your nervous system the support it needs to handle the challenges of life.
- CollaGenius: add 4 tablespoons of CollaGenius® to an 8-ounce glass of water to enhance neurogenesis and BDNF.

The Brilliant Mind Blueprint

We wrote a book called *The Brilliant Mind Blueprint,* which outlines dozens and dozens of tips and strategies to optimize your brain. It's available for free at www.nootopia.com/book/blueprint.

EVENING RITUALS

The evening is the time to downshift your brain. Yes, you can work in the evening if you want to. However, you should stop working at least three hours before bed.

The other major key is not eating for three hours before bed. We've found in ourselves and in clients that it crashes sleep quality on Oura Ring scores.

Three Hours before Bed

You want to start simulating dusk at this time, so dim the lights throughout the house. You can install dimmers that you can automate with smart-home apps.

Two Hours before Bed

It's important to start slowing down your brain waves at this point.

The Brain Dump Process

We often have a bunch of random thoughts working in the background of our minds.

To clear them from yours so you can sleep better, try this great process Matt learned from one of his marketing mentors, John Reese. On paper or in a journal, write down every single thing that comes through your brain—every project, every worry, every thought—and keep going until there's nothing left. Once you go blank, stop. It's that simple. That exercise can be a life-changer for people who struggle to slow down their brains because of the endless stream of thoughts.

One Hour before Bed

No more electronic devices. This is a good time to read spiritual books using dimmed, low-blue-light reading lights.

It's also time to load up on sleep supplements:

- Take two to three capsules of Magnesium Breakthrough.
- Mix two scoops of Sleep Potion with 4 ounces of water and sip it for the next 30 minutes.

You can quiet down your beta brain waves with meditation, so for some people, it's a great time to do that. It's also a good time to do another session of neurofeedback, especially theta training.

Beware of Light

At this time, beware of having bright lights hit your eyes, which reawakens your mind.

WHAT SHOULD YOU EAT FOR PEAK MENTAL PERFORMANCE?

The best mental performance food differs from person to person. Many people thrive mentally on a keto diet. If you feel you've got more energy and brain clarity when you eat that way, then you're probably getting a lot out of ketones.

If you find your energy is low on a ketogenic diet, then carbs are probably better for you. Eating complex carbs, fiber, and protein will help you maintain a stable blood sugar level throughout the day. Blood Sugar Breakthrough will also help you better utilize the glucose from the carbs.

YEARLY MASTER BRAIN OPTIMIZATION PLAN

If you're serious about taking your cognitive abilities to the pinnacle, then this is for you.

For the last few years, we've done several weeklong brain transformation programs. We've gone to several of the top facilities in the world and worked with the brain masters on the cutting edge of brain-enhancing technologies. There is a ground-breaking new headset that allows anyone to train their brains anywhere. All you need is a phone. Visit www.BIOptimizers.com/book/neurofeedback to learn more.

Maximizing the Brain Gains

We innovated and broke dozens of brain-training records at these facilities by hyper-optimizing our brains and bodies for this intense week of training.

The combination of the right amount, intensity, and type of brain training plus loading your body with every brain-boosting compound equals the metamorphosis.

CONCLUSION

The final key point we want to make here is the power of compounding all of these strategies, technologies, and nootropics. We've hammered the power of stacks and synergy throughout this book, and applying this principle to the brain is no exception.

The more of these breakthrough brain enhancers you combine, the better your brain will perform.

Make sure to visit www.nootopia.com to stay up to date on the latest in brain-enhancing supplements and technologies.

SUMMARY

This chapter is for those who need their brains to be at their peak, such as:

- Highly driven entrepreneurs
- High performers
- Business executives
- Creatives

The Perfect Brain Day

We give a 24-hour view of all of the activities, foods, and supplements you can use to be in a peak state all day.

First, it's important to honor your chronotype to know when you should wake up each day:

- Lions are morning people
- Wolves are night people
- Bears are in the middle
- Dolphins are light sleepers who struggle to get a good night's sleep

Upon Waking Up

The main goal is to go from tired to fully optimized within 15 minutes after waking:

- As soon as you wake up, drink 500 ml of water
- Shine light in your eyes
- Meditate
- Follow breathing practices
- Journal
- And more

Stacking Biohacking Technologies and Processes

Stacking various biohacking technologies like the ones below is a major Power Move:

- Photobiomodulation
- Pulsed electromagnetic field therapy (PEMF)
- CVAC
- Neurofeedback
- Grounding
- Sunlight in your eyes

Key Brain Supplements

It's important to choose the best nootropic stack to help you be optimal for your day. Try these:

- kApex
- Cognibiotics
- Magnesium Breakthrough

Nootropic Power Moves

Some nootropic Power Moves include:

- Stack your fats
- Movement is life
- Avoid protein with nootropics
- Time your nootropics so you peak around key events

Evening Rituals

It's super important to downshift your brain at night. You can work in the evening if you want to, but you should stop at least three hours before bed.

GOAL #5:

MAXIMIZING YOUR BIOSPAN AND JOINING THE CENTURY CLUB

The next chapter will show you how you can live a long, strong life and maximize your chances of making it to the Century Club, which means you live a great life to 100+ years old and beyond.

CHAPTER 19

ASSEMBLING THE ULTIMATE BIOPTIMIZATION MASTER PLAN

In this chapter, you'll learn:

- How to know if a diet, supplement, or biohack will bring you toward Biological Optimization
- Our tried-and-true, three-step framework, which has helped thousands of people achieve Biological Optimization against all odds
- Key biological levers to assess and test for Biological Optimization
- How to maximize your health span and life span for a long, healthy life
- The ultimate way you can buy more time and even add decades to your career
- The three physical fundamentals of longevity you must implement if you want to become a centenarian and beyond
- The three nutritional fundamentals of longevity
- Why you need your own Jedi Council to run the Biological Optimization Process successfully

The BIOptimization master plan is primarily about maximizing your life span and your health span. The goal is to live a long, healthy, rich life full of epic adventures. This chapter puts all the puzzle pieces together.

Achieving and maintaining biological optimization is a never-ending process. The structure of this chapter is very different from previous master plan chapters, and it might seem a bit daunting at first, but don't worry. The journey to reach your biological apex and become BIOptimized happens one step at a time.

THE ONLY WAY YOU CAN BUY TIME

A lot of wealthy people will tell you that the most precious asset they have is time, because they can't buy more of it. This isn't true. There is one way you can buy time: by optimizing your health. With biological optimization, you can extend your prime by decades and can add that much high-quality life.

A lot of people retire in their mid-50s or mid-60s. Why? They've lost their drive. Men's testosterone and dopamine is in the gutter. Their mitochondria get weaker and die. They struggle to work for 8 to 12 hours a day, even if they want to.

Some retire because cognitive decline really starts kicking in. In our opinion, decline is completely unnecessary. People can stay sharp and active, work, and be productive until they pass. Following the suggestions in the previous chapter will help you maintain a highly functioning brain.

The Biological Optimization Process can add decades to your career as well. From a purely return-on-investment perspective, it's one of the best investments you can make.

We are seeing this in sports with the longevity of legends like LeBron James and Tom Brady. They're adding years to their careers, which for them is worth tens or hundreds of millions of dollars. If entrepreneurs like Elon Musk added a few extra decades to their lives, how much additional value could they create for the world?

Shift Your Paradigm around Aging

Most people have resigned to the idea that their bodies and brains peak in their late 20s and then the decline begins to happen. And they will live the last few years of their lives in a decrepit state. We challenge you to see life in a new way. If you invest the energy, time, and resources into your brain and body, you can very likely extend your life and more importantly: you will live a better life.

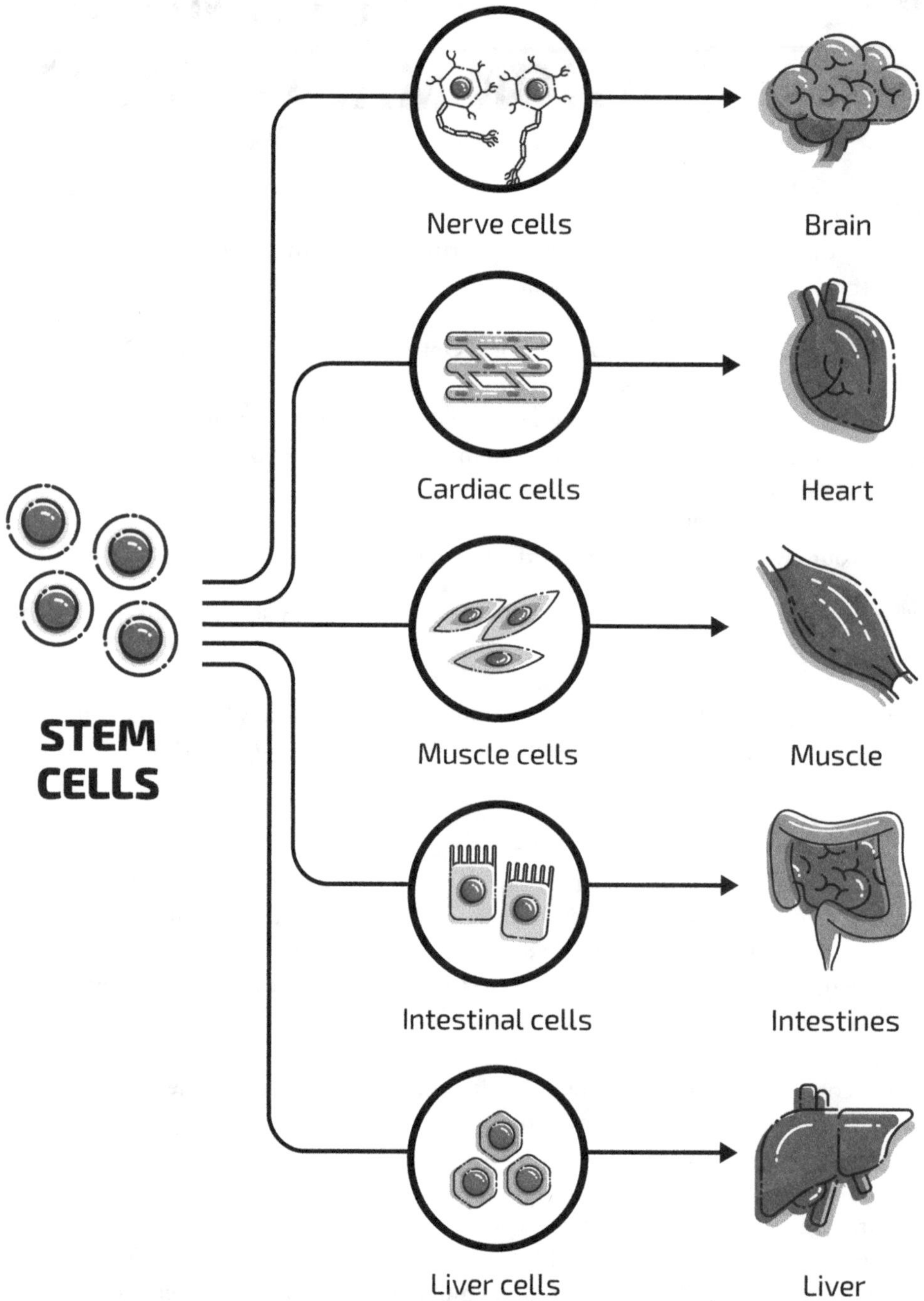

Stem cell therapy is one of the most promising new fields for anti-aging benefits. Stem cells convert into various types of cells and are critical for repair and longevity. We believe that it will be possible within our lifetime to live well beyond 100 years old.

DON'T BURY YOUR HEAD IN THE SAND

A lot of people don't want to look at health data. They're scared that it will reveal something they won't like. A lot of people are scared to go to the doctor. They're scared of looking at their health markers. However, they're really doing a massive disservice to themselves, because often these things can easily be fixed early on.

Your health is like a long boat voyage. If you're off course a few degrees, you'll end up in Africa instead of Paris. A lot of people have minor health issues that are suboptimal, and they don't feel them. There are a lot of things in the body that we don't feel. But when you look at your bloodwork, you can see that it's off.

The sad part is, many disastrous health icebergs that people deal with now could have been avoided. Many degenerative conditions started decades earlier. Instead, people bury their heads in the sand and wait for serious health issues to rear their ugly heads. Sometimes, it's too late. Multiple systems are severely compromised. The transmission was damaged and blew out the motor.

What's the cost of being taken out by a heart attack or stroke in your early 50s? What's the cost to your family? What's the cost to your society? What's the cost to your sense of happiness and satisfaction during the course of your life?

That's why the Biological Optimization Process is so important. Regularly getting high-quality health data and having your Jedi Council make adjustments is the key to optimizing your health.

RUN YOUR BODY LIKE A BUSINESS

You want to manage your body like a well-run corporation. You wouldn't run a business without solid accounting. How do you think you can run your life without solid biological accounting? Your health is your most precious asset. Treat it that way and protect it.

Running blind, without data, is like not paying taxes for a decade and hoping you won't get caught. It's a bad day when the tax man shows up with a bill for back taxes owed *plus* penalties.

HOW THE BODY FALLS APART

The body is incredibly resilient. The proof of that is when you see obese people who constantly consume a wide variety of toxins like excess calories, alcohol, cigarettes, and inflammatory foods for decades, yet their bodies still achieve homeostasis.

However, eventually homeostasis breaks, and their bodies fall apart. The journey to sickness is usually a chain reaction that starts once a key organ or biological system becomes compromised.

Look at the body from a multi-decade perspective. If a system is suboptimal for decades, it can fall apart and activate a cascade of health problems.

A lot of people mistakenly think that if they get surgery on a diseased organ, it fixes the problem. Unless they address the underlying conditions that led to organ failure, they've only gained temporary relief.

Today, the medical industry is designed for acute care just to keep you alive. It's in the business of selling you surgeries and drugs.

THE 10 AGING DRIVERS

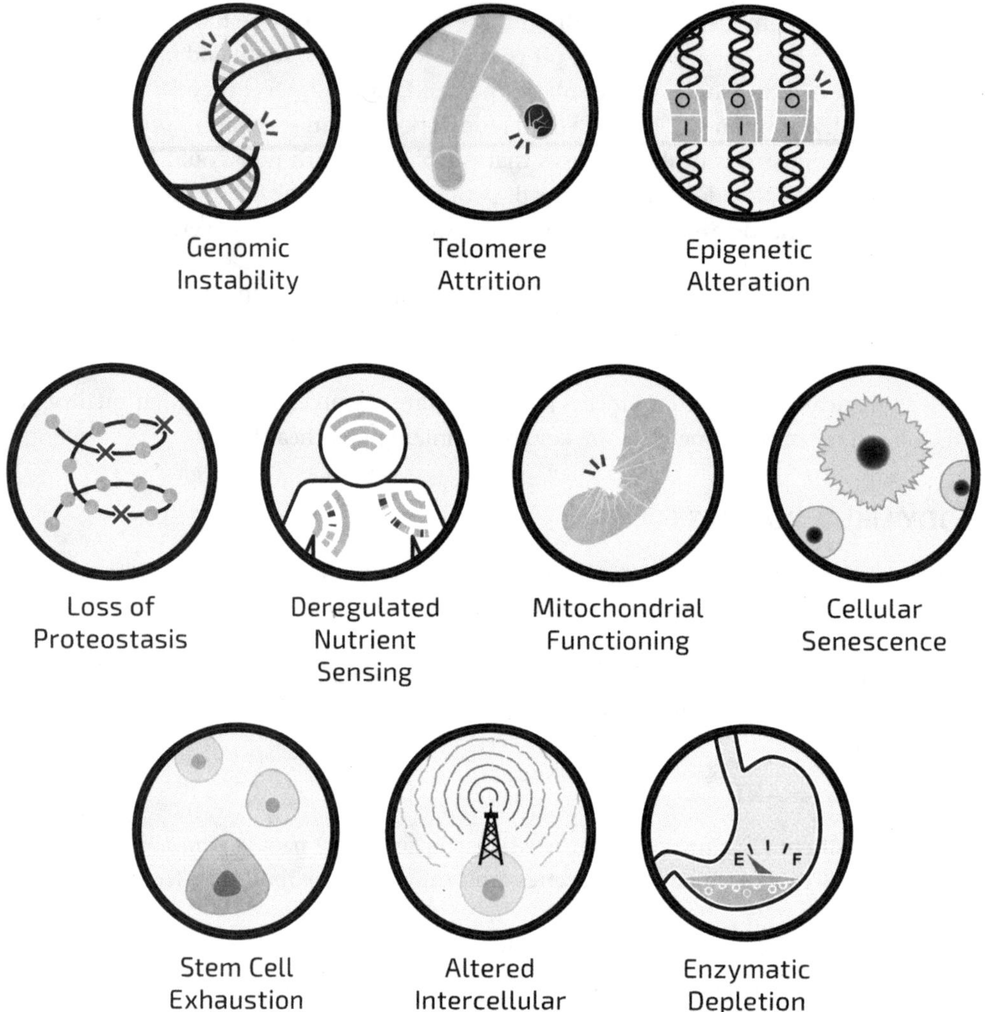

If we look at our DNA as software, we can state that it's designed to have an awesome user experience until we get to our golden age. However, we have the power to upgrade the code, thanks to epigenetics.

If you implement the Biological Optimizers in this book, you'll positively upgrade your code and have a much better user experience of life in your 80s, 90s, and beyond. The way to extend life is to incorporate healthy habits that counter, slow down, and minimize the negative impact of these 10 aging drivers.

1. Genomic Instability
2. Telomere Attrition
3. Epigenetic Alteration
4. Loss of Proteostasis
5. Deregulated Nutrient Sensing
6. Mitochondrial Functioning
7. Cellular Senescence
8. Stem Cell Exhaustion
9. Altered Intercellular Communication
10. Enzymatic Depletion

It's critical to note that the interlink and correlations between these aging drivers are very high. Some of them directly impact other aging drivers. In our book *From Sick To Superhuman*, we dive deep into each one of these.

THE PHYSICAL FUNDAMENTALS OF LONGEVITY

- Get your body fat down to a healthy range and maintain it.
- Build a healthy amount of lean muscle mass and maintain it. This can be accomplished with three weight lifting workouts a week.
- Aim for about two hours of movement a week.

These three objectives are foundational if you want to become a centenarian and beyond.

Goal Shifts over Time

Your teens and 20s are a good time to focus on muscle building, fat loss, and sports performance. When you build lean body mass, you don't lose it very easily. You only need about one-third of the training volume to maintain lean muscle mass. Muscle is valuable because it absorbs and utilizes glucose. Having stable, healthy blood sugar levels is essential for anti-aging.

Excess body fat is not healthy. If you want to live a long, healthy life, then losing excess body fat is crucial. It's not just for aesthetics but for improving health markers, lowering inflammation, and lowering triglycerides.

As you move into your 30s and beyond, brain optimization becomes critical. It's a great time to start doing intensive neurofeedback and meditation, and using personalized nootropics like Nootopia.

As you get into your 40s and beyond, longevity and quality of life are the name of the game. It's time to optimize your health to extend your life span and health span. Read our book *From Sick to Superhuman* to learn about hundreds of ways you can slow down aging and maximize your health span.

THE NUTRITIONAL FUNDAMENTALS OF LONGEVITY

- Optimize your key nutrients and maintain optimal levels.
- Pull toxins from your body and minimize their intake.
- Live in a slight calorie deficit most of the time.

What Are the Key Anti-Aging Mechanisms?

Aging is extremely complex. We have only begun to understand all of the aging pathways. Based on today's science, here are some promising ways to extend your BioSpan:

- Reduce body fat and related inflammatory markers
- Increase autophagy and apoptosis, reducing the accumulation of damaged and zombie cells[1]
- Increase nicotinamide adenine dinucleotide (NAD+)
- Lower IGF-1
- Lower mTOR
- Activate sirtuins
- Reduce metabolic rate (reflected as reduced core temperature and T3) and thus less oxidative damage[2]

For an extensive review of aging science, read Chapter 2 of *From Sick to Superhuman,* Biological Enemy #1: The 10 Aging Drivers.

Immortal Chicken Cells

At the Rockefeller Institute in New York City, French surgeon and scientist Alexis Carrel and his colleagues maintained live heart tissue cultures from chicks between 1912 and 1946. The cells were labeled "immortal," since the culture had lasted far longer than a normal chick's life span. He showed that a cell is possibly immortal if you take care of it long enough.[3]

One thing that can kill cells is toxins. An overload of them disrupts healthy cell function. When toxins accumulate beyond the body's ability to remove them, health issues can occur.

Throughout this book, we've praised the power of protein. However, undigested, unassimilated protein is a form of toxin. In fact, one theory about the primary cause of death in supercentenarians is protein agglomeration. Why? Proteins accumulate in cells, and eventually the cells stop working.

This is why we're big believers in taking a lot of proteolytic enzymes on an empty stomach. We believe they dramatically improve autophagy. A main benefit of autophagy is breaking down proteins and cleaning them from cells. So, taking a lot of MassZymes on an empty stomach is a great anti-aging strategy.

The Cost of Deficiencies

One thing that causes cells to function suboptimally and eventually to stop altogether is nutritional deficiency. We know the immediate consequences of deficiencies in macrominerals like magnesium, sodium, and potassium.

However, what hasn't been researched or documented are the long-term consequences of trace mineral deficiencies. In our opinion, cells function at their best if they have every single essential nutrient, including all trace minerals. These are vital co-factors that optimize the bio conversions within cells. We believe that the consequences of any deficiencies play out over decades and go unnoticed. Read the Magic of Micronutrients in Chapter 27 and incorporate its suggestions.

Living in a Calorie Deficit

Calorie restriction as a form of life extension has been researched for several decades now. In many short-lived species, the life extension benefits of chronic calorie restriction are well documented.[4, 5, 6] However, the implications in humans and other primates are still being debated. That being said, we believe that these anti-aging pathways tend to increase health span and improve metabolic health in humans.

In gray mouse lemurs, 30 percent chronic restriction extends life span by 50 percent. However, while restriction reduced age-related diseases and preserved brain white matter, the restriction group seems to have had accelerated gray matter loss through their cerebrum.[7] This is possibly from a deficiency in healthy fats and/or a lack of key nutrients. This is why supplementation is even more important for people who are focused on lowering calories.

Caloric restriction is scientifically defined as a reduction in energy intake well below the number of calories that would be consumed naturally. The calorie deficit ranges are usually greater than or equal to 10 percent in human studies and usually 20 percent or higher in rodent species.

How much did restriction move the needle? It has ranged as high as 60 percent in the most extensively studied rodent models.[8]

Creating long-term, calorie deficit longevity research on humans is extremely difficult. Most people don't want to subject themselves to multi-year diets.

Some initial evidence of caloric restriction efficacy comes from epidemiologic studies of long-living populations, such as the Okinawan centenarians. They are famous for their Confucius-inspired phrase *hara hachi bu*, which we've seen before. It means to eat mindfully and stop eating at 80 percent full,[9] which is a common practice among centenarians in the Blue Zones.[10]

Okinawans seem to be in a caloric restriction of around 10 to 15 percent throughout their lives. Part of the deficit also comes from physically demanding occupations such as farming and fishing. Also, their diet is nutrient dense, although low in calorie density.[11]

Although long-range caloric restriction studies are difficult, a few have been published. The National Institute on Aging sponsored a comprehensive assessment of the long-term effect of reducing intake of energy (CALERIE) trial, enrolling 218 non-obese participants aged 21 to 50. This study aimed to find both the benefits and side effects of long-term caloric restriction, with eating disorders being a main concern.[12]

The caloric restriction (CR) group was in a 25 percent caloric deficit, half from diet and half from physical activity. The control group ate its normal diet.

No serious adverse events were reported. The main adverse events that were more frequent in the calorie-restricted group than the control group were dysmenorrhea, dizziness, diarrhea, and constipation. Normal-weight participants were more likely to have adverse events than the slightly overweight ones.[13] Also, the following relevant adverse effects were observed:

- 5 of 143 in the CR group vs. 1 of 75 controlled participants developed moderate depression.
- The bone densities of the lumbar spine, hip, and upper leg (intertrochanteric) were significantly lower at months 12 and 24 in the CR group compared to the control. This was probably due to mineral deficiencies.
- The CR group's heart rate also slowed down, possibly due to reduced sympathetic and thyroid function.
- 65.7 percent of CR vs. 52 percent of control groups had Multiaxial Assessment of Eating Disorder Symptoms scores, suggestive of eating disorders at some point during the study, but there were no officially diagnosed cases. The starvation self-defense mechanisms kicked in.

Phase 1 lasted six months, while phase 2 lasted two years. Participants had the expected weight loss, reduction in insulin, and shrinkage of both fat tissues and liver fat cells. Metabolic parameters across the board improved.

The observed benefits included:

- Reduced total-cholesterol-to-HDL ratios
- Drop in serum triglycerides
- Drop in systolic, diastolic, and average blood pressure
- Drop in fasting blood glucose
- Reduced insulin and improved insulin sensitivity (HOMA-IR)
- Drop in hs-CRP concentrations
- Reduction in oxidative stress
- Most of the weight loss was fat, not muscle

These benefits were not without a cost, however. The CR participants had metabolic adaptations, overall burning about 100 calories per day less than the control group. Most of the reduced calorie burn happened during sleep. The CR group also had a significant drop in leptin and overall activity of the thyroid axis, including TSH, T4, and T3.[14]

Based on what we know about long-term caloric restriction and its potential side effects, you can reap the most benefits and avoid the side effects by cycling in and out of the restrictions and following the Optimized Metabolism framework. You also want to work with a professional to monitor your mental health, overall health, and bone mass. Most important, keep track of your nutrient levels to ensure you're optimal.

Aside from actual caloric restriction, fasting, ketogenic diets, and some supplements can stimulate the same biochemical pathways. These are called caloric restriction mimetics and include such substances as NAD+ and its precursors, the epigallocatechin gallate (EGCG) in green tea, spermidine, allulose, and more.[15]

So, what's our opinion? As you grow older, slowly decrease your calories. One of the easiest ways to do this is to incorporate fasting as a lifestyle. Fasting one day per week, three times every quarter are solid longevity habits. However, it's vital to maintain optimal levels of nutrients at all times.

THE BIOLOGICAL OPTIMIZATION PROCESS

This chapter is perhaps the most important, because the Biological Optimization Process is the ultimate tool for constant, never-ending improvements.

You're biologically unique, with your own sets of genes, goals, and life experiences. Even the best clinical studies cannot predetermine the right combination of diet, supplements, exercise, or biohacks that will instantly make you optimal.

Some of these add incremental gains toward your optimization goals, while others subtract. By making random changes without the right system or understanding of biology, you might not reach your goals. Or you could end up in worse shape than when you started.

This chapter will teach you a scientific improvement framework that helps you identify the key things that move you faster to your goals and avoid wasting time and money on the wrong things.

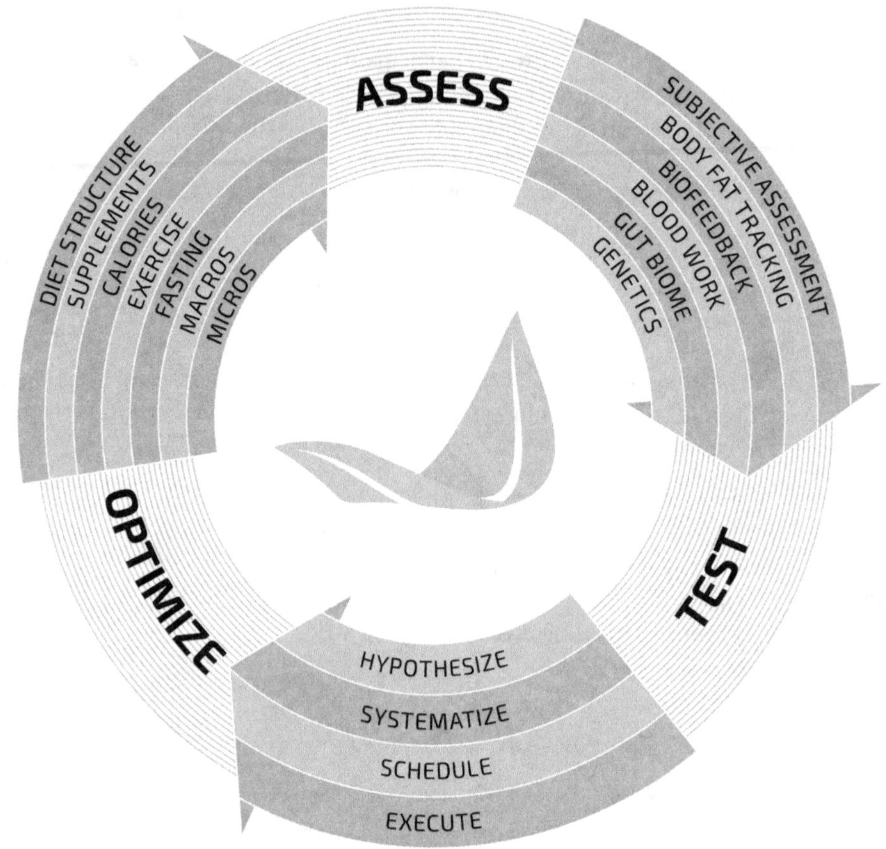

Kaizen Your Way to Superhuman Health

Rather than a "one and done" process, the Biological Optimization Process is our iteration of the kaizen principle, which stands for constant, incremental improvements.

In the past 20 years, we've coached thousands of clients from all walks of life to achieve Biological Optimization against all odds.

The Biological Optimization Process is a three-phase kaizen framework:

1. *Assess.* Evaluate all the relevant objective and subjective data to get an accurate picture of where you are.
2. *Test.* Formulate a hypothesis or a game plan before executing and testing new strategies, diets, exercise programs, and more.
3. *Optimize.* Tweak parameters to optimize your biology with diet, supplementation, exercise, technology, and sleep.

The lifelong journey of Biological Optimization never stops as you improve all three sides of the BIOptimization Triangle: aesthetics, performance, and health. Going through these iterations means you will adapt and reoptimize as your health, environment, and goals evolve.

THE ASSESSMENT PHASE

If you can't measure it, you can't improve it. To optimize, you must assess, measure, and track subjective and objective data.

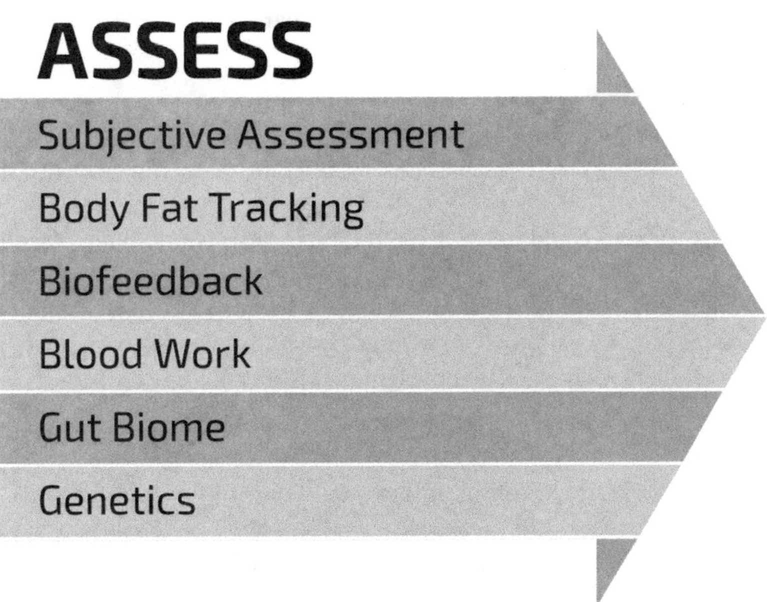

Subjective Assessments

Subjective assessments are your own qualitative assessment of your:

- Current position with respect to your challenges
- Well-being
- Energy levels
- Mental, cognitive, and physical performance
- Mood
- Appearance in the mirror
- Appetite and cravings
- Pain and any other symptoms

Objective Assessments

Objective assessments involve measurable data about what's going on in your body, including measurable biofeedback. You'll measure with:

- Data from your Oura Ring or fitness tracker
- Lab tests
- Body composition measurements
- And much more

Keep in mind that wearables (such as the Oura Ring or fitness tracker) don't come with standard, normal values, because everyone is different. To optimize your biology, first collect and assess your data at baseline. Then, compare your progress to your baseline starting point as you go through the Biological Optimization Cycles.

Biological Levers

The following are key biological levers to assess, because they provide a massive amount of useful and actionable information related to your aesthetics, health, and performance.

1. Body Composition Tracking

Body composition tracking is a critical metric to assess where you're at both from a body fat percentage standpoint and a lean body mass perspective. Dual-energy X-ray absorptiometry (DEXA) scans will also provide bone density assessment, which is important for health span and longevity as you get older.

If you cannot access a DEXA scan, which is the gold standard for body composition assessment, choose the next best option. You may need to use a skinfold caliper, hydrostatic weighing, or Bod Pod. Body circumference measurements and pictures are also helpful pieces of data to track your progress.

2. Heart Rate Variability (Oura Ring)

Heart rate variability (HRV; see Chapter 12) is a real-time measure of your stress and recovery. Persistently low HRV predicts a higher risk of sickness and death from all causes.[16] Therefore, to maximize health span and longevity, aim to maximize your HRV.

What raises HRV for one person could crash it for the next, just as one man's medicine could be another man's poison.

As an example, Matt finds that when he stays on a ketogenic diet or fasts, his HRV shoots up because keto and fasting are compatible with his physiology. However, we know many people who have the opposite HRV response to keto and fasting because these dietary changes are not right for them.

3. Body Temperature (Oura Ring)

Body temperature is a readout of your metabolism, or how well your thyroid is working. A revved-up metabolism keeps your body warm like a hot furnace.

Declining body temperature could be a sign of metabolic adaptation, which precedes a stall in your fitness results. You may need a refeed or diet break to give your body a break.

4. Sleep Tracking

Optimal sleep is the basic foundation for all health goals. If you don't have your finger on the pulse of your sleep quality and quantity to optimize both, you likely will waste years of your life in unrestful sleep.

Matt used to need eight or nine hours of sleep and was still waking up tired.

When he started tracking sleep with the Oura Ring, he was shocked to learn that he was getting no deep sleep at all. After years and thousands of dollars of sleep optimization, he now gets 75 minutes to two hours of deep sleep nightly. Now, he only needs around six or seven hours to wake up refreshed and perform optimally.

5. Physical Performance Tracking

How you feel and how well you perform during your workouts are crucial pieces of biofeedback for how well you've dialed in your nutrification, sleep, stress, and health.

Exercise is a hormetic stimulus to elicit certain responses, such as increasing strength, muscle gain, muscle retention, or neurologic changes. To reap these benefits, you need to be able to recover from workouts. If your performance isn't improving over time, you may need to adjust your program.

If you're in a fat loss program, one of the parameters to monitor is strength. If you're losing strength or if your reps are going down, then you're likely losing some muscle tissue. You may need a refeed, an increase in protein or amino acid intake, or to ease up on the caloric deficit.

6. Lab Tests

Men's health, performance, and aesthetics expert Paul Maximus, N.D., routinely uses the following lab tests, which you can likely get from your medical doctor:

General Screening

- Fasting glucose. A measure of your insulin sensitivity and ability to handle carbs.

- Fasted insulin*. Gives a fuller picture of your blood sugar regulation than fasting glucose alone. For example, it is possible to have normal fasting glucose but very high insulin, which means that you are insulin resistant.
- Cholesterol assesses your metabolic health, risk of heart disease and Alzheimer's disease, and many other conditions.
- Liver function tests include GGT* (gamma-glutamyl transferase), other liver enzymes, and some proteins in your blood. GGT is the best indicator of health and your oxidative stress level.
- Kidney function tests screen for any issues with your kidneys, including diabetes and hypertension.
- Complete blood count screens for anemia, some nutrient deficiencies, blood disorders, and infections.

*In a general checkup, your doctor will typically not order fasted insulin and GGT, so you will have to specifically request them.

SpectraCell Micronutrient Test

This test checks for your micronutrient status over a three-to-six-month time window. They split your blood into 30 different sample tubes to test for micronutrients like vitamin C, calcium, magnesium, chromium, etc. This test also looks at your metabolism, oxidative stress, and immune response.

Protein Unstable Lesion Signature (PULS)

The PULS test estimates your heart attack risk by measuring traces of protein that leak from heart lesions in blood vessel walls, along with HDL, inflammatory proteins, and HbA1c. Based on this, the report estimates your heart age and your likelihood of getting a heart attack in the next five years.

DUTCH: Dried Urine Test for Comprehensive Hormones

DUTCH provides a very illuminating snapshot of your stress response, circadian rhythm, hormone levels metabolism, and toxic hormone metabolites. It is a noninvasive urine test in which you send in dried filter papers that have been saturated with your urine samples.

We recommend the DUTCH Complete, which includes both adrenal and sex hormones. They also now test for neurotransmitters, vitamin, melatonin, and oxidative stress markers in your urine.

The four-point daily cortisol pattern assesses your stress response and circadian rhythm, which could also be abnormal due to inflammation. The ratio of stress hormones to prohormones (DHEAS and pregnenolone) can tell whether your stress is stealing the resources from your sex hormone production, causing hormone imbalances.

Lastly, your toxic hormone metabolites and your hormone metabolism pattern may explain some hormonal symptoms such as hair loss, low libido, weight gain, or acne. Some toxic metabolites increase cancer risks. The DUTCH report also tells you which pathways are responsible for these hormonal issues, so you can address them naturally.

7. Gut Biome

The 100 trillion bacteria in your large intestine work like an extra organ that masterminds all aspects of your health. A rich and diverse microbiota full of friendly species will keep you lean, healthy, happy, and resilient. Conversely, lacking a diverse microbiome and having more unfriendly strains can keep you suboptimal or sick.[17]

Gut health tests can assess the bacteria in your gut. They also tell you which foods are best for good bacteria, and which ones feed the bad ones. Understanding your bacteria can help you optimize your diet for the optimal microbiome. The key is to eat and live right for your microbiome. Go to www.BIOptimizers.com/book/guthealth to do a gut health test—this will help you choose better foods for YOUR gut biome.

Biome Breakthrough is one of the most powerful solutions to optimize your gut health.

8. Genetics

Your genes load the gun, while your environment pulls the trigger. Genetics are not a life sentence. Rather, you can adjust your gene function and mitigate unfavorable genetics with epigenetics.

Genetics is a vast field. You have over 20,000 genes and numerous ways to change your epigenetics. We recommend empowering yourself with a nutrigenomics expert who can help you assess your genes and develop an effective epigenetic optimization protocol. The best way to start is by doing your nutrigenomic test. Go to: www.BIOptimizers.com/book/genes.

Connecting Objective and Subjective Assessments

As you become more experienced in your BIOptimization journey, you will become more in tune with your body. Your subjective assessments will dramatically improve when you connect the body's sensations to hard data.

You will notice that how you feel correlates strongly with certain objective measurements, such as:

- Feeling refreshed after a night of great quality sleep correlates with high deep sleep scores, high HRV, and low resting heart rate.
- Sensations in your body, such as feeling cold or fatigued, indicate your body temperature dropping when you are in an aggressive caloric deficit.
- Feeling extra soreness and inflammation when your HRV is low the day after hard training.
- Having a better mood and cognitive function once your HRV improves.
- Feeling fewer cravings once your sleep and nutrition status become optimized.

TESTING PHASE

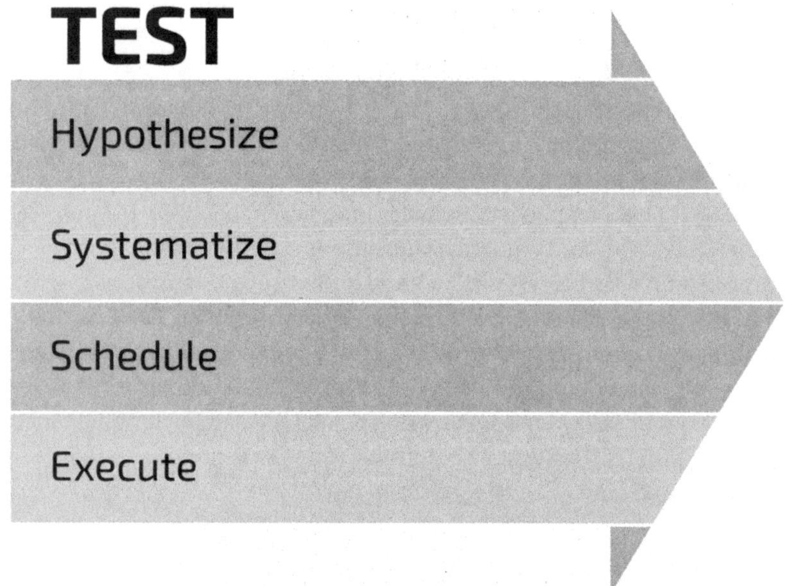

Once we have the data from the assessments, we move on to the testing phase. During this phase, we follow an n = 1 scientific game plan to test out ways to optimize your biology.

You may be self-motivated enough to coach yourself, but we recommend working with a knowledgeable coach to keep you accountable, and troubleshoot as problems arise. See the Jedi Council on page 259 to learn more about this. Or go to www.BIOptimizers.com/coaching.

Hypothesize

Hypothesizing involves formulating an educated guess about changes that will likely lead to the desired outcome. These could be the changes in your exercise, supplement stack, diet, biohacking technologies, lifestyle changes, or other health modalities. An experienced coach will hypothesize based on preexisting science, their clinical experience, and your data from the assessment phase.

Systematize

A guaranteed way to fail is to do whatever you feel like doing or change your plans randomly. The lack of a system will cause confusion and prevent results. Also trying too many changes at once keeps you from knowing which ones produce the results or side effects.

Systematization is all about creating a great game plan. Make sure you have a systematized exercise, nutrition, and supplementation program. Systematize whatever approach you're trying to incorporate in your Biological Optimization journey.

Schedule

Failing to plan is planning to fail. To ensure that implementation happens, you must plan it in your schedule. Scheduling is one of the most powerful ways to ensure that you stick to your plan, and thus guarantee your success.

In other words, plan and build a routine, and stick to it:

- Put your workouts in your schedule
- Plan your diet and prep your food for the week
- Create your supplement stack on paper and stick it on your fridge door or, even better, preload all of your pills in a weekly pill case

Execute

Executing the game plan is the most important part. Even a poorly executed plan is much better than the greatest plan on earth that never gets executed.

OPTIMIZATION PHASE

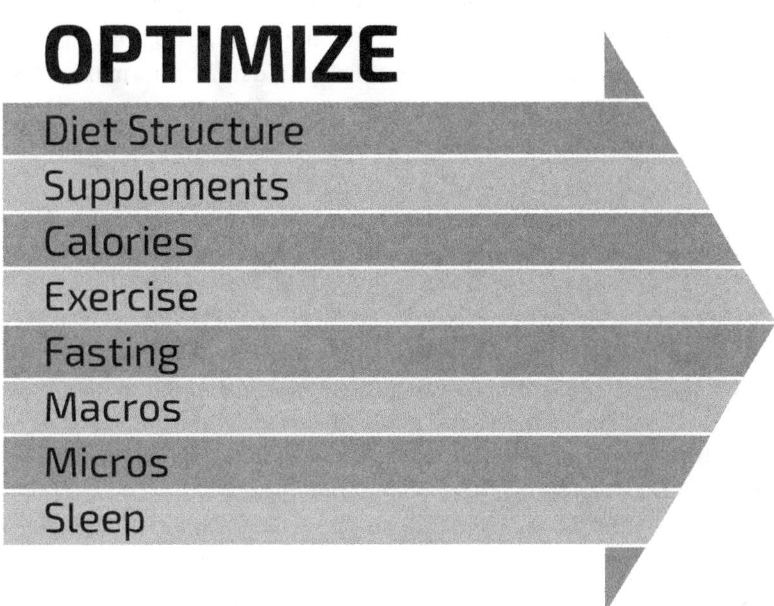

During this phase, we optimize certain parameters for the best results. The biological levers for optimization include diet structure, caloric intake, supplements, and exercise programming.

Diet Structure and Nutrition

Diet structure refers to the kind of diet you will follow. Are you going to follow a ketogenic diet, a high-carb/low-fat diet, a paleo diet, or some other type of diet?

What macronutrient composition will you follow? Typically, high protein along with a caloric surplus will improve muscle anabolism during a muscle-building phase. Whereas when you are in a caloric deficit, the high protein will preserve muscle tissue.

The best macro for you may depend on your genetics and, to some extent, your environment, which is why we reassess.

Micros

Micronutrients, including trace minerals, vitamins, and other nutrients, are essential for your health, aesthetics, and performance. If you can't get optimal levels from your diet, you will need to supplement them.

Feeding/Fasting Window

Fasting overnight every day is important for autophagy and rejuvenation, as mentioned earlier in this book. You may find that extending the fasting window delivers more health benefits, such as fat loss, improved insulin sensitivity, and improved performance. Therefore, the fasting protocol and feeding window are other diet parameters to optimize.

Calories

Your caloric intake is another biological lever with a massive impact on the results you get, be it muscle building, fat loss, or longevity. If you want to gain muscle mass, then you need to be in a caloric surplus. If your goal is to lose body fat, you typically need to be in a caloric deficit. Lastly, if your goal is longevity, then you should be in a slight caloric deficit.

Supplements

We spend a great deal of time talking about supplements in this book. Supplements can have massive impacts on your results, so it is important to optimize your supplement protocol.

Some supplements are beneficial on an ongoing basis. In contrast, others may have more benefits when you start on a high dose or cycle them. Other times, you may find some supplements do nothing or set you back. Therefore, it is essential to reassess the impact of your supplement protocol with data. It's normal for your supplement program to evolve with time.

Exercise

Exercise includes all types of movements we've covered, as well as resistance training. These have massive effects and impact on all three sides of the BIOptimization Triangle: aesthetics, performance, and health goals.

REASSESSMENT PHASE (AND FUTURE ITERATIONS)

After you have implemented the Test and Optimization phases for long enough to affect your physiology, it's time to reassess your bloodwork, body fat, biofeedback, and gut biome to see which changes are happening.

You will then learn whether your hypotheses were true, or whether you need to refine them further or develop alternate ones. Then, you will follow the same process to test and optimize.

One of our core values at BIOptimizers is to test, learn, grow, and evolve. That core value is the process that drives the Biological Optimization Process. We're testing things, we're learning, we're growing from them, and eventually, we will evolve.

Successful BIOptimization requires knowledge, wisdom, discipline, and, often, problem-solving from experienced experts. Studies have also shown that accountability makes people 65 percent more likely to adhere to and follow through with whatever diet and strategy they're using.[18]

This is why we are offering our coaching to those who are serious about their journey into Biological Optimization. Visit www.BIOptimizers.com/book/coaching for more information.

Assembling Your Jedi Council

To do a great job of running the Biological Optimization Process, you need your own Jedi Council. It's almost impossible to be an expert in every aspect of health. The best strategy is to build your own team of health Jedis who can help navigate you through all of your challenges.

We wrote an extensive chapter about this in the appendix of our *From Sick to Superhuman* book, but here's a highly condensed summary of the key experts you want to add to your team.

- *Integrative health coaches* are great "head coaches" for your biological optimization journey. Your best choice is a passionate health expert who is knowledgeable in a wide variety of health topics.
- *Naturopathic doctors* use treatment modalities that can include herbal medicine, counseling, lifestyle medicine, nutrition, homeopathy, manual therapy, and traditional Chinese medicine.
- *Functional* and *precision medicine doctors* are conventional medicine physicians with an expanded toolbox. The best ones use personalized medicine, biofeedback data, and genetic test results.
- *General practitioners* and *medical doctors* are trained to treat diseases and save lives with pharmaceuticals and surgeries. They're important to have on your team, because they can order any standardized lab tests that have been around for a long time. And you may need them in a health crisis.
- *Nutrigenomic experts* can recommend the right genetic tests and interpret the results based on your clinical picture. Then they make recommendations to optimize your genetic expression and address your genetic predispositions for a deficiency, disease, or a metabolic advantage. They can help identify weaknesses and challenges based on your unfavorable mutations and advise you on how to address them.
- *Nutritionists* can help create and optimize your diet over time. Before seeking out a nutritionist, we suggest you decide for yourself the best diet for *you* based on this book. Then find someone who is an expert in the diet type you want to optimize. Ideally, you should find someone who's not stuck in one dogmatic way versus another.
- *Fitness trainers* and *athletic coaches* motivate you and keep you on track with your exercise routines. Do you prefer ass-kickers who pump you up? Or someone who tries to help you resolve emotional blocks? We recommend working with a fitness trainer or coach who has been able to deliver replicable results with multiple people.
- *Yoga practitioners* can help you incorporate exercise that promotes the parasympathetic nervous response. The other key benefits are better posture and increased flexibility.
- *Chiropractors* aren't just people who crack your back. They can help you optimize structural components. Any minor postural issue can also cause problems up and down the kinetic chain. For example, if your back is off by a little bit, it can have ripple effects on other parts of the body, such as the hip, knees, and ankles. It can affect your gait and many other movements.
- *Soft tissue and manual therapy experts* use bodywork, which can be very beneficial as a stress relief and recovery tool—especially the gentler forms such as Swedish massage. The skin-on-skin contact increases oxytocin (the hug hormone) while reducing stress hormones.[19] Massages can also activate the vagus nerve, which relaxes you and reduces inflammation.[20]
- *Physiotherapists* are medical professionals who diagnose and treat injuries, illnesses, surgical recovery, and disabilities. Their toolboxes may include exercises, manual therapy, and other treatment tools.
- *Biohackers* are self-experimenters who leverage technologies, tests, devices, health practices, supplements, and procedures. Biohackers are the best group to follow if you want to keep up with new, cutting-edge breakthroughs in health.

A GREAT ROLE MODEL FOR BIOLOGICAL OPTIMIZATION

We want to praise and highlight the efforts of Bryan Johnson, who is pushing the boundaries of biological optimization perhaps further than anyone ever has. He's spent over two million dollars on his body and has reversed his biological age by five years. He's developed multiple Biological Optimization Processes for various parts of his body. He's relentlessly assessing, testing and optimizing. Google "Bryan Johnson Blueprint" to learn more about what he's doing.

SUMMARY

The BIOptimization master plan is all about maximizing your life span and your health span in the best way possible.

The Physical Fundamentals of Longevity

- Reduce body fat to a healthy range
- Build a healthy amount of lean muscle mass
- Do two hours of movement a week

The Nutritional Fundamentals of Longevity

- Make sure your key nutrients achieve and maintain optimal levels
- Make sure to pull toxins from your body
- Live in a calorie deficit most of the time

Anti-aging Mechanisms Include:

- Reducing body fat and related inflammatory markers
- Increasing autophagy and apoptosis
- Increasing NAD+
- Lowering IGF-1
- Lowering mTOR
- Activating sirtuins
- Reducing metabolic rate

The Biological Optimization Process Is a Three-Phase Kaizen Framework

1. Assess: You must assess, measure, and track subjective and objective data.

- Subjective assessments are your own qualitative assessment of your:
    - Current position with respect to your challenges
    - Well-being
    - Energy levels
    - Mental, cognitive, and physical performance
    - Mood
    - Appearance in the mirror
    - Appetite and cravings
    - Pain and any other symptoms

- Objective assessment involves measurable data such as:
    - Data from your Oura Ring or fitness tracker
    - Lab tests
    - Body composition measurements
    - And more . . .

2. Test: Formulate a hypothesis or a game plan.
    - Hypothesize: Formulate an educated guess about changes that will lead to the outcome
    - Systematize: Build a system to avoid confusion and inaccurate result
    - Schedule: Failing to plan is planning to fail
    - Execute: Executing the game plan is the most important part
3. Optimize: Optimize certain parameters for the best results. The biological levers include:
    - Diet structure and nutrition
    - Feeding/fasting window
    - Calories
    - Supplements
    - Exercise

After those phases, it's time to reassess your bloodwork, body fat, biofeedback, and gut biome to see which changes are happening.

Finally, to run the Biological Optimization Process successfully, you need your own Jedi Council. This could include:

- Integrative health coaches
- Naturopathic doctors
- Functional and precision medicine doctors
- General practitioners and medical doctors
- Nutrigenomic experts
- Nutritionists
- Fitness trainers and athletic coaches
- Yoga practitioners
- Chiropractors
- Soft tissue and manual therapy experts
- Physiotherapists
- Biohackers

EVERY DIET DECODED

The next six chapters cover the core fundamental diets. Ninety-nine percent of diet books are simply slight variations of these core diets.

CHAPTER 20

BIOPTIMIZING THE KETOGENIC DIET

by Matt Gallant

My first foray into keto started when I was 15 and my uncle told me I was fat. I was upset and hated my spare tire, so I decided to try the Atkins Diet to lose the excess body fat. I started doing keto and jogging, going from 190 pounds down to 147 in about six months.

Then I felt too skinny, especially after seeing two huge professional bodybuilders at the beach (fortunately, they didn't kick any sand in my face). Being an impressionable 16-year-old, I was inspired to be less of a scrawny teenager. So, I got bitten by the bodybuilding bug.

Using a cyclical keto diet (CKD) called the Anabolic Diet, plus training twice a day, I bulked up from 147 to 235 pounds in three years. It wasn't all muscle; I gained fat along with it. But back in the day, bulking was the way. (You'll hear more about cyclical keto strategies for building lean muscle and other benefits later in the chapter.)

Then, I decided to compete in my first bodybuilding show. From 235 pounds, I went down to 171 in 14 weeks. That's a 64-pound drop in three and a half months—and I made almost every mistake in the book. But for me, keto was an effective way to build muscle and lose weight.

At 19 years old, I helped my 400-pound best friend lose 191 pounds in 18 months on a cyclical ketogenic diet. At 20 years old, he had never had a date. He became a new man. His transformation was not just physical but also mental and emotional—he got married soon after. Seeing this whole transformation was so rewarding that I knew I wanted to create the same for others for a living.

I became a passionate keto advocate . . . a keto zealot, in fact. I erroneously believed that ketogenic diets were the ultimate solution for everyone. I put all my clients on one and argued with anyone who didn't agree that keto was the best diet ever. However, 30 to 40 percent of my clients didn't do well.

Some had digestive problems. Some lost lean muscle. Some didn't have energy, or they had fatty stools and skin problems. I didn't understand the importance of nutrigenomics at the time. Today, we know that some people aren't genetically built to thrive on keto. To help you find out, go to: www.BIOptimizers.com/book/genes.

That being said, being in ketosis does provide some advantages. Some, who have the appropriate genetics, *thrive* on keto and find it easy to follow. Their food cravings are lower, they have more energy, and their skin complexion improves. And they can easily achieve their goals.

In this chapter, you will learn:

- How to know if the ketogenic diet is right for you—and when *not* to do a ketogenic diet
- How to smoothly transition into ketosis and reap the benefits while avoiding common keto pitfalls and side effects
- Strategies to maximize benefits and metabolic flexibility for lifelong benefits from keto while living an awesome lifestyle without sacrifices or compromises
- How you can use the ketogenic diet as a short-term nutritional strategy for longevity and metabolic benefits
- The four phases of keto adaptation and how to adapt to fat burning so your body never loses the ability (and it becomes easier the next time)
- How to avoid digestive issues (like constipation, acid reflux, or even "disaster pants") when you start on a ketogenic diet

- Why optimizing your fats *and* getting nutrigenomic and blood tests can make a big impact on your health results
- Why you might want to consider the carnivore diet if you get inflammation, gut problems, or immune system triggers from plant-based substances
- The potential downsides to the ketogenic diet and what to consider before you begin that lifestyle and plan out your unique goals

WHAT IS A KETOGENIC DIET?

Traditional ketogenic diets (aka keto) are very low carb (5 percent or less), moderate in protein (20 to 30 percent), and high fat (65 to 75 percent). Your goal in this diet is to enter nutritional ketosis, in which your body is fueled primarily by ketones. Ketones (ketone bodies) are made from short snippets of the fatty acids you eat, or from your own body fat.

Our bodies are adapted to handle:

- Low-to-no-carb diets. Carl the Caveman didn't have access to fruits and veggies during long, cold winters. Eating animal meat and organs was the only way to survive.
- Starvation phases. When one stops eating for long enough to run out of glycogen reserves, the body converts fat stores into ketones. This type of ketosis is called "starvation ketosis" or "fasting ketosis."

Ketosis is *not* the same as ketoacidosis. The latter is the dangerous state of having extremely high blood ketones, which only happens in uncontrolled type 1 diabetes. You don't have to worry about this if you're not a type 1 diabetic.

Keto is a type of low-carb diet, but not all low-carb diets are keto. You can eat a low-carb diet without being in ketosis if you eat too much protein. Your body can convert amino acids into sugar, which can kick you out of ketosis. Atkins Diet is generally low-carb but not necessarily keto. However, once you're highly fat adapted, you can stay in ketosis even when you lower fats and increase proteins (more on this later in the chapter).

On a ketogenic diet, you deliberately cut out all carbs and eat mostly fats, causing the following to happen:

1. Your body uses up all its stored glycogen.
2. Your liver starts producing ketones from the fat you eat.
3. Your brain, muscles, and internal organs increase mitochondria and cellular enzymes that are involved in using ketones for energy.
4. Your anti-aging pathways, such as autophagy and sirtuins, are activated.
5. Your cells learn to shift back and forth between burning sugar and ketones for energy.

UNIQUE HEALTH BENEFITS OF KETO

One of the reasons that ketogenic diets have taken the Internet by storm is that they offer an antidote to the high-carbohydrate standard American diet with the health benefits we discuss below.

Boosted Brain Function and Cognitive Clarity

Ketones are a preferred fuel for the brain, especially in older adults.[1] Ketosis also protects neurons and boosts mitochondrial function in the nervous system, which is why it has been a successful treatment for epilepsy for over 80 years.[2] Therefore, if you enter ketosis, even temporarily or with ketone supplements, you'll experience brain-enhancing benefits.

Some people find that it stabilizes their mood or helps with psychiatric disorders, but individual responses vary.[3]

Reduced Blood Pressure

Ketogenic diets cause your kidneys to excrete more salt and water. Therefore, if you have hypertension, your blood pressure may normalize on a ketogenic diet. For people who naturally have low blood pressure, it's worth monitoring. When Matt was 20, he wasn't consuming enough salt on his strict keto diet, and his blood pressure got too low.

This is why it's critical, especially on a ketogenic diet, to properly mineralize with sodium and potassium to help optimize cellular hydration.

Power Move: Optimizing Hydration on a Keto Diet

Your potassium intake should ideally be around three times your sodium intake. Most people's ratio is out of whack because their sodium is too high and their potassium is too low.

Adding ¼ to ½ teaspoon of high-quality salts (we recommend Himalayan or sea salt) to your water is an inexpensive way to get more minerals into your body. The sodium will help you better absorb the water.

For people on ketogenic diets, we also recommend adding ½ teaspoon of cream of tartar, with the salt, to 2 liters of water once a day to get the necessary amounts of potassium. We also recommend using trace minerals.

Better Insulin Sensitivity and Stable Blood Sugar

Reducing carbohydrate intake typically reduces insulin, which improves insulin sensitivity. Ketogenic diets have also been shown to improve blood lipid profiles and overall metabolic health.[4]

Diminished Appetite and Cravings

Ketosis reduces appetite, even in caloric restriction during a weight loss program.[5] Even after weight loss, ghrelin (the hunger hormone) remains low in people who stay in ketosis.[6]

On a standard American diet, the high carbohydrate content often triggers insulin and blood sugar fluctuations. The blood sugar lows can cause "hangry-ness," which drives people to overeat and crave sugary foods. In ketosis, such fluctuations are virtually eliminated.[7]

For these reasons, many people find it easier to lose weight and keep it off on keto than on other types of diets. Keep in mind that if your goal is weight loss, calories out still need to exceed calories in.

Reduced Inflammation

Ketone bodies have anti-inflammatory and antioxidant properties.[8] Therefore, some people may experience some reduction in pain or remission of a chronic condition.

Chronic low-grade inflammation can cause leptin resistance and increase hunger, and lead to weight gain.[9, 10]

Chronic inflammation goes hand in hand with mitochondrial dysfunction.[11] Ketone metabolism often boosts the mitochondria, which may reduce chronic inflammation.[12] A study compared low-carb/high-fat (56 percent fat, 33.5 percent protein, 9.6 percent carb) with high-carb/low-fat eaters (22 percent protein, 25 percent fat, and 55.7 percent carb). They found that the first group had lower inflammation markers and an improvement in blood lipids than the latter group.[13]

Ketosis stimulates the production of more mitochondria and increases overall mitochondrial function.[14] In some cases, the boost in mitochondria increases metabolism.[15]

A clinical study compared the effects of ketogenic and calorie-counting diets on weight loss for six months. Both groups lost a significant amount of weight, but the keto group lost more and had better insulin sensitivity.[16] In another study from Boston University, 20 obese subjects lost 44.5 pounds within four months on a very low-calorie ketogenic diet. No reduction of resting metabolic rate was observed.[17]

While it doesn't mean you can eat more food, a ketogenic diet might mean that you will find it easier to lose weight and keep it off.

HOW TO START A KETOGENIC DIET

Simply put, to enter ketosis:

1. Cut out all sources of starch and sugar. In the beginning, your overall carb intake should be as low as possible, ideally under 30 grams per day, excluding dietary fibers. This can change in Phases 2, 3, and 4, as we will discuss below.
2. Eat good fats liberally within your calorie limit.

3. Eat just enough protein to preserve your muscles and support your training, but not enough that they kick you out of ketosis. That's usually within 20 to 35 percent of total calorie intake. This too will change as you adapt (more on that below).

MASTERING KETOSIS: THE FOUR PHASES OF KETO ADAPTATION

To be able to efficiently generate and burn ketones for energy, you need to get fat adapted. Fat adaptation can be divided into four phases. You might feel a drop in energy the first 7 to 14 days, but once you become fat adapted, you will reap all the benefits of keto and enjoy diet breaks from time to time. Once you've gone through the process of fat adaptation, your body never loses the ability. It's far easier the second time, and so on.

Phase 1: Getting into Ketosis (First 14 Days)

This phase is about forcing your body to use fat for fuel by depleting your glycogen stores and feeding it with mostly fat. Your liver will ramp up ketogenesis while your cells ramp up mitochondrial activities to burn ketones for energy.

During this phase, start with at least 65 or 75 percent of your calories as fat and 25 to 35 percent protein. Aim for fewer than 30 grams of carbs a day.

Once you deplete glycogen stores, your body might feel "out of fuel." You may experience "keto flu," which could include fatigue, irritability, brain fog, headache, nausea, and sugar cravings. Your exercise performance may also drop significantly. Your body isn't effective at using fats as a primary fuel . . . *yet.*

These symptoms may last from a few days to a week, so plan to take it easy during this phase. Don't stack Phase 1 with your hardest workout weeks and work deadlines.

Power Move: Hacking the "Keto Flu"

Here are some hacks that solve any keto flu issues. Medium-chain triglyceride (MCT) oil, ketone salts, and ketone esters can quickly increase your blood ketones, which will help eliminate most if not all keto flu symptoms. Note that too much MCT oil can cause "disaster pants" (aka flushing diarrhea), so start slowly (1 teaspoon at a time) and gradually increase the dose.

Your appetite might be different from usual, because your blood sugar will be low and your gut microbes still want carbs. During this phase, we usually eat keto-compliant foods to our heart's content. The primary goal is to become fat adapted, not to lose weight (although that usually happens naturally due to the shift from a standard American diet to a regimented diet).

It's not unusual for people to lose 8 to 10 pounds in the first two weeks on a keto diet. The majority of that is a loss of glycogen and water.

Phase 2: Becoming a Fat-Burning Machine (2 Weeks to 3 Months)

After two weeks, your body learns to generate and burn ketones, so you start to feel more energized. Your cravings and keto flu will be gone. Your body will literally become a fat-burning machine. Your lipolytic (fat-burning) pathways are improving. Fat will be your body's primary fuel source.

During this phase, you can start tweaking and optimizing your diet. You want to find out what kinds of foods work best for you and which foods don't work for you.

Humans have genetically evolved to handle feast and famine cycles, rather than having abundant food all the time. During extended famines, our bodies entered ketosis to harness energy from fat. While we're not busy digesting and assimilating nutrients, our cells self-clean (autophagy) and upregulate many rejuvenation processes.[18]

Phase 2 is a good time to start experimenting with intermittent fasting (IF), because it will accelerate your results and force your body deeper into ketosis. Also, already being in ketosis will reduce much of your hunger. The easiest fasting protocol to start with is 16:8—that is, 16 hours of fasting and 8 hours of feeding window. You can start by skipping breakfast and eating most of your food during lunch and dinner. For more information on fasting, see Chapter 30.

Power Move: Experiment with Fasting

Fasting and keto are like peanut butter and jelly—they work great together. Why? Because your body is already in a fat-burning state, so it's easy to start using stored body fat for energy.

This means there are usually very few dips in energy when fasting on keto.

When people fast on a high-carb diet, they might experience what Wade calls "the carb toilet," which means their glycogen levels drop and they lose their energy because they aren't fat adapted.

When you start intermittent fasting or skipping meals, your body releases ghrelin (the hunger hormone) an hour before your daily mealtime. Because you've been eating regularly and your body expects that according to your circadian rhythm, you may feel hunger pangs for at least four days as your body starts to adjust to the new eating schedule.[19]

We don't recommend doing intermittent fasting every day. Why? We believe it's too catabolic, especially if you're training hard. Many people, including well-known health expert Peter Attia, have reported that their lean body mass dropped when they did a lot of fasting. Remember, one of our key objectives is to maintain lean body mass. Instead, do IF two or three days a week. This should lessen metabolic adaptation compared to doing IF every day.

Another option is to fast one day a week. This is a powerful tool that we recommend using as you get deeper into your diet. It's a simple way to reduce your weekly calories by about 15 percent.

When you break your fast and eat large meals during your feeding window, you may experience some digestive issues. We suggest having Biome Breakthrough as your first meal. This will help rebuild your biofilm, which can get thinner after extended fasts. Then, use kApex, HCL Breakthrough, and P3-OM to optimize your digestion.

Phase 3: Metabolic Flexibility (4th to 12th Month)

The longer you stay in ketosis, the better you can generate ketones and utilize them for energy. This is called fat adaptation—your lipolytic pathways get stronger. Your body also gets better at preserving and refilling its glycogen stores if you're doing refeeds, so your strength and exercise performance will improve.

At this stage, we recommend increasing proteins and decreasing fats. Your body will stay in ketosis even with the increased protein, because it's become more efficient at using fat. The increased protein will increase anabolism and also increase your overall calories out from food due to the thermic effect of protein. This makes it easier to lose body fat and maintain lean muscle mass in a caloric deficit.

One of Matt's coaches, Kevin Weiss (a natural bodybuilding and powerlifting champion), used this strategy to get into phenomenal shape and win several championships.

At this point, we suggest decreasing fats to 40 to 60 percent, increasing protein levels to 30 to 50 percent, and raising carbs to 10 percent. The process is to progressively shift your meat selection from those with higher fats to those with lower fats. Here's a chart to help you select lower-fat animal proteins.

Animal Fat and Protein Percentage Chart

FOOD	TOTAL CALORIES	FAT GRAMS	% OF FAT CALORIES	TOTAL PROTEIN	% OF PROTEIN CALORIES
Beef Ribs	351	28.8	74%	23	26%
Prime Rib	341	27.7	73%	23	27%
New York Strip	310	22.9	66%	26	34%
Beef Short Rib	305	22.8	67%	25	33%
Pork Shoulder	292	22.2	68%	23	32%
Lamb Chops	305	21.4	63%	28	37%

T-bone	289	21.0	65%	25	35%
Ground Lamb	283	20.3	65%	25	35%
Pork Rib	261	19.7	68%	21	32%
Rib Eye	271	19.0	63%	25	37%
Lamb Burger	228	18.7	74%	15	26%
Ground Beef	272	18.2	60%	27	40%
Filet Mignon	267	18.1	61%	26	39%
Ground Turkey	258	17.6	61%	25	39%
Ground Bison	238	15.8	60%	24	40%
Top Sirloin	243	15.0	56%	27	44%
Dark Meat Chicken	214	13.6	57%	23	43%
Lean Ground Beef	230	13.1	51%	28	49%
Veal	231	12.3	48%	30	52%
Pork Loin Chop	209	11.7	50%	26	50%
Lean Ground Turkey	213	11.7	49%	27	51%
Ground Chicken	189	10.8	51%	23	49%
Pork Loin	192	9.8	46%	26	54%
Flank Steak	192	8.9	42%	28	58%
Turkey	189	8.1	39%	29	61%
Beef Chuck	191	7.0	33%	32	67%
Extra Lean Ground Beef	175	6.6	34%	29	66%
Ham	139	5.7	37%	22	63%
Pork Tenderloin	147	4.8	29%	26	71%
Skinless Chicken Breast	165	4.6	25%	31	75%
Venison	150	3.3	20%	30	80%
Turkey Breast	147	3.0	18%	30	82%
Extra Lean Ground Turkey	151	2.6	15%	32	85%

Leptin, the well-fed hormone, typically increases with insulin. On ketogenic diets, insulin and leptin are kept perpetually low, like in prolonged fasting.[20] So, if you stay on keto nonstop, you may experience a stall in fat loss and some survival mechanisms kicking in. The following survival mechanisms could cause fatigue, feeling cold, reduced sex drive, or compromised immune function. Also, glycolytic (carb-burning) pathways get weaker over time if you don't eat carbs.

This is why we strongly recommend incorporating refeeds, or what some people call "cyclical keto."

Power Move: Refeeding Carbs to Your Body

Carb refeeding on a ketogenic diet is a powerful strategy. You consume an optimal amount of carbohydrates for one or two days. This will replenish your muscles and liver with glycogen. It will give your brain the pleasure of enjoying some of your favorite carbs again. Your workout performance will improve for two or three days, and you'll look better (if you're lean) because your muscles will be harder and fuller.

Another reason for carb refeeding is that it helps build muscles, and—if you're in a major caloric deficit—maintain lean muscle mass.[21]

This approach is also one of the ultimate lifestyle diets. This means that if you want to go out and enjoy restaurants during the weekends, you can be on strict keto during the week (and in a deficit) and then eat your favorite carbs during the weekend. It's usually pretty easy for people to stay at maintenance (meaning their weight doesn't go up or down) using this model. This isn't a license to go bonkers at the buffet. Matt made that mistake, and it compromised his results.

CYCLICAL KETO DIET STRATEGIES

CKD Strategy #1: Weekend Refeeds

Anabolic Diet

This was the strategy we started with. The Anabolic Diet was developed by Dr. Mauro DiPasquale, a brilliant physician and professional powerlifter. He built it to help bodybuilders get lean and build lean muscle mass. This diet includes five days of low-calorie ketogenic diet and two days of high-calorie, high-carb days.

- If your goal is to lose body fat, do a one-day refeed with weekly calories below maintenance.
- If your goal is to recomp, do a two-day refeed with weekly calories at maintenance.
- If your goal is to gain lean muscle, do a two-day refeed with weekly calories at a slight surplus.

Whether your goal is to gain, maintain, or lose weight, it will come down to your weekly energy balance.

The original Anabolic Diet protocol was two days of carb refeed. Keep in mind that if you want to keep losing body fat, what matters is a weekly caloric deficit. So, if you're eating at a surplus on the weekends, you need to do the math and be in a deeper caloric deficit during the week.

Many studies have shown that people who do carb refeeds or cycle their caloric intake achieve better weight loss results, even though they eat the same total number of calories. A study compared between refeeding and no refeeding among 27 young, well-trained subjects who ate a net 25 percent caloric deficit each week. The group who did two days of carb refeeds weekly, and ate less during the next five days, maintained more muscle mass and metabolic rate than the group that did not do refeeds.[22]

Continuous Group

MON	TUE	WED	THU	FRI	SAT	SUN	AVG
-25%	-25%	-25%	-25%	-25%	-25%	-25%	-25%

For Seven weeks

Refeed Group

MON	TUE	WED	THU	FRI	SAT	SUN	AVG
-35%	-35%	-35%	-35%	-35%	100%	100%	-25%

For Seven weeks

This is also the ultimate recomping strategy (your bodyweight stays the same, but you're getting leaner and adding muscle). Matt has been able to build 4 to 10 pounds of lean muscle mass while losing that many pounds of body fat over the past five years with this strategy.

Your muscle mass expands all three sides of the BIOptimization Triangle: health, aesthetics, and performance. Refeeds help you maximize your lean muscle gains on a keto diet.

CKD Strategy #2: Targeted CKD

Ingest Carbs as a Performance Enhancer

Dom D'Agostino said on our podcast, *The Awesome Health Show,* that if you're fully adapted, you can use carbs as a performance enhancer. Here are some recommended doses based on activity:

- 30 grams of carbs: easy weight lifting workout (arms, abs), or a HIIT workout
- 45 grams of carbs: moderately hard weight lifting workout, or a HIIT workout
- 60 grams of carbs: hard workouts—back, chest
- 80 grams of carbs: brutal workouts—squats, deadlifts

Because you're at Phase 3 fat adaptation, it means you can readily enter ketosis even after a high-carb meal. At this stage, you can start trying carb refeeds to reap the metabolic and psychological benefits.

However, there are pros and cons to carb refeeds that you should understand.

Reasons to Do Carb Refeeds

1. Psychological break. You may enjoy some non-keto foods or the emotional memories associated with them. Even Dr. Peter Attia found it hard to stay on keto, because he missed rice. Being able to take a break from a restrictive diet can be a huge psychological plus. Last, programming in the refeed allows you to enjoy holiday and social gathering meals without feeling like you're "failing" or "cheating."
2. Anabolic response. A temporary increase in calories and insulin can help build and maintain muscle mass.
3. Leptin reset. You get this from eating carbs and eating above maintenance, which helps avoid metabolic adaptation.
4. Improved exercise performance. Your workout will be better, even if you return to ketosis for the next few days. We suggest doing your toughest training on your carb-load days.
5. Metabolic flexibility. Doing carb refeeds regularly helps maintain your ability to burn carbs, even though you stay in ketosis most of the time.

Reasons Not to Do Carb Refeeds

1. Medical contraindications. If you have a medical condition that is best managed by ketosis and may worsen with a carb refeed, then it is best not to do refeeds.
2. Emotional eating, food addiction, or disordered eating. This is a tricky one. If you have one of these issues, you need to keep your refeeds structured and planned. Instead of having a refeed be a free-for-all, create a meal plan for your carb days. We suggest eating only unprocessed carbs, such as fruits, potatoes, sweet potatoes, and white rice.

Do not use your refeed days to gorge on tubs of ice cream. Matt had a client who would eat three pints of Ben & Jerry's for breakfast on carb days. Refeed days weren't good for him because he had emotionally fueled food issues. If you can't control yourself or get back to eating keto the next day, maybe refeeding won't work for you.

Refeed Optimization Supplements

1. Blood Sugar Breakthrough can help control blood sugar and make your cells more sensitive to insulin. Take two capsules, 20 minutes before *every* carb meal.
2. Gluten Guardian contains both gluten and carb-digestive enzymes for high-carb meals. It will help eliminate any gas and bloating from carbohydrate-rich foods, especially anything with gluten. The gluten-digesting enzyme also helps you fully break down A1 casein to reduce inflammation from it.
3. MassZymes has transformed the digestive health of thousands of our clients. Adjust your dosage based on your calories. We suggest using three to five capsules with each meal.
4. HCL Breakthrough can improve your stomach acid levels and ensure overall smooth digestion. We suggest two to three capsules with each meal. It synergizes with MassZymes.
5. P3-OM will also help break down gluten and other proteins. Take two to four capsules with each meal. It synergizes with MassZymes and HCL Breakthrough.

Gluten Guardian and HCL Breakthrough will ensure that you have zero digestive distress, no matter what you eat when you are carb loading.

Phase 4: Total Fat Adaptation (12+ Months)

During this phase, you will have achieved full metabolic flexibility if you've been cycling in and out of ketosis. At this point, you've been going back and forth from carbs to fats for months. You are now a full-on fat-and-carb-burning machine.

Signs that you are in Phase 4:

- You can bounce back into ketosis relatively quickly, even after eating carbs. Matt measures his ketones after a full day of carb loading, and he'd still be in ketosis with 0.5 millimolar of blood ketone. He did an experiment of eating more than 250 grams of carbs a day for 10 days, and he was still at 0.5 millimolar (which is considered ketosis) on his blood ketone monitor on the 10th day.
- Your body learns to hold on to glycogen stores better and upregulate glycolytic pathways, so your strength and explosive performance will be closer to peak. However, if you're a strength or power athlete, carbs are the way (more on this in a moment).
- Your muscles will also look fuller due to replenished glycogen stores.

Now is when you reap the most benefits from being in ketosis and enjoy the freedom from carb dependency. Your metabolic flexibility to go back and forth between carbs to ketones is at its peak.

Ketogenic Food Staples

- Avocados
- Coconut and unsweetened coconut products (not coconut water or sugar)
- Olives and olive oil
- Pork rinds/cracklings
- Rendered lard and tallow (unhydrogenated only)

- Grass-fed, organic, and fatty cuts of meat
- Sugar-free, high-fat sausages, pepperoni, and other deli meats
- Fatty wild-caught or organic fish such as salmon or sardines
- Seafood
- Butter and ghee (if tolerated)
- Sugar-free mayonnaise made from avocado oil, MCT oil, olive oil, bacon fat, or lard
- Greens and other low-carb veggies, such as salad leaves, peppers, mushrooms, asparagus, kale, arugula, lettuce, spinach, cabbage, broccoli, cucumbers, and celery

Include these only if you are *not* sensitive or allergic to them (see Chapter 31, Eliminating Food Toxins, for more detail):

- Pork, bacon, lard, and pork-derived products
- A1 cream, cheese, and butter
- Fish and seafood
- Low-carb nuts and seeds such as chia, flaxseed, sunflower

Eat in reasonable amounts:

- Macadamia nuts
- Pecans
- Walnuts
- Low-carb spices and condiments

Drink:

- Water
- Plain coffee, tea, and herbal tea
- Unsweetened soda

Avoid or minimize:

- Peanuts
- Cashews
- Almonds
- All grains and pseudograins (quinoa)
- Legumes and beans
- High-carb vegetables such as winter squashes, carrots, tubers, and potatoes
- Sugar
- Sugar-containing foods and condiments
- High-omega-6 vegetable oils such as canola, sunflower, rice bran, soybean, peanut, and sesame oil (because they're pro-inflammatory)
- Processed and charred meats, which are sources of advanced glycation end products that age your cells and cause heart diseases and cancers
- Fruits

BIOPTIMIZING YOUR KETOGENIC DIET

In the past 26 years, Matt has made many mistakes in his ketogenic diet journey. He also witnessed many problems with some of our coaching clients. The tips below will help you enter ketosis smoothly while avoiding painful and costly mistakes.

1. Using Nutrigenomics

Do you have the right genes for the keto diet? Which keto foods are optimal for your body? Which ones should you minimize? Nutrigenomics can shine the light on those questions.

AMY1: The AMY1 gene provides instruction for amylase, an enzyme that digests starch in your saliva. If you have fewer copies of AMY1, you are more likely to do better on a low-carb or ketogenic diet.[23]

The **CPT1A** gene is a key enzyme in mitochondrial fatty acid oxidation. The variant A (rs80356779) reduces ketogenesis, while T increases it. Surprisingly, the A variant is present in 68 percent of Northern Siberian Inuits and many Canadians.[24] If you have the A variant, you're likely to do better on a ketogenic diet.

PPAR-alpha activates other genes that are involved in lipid metabolism. Better PPAR-alpha function means that you will do better with fasting. There are multiple known variants within this gene. Weak versions of PPAR-alpha may reduce fatty acid metabolism, apolipoproteins, HDL, LDL, and ketone body production, making it harder to enter ketosis.[25] So, if you have weak PPAR-alpha, the ketogenic diet might not be for you.

ADRB2 (rs1043713 A) and **ADRB3** are thrifty genes. Certain variants of these genes are associated with belly fat and type 2 diabetes.[26, 27] People with weaker versions of these genes may need to be more careful with calories and saturated fats. So, if you have the weak versions of these genes, you may do better with a caloric deficit on a ketogenic diet low in saturated fat.

APOA2 is the "eat fat, get fat" gene, especially if it's saturated fat. Saturated fats tend to increase ghrelin, the hunger hormone, in people with weaker versions of this gene.[28] If you have the strong version of APOA2, you're more likely to do well on a ketogenic diet. If you have the weak version, you may be able to do a ketogenic diet but with fewer saturated fats.

2. Optimize Your Digestion

Many people experience digestive issues when they start on a ketogenic diet. For some, high-fat meals and MCT oils cause disaster pants, while others struggle with constipation due to the lack of fiber. Belching and acid reflux are also common.

When you first start keto, your gut biome changes, and high-fat meals demand a lot of lipase and bile. You may also experience digestive distress from fat indigestion. We built a special digestive enzyme called kApex for keto eaters. It has a lot of lipases and proteases, which help digest fats and proteins. The dandelion root in it also stimulates bile flow, which is important for fat digestion. In addition, kApex contains some energizing ingredients, which help you get through keto adaptation fatigue.

All the bacteria strains that were feeding off your carbs and processed foods starve, which can cause digestive distress. P3-OM—one of our probiotic products—can help alleviate the issue.

Stomach acid is also crucial for overall digestion and to stimulate your natural bile flow. If you have heartburn and belching, HCL Breakthrough can help you with this.

3. Minimize Inflammation

If you're eating something that causes your body to feel off due to inflammation, it's going to be difficult, if not impossible, to stay on your diet long term. Inflammation can derail your weight loss goals. It makes keto adaptation harder because it worsens keto flu and makes you hungrier due to increased leptin resistance.[29]

Don't Rely on A1 Dairy for Your Fat Intake

A1 dairy, which is 80 percent of all cow's milk in North America, can cause gut inflammation and other inflammatory symptoms for many people.[30] It's also hard to digest. Some dairy has minute amounts of carbs as lactose. However, the proteins in dairy can trigger insulin spikes.[31] Some people who may have leaky gut can have inflammatory responses from A1 milk protein.

A common mistake is to start out keto by gorging on A1 cream, butter, and cheeses. If you're sensitive to A1 casein, which is different from a lactose sensitivity, it will cause a lot of inflammation and make you feel sick. Note that lactase (the lactose-digesting enzyme) does not help with casein sensitivity. Gluten Guardian can help digest the A1 casein, but it doesn't eliminate 100 percent of inflammation from casein.

Therefore, if you consume dairy, it's better to focus on dairy products from other animals, such as sheep, goats, bison, or camels. You can test these different types of dairy separately and see how your body responds.

4. Support Your Microbiome and Gut Barrier

Which foods does your gut biome easily digest and thrive on? And which foods can impact your health? You want to know, so doing a gut health test every six months is smart. Go to www.BIOptimizers.com/book/guthealth to do a gut health test—this will help you choose better foods for YOUR gut biome.

Very high-fat meals can reduce the protective mucus that coats your gut barrier and reduce gut bacteria diversity, which may compromise the barrier.[32] Therefore, we don't advise doing highly restrictive ketogenic diets long term unless you need it to manage medical conditions. Either way, you'll have to work harder to support your microbiome and gut barrier on a ketogenic diet with the following tips.

Add more polyphenols and gut bacteria–friendly micronutrients. Use a gut health test to see the current status of your microbiome. It also provides you with a list of superfoods that are best for feeding your gut bacteria. Go to www.BIOptimizers.com/book/guthealth to do a gut health test—this will help you choose better foods for YOUR gut biome.

Consider dietary fibers, which are important foods for your microbiome—and their fermentation products are great for your gut.[33] If you do well on low-carb vegetables and some prebiotics, then they are good to include in your diet.

Test vegetables and fruits to see if they kick you out of ketosis. Doing ketone and blood sugar tests can be helpful for choosing the best vegetables and fruits for you. As far as fruits go, once you're in Phases 3 and 4, you can start to enjoy low-carb berries such as strawberries, blueberries, and raspberries in moderation.

Biome Breakthrough contains IgYmax and a synergistic blend of probiotics, prebiotics, and collagen. It effectively reduces bad bacteria and improves the colonization of good bacteria. It also helps promote a healthy gut barrier.[34]

5. Add Salt and Minerals

You may experience dizziness and other symptoms of low blood pressure as your kidneys dump minerals. Make sure you eat plenty of high-quality salt and mineral sources.

- Salt your food liberally with Himalayan or sea salt
- Take Magnesium Breakthrough, as keto diets are typically low in magnesium
- Use trace minerals

Matt consumes about 10 grams of salt a day, which might seem high. However, he feels much better with a higher salt consumption. When his salt intake is too low, he loses too much water on keto. His hack to solve this is to put half a teaspoon of Himalayan pink salt and a quarter teaspoon of cream of tartar (a potassium source) into two liters of water and drink it throughout the day. This helps his body keep more water and prevent dehydration. Consult with your doctor before making any drastic changes to your diet.

6. Optimize Your Fats

Matt believes that optimizing your fats based on your nutrigenomics and gut biome can make a big impact on your health. This is where doing a nutrigenomic test and looking at your bloodwork with the guidance of a professional can pay big dividends.

Here are some of the main considerations:

Increase your omega-3 fatty acids.[35] Get as much omega-3 as possible from seafood and red meat. If it's not possible, due to reasons such as food allergies or other dietary restrictions, use a supplement to make sure you get 1 to 2 grams of DHA or EPA daily. DHA is critical for optimizing your brain function. See more on this in Chapter 26, Redefining Nutrition.

Test nuts and seeds. Check to see if they cause inflammation or pull you out of ketosis before consuming ample amounts of them. The best nuts for keto diets are Brazil nuts, macadamias, walnuts, and pecans due to their high-fat and low-carb content. Many nuts are high in phytic acids (such as almonds), which become problematic if too many are consumed. The biggest potential pitfall with nuts is overeating them. It's very easy to sneak in an extra 300 calories when you grab a handful of nuts. This is where measuring matters.

Be mindful of saturated fats: Many animal studies show that saturated fats are highly inflammatory. Still, the effects on humans are more subtle and may vary from person to person.[36, 37, 38] Genetics play a role here. Some genotypes do better with mostly monounsaturated fats. To get a genetic report for the best fats for your body, go to: www.BIOptimizers.com/book/genes.

Before you drink ample amounts of fat coffee and gorge on coconut oil like they're superfoods, check your biofeedback to see how your body responds to them. My triglycerides skyrocket on coconut oil, so it's not a superfood for me.

Avoid trans and hydrogenated fats. These bad fats can be found in shortening, margarine, hydrogenated lard, and many processed foods. Trans and hydrogenated fats are very inflammatory and promote dysbiosis.[39, 40] Avoid them and any processed foods that contain them.

Minimize processed keto foods. They can often contain too many carbs, chemicals, insulinogenic, or inflammatory ingredients. Matt made the mistake of eating lots of low-carb foods that supposedly had low net carbs, and sabotaged his success. Monitoring your blood sugar response to packaged keto foods is one of the best ways to see how your body handles them.

7. Experimenting with a Carnivore Diet

Many years before the term *carnivore diet* was thrown around, Matt would do phases of eating just meat and fish and cutting out all carbs from his diet. He usually did this when he wanted to lose body fat. He found it helpful to reduce food cravings even further and cut calories.

In the last couple of years, carnivore diets have become increasingly popular. For some people who have severe autoimmune issues, it's a potential answer. Some can experience relief by going carnivore because they get inflammation, gut biome problems, or immune system triggers from plant-based substances.

Figure out which types of meat work best for you. Some of them could cause inflammation and stress in your body. Also, you may not have the ideal gut bacteria for certain foods. As an example, Matt never digested chicken well, and the gut health test revealed that he should minimize or avoid it. On the other hand, Matt always felt great eating beef, and the data says it's a superfood for his gut biome.

Very high-fat meals can reduce the protective mucus that coats your gut barrier and reduce gut bacteria diversity, which may compromise the gut barrier.[41] Therefore, we don't advise doing highly restrictive ketogenic diets long-term unless you need it to manage medical conditions. Either way, you are going to have to work harder to support your microbiome and gut barrier on a ketogenic diet with the following tips.

Check out our *Ultimate Carnivore Cookbook* and download the Me Diet app to get started. Of course, we take out all of the guessing and use our formulas to design your personalized journey designed with the Me Diet app. Go to www.BIOptimizers.com/book/dietapp to download our app to make your Me Diet journey simple and easy to follow.

8. Don't Guess, Test

As we keep stressing, data shapes destinies. You can't manage what you can't measure, and that's why we want to use data to optimize a ketogenic diet.

Biofeedback is one of the most important things that lets you find out if a food (or the ketogenic diet itself) is working for you. However, subjective biofeedback has its limitations. This is where hard data coming from bloodwork, urine tests, and other technologies comes into play.

If you've read other keto diet books, not much we've said so far is new. But now, it's time to take your keto diet to its full potential.

HOW MUCH TO EAT ON KETO

Although a lot of keto zealots want you to believe that you can eat however much you want on a ketogenic diet, it isn't magical. Keto doesn't bypass the laws of thermodynamics. Eating too many calories on keto can cause body fat gain and blood lipids to go off the rails.

Most people will naturally be in a caloric deficit when they start keto, and thus lose weight. The elimination of processed foods combined with the satiating nature of high-fat foods makes it easier for many people to eat fewer calories. That being said, most people on an extended weight loss journey will hit a plateau, and at that point, calories should be tracked. See more on this in Chapter 26, Redefining Nutrition.

A good starting-point formula for a diet is consuming around 12 calories per pound of bodyweight per day. Follow this for two weeks, and monitor your weight and the tape measurements. If they go down, you're in a deficit. If you're not, target a 500-calorie daily deficit. You can achieve this by increasing exercise, increasing anabolism, or decreasing calories. Read Chapter 7, The Optimized Metabolism System, for more insights, and read Chapter 8, Advanced Cycling Strategies, to get deeper breakdowns of how to optimize your calories. You could also download our Me Diet app and use our awesome Optimized Calorie Calculator.

Of course, we take out all of the guessing and use our formulas to design your personalized journey designed with the Me Diet app. Go to www.BIOptimizers.com/book/dietapp to download our app to make your Me Diet journey simple and easy to follow.

After Phase 1, your calorie needs depend on your goals:

Goal	Calories
Longevity and health span	Maintenance or slight caloric deficit (up to 15%)
Maximize athletic performance	Maintenance, or up to 10% above maintenance
Build lean muscles	300–500 calories above maintenance
Fat loss	500-calorie deficit per day

WHAT DOES A KETO DIET LOOK LIKE?

You can still enjoy a variety of foods on keto. Here are some examples:

Day 1: 3,000-Calorie Menu

Breakfast

1 medium avocado
2 large eggs fried in 2 tablespoons ghee
2 fatty beef sausages
1 large plate of spring mix salad
3 tablespoons olive oil to drizzle
Plain coffee

Lunch

2 cups roasted broccoli drizzled with 2 tablespoons olive oil
6 ounces grass-fed ribeye steak
2 tablespoons fat to cook your steak (ghee, coconut oil, or tallow)
6 tablespoons fat to top your steak (olive oil, butter, marrow butter, or coconut butter)

Dinner

4 ounces wild-caught salmon
3 cups cauliflower mash with ¼ cup fat and ½ cup coconut cream
2 tablespoons coconut butter for dessert

Day 2: 3,000-Calorie Menu

Breakfast

Bulletproof coffee with 1 tablespoon MCT oil, 3 tablespoons butter, and 2 tablespoons collagen

Lunch

Shrimp curry with 6 ounces shrimp, 2 cups coconut cream, and low-carb vegetables
2 cups cauliflower rice sauteed in 2 tablespoons coconut oil

Dinner

Keto Shepherd's Pie:
6 ounces grass-fed ground beef
4 cups cauliflower mash with at least ½ cup of fat (butter, coconut cream, or high-fat cheese)

Day 3: 3,000-Calorie Menu

Breakfast

4-egg omelette with ¼ cup fat and 1 ounce mozzarella
1 large plate of salad leaves
Optional: peppers, mushrooms, tomatoes
2 strips bacon

Lunch

Zucchini noodles with 1 cup coconut cream alfredo and 8 ounces seafood
2 tablespoons butter

Dinner

9 ounces grass-fed short ribs
4 tablespoons fat (olive oil, marrow butter, or butter)
Mixed low-carb vegetables

OPTIMIZING YOUR KETOGENIC DIET

As we covered in previous chapters, getting high-quality data is critical for making sure that the diet you're following is working well for you. When deciding if keto is right for you, there are a few factors to consider and various ways to test if a ketogenic diet is for you. These tests include:

Blood Tests

Ask for the following tests from your doctor before and during your keto journey:[42]

- Fasting blood glucose
- HbA1c
- Triglycerides
- High-density lipoprotein cholesterol
- Low-density lipoprotein cholesterol with particle size
- Lipoprotein(a)
- Fasted insulin
- High-sensitivity C-reactive protein
- Uric acid
- Liver enzymes, including GGT
- Thyroid panel
- Sodium and potassium

We suggest doing bloodwork every three months when you do drastic dietary changes. Your doctor may also order lab tests to screen for kidney problems if they suspect that could be an issue.

Hormone Tests

The DUTCH Complete test measures all the different hormone metabolites in your urine. It's an excellent way to track how the ketogenic diet affects your hormones and stress responses.

Wearable Biofeedback Devices

At-home monitors like your Oura Ring or similar devices can track:

- Body temperature
- Heart rate
- Heart rate variability

Matt has seen lower HRV and readiness scores in Oura readings with many clients who don't have the ideal genetics for keto. Does that mean they shouldn't do a keto diet short term to reach specific goals? No. It's just another data point to consider.

Ketone and Blood Glucose Levels

To enter ketosis and monitor factors that bring you in and out of it, you need to track your ketones. Three different ketone bodies—beta-hydroxybutyrate, acetoacetate, and acetate—are present in your blood in varying amounts. Some ketone tests detect one but not another, which makes them less accurate.

On a ketogenic diet, you want to shoot for ketone bodies between 0.5 and 3.0 millimolar. Above 0.5, you are considered in ketosis.

Measuring Ketones

- Avoid urine ketone strips, which are the least expensive way to test your ketones. They test only for excess acetoacetate excreted in the urine and are therefore the least accurate.
- Breath ketone tests measure acetone, the breakdown product of acetoacetate and acetate. This is the most convenient and least invasive option, as you only need to blow into the device. However, many other factors, such as what you eat and your respiratory rate, can affect your results—making it rather inaccurate.
- Blood ketone tests are the most accurate. However, for them you need to prick your finger or get a blood draw. The tests measure beta-hydroxybutyrate, the most active ketone body in your blood. The home devices measure both blood ketones and sugar using the same strips. This is the gold standard.
- Matt suggests you avoid carbon dioxide breath testing. It can estimate the amount of carbs and fats you're burning based on oxygen you inhale and carbon dioxide you exhale. While this may be helpful to track your ketosis, it is not a direct measure of ketones.

We recommend the Keto Mojo as the main tool to track both ketosis and blood glucose. It also has the lowest price per test strip and comes with an app that makes it easier to record and track your results.

Don't get too caught up with ketone levels, though. What typically happens is higher ketone levels in the beginning of someone's keto journey that lower over time. This is a positive sign that your body is more efficient at using ketones for energy.

As noted earlier, Matt suggests measuring your ketone and blood sugar response to various foods, which can help you identify which are ideal for you and which you should minimize or avoid. Once you've gathered data for a few weeks, testing your ketone levels becomes less useful.

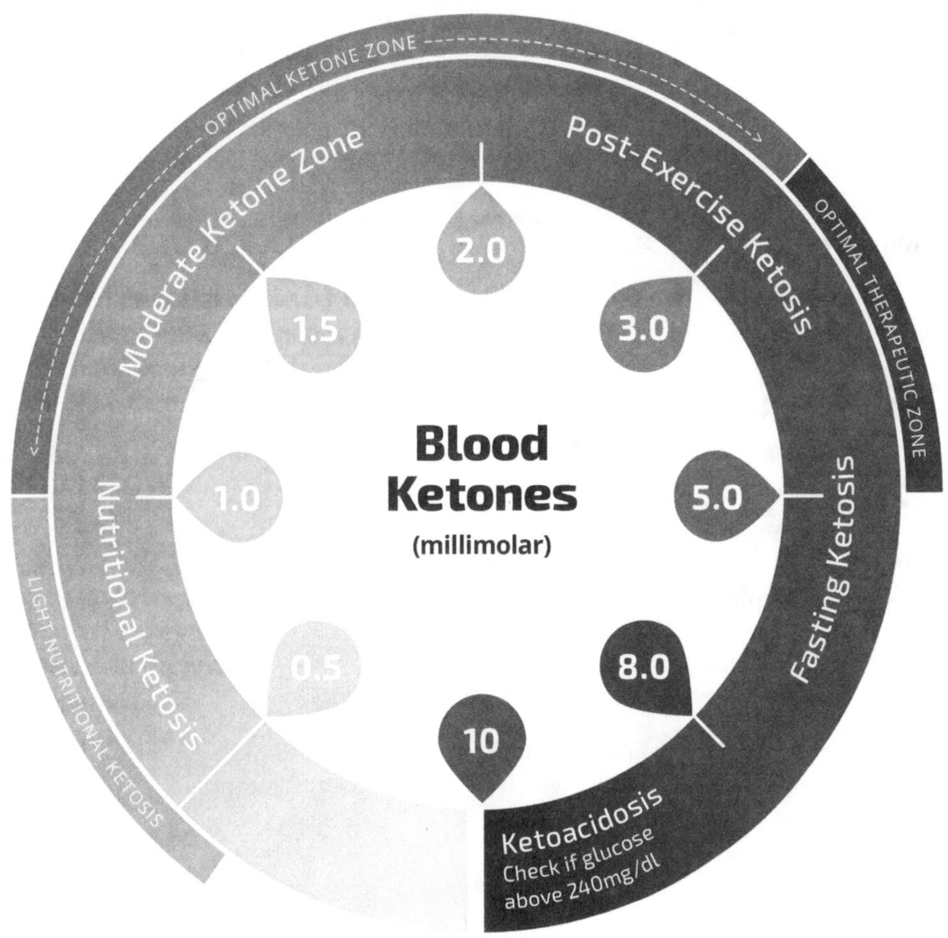

PROS AND CONS OF A KETOGENIC DIET

With every diet comes a set of trade-offs. To determine if a diet is right for you, you should find its pros very attractive and its cons tolerable. Fortunately, most of the cons of keto can be managed or avoided altogether if you follow the tips in our Keto Diet Considerations section.

Potential Upsides and Downsides of a Ketogenic Diet

Health

Pros

The ketogenic diet can improve biological markers of longevity, reduce blood pressure, and promote insulin sensitivity for many people.

Cons

Reduced thyroid hormone. Free active thyroid hormone (T3), a mastermind of your metabolism, starts to drop, causing you to feel cold and lethargic.[43]

Increased sex-hormone-binding globulin (SHBG) and increased free testosterone. Dr. Paul Saladino, a carnivore diet expert, finds that SHBG significantly increases for both him and his male patients on that diet. High SHBG can reduce free testosterone, which affects your overall well-being and exercise response.[44]

It also has the potential to cause some side effects such as:

1. Too-low blood pressure
2. Kidney stones
3. Gallbladder issues
4. Digestive problems
5. Constipation
6. Nutrient deficiencies (e.g., of vitamin C)
7. May throw off blood lipids for some

Aesthetics: Lean Muscle Mass

Pros

Many people find it easier to lose body fat and maintain weight because they're less hungry and thus it's easier to manage calories. Some cyclical keto-style diets, such as anabolic diets, can help optimize muscle growth. In Matt's opinion, it's the best way to recomp. Go for fat loss for five days by doing a calorie deficit in a keto diet. Then, refeed with carbs and focus on gaining lean muscle for two days.

Cons

Because your insulin will be perpetually low, you may find it harder to gain muscles on keto unless you do carb refeeds. If you're obsessed with putting on as much lean muscle mass as possible, Matt suggests following a high-carb, high-protein, low-fat diet.

Aesthetics: Losing Body Fat

Also, because being keto adapted allows you to tap into your body fat stores, you can just fast if you can't find the food or the time to eat. Ketosis is muscle-sparing, which helps prevent losing lean muscle mass.

Athletic Performance

Pros

Nutritional and supplemental ketosis can also potentially be a great tool to support endurance performance.

Cons

You have a reduced ability to handle carbs. Being in ketosis makes you slightly insulin resistant, as your body wants to conserve all the glucose for the brain.[45] Also, once ketones become the preferred fuel, your cells dial down pathways that are involved in burning glucose.[46]

Power sport athletes should avoid ketogenic diets weeks before and during competitions.

Strength, speed, and agility have been shown to drop when using a ketogenic diet. We suggest using a carb-based diet for competitive events. More specifically, start using carbs several weeks before the sporting event, because you need to rebuild and strengthen your glycolytic pathways.

Mental Performance

Pros

For many, this is the main edge. Ketosis boosts mental performance and balances out the brain and cravings.

Cons

Some people who don't have the right genes for keto and thrive on carbs may experience significant drops in mental energy and focus.

Lifestyle

Pros

In Matt's opinion, a cyclical keto diet is one of the best lifestyle diets. Even though you're carb restricting for five days, the two days of eating whatever you want (within your caloric allotment) is great for a foodie lifestyle.

Cons

It can be socially isolating to be on such a restrictive diet.

Psychological Considerations

Pros

Keto works well if you find a diet with fewer options easier to stick to. Matt is one of these people. It also stabilizes mood and mental health for some.[47]

Cons

You may miss your favorite non-keto foods. For some people, the lack of variety makes it psychologically impossible to stick to.

SHOULD YOU TRY A KETOGENIC DIET?

Here are the factors to take into account to decide whether or not to try a ketogenic diet:

1. Your Mother's and Grandmother's Metabolisms

Everyone inherits their mitochondria from their mother. Human and mouse studies have shown that females with obesity and insulin resistance develop abnormal mitochondria and then transmit these to their children and grandchildren. These generations also inherit epigenetic changes that make them glucose intolerant and insulin resistant. As a result, they are at an increased risk of obesity, cardiovascular disease, and diabetes.[48]

So, if obesity and insulin resistance run in your family, there's a chance that a ketogenic diet could be the healthiest diet for you.

2. Your Genetics

Your genes create genetic tendencies, but tendencies don't always play out. However, understanding your genes will provide you with powerful knowledge to control outcomes.

As a generalization (not a hard rule), Northern European genetics are great for ketogenic diets. Why? Because those ethnic groups had to endure hard winters and usually lived off wild animals. A lack of fruits and vegetables forced people to switch to animal fat and protein to survive. To find out how good your genes are for keto, go to: www.BIOptimizers.com/book/genes.

3. Insulin Resistance

Many people with health conditions involving insulin resistance, such as type 2 diabetes and polycystic ovarian syndrome, find it easier to manage their conditions on ketogenic diets. Some others, however, find that plant-based diets work better for the same goal. Therefore, you should work with your doctor and coaches to monitor your biofeedback and bloodwork.

Even if you don't have diagnosed conditions, subclinical insulin resistance is extremely common. If you crave carbs, suffer from hormonal imbalances, or have mood swings, you may find that ketosis stabilizes or eliminates these symptoms altogether.

4. Brain Health Issues or Neurological Disorders

Ketogenic diets have been used to treat refractory epilepsy for over 80 years.[49] Ketones protect neurons and boost mitochondrial function, which often jump-starts healing processes.

Recent studies confirm that ketosis may help with other neurological conditions, such as multiple sclerosis, Alzheimer's disease, and mild cognitive impairment.[50, 51]

5. Athletic Goals and Recovery

Many superhuman athletes find that ketogenic diets boost their performance, improve their recovery, and help them stay lean.

For endurance sports, nutritional ketosis is emerging as a viable option. Competing in ketosis taps into an athlete's fat stores, which eliminates the need to carb load pre-event. They no longer bonk or need to eat when they run out of glycogen during competition.

Endurance athletes may find it easier to enter ketosis, as they already have more efficient mitochondria.[52] A 2016 clinical trial in *Cell Metabolism* found that muscles can shift to burn ketones even at high-intensity efforts among professional cyclists.[53] Also, the cyclists in ketosis outperformed those who ran on carbs.

Ben Greenfield, a professional ultra-endurance athlete, has found that ketosis gives him the extra edge. He's also found that it counteracts a lot of oxidative damage and inflammation from training and competing in these events.[54]

Peter Attia, M.D., is a prominent longevity physician and extreme endurance athlete. He swam 20 miles across the Catalina channel within 12 hours while on a ketogenic diet.

6. You Do Better with More Rules and Fewer Options

A keto diet can be very restrictive. Unless you're on a carb refeed day, then you'll have to skip things like french fries and bread at restaurants. However, you can still consume your favorite tasty carbs at the right times if you do a cyclical keto diet like the ones shared in this chapter.

One of the main reasons Matt loves keto is that he's not naturally disciplined. That's why he's better with rigidity and fewer options. The natural structure (to a certain degree), combined with fewer cravings, helps him stay compliant.

7. You Enjoy Meat

A nutritional strategy only works if you can follow it. To stick to a ketogenic diet, you have to enjoy keto foods. Meat lovers can usually thrive on keto or carnivore diets. People who don't love meat and fish usually struggle. Is it possible to go keto as a vegetarian or vegan? Yes, but, in our observation, it tends to be a fail.

However, food preferences can change over the course of a few weeks as your gut bacteria changes.[55] If you think you may benefit from keto but dislike the foods, you can try it over a few weeks to see if you grow to like them.

8. Favorable Biofeedback

If a ketogenic diet is right for you, your blood markers and heart rate variability will show a favorable response in the right direction.

REASONS NOT TO DO A KETOGENIC DIET

Keto zealots will try to convert everyone to it because they think it's the greatest diet for everyone. Matt was once a keto zealot. But the truth is, keto is not the greatest diet for all humankind. For Matt, it is. But you need to use data and science to find out if it's for you.

1. The Wrong Genetics

Some people, especially those from tropical climates, may have genes that do better on a higher-carb diet. Also, if you have weaker keto genes, then maybe a keto diet isn't right for you.

2. Medical Contraindications

Avoid a ketogenic diet if you have pancreatitis, liver failure, and disorders of fat metabolism.[56] Also, if you don't have a gallbladder, you may be able to do a ketogenic diet but only under medical supervision and plenty of digestive support.

3. Major Hormone Imbalances or Severe Adrenal Burnout

Going through keto adaptation can be stressful to your body and demands a lot from your stress response system. If you have major hormone imbalances, you should address those issues first before trying to get keto adapted. One exception would be if insulin resistance and blood sugar problems are driving the hormone imbalances.

4. Needing Carbohydrates for Maximum Power

When you attempt ketosis, your overall strength and physical performance will go down significantly, even if you use ketone supplements. It can take up to a year for peak athletic performance to return. Therefore, if you need to perform at your peak in the near future, a ketogenic diet may not be a good idea.

5. Unfavorable Biofeedback

Some people have the genes to reverse their insulin resistance better with whole grains and legumes than with ketogenic diets.

If your cholesterol and inflammation markers skyrocket while your HRV crashes on a ketogenic diet, then the diet might not be right for you.

SUMMARY

Traditional ketogenic diets (aka keto) are very low carb, moderate protein, and high fat. The goal of this diet is to enter "nutritional ketosis," or the state where your body is fueled primarily by ketones. Ketones or ketone bodies are made from short snippets of the fatty acids you eat or from your own body fat.

Our bodies are adapted to handle low-to-no-carb diets and starvation phases.

On a ketogenic diet, you deliberately cut out all carbs and eat mostly fats, causing the following:

- Your body uses up all stored glycogen
- Your liver starts producing ketones from the fat you eat
- Your brain, muscles, and internal organs increase mitochondria and the cellular enzymes involved in using ketones for energy
- Your anti-aging pathways, such as autophagy and sirtuins, are activated
- Your cells learn to shift back and forth between burning sugar and ketones for energy

Unique Health Benefits of Keto

- A boost in brain function and cognitive clarity

  If you enter ketosis, even temporarily or with ketone supplements, you will experience brain-enhancing benefits.

- Reduced blood pressure

  Properly mineralizing with sodium and potassium to help optimize cellular hydration is critical.

- Better insulin sensitivity and stable blood sugar

  Reducing carbohydrate intake typically reduces insulin, which improves insulin sensitivity.

- Diminished appetite and cravings
  Ketosis reduces appetite, even in caloric restriction during a weight loss program. Even after weight loss, ghrelin (the hunger hormone) remains low in people who stay in ketosis.

- Reduced inflammation
  Ketone bodies have anti-inflammatory and antioxidant properties. Therefore, some people may experience some reduction in pain or remission of a chronic condition.

The following tips will help you enter ketosis smoothly while avoiding painful and costly mistakes:

- Use nutrigenomics
- Optimize your digestion
- Minimize inflammation
- Support your microbiome and gut barrier
- Add salt and minerals
- Optimize your fats
- Experiment with a carnivore diet
- Test, don't guess

Factors that Affect Whether the Keto Diet is Right for You:

- Your mother's and grandmother's metabolism
  If obesity and insulin resistance run in your family, there is a chance that a ketogenic diet could be the healthiest diet for you.

- Your genetics
  Your genes create genetic tendencies, but they don't always play out. However, understanding your genes provides you with powerful knowledge to control your outcomes.

- Insulin resistance
  Many people with health conditions involving insulin resistance find it easier to manage their conditions on ketogenic diets.

- Brain health issues or neurological disorders
  Ketones protect neurons and boost mitochondria function, which often jump-starts the healing processes.

- Athletic goals and recovery
  Many superhuman athletes find that ketogenic diets boost their performance, improve their recovery, and help them stay lean.

- You do better with rules and fewer options
  The ketogenic diet can be very restrictive, but that might work for you.

- You enjoy meat
  To stick to a ketogenic diet, you have to enjoy keto foods.

Reasons *Not* to do a Keto Diet:

- The wrong genetics
- Medical contraindications
- Major hormone imbalances or severe adrenal burnout
- Needing carbohydrates for maximum performance
- Unfavorable biofeedback

CHAPTER 21

THE KEYS TO SUCCESS FOR VEGAN AND VEGETARIAN DIETS

by Wade T. Lightheart

In this chapter, you'll learn:

- The most effective way to follow veganism and vegetarianism as nutritional strategies for maximal health and longevity
- The right and wrong ways to do a plant-based or vegetarian diet
- The 11 symptoms to watch for while on a plant-based diet that warn of nutritional deficiencies
- The health risks of a vegan or vegetarian diet, and how to thrive despite them
- How seasonality and climate can affect your success on a vegan or vegetarian diet plan, and why sourcing food locally throughout the year can provide you with extra benefits
- How to determine the ideal macronutrients for vegetarians and vegans
- The cons to the vegetarian diet that you should consider before you begin

Let us start with a key point (which is true for all diet types). Going vegan or vegetarian isn't ideal for everyone, genetically speaking. Some people have better genes than others for thriving on a plant-based diet.

That being said, if you've decided to follow a vegan or vegetarian diet for spiritual or ethical reasons, we respect that, and we're here to help you.

SPIRITUAL AND ETHICAL FACTORS

Many people decide to forgo meat for spiritual or ethical reasons. You may want to become vegan from a deep compassion for animals. Many vegans oppose all things that put animals through suffering and death, so they may also avoid honey and leather products.

How the Meathead, Mr. Universe, Turned Vegan

Wade was a meat-eating bodybuilder until he read the book *Holy Science* by Swami Sri Yukteswar. The book described how form and function differ between carnivores versus omnivores, herbivores, and frugivores (raw fruit eaters).

Convinced, Wade tried going vegan for two weeks as an experiment. It agreed with him so well that he just kept extending the experiment. Eventually, he just abandoned meat and animal products altogether. It's been over 20 years now.

The key differences and benefits Wade observed in his body included:

- Improved digestion. He no longer feels the post-meal bloat that many people associate with meat
- Reduced aggression
- Reduced sleep by about an hour a day, from eight to six or seven hours, which was manageable
- Significantly changed sweat and body odor
- Resolved skin conditions, less earwax, and less crust in the eyes
- Less inflammation in the joints, especially after training

On the other hand, he struggled with:

- Sourcing a gut-friendly, high-quality protein source to support his training and muscle building.
- His muscles and connective tissues became softer, which his massage therapist and chiropractor both noticed. This was good for flexibility but not for physique or aesthetics.
- Going to the bathroom a lot more than he used to.
- Making sure he ate enough protein for satiety so he didn't overeat carbs.
- Reduced testosterone. He had to make sure he got enough saturated fats and essential fatty acids.

What Wade Learned as a Vegan Bodybuilder (and Why That's Important for Every Vegan and Vegetarian)

Getting Enough Protein

Prior to becoming vegan, Wade stuck to the myth that he needed to consume 1 gram of protein per pound of bodyweight to build and maintain muscles as a professional bodybuilder. This notion is widespread among both professional and amateur bodybuilders.

Once Wade switched to a plant-based diet, he found that trying to eat that much protein per pound of bodyweight on a plant-based diet was close to impossible without protein powder. Wade then consumed a whole pile of whey protein, which really negatively impacted his gut health.

Once Wade supercharged his digestion with MassZymes, he only needed 85 to 100 grams of high-quality protein to recover from his workout and maintain his muscle mass.

For people who are all-in on building lean muscle mass or focusing on weight loss for a limited time, a gram of protein per pound can make sense. However, we strongly advise using MassZymes or VegZymes with it. A good target for someone with those goals is 0.7 grams of protein per pound of bodyweight.

It's very difficult to eat enough protein from plants, so sophisticated vegans and vegetarians should use a plant-based protein powder to help them hit their macro goals. Check out our 100 percent plant-based Protein Breakthrough. It tastes absolutely amazing and will help you hit your macro goals.

Expect an Adjustment Period

When you switch to a substantially different diet, there will be an adjustment period with your microbiome. The key is to be mindful of this transition and not react prematurely to short-term changes.

Studies show that the microbiome changes the most in the first 24 to 72 hours after switching to a plant-based diet.[1] Wade has found that it can take 21 to 90 days to adapt psychologically.

Avoid the Vigilante Veganism Mindset

We've covered how people who get phenomenal results using a diet type often become diet elitists. Vigilante vegans are so passionate about advocating for their diets that they want the entire world to follow in their footsteps.

Wade realized this when he attended a raw vegan festival and was shunned because he wasn't "100 percent raw." The dietary elitism mentality can be extremely strong in veganism, and its members often resort to spiritual and emotional shaming of others. We suggest avoiding this kind of zealotry. Focus on what's best for you and ignore the fanatics.

HEALTH BENEFITS OF VEGAN AND VEGETARIAN DIETS

Many aspects of vegan and vegetarian diets are perfect antidotes to the harmful effects of the standard American diet. As a result, many people experience significant improvements in their health and body composition when they switch over to a plant-based diet. Salads are a big upgrade from super-sized Happy Meals.

1. Potential Beneficial Shifts in the Gut Microbiome

A Harvard University study put subjects on vegetarian and carnivore diets for five days. Their fecal microbiome underwent major shifts within one to two days.[2, 3, 4] Compared to a meat-based diet, the plant-based diet grew more Firmicutes bacteria, which fermented the fibers and increased the overall diversity of the gut flora community. The meat-based eaters in the study had microbiome genetic expression (gene readouts) that were more similar to those of carnivorous mammals, whereas the vegetarians' microbiome gene readouts were more similar to those of herbivores.[5] The meat-based diet, which was higher in fat, grew more bile-tolerant bacteria.[6]

2. Increase in Dietary Fiber

Many modern diseases are exacerbated by a lack of dietary fiber.[7] Most people simply don't eat enough plant matter. According to the CDC, only 1 in 10 adults gets five servings of fruits and vegetables a day.[8]

Even epidemiologic studies that demonstrate the benefits of fiber intake typically report the highest intakes as well under 30 grams per day. Our ancestors ate perhaps over 100 grams per day of dietary fiber,[9] suggesting that the optimal fiber intake for health and longevity should be much higher than 30 grams.

What's even more important than fiber are ferments (more on this in a moment).

How a High-Fiber, Plant-Based Diet Improves Your Health

It binds up and eliminates toxins.

Fibers help bind toxins, hormone metabolites, and cholesterol, which improves their excretion. By increasing stool volume, fibers dilute these substances and reduce their harmful effects on your body.

It improves satiety and blood sugar control

They also bulk up your meals, slowing down carbohydrate absorption and making the foods more filling. As a result, the increase in fiber tends to improve blood sugar control and help with weight loss.

It feeds your gut bacteria and creates postbiotics.

The fibers do a lot more than just bulking up stool, because they're also excellent foods for your gut bacteria. A high-fiber diet allows good bacteria to thrive. The bacteria then ferment the fiber into beneficial postbiotics, such as:[10, 11]

- Short-chain fatty acids: acetate, propionate, and butyrate
- Cellular components of the bacteria, which may have anti-inflammatory and immunomodulating properties
- Neurotransmitters and hormones, and their metabolites[12]
- Secondary bile acids, which influence your metabolism and overall microbiome composition[13,14]

Among all postbiotics, butyrate is the most studied and perhaps the most beneficial one. It boosts mitochondrial function, balances the immune response, and activates gut repair epigenetics.[15, 16, 17] Historically, butyrate has been used as an antifungal and antimicrobial. It may also help with blood sugar control and obesity.[18, 19] Through its epigenetic activity, it inhibits cancer formation, especially colon cancer.[20]

It even enhances deep sleep and stimulates muscle stem cells in animal studies.[21, 22]

Health benefits of dietary fiber intake include:[23]

- 29 percent reduction in risk of heart disease
- 26 percent reduction in risk of stroke
- 19 percent reduction in risk of diabetes
- 30 percent reduction in risk of obesity
- Net reduction in cholesterol (depending on the type of fiber)

The highest fiber intake is great for your gut, as it is associated with a reduced prevalence of esophageal cancer, GERD, stomach cancer, stomach ulcers, gallbladder diseases, diverticular disease, constipation, and hemorrhoids.

Meta-analyses on dietary fiber supplements found that each 11.5 grams per day of fiber intake was associated with a 1.1 mmHg reduction in systolic blood pressure and a 1.3 mmHg reduction in diastolic pressure. By diluting the carcinogens in the gut, reducing the transit time, and increasing short-chain fatty acids, dietary fiber intake was associated with a 6 to 14 percent reduction in colon cancers.[24]

3. Filling Our Holes: Increased Phytonutrients, Vitamins, and Minerals

Hunter-gatherers have consumed over 100 plant species, although only a small percentage of them have been available at any given time.[25] These wild plants were much higher in phytonutrients, vitamins, and minerals, as they grew in fertile soil and had more positive stressors compared to modern farmed versions.

By eating more fruits and vegetables, you will get more phytonutrients, vitamins, and minerals.[26] We are still very early in discovering all of the potential benefits of various polyphenols and phytonutrients in plants.

Potential benefits of phytonutrients and polyphenols include:[27]

- Improving your gut microbiome composition toward a healthier metabolism
- Supporting and protecting your mitochondria
- Protecting your cells, especially your eyes, nerves, and blood vessels from oxidative stress
- Balancing your immune system
- Helping balance your hormones
- Supporting your detoxification pathways
- Promoting autophagy, which has a potent anti-aging and anti-inflammatory effect

Sensibly, higher phytochemical intake is associated with reduced risk of heart disease, cancers, diabetes and diabetic complications, osteoporosis, and cataracts.[28]

Plant-based diets are higher in some nutrients that omnivore diets tend to lack.[29] They have higher magnesium, vitamin C, vitamin E, niacin, and folate intake, although both groups are deficient in vitamin B_6 and niacin.[30]

4. Reduced Insulin Growth Factor (IGF-1)

Insulin growth factor (IGF-1) is a hormone that promotes growth overall. But having too much of it can promote diseases of excessive tissue growth such as cancer, endometriosis, and obesity.[31, 32] To maximize your BioSpan (health span + life span), we believe that your body needs to cycle between high-autophagy (low IGF-1) and anabolic (high IGF-1) states.

The modern lifestyle, with its constant availability and abundance of foods and animal products, tends to lead to chronically elevated IGF-1 levels. However, the vegan diet is associated with a 13 percent reduction in blood IGF-1,[33] which may explain why vegans have a lower risk of diseases linked to high IGF-1. In some cases, plant-based diets are somewhat effective experimental treatments for cancers and endometriosis.[34, 35]

Dairy proteins in particular increase insulin and IGF-1, so if you do a lacto-vegetarian diet, you may not reap these benefits.

5. Reduced Toxins from Food

Toxins such as pesticides, heavy metals, antibiotics, and pollutants tend to bioaccumulate up the food chain. Herbivorous animals accumulate more of these toxins throughout their lifetimes. Then carnivorous animals that eat the herbivores accumulate even more toxins. Bioaccumulation happens more with fat-soluble toxins, which tend to get stored in fat tissues.[36]

Therefore, some people initially feel much better once they transition to a plant-based diet as it significantly cuts down their toxic loads.

6. Reduced Processed Foods

A plant-based diet significantly cuts down your processed food options, so you'll have to think more about cooking from scratch. Therefore, you'll avoid unhealthy amounts of added sugar, sodium, fats, and food additives. Be careful not to eat too many processed vegan snacks. These can be loaded with sugar and fats and impact your goals. Read the label! Watch the macros.

7. Increased Enzymes

By focusing more on raw and fermented plant-based foods, you'll consume more enzymes. These enzymes support digestion and help reduce inflammation.

HEALTH RISKS OF A VEGETARIAN AND VEGAN DIET (AND HOW TO THRIVE DESPITE THEM)

Vegan and vegetarian diets are not for everyone. As you transition into a new diet, it's critical to monitor your biofeedback such as energy, bowel movements, skin health, blood sugar response, triglycerides, and nutrient levels.

The first three to six months on any new diet will reveal the places you need to supplement to offset your epigenetic responses. It's crucial to get bloodwork to monitor how your body is responding to the diet. Long-term deficiencies can lead to serious health problems if they're not addressed.

How to Know if Nutrient Deficiencies Are Catching Up to You

When transitioning to a new diet, especially a restrictive one, it's essential to test your nutrient levels on a regular basis—every three to six months. Correlate the test results with how you feel and whether your supplements are improving you in that area.

The following symptoms could mean that you might be developing nutritional deficiencies, which should be investigated.

- Symptoms of anemia (fatigue despite getting enough sleep, malaise, and looking pale)
- Hair loss
- Reduced immune function (may present as frequent colds and flus, poor wound healing)
- Dry skin or skin breakouts
- Brain fog, reduced cognitive function, and problems with your mood
- Muscle loss
- Body fat gain
- Joint pain and other inflammatory symptoms
- Reduced appetite, bloating, and poor digestion
- Reduced sex drive and overall vitality
- Poor sleep or reduced sleep quality

TROUBLESHOOTING GUIDE FOR VEGANS AND VEGETARIANS

1. Nutrient Deficiencies

Common nutrient deficiencies among vegetarians and vegans include:[37, 38]

- Protein
- Zinc
- Preformed vitamin A (retinol)
- Vitamin D
- Iodine
- Selenium
- B vitamins (especially vitamin B_{12}, which needs to be supplemented)
- Iron

It is, therefore, a good idea to routinely test for these nutrient levels with the SpectraCell test and supplement, if you need to.

Wade tries to get most of his vitamin D through sun exposure. When he's in a cold climate, though, he uses vegan vitamin D_3 to ensure that his levels are optimal.

Poor Absorption and Low Stomach Acid: Why Vegetarians and Vegans Develop Deficiencies

Zinc from animal sources, such as meat, tends to be more bioavailable than zinc from plant sources. Also, plant-based sources of minerals tend to be higher in copper. Therefore, zinc deficiency is common among vegetarians.

Zinc deficiencies and the lack of meat tend to lower stomach acid, reducing the absorption of key minerals such as iron, magnesium, and vitamin B_{12}. Also, the high anti-nutrient content of the diet can block even more minerals from these foods. It is, therefore, important to support your stomach acid levels with HCL Breakthrough and take steps to reduce your food's anti-nutrient content (see below).

Saturated and Preformed Essential Fatty Acids: Hormones, Brain Function, and Immune Balance

Saturated Fats. Plant-based diets also tend to be lower in saturated fats. Wade found that he needed to deliberately add saturated fats, such as coconut oils, to support his testosterone levels.

Omega-3. Most plant-based sources of omega-3 are in the short-chain form, alpha-linolenic acid (ALA), found in flaxseed, walnuts, and hempseed. You need long-chain omega-3s, such as docosahexaenoic acid (DHA) and eicosapentaenoic acid (EPA), for your brain function, healthy cell and mitochondrial membranes, and balanced inflammatory responses.

The conversion of ALA to EPA and DHA is not very effective. Also, testosterone inhibits this conversion, so men are naturally worse at it than women.[39] Many people who do well on plant-based diets are genetically better at the conversion.[40] To learn more about your plant-based genetics, go to: www.BIOptimizers.com/book/genes.

Given how important omega-3 is for health, you should test your genes and monitor your red blood cell omega-3 index. We strongly recommend supplementing with algae oil to ensure you get enough long-chain omega-3.

Arachidonic acid (ARA) is a long-chain omega-6 fatty acid created from short-chain omega-6 fatty acids with the same enzymes you need to make EPA and DHA. Although ARA is a pro-inflammatory fatty acid because it's a precursor to inflammatory prostaglandins, it also has many other essential roles. You need arachidonic acid for your brain and memory, and for cellular suicide (apoptosis), which kills cancer cells.[41]

Importantly, 15 to 17 percent of fat in your muscles consists of arachidonic acid. It controls neuromuscular signaling, making it an important fatty acid for strength and muscle building. If your goal is to build or retain muscles and gain strength, you need to consume enough arachidonic acid.[42] ARA also stimulates testosterone production in the testicles.[43]

The only food sources of arachidonic acid are animal products.[44] If you have trouble making EPA and DHA from plant-based sources, you're also going to have trouble making ARA from plant-based omega-6. On a plant-based diet, you won't be getting any ARA from food. If you need more ARA, one option is to supplement with a fungal-based arachidonic acid[45] to help you achieve your muscle-building goals.

Protein Deficiency: Muscle Mass and Brain Function

Many vegans and vegetarians don't consume enough proteins to support the bare minimum for their health. As a result, they lose a lot of muscle mass, and their brain function starts to suffer. Therefore, we recommend supplementing with a complete plant-based protein powder, such as Protein Breakthrough, to prevent protein deficiencies. Aim for at least 0.5 gram per pound of lean body mass, or maybe more if your goal is to lose weight or gain muscle.

Other Vital Nutrients to Pay Attention to

Vegetarian diets tend to be low in the following nutrients, even though your body can produce some of them. Many vegetarians find it beneficial or performance-boosting to intentionally increase them. These may help with weight loss, brain function, exercise performance, and exercise recovery.

- **Choline** provides a building block for acetylcholine, a very important neurotransmitter. It is also an important methyl donor in liver detoxification.[46] Food sources of choline include eggs and lecithin from soy or sunflower. We suggest supplementing with Nootopia's brain-enhancing stacks to truly optimize your mind.

- **Creatine** is important for cellular energy production, and you may recognize it as a strength-boosting pre-workout supplement. Vegetarian diets tend to lack creatine because it's mostly found in meat and fish. Creatine is one of the best overall supplements anyone can take due to its various health-boosting benefits.
- **Carnitine** helps bring fatty acids into your mitochondria to jump-start fat burning. Vegetarians have lower blood carnitine than meat eaters.[47]
- **Cholesterol** provides a backbone for your steroid hormones, like testosterone and cortisol. Plant-based foods are devoid of cholesterol, and many plant sterols lower cholesterol. So, you want to make sure your cholesterol and steroid hormones are in optimal ranges—not too high or too low. Wade personally needs to eat some plant-based saturated fats to maintain his testosterone levels.

Anti-Nutrients and Gut Irritants

Plants can't run away from their predators, so they produce substances to deter or kill them.

Many people who do well on a plant-based diet have genetics and epigenetics that allow them to better tolerate or derive benefits from these substances. Some nutrition experts promote the idea that "lectins" are dangerous for everyone. This is not accurate. There are many ways to mitigate their downsides.

In fact, the majority of the population tolerates these substances in food doses and feels better eating more plants. On the other hand, the minority that feels better by avoiding grains and beans may have the genetics, epigenetics, and microbiome that make these substances dangerous for them (see Chapter 33).

If you're susceptible, plant anti-nutrients can irritate the gut, block digestive enzymes, neutralize stomach acid, and prevent effective nutrient absorption.

Phytates

Phytates are found in plant seeds, roots, and tubers. They bind to minerals like iron, zinc, and magnesium, impairing the absorption of these minerals. You can reduce phytates by soaking, sprouting, and fermenting your grains and beans.

Tannins

Tannins are water-soluble polyphenols that make tea, coffee, and vegetables bitter. Plants make tannins to deter you from eating them.

In animal studies, tannins reduce feed intake, growth rate, feed efficiency, net metabolizable energy, and protein digestibility.[48] They neutralize stomach acid and impair the absorption of zinc, magnesium, copper, and iron, especially non-heme iron.[49, 50, 51] They may also precipitate proteins and inhibit digestive enzymes.

Most human studies that demonstrate the anti-nutrient effects of tannins are based on tea. So, you should avoid drinking coffee and tea with meals, especially if you are concerned about mineral deficiency.

Enzyme Inhibitors

Enzyme inhibitors are substances that block the function of enzymes, which are meant to protect seeds against predators. Most of these can be reduced by soaking, sprouting, fermenting, and cooking.

Oxalates

Oxalates can be found in leafy greens, cruciferous vegetables, rhubarb, black pepper, chocolate, tea, nuts, and berries. These can cause kidney stones and pain in people with oxalate intolerance. In healthy people, they can bind minerals in the gut and prevent absorption. Boiling vegetables and discarding the water may reduce oxalates by 30 to 87 percent.[52]

If you have severe oxalate sensitivity that causes excruciating pain, you may have to be very careful with a plant-based diet.

Goitrogens

Goitrogens are substances that prevent healthy thyroid function by blocking iodine entry, interfering with thyroid peroxidase, or interfering with thyroid-stimulating hormone. These are found in unfermented soy products such as tofu, soy milk, and edamame, and fresh or fermented cruciferous vegetables. For this reason, you should limit your soy consumption and avoid relying on it for protein.

Lectins

Lectins are proteins that help cells recognize each other, a mechanism that's present in all species.[53] Many plant lectins have protein structures that are difficult to digest, so high-lectin plant foods are common causes of food sensitivities.[54] They also tend to activate your immune system,[55] leading to the production of antibodies, although this only rarely leads to autoimmune diseases.

Some lectins are just outright toxic whether you're sensitive or not. For example, raw white kidney bean lectin causes food poisoning in everyone.[56] Ricin (nefariously used in the TV show *Breaking Bad*), the castor bean lectin, has been used as a toxic weapon.[57]

Legume lectins can be degraded just by cooking or sprouting, but grain lectins don't fully degrade through these processes. If your grains, nightshades, squashes, and legumes cause you inflammation, it is likely you're sensitive to lectins.

If you are sensitive to lectins or have the genes for lectin sensitivity, it may be extra challenging to do a plant-based diet. Some people may be able to do plant-based despite lectin sensitivity by maximizing protein digestion with VegZymes and ensuring that their lectin-containing foods are cooked properly.

Glycoalkaloids and Saponins

Glycoalkaloids are nitrogen-containing toxins found in nightshade plants. Plants in this family include:

- Tomatoes
- Tomatillos
- Potatoes
- Tobacco
- Eggplant
- Peppers and pepper products such as cayenne, chili pepper, paprika, and dried red peppers

Saponins are soap-like glycoalkaloids that can poke holes in cell membranes, causing cells to burst. They're found in legumes, quinoa, onions, garlic, asparagus, oats, spinach, sugar beets, tea, and yams.[58] Saponins may also inhibit digestive enzymes.[59]

FODMAPs

Fermentable oligosaccharides, disaccharides, monosaccharides, and polyols (FODMAPs) are fermentable fibers that are poorly absorbed in the gut. If you are sensitive to FODMAPs, you likely have an overgrowth of gut bacteria that ferments them in your small intestine. It can cause abdominal pain, bloating, constipation, and diarrhea.

Although low-FODMAP diets help with many cases of IBS, in the long term, they can starve the good gut bacteria. Therefore, complete avoidance of FODMAPs remains a very controversial approach.[60] The best strategy is to do the BIOptimized Gut Health test to see which type of plants are optimal for *your* digestive system. Go to www.BIOptimizers.com/book/guthealth to do a gut health test—this will help you choose better foods for YOUR gut biome.

Keep in mind that if you have a severe sensitivity to major categories of plant-based foods, such as oxalates (present in all leafy vegetables), FODMAPs, or lectins, it can make a plant-based diet very restrictive for you. In these cases, you may need to heal the gut and address these food sensitivities first before transitioning out of animal products. However, sensitivities to smaller categories of foods such as those with gluten or nightshades may be manageable on a plant-based diet.

Genetic tests can help reveal these potential issues.

HOW TO THRIVE ON A PLANT-BASED DIET DESPITE THE ANTI-NUTRIENTS

Becoming plant-based means it becomes much more important to pay attention to your nutrient absorption and levels to avoid deficiencies. It's less about how much iron, magnesium, and zinc you consume and more about how much you actually absorb.

1. Use Digestive Support

Concentrated plant-based digestive enzymes like VegZymes are designed to optimize the body's breakdown of plants. VegZymes can help you break down many anti-nutrients and overcome the enzyme inhibitors that are naturally in your food.

More importantly, it has alpha-galactosidase and other sugar-digesting enzymes to break down carbohydrates in legumes that can cause gas and bloating. And it contains multiple cellulases, which help break down plant cell walls.

Avoiding meat and being in zinc deficiency tend to reduce stomach acid over time, but stomach acid is still critical for your overall digestive health and nutrient absorption, and for preventing infections. You can get parasites on a vegan diet, as Wade did in Bali. Therefore, we recommend that all vegetarians and vegans support their stomach acid levels, such as with HCL Breakthrough. HCL Breakthrough is a synergistic blend of plant-based digestive enzymes and HCL (hydrochloric acid, the same acid your stomach releases). HCL can help kill parasites before they take hold in your intestinal system.

2. Pay Attention to Nutrient Forms, Synergy, Effective Dosages, and Competition to Maximize Absorption

Anemia from iron and vitamin B_{12} deficiencies are more common among vegetarians than meat eaters.[61] When you supplement to prevent or correct nutrient deficiencies, you need to pay attention to how nutrients are absorbed together, or how they compete with each other for absorption.

All plant-based iron is non-heme iron, which requires vitamin C or acid to help you absorb it, so it's important to pair sources of vitamin C with high-iron foods.[62] If your iron is too low, we strongly suggest using supplements to compensate.

Multivalent minerals include zinc, magnesium, copper, and calcium. They use the same absorption pathways, so they compete with each other for the same absorption proteins in the gut.[63] A deficiency in zinc can also increase your absorption of toxic heavy metals as your body tries to replenish the zinc.[64] Therefore, if you're working to correct any of these mineral deficiencies, you want to take their supplements separately, perhaps a few hours apart.

Fulvic and humic acid can greatly improve mineral absorption,[65] so we incorporate these in our Magnesium Breakthrough.

Keep in mind that calcium requires vitamins D and K for absorption and assimilation. When you take vitamin D, you also need magnesium for the vitamin D to work.[66]

B vitamins work together, even though the only B vitamin that you supplement may be vitamin B_{12}.

3. Eat Ferments

Fermented foods are some of the best things you can eat.

We suggest eating fermented foods at least once a day. Ideally build up to adding a bit to each meal.

Raw fermented foods are a rich source of not only probiotics, but also antioxidants, enzymes, and other beneficial bacterial metabolites.[67]

These components of fermented foods work together to both modulate and strengthen the immune system.[68] By modulating the immune system, they inhibit excess chronic inflammation, allergies, and autoimmunities. At the same time, they keep your immune system ready to fight off germs you're exposed to.[69]

In a Spanish clinical study, healthy volunteers deprived of fermented foods started to have weakened innate immune response within about two weeks.[70]

Here are the foods richest in probiotics:

- *Real yogurt.* Most commercial yogurts are filled with dead probiotics and an overload of sugar. Real yogurt is incredibly sour to the taste because the live probiotics have consumed the sugar and produced beneficial acids.
- *Kefir.* Closely resembles yogurt. It provides a good dose of calcium as well as healthy bacteria. Choose unflavored kefir, since any added sugars may prevent healthy bacteria from thriving inside your body.
- *Sauerkraut.* The primary bacteria in this type of food is Lactobacillus, and in concentrations even higher than found in yogurt. Prepare sauerkraut yourself rather than purchase a store variety, because they are typically prepared using vinegar, which kills off much of the beneficial bacteria.
- *Raw fruits and vegetables.* Raw fruits and vegetables are a great natural source of probiotics and have a very diverse range of live bacteria.
- *Kimchi.* Kimchi is prepared using cabbage, radishes, and scallions, and it may also contain red pepper. The probiotic strain found in kimchi is called *Lactobacillus brevis*, which may help promote greater weight loss.
- *Miso.* Miso soup is made from fermented soybeans along with salt and koji, which is an edible fungus. Miso helps to boost your digestive system and enhance your immune system, and may also help to lower your overall risk factor for cancer as well.[71, 72]
- *Kombucha.* Kombucha is a fermented probiotic drink made with black or green tea, along with the yeast that helps to ferment it.
- *Pickles.* You want fermented pickles, which are usually best made yourself. You don't need any ingredients besides cucumbers (or any other vegetable you desire), salt, and water.

  The good news is that if you choose to make your own, you can sidestep many of the additives that are included in supermarket pickles.
- *Natto.* This is a Japanese dish made from fermented soybeans and has a sticky sort of texture. This dish is very rich in vitamin K and has been known to help with skin health as well, preventing wrinkles and boosting skin elasticity.[73]

Research has shown that bacteria help nutrient absorption—from macronutrients like protein and fats to micronutrients.

4. Biomimic Your Food Preparations

Many plant-based minerals are already bound to anti-nutrients as stored nutrients in dormant plant seeds. So, you may not absorb them unless you prepare your foods specifically to activate them. Traditional cultures that consume such seeds take the time to prepare them properly, as they've discovered that skipping these processes can make people sick.

Preparations that increase nutrient bioavailability in plant foods include:

- Soaking or submerging grains or beans under water overnight or until they soften. Soaking legumes can also remove gas-producing sugars and make the legumes much easier to digest.
- Rinsing a food and discarding the water can remove some anti-nutrients (such as saponins from quinoa).
- Sprouting involves soaking seeds overnight, then draining and regularly rinsing them two to three times per day until they grow into sprouts. Sprouting activates the life force and releases stored nutrients. Sprouts have fewer anti-nutrients but more enzymes and vitamin C.
- Fermenting may involve adding a fermentation starter culture to a prolonged seed soak, or doing lacto-fermentation with salt water.
- Cooking legumes and grains sufficiently is needed to break down harmful components and gut irritants. One exception is if they've been sprouted to the point that they resemble vegetables more than seeds.

HOW TO DO A PLANT-BASED DIET

The concept of a plant-based diet is simple: just give up meat and animal products. However, to harness the power of the diet to maximize the three sides of your BIOptimization Triangle, you need to do it right.

Consider including the following foods on a regular basis if they don't cause inflammatory reactions (see below) or excessive blood sugar fluctuations.

Foods to Include on a Regular Basis

Vegan Food List

The definition of a vegan or plant-based diet is to exclude all animal products—i.e., meat, fish, seafood, dairy, and eggs. You can eat any food in the following categories. Please note that we give a few examples; the lists are not exhaustive.

- Vegetables: leafy greens, tubers, cruciferous vegetables, tomatoes, carrots, rutabaga, onions, garlic, eggplant
- Fruits: citrus, apples, pears, bananas, melons, avocados, peaches, coconut
- Legumes and lentils: red beans, mung beans, black beans, kidney beans, lima beans, peas, chickpeas, lentils
- Mushrooms and fungi: nutritional yeasts, shiitake, crimini, white button mushrooms
- Grains: rice, oats, wheat, barley, millet, rye, and their products
- Pseudograins: quinoa, kaniwa, buckwheat, and amaranth
- Nuts: macadamias, walnuts, cashews, almonds, Brazil nuts, hazelnuts, pine nuts
- Seeds: chia, flax, sunflower, pumpkin, hemp, sesame, watermelon
- Marine plants: seaweed, kelp, chlorella, spirulina, kombu, nori, sea grapes
- Fats: oils extracted from avocados, coconut, palm, nuts, and seeds

We believe that it's probably better to eat organic and local foods that are of heirloom origin rather than genetically modified versions.

THREE-DAY VEGAN MEAL PLAN

We suggest starting with 12 calories per pound of bodyweight for two weeks. And if you're not losing weight, then lower your calories to 11 calories per pound. And if that's not working, lower it to 10 calories per pound.

Here we present various meal options, which you can access in our resource section for the book: www.BIOp timizers.com/book/resources.

Day 1

- Superfood oatmeal (285 calories)
- Seaweed kale salad (420 calories)
- Macrobiotic bowl (478 calories)

Day 2

- Carrot cake breakfast muffins (553 calories)
- Spring salad with raspberry vinaigrette (358 calories)
- Maitake stakes with saffron cauliflower rice (438 calories)

Day 3

- Superfood buckwheat kasha (287 calories)
- Summer jicama picnic salad (682 calories)
- Spicy pad Thai veggie noodles (573 calories)

THREE-DAY VEGETARIAN MEAL PLAN

Day 1

- Protein Breakthrough Seed Breakfast Bar (507 calories)
- Fruit salad (280 calories)
- Raw vegan lasagna (433 calories)

Day 2:

- Sweet potato toast (243 calories)
- Collard spring rolls (643 calories)
- Vegetable Cambodian lemongrass curry with spirulina shirataki noodles (711 calories)

Day 3:

- Rainbow chia pudding (472 calories)
- Nori roll-ups (550 calories)
- Zaatar veggies tacos (721 calories)

You can find all of these recipes in our *Plant-Based Superfood Delights Cookbook.*

LACTO-VEGETARIAN

The advantage of going lacto-vegetarian is the access to good protein sources. Lacto-vegetarians consume all plant-based foods and also dairy products, which may include milk, butter, cream, cheeses, and their byproducts.

Many vegetarians keep dairy and/or eggs in their diets either due to preference or to continue getting animal sources of nutrients. We recommend trying an elimination diet first to see if these foods cause any inflammation before eating them on a regular basis.

These are excellent sources of complete protein and animal-based nutrients. However, the high leucine content of dairy proteins also tends to stimulate insulin releases.

Because A1 milk can cause inflammation (especially if someone has a leaky gut), causing digestive issues and increasing mucus,[74] we recommend finding A2 dairy products or dairy products from animals other than cows.

If you're sensitive to A1 but not A2 dairy, Gluten Guardian, which contains the enzyme that can completely digest casein, can typically help fully break down the A1 peptide.

OVO-VEGETARIAN

Ovo-vegetarians consume all the plant-based foods, along with eggs and their products. Eggs make an excellent source of complete protein and animal-based nutrients. Wade does occasionally incorporate eggs into his diet.

PLANT-BASED PROTEIN SOURCES

While it's possible to get enough protein from plant-based sources, it's crucial to pay attention to creating complete proteins.

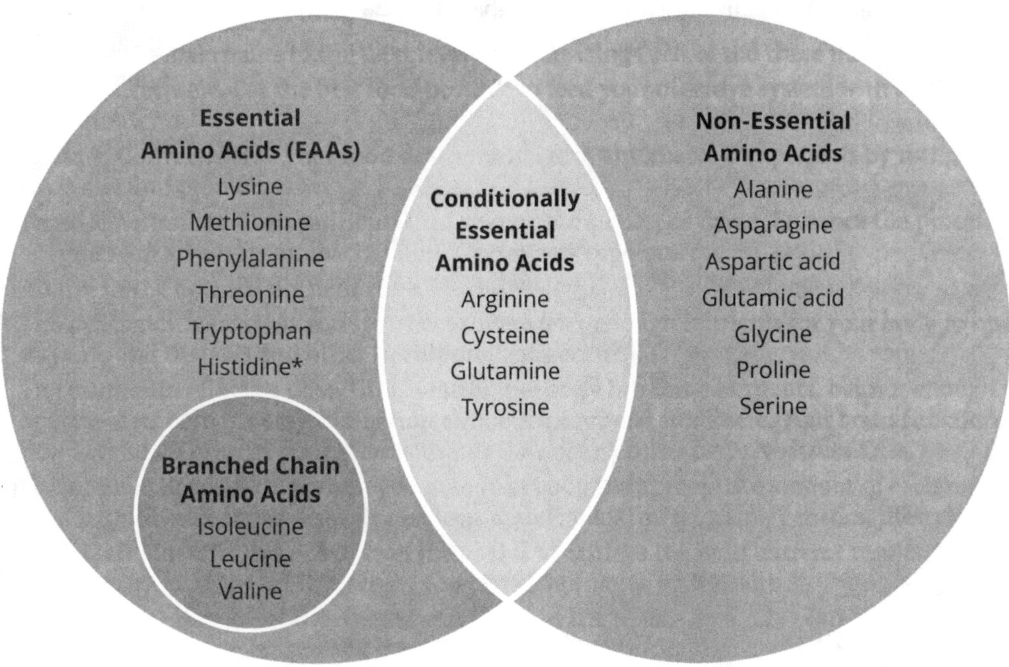

*Histidine is a special case, as it's sometimes listed as an essential amino acid. However, histidine deficiency takes a longer period of time to cause problems than deficiency in other EAAs.

Complete Protein

Of the 20 amino acids, seven of them are nonessential because your body can create them on its own. Four of them are conditionally essential, meaning your body can usually make them but may struggle to catch up with the demand during sickness or stress. The remaining nine are essential because you can only get them from food.

You need all 20 amino acids to build muscles and construct other proteins in your body. If you don't have all the essential amino acids, then your body is more likely to burn amino acids for energy rather than use them to make more proteins.[75, 76] This means you're catabolic and losing lean muscle.

It's a common misconception that you can't get complete proteins from plants—all plant sources have complete proteins. However, grains are very low in lysine, whereas legumes are low in methionine and cysteine. If you consume only one protein source, you may not be able to fully utilize the protein. The key is to eat a diverse diet that consists of both categories of food within 24 hours of each other. Score another one for the "big-ass salad"!

Some plant-based protein sources provide complete proteins or a relatively well-rounded combination of amino acids. These include:

- Hemp
- Pea
- Pumpkin
- Soy and soy products
- Buckwheat
- Quinoa
- Potatoes
- Chia seeds
- Spirulina
- Spinach
- Quorn (protein from fungi)

IS IT HARDER TO BUILD MUSCLE ON A PLANT-BASED DIET?

Plant-based proteins are also lower in leucine than animal proteins,[77] so they activate mTOR to a lesser extent. In theory, this can make it harder to gain muscles on a plant-based diet. The lower mTOR activation also contributes less to your cancer risk. If your goal is to activate mTOR and you don't consume dairy, you can simply supplement with leucine. Aim for more than 3 grams of leucine per meal to maximize the anabolic response.

DETERMINING THE IDEAL MACRONUTRIENTS FOR VEGETARIANS AND VEGANS

At first, you may find it less satisfying to cut out meat and animal products. Therefore, you'll have to find the right combination of protein and fats that will keep you satiated. Be mindful that there's a tendency to gravitate toward refined carbs when starting a plant-based diet. This can leave you feeling hungry and drive you to overeat.

You do need regular servings of high-quality protein. We recommend starting with 20 to 30 percent of your daily protein. Often, to achieve this level, you'll need to supplement with a protein powder.

Then you can allocate about 20 to 40 percent of your daily calorie intake on fats and carbs each, depending on your goals and biofeedback.

People who feel better eating frequently, like Wade, do better on more carbs, but those who do better on lower carbs tend to do better eating less frequently.

Seasonality and Climate

You may find that your body has different needs in different climates or seasons.

Wade has found that his appetite drops significantly when he gets more sun exposure, even though he feels more energized. Once it gets colder or he gets less sun, his appetite goes up.

Studies confirm this pattern. In people who live in temperate climates with four seasons, their bodies go into thrifty mode in the fall. When the days get shorter and the weather gets cooler, the body becomes more insulin resistant and appetite goes up, causing it to store more fat.[78] At the same time, food is most available in the fall after it grows all summer.[79]

Therefore, we think it's important to structure your diet around the seasons and eat locally as much as possible. Fresher seasonal and local produce are richer in nutrients. You may crave more raw foods in the summer and more hearty, cooked foods when it gets colder. Because insulin sensitivity is highest in the summer, it might be a good idea to eat more carbs at that time, and then more fats in the winter.

HOW *NOT* TO DO A VEGAN OR VEGETARIAN DIET

Eating Too Much Processed Food

Potato chips are vegan, but it doesn't mean they are a good diet option. Of course, you can enjoy occasional treats as long as they are within your macro and calorie targets. Without paying attention to nutrition, it's easy to fall into the habit of relying on processed or hyper-palatable vegan foods. Learn to read the labels and watch your macros.

A well-rounded vegetarian diet should consist of mostly whole foods and plenty of vegetables. Even then, you should routinely monitor for micronutrient, fatty acid, and amino acid deficiencies.

Not Paying Attention to Your Genes and Ancestral Heritages

Many people who desire to do a vegetarian diet have ancestors who evolved in cold climates. So, they may have genes that are not ideal for a plant-based diet. However, the more you understand your body and genetic tendencies, the better you can find ways to thrive despite your tendencies. Even though Wade has Northern European genes, he's found a way to make a vegetarian diet work.

Pros of a Vegetarian Diet

Health

- Potentially improves longevity and metabolic health[80]
- Improves gut microbiome[81]
- High in fiber, phytochemicals, and certain nutrients
- Reduced exposure to carcinogens and thus cancer risk[82]
- May eliminate some food sensitivities

Aesthetics

- Some people may find it easier to lose weight and maintain it[83]
- Some may experience better skin from the overall reduction of IGF-1 and androgens[84]

Performance

- Some people may find that they perform better physically or cognitively

Lifestyle

- Reduced grocery budget and food costs

Psychological

- Some believe it's more ethical to avoid eating animals

Cons of a Vegetarian Diet

Health

- Increased risk of nutrient deficiencies
- Increased risk of cognitive impairment, depression, and anxiety[85]

Aesthetics

- It may be more difficult to gain and maintain muscles or recomposition on this diet

Performance

- Some may find that their cognitive and physical performance drop on this diet

Lifestyle

- The diet can be restrictive, making it harder to go to restaurants or enjoy social occasions

Psychological

- If nutrient deficiencies are not addressed, they can contribute to depression and anxiety[86]

SUMMARY

Going vegan or vegetarian isn't ideal for everyone, genetically speaking, although some people may have stronger genes for thriving on a plant-based diet.

That said, some of the health benefits of a plant-based diet may include:

- Beneficial shifts in the gut microbiome
- Increase in dietary fiber
- Filling holes: increase in phytonutrients, vitamins, and minerals
- Reduced insulin growth factor (IGF-1)
- Reduced toxins from food
- Reduced processed foods
- Increase in enzymes

Here are some of the risk factors that come with a plant-based diet:

- Nutrient deficiencies
- Anti-nutrients and gut irritants

You can still thrive on a plant-based diet despite anti-nutrients by:

- Using digestive support
- Paying attention to nutrient forms, synergy, effective dosages, and competition to maximize absorption
- Eating ferments
- Biomimicking your food preparations

The concept of a plant-based diet is simple—just give up meat and animal products. However, to harness the power of the diet to maximize the three sides of your BIOptimization Triangle, you need to do it right.

CHAPTER 22

HOW TO SUCCEED ON A PALEO DIET

In this chapter, you'll learn:

- Why a paleo diet often results in effortless fat loss and improved health
- Common mistakes new paleo dieters often make, and how to avoid them
- What exactly a paleo diet is, what foods it includes, and what its restrictions are
- The significant beneficial nutritional changes in a paleo diet and the six health benefits that most paleo followers experience as a result
- How to start a paleo diet
- The five keys to succeeding on a paleo diet
- Supplements you can use to optimize your results on a paleo diet
- How to optimize paleo for achieving aesthetic goals and maximizing athletic performance
- Seven factors that could lead to failing on your paleo diet
- How to decide if the paleo diet is right for you, based on its pros and cons

WHAT IS A PALEO DIET?

The original paleo diet concept, popularized by Mark Sisson and Loren Cordain, was based on the idea that our human genes have not significantly changed in 10,000 years. The theory is that we should eat like hunter-gatherers, since it assumes that they were free of modern chronic diseases such as cardiovascular problems, diabetes, high blood pressure, and cancers.

The diet excludes foods that presumably did not exist 10,000 years ago, such as processed foods, grains, legumes, dairy, and vegetable oil. It advises people to focus on high-quality grass-fed, organic meat, plus organic fruits and vegetables, as much as possible.

One of the best things about paleo diets is that the rules of engagement are clear and straightforward. The original version took the world by storm with its simplicity, health benefits, and eco-consciousness.

More hardcore paleo enthusiasts may focus on wild game meat and foraging for wild plants and mushrooms. Many seek out produce from farms that practice biodynamic farming or regenerative agriculture.

Many paleo followers also are motivated by strong environmental concerns. They examine the impact of their diet and actions on the environment. However, the logistics are different from what some other eaters believe. Vegans think meat is the worst thing for the environment, but paleo dieters believe that industrial agriculture and feedlot meats are the worst things for the environment. They feel that what's best for the environment is regenerative agriculture that supports the topsoil with its grass-fed animals that are allowed to roam freely. Again, we're not here to debate these things. You can form your own ethical, spiritual, and political opinions.

Overall, the paleo diet has attracted some of the biggest groups of online and global dietary enthusiasts. There are many great things about this diet, but there are also pitfalls. This chapter is about harnessing the power of paleo principles to maximize your BIOptimization Triangle without falling for any dogma.

A Strict Paleo Diet Includes:

- Grass-fed or wild meat, especially organ meats and fattier cuts
- Wild-caught or responsibly raised fish and shellfish
- Pastured eggs
- Nuts and seeds
- Herbs
- Spices
- Sugar-free fermented vegetables, meat, and fish
- Healthy fats, including avocados, coconuts, lard, tallow, olive oil, and animal fats
- Fruits and vegetables, including tubers but excluding white potatoes
- Small amounts of natural sweeteners such as stevia and monk fruit

A Strict Paleo Diet Excludes:

- Grains and pseudograins
- Legumes
- Processed foods
- Sugar in all forms
- Soft drinks
- Dairy products
- Artificial sweeteners
- Vegetable oils
- Margarine
- Hydrogenated or trans fats

Many long-term paleo dieters eventually bring back some gluten-free grains, legumes, and dairy such as butter, ghee, or heavy cream. Some only consume non-cow or A2 dairy.

The Autoimmune Paleo Protocol

The Autoimmune Paleo Protocol (AIP) is the stricter version of paleo. Its aim is to manage autoimmune diseases, and it removes immune-stimulating components by cutting out the following foods:

- Nuts and seeds
- Nightshades (such as tomatoes, potatoes, peppers, and tomatillos)
- All spices, herbs, and fats that come from seeds
- Eggs
- Coffee
- Chocolate
- Sweeteners and all sugar substitutes
- Alcohol

HEALTH BENEFITS OF A PALEO DIET

As with most diets, a paleo diet is an excellent antidote to the standard American diet. It removes processed and inflammatory foods while significantly cutting down on toxins. At the same time, it increases satiating, nutrient-dense foods such as vegetables, fruits, and organ meats. As a result, it usually lowers overall calories, which can lead to weight loss.

Many paleo dieters have successfully achieved their weight loss goals and resolved their chronic health issues and so have become evangelists for the diet. Currently, many functional medicine doctors follow the paleo nutrition approach as a therapeutic diet.

The significant and beneficial nutritional changes in a paleo diet include:

- Reduction in dietary lectins, which may reduce inflammation for those who are sensitive to them[1]
- Increased micronutrient and antioxidant intake due to vitamins and minerals from food selection, choosing foods grown in healthy soil, and sourcing food locally
- Reduced omega-6 intake and increased natural omega-3 intake[2]
- Reduced food-based toxins, such as pesticides, damaged fats, and antibiotics
- Reduced overall carb intake by cutting out grains and other processed carbs
- Increased overall intake of saturated and monounsaturated fats, along with fat-soluble vitamins
- Increased fiber and polyphenol intake from eating more vegetables and fruits, which is good for your gut bacteria[3]
- Reduced hedonic eating from cutting out processed foods (with some exceptions), which typically reduces caloric intake[4]
- Increased awareness of how food affects one's health and body, including hunger and satiety

As a result, many paleo eaters experience the following health benefits:

1. Reduced Inflammation

The ideal ratio of omega-6 to omega-3 intake is between 1:1 to 4:1, but with ubiquitous use of vegetable oils, most people consume more than 10:1.[5] Excess omega-6 is a major contributor of inflammation for people consuming the standard American diet.

Improving the quality of your fats on any diet is a Power Move. Seafood is the richest source of omega-3s: mackerel, salmon, cod liver oil, herring, oysters, sardines, anchovies, and caviar are the top sources. For plant lovers, flax seeds, chia seeds, and walnuts are the winners.

Omega-6 fats are fragile molecules that are easily damaged by oxidative stress, so consuming a lot of them leads to cellular components that are more susceptible to oxidative damage. Overall, it increases all kinds of disease risks, including fatty liver, heart disease, rheumatoid arthritis, and Alzheimer's disease.[6]

Many people have food sensitivities that they are unaware of (see Chapter 31). The common ones are to gluten, dairy, lectins, eggs, coffee, and nightshades. When eaters experiment with removing these foods, they often feel significantly better, with fewer aches and pains and clearer thinking. Sometimes the diet even puts their chronic health conditions into remission.

2. Better Blood Sugar Control

Sugar cravings are often signs of major blood sugar fluctuations. Elevated blood sugar accelerates aging by increasing advanced glycation end products (AGEs). These are proteins or lipids that become glycated (bonded with sugar molecules) as a result of exposure to sugars. By cutting out processed foods, grains, legumes, and refined carbs, the paleo diet is naturally a lower-sugar diet by default. This leads to more stable blood sugar levels.

The increase in micronutrients and omega-3, and the reduction in inflammation, also help improve glycemic control. This often accompanies improvements in overall heart health markers, including cholesterol and triglycerides. For those who want to optimize their blood sugar levels even further, we suggest using Blood Sugar Breakthrough.

3. Reduced Cravings

We've already noted that cravings can often be a sign of nutrient deficiency. Because paleo is a more nutrient-dense diet, those types of cravings are often lowered.

Paleo emphasizes whole-food sources of cellular carbs, such as sweet potatoes and squashes, which typically are better for satiety and glycemic control. You'll feel more satisfied and have fewer cravings as a result.

When you try a new diet, your palate and microbiome adapt to it. As a result, some people experience lower cravings for processed food items after a while.

4. Weight Loss

Many people naturally lose weight on the paleo diet without rigorous calorie counting for many reasons, a number of which we've mentioned. First, it reduces inflammation and cravings. Second, it improves blood sugar control. Third, it is higher in satiating fibers and polyphenols that feed the lean gut bacteria. Fourth, it reduces a lot of the factors that cause people to overeat, such as the hedonic response to processed foods. Fifth, you're eliminating calorie-dense food. Sixth, it's naturally higher in protein, which helps anabolism and satiety. Last, it teaches people to be aware of their appetite and how foods affect their bodies.

All of these factors tend to reduce caloric intake and increase calorie expenditure, naturally leading to weight loss.

5. More Energy and Better Mood

Fatigue and low mood are often signs of poor blood sugar control and poor mitochondrial function, which can come from inflammation, toxicity, or nutrient deficiencies. By correcting all three of these problems, many paleo dieters experience better energy and mood.

6. Remission of Chronic Diseases

Many paleo eaters started the diet to see if it could help them manage their inflammatory conditions or put them into remission. Some of these are autoimmune, while others may include chronic pain, allergies, or migraines.

Removing gluten and other gut irritants may help reduce autoimmunity by reducing intestinal permeability.[7] More and more clinical studies are demonstrating that either a paleo or AIP diet can help reduce inflammation and improve quality of life.[8, 9]

HOW TO DO A PALEO DIET

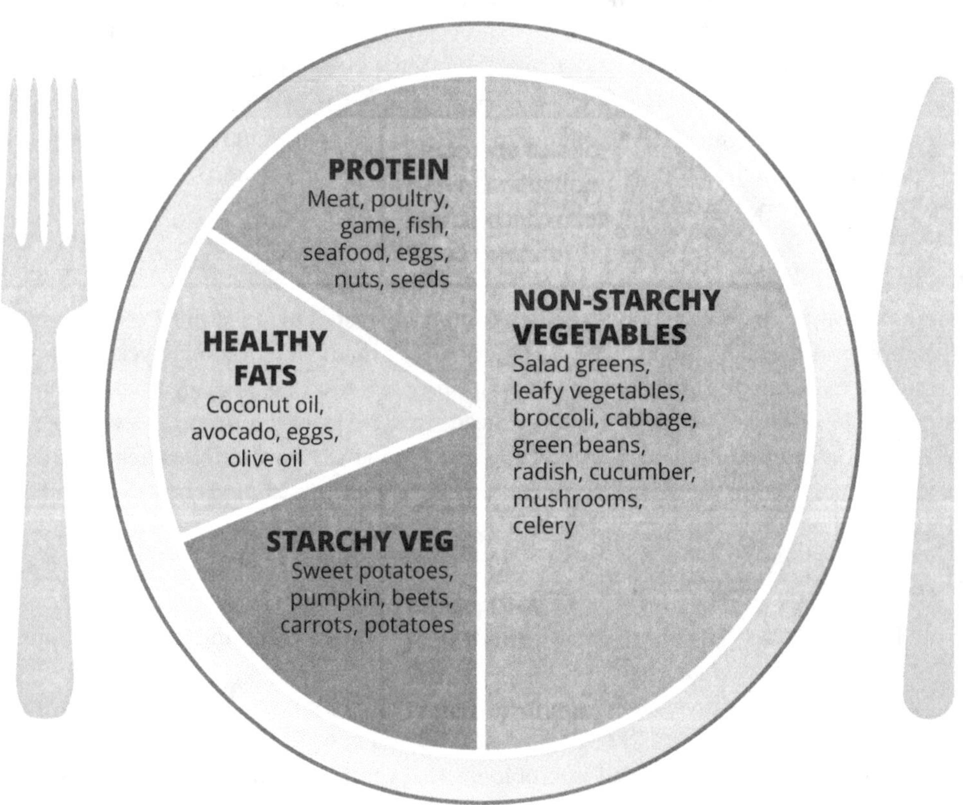

- Cut out all grains, legumes, sugar, and vegetable oils
- Fill half your plate with non-starchy vegetables
- Fill about one-sixth of your plate with protein, another sixth with healthy fats, and another sixth with starchy vegetables. The ratios can be adjusted based on your physique and athletic goals
- Eat slowly to satiety

Typical Paleo Macros

A paleo diet is usually 30 percent of total calories from protein, 40 percent fat (from mostly monounsaturated and polyunsaturated fats), and 30 percent carbohydrates.[10]

Our usual suggestion for people starting a paleo diet is just to stick to the foods that they're attracted to that fit within paleo constraints. Based on the results or lack thereof, you make modifications. Tracking calories and macronutrient intake from the beginning will give you the data you need to troubleshoot.

Paleo principles can be adapted to improve physique and athletic goals. Many of the top CrossFit athletes also follow a paleo diet. However, for these goals, it's important to monitor your macronutrients and calories beyond just how you feel.

Optimizing Paleo for Aesthetic Goals

If you have physique goals such as fat loss or muscle gain, then you probably need to track calories and macros to ensure that you reach them.

For fat loss, some people may lose weight in the beginning without tracking, but then metabolic adaptations occur and they plateau. When plateaus happen, you need to break homeostasis. Increasing overall protein intake while decreasing fats and carbs is one of the main moves. This decreases your net calories. Review Chapter 7, The Optimized Metabolism System, and Chapter 13, The Ultimate Fat Loss Master Plan, for more instructions.

If your goal is to achieve extreme leanness, such as cutting for physique competition preps, calorie cutting and increased exercise are mandatory. You may need to focus most of your non-protein macro on either fats or carbs. So, a paleo diet can evolve into a keto-ish diet during these fat loss cycles.

For muscle building, simply increase your calories 300 to 500 above maintenance and follow a well-structured weight training program. Read Chapter 16, The Ultimate Muscle-Building Master Plan, for more guidance.

Paleo for Athletic Performance

If you train in a strength or glycolytic sport such as powerlifting or sprinting, you may need to add more carbs than the typical recommendation for optimal performance in paleo. Remember, one of our core suggestions is to let go of all dietary dogma. Listen to your body.

Some athletes do need to use non-paleo carb sources or supplements to support their training and nutritional needs. The key is to continue to track your performance and biofeedback to make sure your changes are supporting your goals.

Three-Day Sample 2,500-Calorie Paleo Menu

You can find all of these delicious recipes in our *Primal Paleo Cookbook*. And you can access these recipes in our book resource section: www.BIOptimizers.com/book/resources.

Day 1

- Maduros (246 calories)
- Japanese Salmon Salad (276 calories)
- Salmon with Blueberry (761 calories)
- Gooey Butter Cake (656 calories)

Day 2

- Cauliflower Fry Bread (222 Calories)
- Poke Bowl (587 calories)
- Dan Dan Noodles (851 calories)
- Vanilla Honey Cake (580 calories)

Day 3

- Chopped Liver with Crudités (288 calories)
- Cauliflower Pizza (546 calories)
- Steak Fajitas Burrito Bowl (891 calories)
- Tiramisu (391 calories)

Check out our YouTube channel, BIOptimized Paleo: https://www.youtube.com/@bioptimizedpaleo4065, to see some of the recipes from this cookbook in action.

KEYS TO PALEO SUCCESS

1. Go All-in for a Manageable Period before Reintroducing Additional Food

A paleo diet can work like an elimination diet, but it takes building habits and systems around it to be able to execute it successfully. To succeed on a paleo diet or reap the benefits from its principles, it's a good idea to commit to the strictest and cleanest foods for at least a month before reintroducing additional foods.

2. Start from All-Natural Foods in Their Natural States

The paleo blogosphere is full of recipes that help nostalgic dieters get their fix of cakes, cookies, and saucy orange chicken. But cave people did not have these foods, and they tend to defeat the purposes of a paleo diet.

To reap the most benefits from this way of eating, focus on foods that are closest to their natural states—perhaps just meat and vegetables to start. It's even better if you can focus on local meats and produce, since eating out of season can throw off your healthy gene expression.

Once your palate adapts and you figure out your food sensitivities, you can reintroduce ingredients like almond flour and dates. But even then, these foods should be treats rather than staples on your paleo diet.

3. Be Prepared and Well Stocked

It's a good idea to make sure that your home is well stocked with the right groceries. It's usually less expensive to buy an extra freezer so you can buy high-quality proteins in bulk—such as quarter, half, or whole animals from a local farmer. You'll have to learn to cook the organs and odd cuts, which are nutritious.

4. Have Backup Options

It's also a good idea to identify local restaurants or catering options that use paleo-compliant ingredients as your go-to places for gathering or backup plans. Having nuts on hand is a smart move. There are also some decent off-the-shelf paleo bar options from companies like Epic and Primal Kitchen.

5. Monitor Your Bloodwork and Biofeedback

A paleo diet isn't for everyone. For example, some people really don't do well on a lot of saturated fats, which can cause their inflammation and cholesterol to skyrocket. In some cases, people feel worse on the diet because they're sensitive to common paleo items. It is, therefore, important to monitor your bloodwork and biofeedback.

Although the diet is nutrient dense, it's still possible to become depleted in key nutrients on it. Avoiding processed foods means you're on your own with respect to nutrients that are typically fortified by the food industry, such as folate, vitamin D, calcium, and iodine. Magnesium is still low in the food chain. So, we suggest you regularly get tested for these nutrients and supplement accordingly.

PALEO DIET PITFALLS

1. Adding Too Much Fat

Paleo diets promote the idea that fats are healthy and that you should be adding fat to everything. However, it's possible to overdo the fat. Many people become more inflamed with saturated fats, while others just put on body fat due to the excess calories. You also may have genetic mutations that make certain fats suboptimal for *you*. That's why we suggest doing a nutrigenomics test.

2. Eating Too Many Processed Paleo Recipes

Eating paleo, or like cavemen, includes nothing like "paleo" cakes, cookies, pancakes, or even paleo-compliant processed foods. Despite being paleo compliant, these hedonic treats may not be nutritious or even healthy. Although they might be upgrades compared to the originals, they should be seen as treats for special occasions, not as staples.

3. Not Listening to Your Body

Many paleo eaters simply follow the group rather than listening to their bodies. If, for any reason, you don't feel well on this diet or your biofeedback starts to go haywire, it's time to make adjustments. Do regular bloodwork to make sure your nutrients are in the optimal range.

4. Not Being Prepared

Due to this diet's many restrictions and special grocery requirements, it's going to be difficult to stay on the diet if you're not prepared with compliant groceries and resources.

5. Too Much Muscle Meat, Not Enough Fatty Cuts or Organ Meats

Most people nowadays are more familiar with muscle meats, but hunter-gatherers treasured organs as the most nutritious parts of animals. Therefore, a true paleo diet should involve consuming and using most of the animal. Organ meats, such as liver, are higher in certain vitamins and minerals than muscle meats.

Consuming too much muscle meat can also cause amino acid imbalances because muscle meats, especially lean cuts, are higher in methionine and lower in glycine. Consuming so much methionine on a high-protein diet such as this one may raise your homocysteine level, which can be inflammatory.

Fattier cuts of meat are higher in amino acids like proline and glycine. Glycine is important for many physiologic processes and can help lower homocysteine. Many paleo dieters also use gelatin and collagen supplements to balance out their amino acid intake.

6. Too Many Charred or Processed Meats

The charring, smoking, and processing of meat creates toxic substances that can cause inflammation and raise oxidative stress, possibly leading to cancer.[11] While you can enjoy these once in a while, it is an unhealthy mistake to fill up every meal with grill-marked steaks, charred burgers, and fried bacon.

To minimize your health risks and inflammation, cook most of your proteins at reasonable temperatures. The paleo diet is not necessarily a barbeque-and-bacon diet—you can also enjoy stews, pot roasts, soups, and baked and steamed proteins.

7. Being Too Strict

This might sound counter to most of the chapter; however, many people do much better following a paleo structure 80 to 90 percent of the time and then giving themselves the freedom to enjoy other foods the other 10 to 20 percent. Maybe the Paleo Police will arrest you, but don't worry—the BIOptimized Diet-Dogma-Buster Squad will set you free!

PALEO DIET PROS AND CONS

Health

Pros

Reducing dietary toxins and inflammatory components can often result in improved health, reduced toxic load, and reduced inflammation. The diet also tends to help with blood sugar regulation, and thus overall metabolic health. It's also rich in many nutrients that are lacking in the standard American diet.

Cons

Some people may not do well with so much meat and fat in their diet. However, it is possible to adjust the diet within the paleo framework to make it healthy for them. Nutritional deficiencies may occur on a paleo diet, especially for the nutrients that are fortified in processed foods. This is why looking at your nutrigenomics is key.

Aesthetics

Pros

The reduced toxicity, inflammation, and food palatability in paleo can make it easier to lose weight if you come from a standard American diet or have not taken these factors into account before.

Cons

The default paleo diet may be too high in both carbohydrates and fats, making it difficult to achieve a very lean physique without manipulating the macros. This is easy to overcome with the Me Diet app.

Athletic and Mental Performance

Pros

By reducing toxicity and inflammation, while increasing some macronutrients, many people find that paleo improves their cognitive performance.

Cons

Some people do experience symptoms of carb withdrawal and keto adaptation on a paleo diet. Many athletes, especially those in strength and explosive sports, need additional carbs to support their training and performance.

Lifestyle

Pros

If your inflammatory conditions are better managed with the paleo diet, it can make your life easier.

Cons

Paleo can be a very restrictive diet, which makes it hard to enjoy social events and travels. However, since it's become more popular, there are now more restaurants and online options available. Again, as long as you stay within your calorie allotment, you can enjoy a plate of tasty processed carbs once in a while, and God won't zap you off the earth.

Psychological

Pros

Having the group support of people who have similar health and diet struggles can make you feel like you belong.

Cons

You can feel isolated from people who are not on the same diet. And many paleo eaters miss their old favorite foods, though some can be replaced with a paleo-modified version.

Optimization Supplements

- MassZymes and P3-OM can help support your digestion
- kApex can help digest fat and maintain energy levels. This is the best digestive aid for high-fat meals
- Biome Breakthrough is an important supplement to help you repair your gut as you eliminate inflammatory foods
- Magnesium Breakthrough can help ensure that you get enough magnesium levels to support your metabolism and stress responses

SUMMARY

Paleo diets are based on the idea that our human genes have not significantly changed in 10,000 years. The theory is, we should eat like hunter-gatherers, assuming that they were free of various modern chronic diseases. These diets exclude foods that didn't exist 10,000 years ago.

Many Paleo Eaters Experience These Benefits:

- Reduced inflammation
- Better blood sugar control
- Reduced cravings
- Weight loss
- More energy and better mood
- Remission of chronic diseases

How to Do a Paleo Diet:

- Cut out all grains, legumes, sugar, and vegetable oils
- Fill half your plate with non-starchy vegetables
- Fill about one-sixth of your plate with protein, another sixth with healthy fats, and another sixth with starchy vegetables. The ratios can be adjusted based on your physique and athletic goals
- Eat slowly to satiety

Keys to Success on Paleo:

- Go all-in for a manageable period before reintroducing additional foods
- Start with all-natural foods in their natural states
- Be prepared and well stocked
- Have backup options
- Monitor your bloodwork and biofeedback
- Set your calories based on your goals
- Make caloric and macro adjustments if you hit plateaus

Paleo diet pitfalls:

- Adding too much fat
- Eating too many processed "paleo" recipes
- Not listening to your body
- Not being prepared
- Too much muscle meat and not enough fatty cuts or organ meats
- Too much charred or processed meat
- Being too strict

CHAPTER 23

HOW TO SUCCEED WITH A RAW FOOD DIET

In this chapter, you'll learn:

- The detoxification, digestion, and sensory awareness benefits of the raw food diet
- Raw food diet pitfalls people often fall into from cults and dietary dogmas
- How to employ the raw food diet as a periodic nutritional strategy to maximize your overall nutritional results
- The six potential health benefits of doing a raw food diet
- Four possible health risks of a raw food diet and the Power Moves to help avoid them
- Seven preparation processes that can maximize the enzymes, nutrient availability, and life force of raw foods
- The top EFA options for vegetarians and vegans so you can optimize your fats
- What a typical day looks like on a raw food diet, with a three-day sample menu

THE SKINNY RAW VEGAN BECOMES A TONED BIKINI CHAMPION

As one of the first plant-based athletes ever to compete in Mr. Universe, Wade gained a bit of publicity online. When he won two of his three national championships on a completely raw food diet, most people refused to believe that he did it.

That being said, many skinny vegetarians, vegans, and raw food vegans used him as an example in a variety of arguments when confronted by meat eaters who suggested plant-based athletes couldn't build muscle, let alone compete successfully in bodybuilding. He was on a completely raw food vegan diet for two years before he moved to a more moderate vegetarian diet.

Wade shares one of his stories of helping a woman build muscle on a raw food diet below:

Jennifer was a classic skinny raw vegan. She was determined and willing to put in the work for her program despite its challenges for building muscle.

Jennifer's Story

A model student, Jen followed the raw food diet I designed to a T—prepping her food, hitting her workouts, and studying the holes in her diet relative to performance. In short order, her skinny body transformed first into that of a competitive athlete, and then she became a national bikini and bodybuilding champion. She also became a black belt in jiujitsu, a nutritionist, and a world-class coach herself.

Jennifer is the perfect example of transcending stereotypes, limiting beliefs, and the conventional wisdom of other people. She was determined not to be limited by her obstacles or her chosen diet. Interestingly enough, years later as she advanced in epigenetic understanding, she began to reintroduce animal-based products into her diet.

Today, in her 40s, Jennifer maintains an extraordinary level of fitness while practicing both her training and her martial arts, and being a mom.

Now, let's get into the chapter.

WHAT IS A RAW FOOD DIET?

In this diet, essentially you avoid all cooked food. It was first documented in the late 1800s when a doctor discovered that he could cure jaundice with an apple.

The diet didn't become popular until Edward Howell, M.D., popularized the idea that enzymes and life force from food are important for health. He started a facility that treated patients with raw food. When food isn't heated past 114 degrees (give or take), all of the enzymes in the food are still active. This allows you to maximize your digestive capabilities.

According to Dr. Howell, enzymes are a critical component to life—they're the bio-workers that make over 25,000 functions in the body happen. Howell hypothesized that everyone has an enzyme bank account or reserve that can be depleted or replenished.

Eating mostly cooked foods drains more of your own enzyme bank account, says Howell, which could lead to enzyme depletion and eventually diseases. Therefore, he uses the raw food diet, especially with high-enzyme produce, to treat diseases.

Some of Dr. Howell's claims have been disproven with better understanding of biology. However, based on our personal and professional experience, we believe the diet can still be a powerful nutritional strategy if implemented correctly.

This chapter is, therefore, about how to successfully reap the most benefits from the raw food diet without the dogmas and pitfalls. We also share anecdotal evidence, theories, and science.

The raw food community is one of the most intense dietary groups. It usually holds strong spiritual beliefs and often frowns upon dietary supplements or anything even remotely artificial.

This group can also be one of the most dogmatic. At a raw food festival, one of the waif-like characters with glazed eyes looked at Wade and asked, "What percentage of raw are you?" Wade could tell that if his answer wasn't "100 percent raw," he'd be thrown out of the group and exiled for all eternity.

Similar to many other restrictive diets, people became evangelists for it after the diet cured their or their loved one's serious health conditions. As with many diets we've covered, it's a strong antidote to the modern standard American diet, which can explain why it restored their health.

WHAT RAW DIETS INCLUDE

For the purpose of this chapter, we're going to focus on raw veganism. However, it's worth noting that it is possible to eat raw meat, eggs (it worked for Rocky), dairy, or fish (just eat sashimi). Weston Rowe went viral a few years ago when he shared that he had been eating raw meat 99 percent of the time and experienced great results.

Now, back to plants . . .

Raw eaters base their diets on fruits, vegetables, nuts, and seeds that are natural, organic, and free of preservatives. They also avoid heating their foods above 104 to 118°F (40 to 48°C). Rather, their food prep includes soaking, sprouting, juicing, blending, fermenting, dehydrating, or just eating plants in their natural state.

If you've never eaten a good raw dish, then this might sound stranger than Weird Al's music, but this way of eating can offer some of the most delicious meals you've ever experienced.

POTENTIAL HEALTH BENEFITS OF A RAW FOOD DIET

The raw food diet is high in all plant-based nutrients, phytonutrients, enzymes, probiotics, antioxidants, and fiber. By focusing on organic or naturally grown fruits and vegetables, the diet is also lower in pesticides, antibiotics, and other toxins you can find in foods.

Warning about Raw, Non-Organic Fruits and Vegetables

All fruits and vegetables that are not organic are most likely low in, or have zero, enzymes. Why? Because they're sprayed with pesticides, fungicides, and herbicides (such as glyphosates). These chemicals negatively impact the enzymes in the soil, bugs, and plants.[1]

1. May Reverse Modern Chronic Diseases

Many raw foodies are cultists about the raw food diet because it cured their chronic health conditions, or they started to feel amazing on it.

The raw food diet is rich in nutrients, life force, and enzymes that are lacking in the standard American diet and most bodybuilding diets. As a result, many people see improvements in their health markers, and some even reverse their illnesses.

We believe that the core reason a raw food diet has helped many with their health is because it's often low in calories and protein. This can help decrease IGF-1 and increase autophagy. The body can then heal itself of various ailments.

For some, the raw food diet also has big spiritual and community components, which can have some health benefits. Research has shown that having spiritual beliefs makes the immune system stronger.[2]

However, the spiritual and group components can also cause people to turn a blind eye to obvious health problems that arise later on due to nutrient deficiencies.

2. Improved Energy and Vitality

The raw food diet may be lower in toxins that interfere with mitochondrial energy production. In addition, its plant-based antioxidants neutralize oxidative stress that jams the mitochondria. The diet is also high in vitamins, minerals, and life force that other diets lack.

If you eat significantly more green vegetables or algae, you'll also get a lot of B vitamins and chlorophyll that support the mitochondria.[3] Therefore, most people feel more energized—at least in the beginning phases of the raw food diet.

3. Improved Digestion

Almost across the board, raw foodists experience improved digestion on a raw food diet. Possibly, the higher enzyme and probiotic content of the meals support digestion. Also, the diet tends to be significantly lower in fat and proteins, thus requiring less energy to digest.

4. Enhanced Sensory Perception from Food

Many raw foodists become more acutely aware of how foods affect their bodies. Wade noticed a dramatic increase in his sensory perceptions. His palate changed along with his sense of smell[4] and awareness of how food affected him. He started being able to taste if a food contained any pesticides or unhealthy chemicals, or if certain foods disrupted his digestion or sleep.

5. Detoxification

Raw foodists claim that the raw food diet improves health by detoxifying the body, possibly due to the increased fiber, antioxidants, and micronutrient levels.

In Chinese and Ayurvedic medicine, anger is a sign of liver congestion. Wade noticed that he became a lot less angry.

6. May Help with Weight Loss

With the diet being so restrictive, many people end up consuming significantly fewer calories. Raw vegan diets are naturally low in fats and protein.

The higher fiber and polyphenol content may also promote a lean microbiome, which is higher in Bacteroidetes and lower in Firmicutes.

However, it is still possible to overeat the dehydrated nuts and treats. Many of the packaged ones are hyper-palatable with high-fructose sweeteners, crunch, and salt.

HEALTH RISKS ON A RAW FOOD DIET

The biggest risk with a raw food diet—and why we typically don't advise anyone to follow one for more than a few months—is deficiencies. Due to the restrictive nature of the diet, it's easy to develop multiple nutrient deficiencies that can impact your health.

We are not saying this is the case for everyone. If a person eats raw intelligently and focuses on making sure they feed their bodies the following key nutrients, then continued good health can be possible. Matt's friend and legendary raw food master Dr. Aris LaTham has been raw for 37 years. He's in his 70s and one of the most vibrant men you'll ever meet.

1. Amino Acid and Protein Deficiencies

Amino acid deficiency causes a number of disease states, nutritional deficiencies, fatigue, accelerated aging, and even premature death.[5]

A raw vegan diet tends to avoid grains and legumes, so it can be difficult to get enough protein. Also, a lot of plant-based proteins are less bioavailable than animal-based proteins.

Based on our observations, most raw foodists lose an average of 15 to 20 pounds of lean muscle in three to six months. They often lack the amino acids needed to build muscle.

Although Wade felt great on a raw food diet, he needed to supplement with a plant-based protein powder so that he could train hard, maintain muscle mass, and recover from his workouts.

Power Move: Optimize Your Raw Plant Protein Intake

Here are the 12 best raw plant-based protein sources:

1. Spirulina: 57 grams of protein per 100 grams
2. Hempseed: 31.5 grams of protein per 100 grams
3. Pumpkin seeds: 25 grams of protein per 100 grams
4. Chickpea sprouts: 25.7 grams of protein per 100 grams
5. Adzuki bean sprouts: 23 grams of protein per 100 grams
6. Sunflower seeds: 22 grams of protein per 100 grams
7. Flaxseed: 18.3 grams of protein per 100 grams
8. Lentil sprouts: 8.5 grams of protein per 100 grams
9. Pea sprouts: 9.1 grams of protein per 100 grams
10. Sprouted mung beans: 7 grams of protein per 100 grams
11. Alfalfa sprouts: 4 grams of protein per 100 grams
12. Spinach: 2.9 grams of protein per 100 grams

Many plant-based proteins, such as lectins, are more difficult to digest due to their chemical structures. To improve protein bioavailability on any plant-based diet, Wade recommends supplementing with a full-spectrum digestive enzyme like MassZymes and VegZymes. MassZymes is the strongest proteolytic digestive enzyme on the market. VegZymes is designed to optimize plant digestion.

2. Fat-Soluble Vitamin Deficiencies

The nutrients that are generally nonexistent on the raw vegan diet and may require supplementation include:

- *Long-chain omega-3 fatty acids, such as EPA and DHA.* These are important for the brain and balancing inflammation levels. Many people, especially men, are very bad at converting short-chain omega-3, such as ALA, into the long-chain ones. Algae is the best source.
- *Preformed vitamin A, such as retinol and retinoic acid.* This is found only in animal products. Vitamin A is important for mucosal and tissue barrier function, such as the skin and the gut. It's also important for many hormones, such as thyroid and vitamin D, to function correctly.
- *Vitamin D.* This is critical for all aspects of health, especially hormones, immune, and metabolic functions. You may get it from the sun, but most people in temperate climates need to supplement during the colder months.

These nutrient deficiencies, along with a lack of amino acids, may explain the high rates of mental health issues among long-term raw vegans. Vitamin B_{12} is another common deficiency for raw vegan followers, because it's not available in plants.

Genetics may also play a role here (see Chapter 34, Your Genetics Are Not Your Destiny). Those who can stay on the diet healthily without supplementing are genetically more efficient at converting short-chain into long-chain omega-3, and beta-carotene into retinol. We recommend supplementing with these on a raw food diet.

Power Move: Optimize Your Fats

Here are the 7 top EFA options for vegetarians and vegans:

1. Algal oil (derived from algae): 500 mg of EFA per dose
2. Perilla oil (derived from perilla seeds): 9,000 mg of ALA omega-3 per tablespoon
3. Flaxseed: an epic 6,388 mg of ALA omega-3 per ounce
4. Hempseed: a whopping 6,000 mg of ALA omega-3 per ounce
5. Chia seeds: 4,915 mg of ALA omega-3 per ounce
6. Brussels sprouts: over 125 mg of EFAs per half cup
7. Walnuts: 2,542 mg of ALA omega-3 per ounce

A few foods have come up in Power Moves for *both* protein and fats: spirulina, flaxseed, and hempseed. These should be staple foods on a raw food diet.

3. High in Anti-Nutrients and Gut Irritants

Although raw food preparations take great care to soak and sprout foods, you may still end up eating a lot of anti-nutrients and gut irritants such as:

- Oxalates
- Alkaloids
- Saponins
- Salicylates
- Phytates
- Protease inhibitors
- Lectins

Review Chapter 31, Eliminating Food Toxins, to learn more.

Power Move: Soak Your Nuts

Most nuts and many vegetables have enzyme inhibitors, lectins, and other potential gut health disruptors. One of the ways to counter this is to learn how to soak your nuts.

Nuts and Seeds	Soaking Time
Almonds	10 to 12 hours
Brazil nuts	Avoid soaking
Cashews	2 to 3 hours
Flaxseed	Avoid soaking
Hazelnuts	10 to 12 hours
Hempseed	Avoid soaking
Macadamia nuts	2 hours
Pecans	Avoid soaking
Pine nuts	Avoid soaking
Pistachio nuts	6 to 8 hours
Pumpkin seeds (hulled)	8 hours
Sesame seeds	8 hours

4. Too Few Calories

The raw food diet can be low in calorie density because it's higher in fiber, so it's easy to not eat enough calories. Also, cooking allows your body to extract more energy from food.[6]

Therefore, the raw food diet can lead to severe undernutrition, which can lead to fatigue, hormone imbalances, and weight loss. If you're struggling with eating enough on a raw food diet, pay attention to the next Power Move.

Power Move: The Easy Way to Add More Calories

The easiest way to add more calories to a raw food diet is to focus on fats. Here are some of the best high-fat, raw options:

- Cold-pressed olive oil and olives
- Nut butters
- Avocado
- Nuts and seeds:
  - Almonds
  - Brazil nuts
  - Cashews
  - Flaxseed
  - Hazelnuts
  - Hempseed
  - Macadamia nuts
  - Pecans
  - Pine nuts
  - Pistachio nuts
  - Pumpkin seeds (hulled)
  - Sesame seeds
  - Sunflower seeds (hulled)
  - Walnuts

HOW TO DO THE RAW FOOD DIET

Source Your Food Right

The raw food diet is a detoxifying diet where your body will become hyper-aware of how your body responds to various foods. Therefore, to reap the most benefit from the raw food diet, you need to pay attention to the quality of your foods, both tangible and energetic.

The best option is to grow your own organic produce. When you can, harvest right before eating. This will give you the most life force. Consuming produce right after harvest minimizes the nutrient loss from transport and gas ripening.

The second-best option is to source from a local Mennonite or biodynamic farm, or wild foraging. These may not be certified organic, but they could have better quality than an organic farm with otherwise conventional practices.

The third-best option is to visit your farmer's market. If you can't grow your own produce (and it's unlikely you'll be able to grow everything), get organic produce from a local farmer's market. You'll find fresh and local options that are harvested close to the day of sale.

The fourth-best option is mass-market organic. At a minimum, you'll want to seek out organic fruits, vegetables, nuts, and seeds that are ethically grown, especially for items that tend to accumulate toxic pesticides.

However, keep in mind that even certified organic produce could still have pesticides, been gas ripened, and coated with fungicides and wax. In many cases, your organic produce may have traveled from thousands of miles away, which depletes its nutrients and enzymes.

Careful Sourcing of Raw Animal Products

Some people are choosing to experiment with raw meat diets. If you decide to include raw animal products, the quality becomes even more important, since the risk of food-borne illness is significantly higher with them.

Raw poultry and pork are not safe to eat, because they tend to have parasites and harmful bacteria.

Cattle—such as beef, bison, buffalo, sheep, and lamb—can be eaten raw because the pH and texture of the meat inhibit the growth of dangerous bacteria. Cattle are also less likely to carry dangerous parasites. They can even be fermented or dry-aged.

Ideally, get meat and milk from free-range, organic cattle where you know the farm and trust the farmer. Animals grown in tropical climates are more likely to carry dangerous parasites and bacteria than those grown in temperate climates.

Full-fat and grass-fed raw A1 cow's or other animal's milk can have many health benefits if you tolerate it. The farm needs to be very hygienic, while the milk has to be kept very cold and fresh at all times.

If you do a raw carnivore diet, it's important to also include raw organ meats, as these are key sources of vitamins C and B, enzymes, and other nutrients.

Stocking Up and Preparing

The bulk of your raw diet should consist mostly of sprouted veggies, nuts, green vegetables, and fruits. You'll be eating as much as 25 to 30 cups a day, which is easily 5 to 10 times what most people are used to.

Most of your calories will come from sprouts, nuts, and seeds. These need to be soaked, allowed to sprout, and dehydrated, which takes days. Therefore, you'll need to adopt a food prep routine so that you have the foods ready to eat.

You can also find presoaked and dehydrated seeds, vegan juices, dehydrated items, and raw vegan snacks in health food stores.

Different Food-Prep Methods for a Raw Vegan Diet

The following preparation processes can maximize the enzymes, nutrient availability, and life force of your food.

Soaking

Soaking involves submerging the seeds of interest (grains, legumes, seeds, and nuts) into water from a few hours to 24 hours. The moisture typically brings the seeds back to life, so they will release many anti-nutrients into the water and start to produce enzymes.

To deactivate enzyme inhibitors, you can add a tablespoon of salt or apple cider vinegar to a liter of water in the soak. Be sure to discard the soak water rather than use it for future recipes.

Sprouting

After soaking, seeds can be drained and left exposed to air to allow them to sprout. The sprouts may need to be rinsed multiple times a day to remove potential bacteria growth on them and provide the sprouts with enough moisture to continue growing.

Sprouts are more like vegetables than seeds the longer you allow them to grow. Some sprouts, such as broccoli sprouts, have 10 times more sulforaphane than mature broccoli. Sulforaphane is being highly researched for its potential anticancer properties,[7, 8] heart health benefits,[9] and anti-diabetic effects.[10, 11, 12]

Power Move: Sprout Your Seeds

Seed Type	Dry Measure	Soak Time	Sprout Time	Yield
Alfalfa	3 tablespoons	5 hours	5 days	4 cups
Buckwheat	1 cup	6 hours	5–7 days	3 cups
Clover	3 tablespoons	5 hours	5 days	4 cups
Fenugreek	¼ cup	6 hours	5 days	4 cups
Kale	¼ cup	5 hours	5 days	4 cups
Mustard	3 tablespoons	5 hours	5 days	4 cups
Pumpkin	1 cup	4 hours	24 hours	2 cups
Radish	3 tablespoons	6 hours	5 days	4 cups
Sunflower	1 cup	4 hours	24 hours	2.5 cups
Amaranth	1 cup	3 hours	24 hours	3 cups
Barley	1 cup	6 hours	5–7 days	3 cups
Kamut	1 cup	6 hours	5–7 days	3 cups
Millet	1 cup	3 hours	12 hours	3 cups
Quinoa	1 cup	3 hours	24 hours	3 cups
Rye	1 cup	6 hours	5–7 days	3 cups
Spelt	1 cup	6 hours	5–7 days	3 cups

Wheat	1 cup	6 hours	5–7 days	3 cups
Adzuki	1 cup	8–12 hours	2–4 days	2 cups
Garbanzo	1 cup	8–12 hours	2–3 days	2 cups
Lentil	1 cup	8–12 hours	2–3 days	2 cups
Mung	1 cup	8–12 hours	2–5 days	2 cups
Peas	1 cup	8–12 hours	2–3 days	2 cups

Blending

A high-powered blender such as a Vitamix is one of your best friends on a raw vegan diet, because you'll be blending not just vegetables but also nuts and seeds. Blending allows you to break the plant cell walls and access nutrients more easily.

You can make soups, sauces, dips, smoothies, puddings, salad dressings, and ice cream with your blender. Soaked nuts can be blended and strained to produce nut milks.

Juicing

A strong juicer that doesn't overheat is also important for a raw vegan diet, so you can have detoxifying fresh juice that is packed with nutrients without the roughage.

Dehydrating

Dehydrators are small, low-heat ovens with fans to dry your food, which is an important tool for raw eaters. The dehydration process often takes up to 24 hours, depending on how dry you want your end products to be.

Dehydrated foods usually have a different texture and more intense flavor. Completely dehydrated foods can be stored at room temperature.

The possible things that can be dehydrated are endless, such as:

- Any produce or herbs, fresh or fermented
- Soaked nuts or seeds
- Sprouts
- Concentrated smoothies or fruit pastes can be dehydrated into fruit leathers
- Juicing or nut milk pulps into "flours," which can be made into crackers, bars, and cookies by mixing with gelling seeds such as flax or chia seeds, and dehydrating them

Marinating and Pickling

Any produce can be marinated or pickled in acid, such as vinegar and citrus juice, which changes the texture and unlocks new flavors.

Fermenting

Most raw produce can be lacto-fermented in a salty solution, such as sauerkrauts or krauts made with other vegetables. Fermented foods are rich in gut-supporting probiotics and postbiotics (beneficial substances that probiotics produce). The fermentation process also unlocks many beneficial nutrients and phytochemicals.

Many nuts and seeds, and their milks, can also be fermented into yogurts or cheeses.

You can also enjoy raw fermented beverages such as kombucha or beet kvass, or just drink the liquid from your fermented vegetables.

You can do a wild ferment where you put out the fermentation mix and allow the existing bacteria on your produce and from the air to grow. Alternatively, some people add the content of probiotic capsules to start a fermentation culture so that they can control the bacteria strains in their ferments. Some of our customers use P3-OM for this purpose.

THREE-DAY SAMPLE RAW FOOD DIET

Day 1:

- Protein Breakthrough Seed Breakfast Bar (507 calories)
- Summer Jicama Picnic Salad (682 calories)
- Spicy Pad Thai Veggie Noodles (573 calories)

Day 2:

- Superfood Buckwheat Kasha (287 calories)
- Collard Spring Roll Wraps (643 calories)
- Raw Vegan Lasagna (433 calories)

Day 3:

- Dragon Fruit Parfait with Superfood Granola (778 calories)
- Fruit Salad (280 calories)
- Nori Roll-Ups (550 calories)

Go to www.BIOptimizers/book/resources to get these recipes and much more.

Raw Diet Pitfalls

Most raw food eaters feel great initially before their health falls apart. It's important to keep in mind that the raw diet is not the end-all, be-all of health. The following pitfalls should serve as cautions:

- Not replacing their missing nutrients can be the biggest reason people lose muscle mass and deplete their EFAs and vitamin B_{12} stores.
- Listening to dogma instead of their own bodies can cause people to ignore signs and symptoms that something is going wrong. Some people experience detox reactions when they start a raw food diet, which might be a sign that they need to ease up or add a few supplements.
- Focusing on hyper-palatable foods. A raw diet strips down a lot of hyper-palatability, but it's possible to overdo the nuts and packaged raw vegan snacks. Even though these are raw compliant, they have the right mix of salt, sugar, and fat to cause you to overeat, which defeats the purpose. The raw vegan diet should help you reset your palate to enjoy the most natural states of food.
- Overdoing the superfoods. Raw foodists tend to get fanatical about ancient superfoods from traditional cultures, and these tend to take up aisles of health food stores. Keep in mind that if plants have medicinal properties, they can also have side effects even if they're natural. In most cases, you don't need them.

Power Move:

Work with a coach to monitor your biofeedback on a raw diet.

Pros of a Raw Vegan Diet

Health

A raw vegan diet, especially in the short term, can have many health benefits, including:

- Detoxifying
- Resetting your gut bacteria
- Improved digestion and enzyme reserves
- Weight loss

Performance and Aesthetics

Some people find that raw food can help them bust through their fat loss plateau or make it easier to stick to their other diets in the long term. In some cases, the short-term detoxifying, and the replenishing of nutrients and enzymes, may have performance-enhancing benefits.

Psychological Benefits

The raw vegan diet may serve as a mental exercise to remind you of what you don't need to survive. For many people, practicing the raw diet enhances their spiritual or religious practices.

Cons of a Raw Vegan Diet

Health

The raw diet can be very risky to do long term, so few people have been able to sustain their health on raw food, especially without supplements. You run the risk of depleting important nutrients and eventually developing chronic health problems.

Aesthetics

Even though Wade was able to pull it off, we don't advise people to follow a raw food diet if their goal is to build lean muscle mass.

Performance

Wade finds that he needs to supplement with protein powder to maintain his training intensity and recovery. Many nutrients that are nonexistent on a raw vegan diet are also important for brain health and cognitive performance.

Lifestyle

The raw diet can be very restrictive socially. It's also very difficult to do in a cold climate. Last, the diet requires a lot of preparation and forethought.

Optimization Supplements

- MassZymes and VegZymes, full-spectrum digestive enzymes that help break down difficult-to-digest plant proteins and overcome some anti-nutrients
- Protein Breakthrough, a 100-percent plant-based, complete protein source that tastes great
- HCL Breakthrough, which ensures that you don't pick up parasites from your raw produce and meat
- Vitamin D
- Magnesium Breakthrough, which prevents deficiencies, as the soil is quite depleted of magnesium
- Algae oil, as a plant-based source of long-chain fatty acids

SUMMARY

A raw food diet essentially means that you avoid all cooked food. This is to keep all the enzymes in the food active, which is the case if it's not heated above 114°F.

During a raw food diet, most of your calories come from sprouts, nuts, and seeds. These all must be soaked, sprouted, and dehydrated, which can take days.

- Soaking. This involves submerging the seeds under water for a few hours to 24 hours.
- Sprouting. This occurs when seeds are drained and left exposed to air.

Optimize Your Fats

The top EFA options for vegetarians and vegans are:

- Algal oil (derived from algae)
- Perilla oil (derived from perilla seeds)
- Flaxseed
- Hempseed
- Chia seed
- Brussels sprouts
- Walnuts

Add fermented foods to your diet. They're rich in gut-supporting probiotics and postbiotics.

While on a raw food diet, make sure you monitor your bloodwork and biomarkers to spot deficiencies and make changes quickly.

CHAPTER 24

HOW TO SUCCEED WITH A SLOW-CARB, LOW-GLYCEMIC DIET

In this chapter, you'll learn:

- How stabilizing blood sugar can curb cravings, improve mood, reverse insulin resistance, and lead to effortless fat loss
- How to find your personalized blood-sugar-stabilizing diet based on your glucose response and microbiome
- The secrets to manipulating your blood sugar for maximum muscle gain and minimal fat gain, even on refeed meals
- The difference between glycemic index and glycemic load, and why it's important to consider for your meals
- How a slow-carb diet is different from a keto diet, and how you can follow one simply and effectively
- Why you should start out "eating to your appetite" instead of counting calories, and when to eventually start tracking calories and macro breakdown as you progress with your diet
- Why the *combination* of the foods you eat has a massive impact on the glycemic response and you can't eat whatever you want
- The three steps to successfully follow a slow-carb diet
- What a 2015 study found about different blood sugar responses to the same meal, and what that means for your own journey to discover which foods keep your blood sugar stable

WHAT IS A SLOW-CARB (OR LOW-GLYCEMIC-IMPACT) DIET?

A low-glycemic-impact diet focuses on food that minimizes the impact on blood sugar. The original version of this diet was based on the glycemic index, which was invented in the 1980s. Later on, these diets evolved to take into account the total amount of carbohydrate, or glycemic load, in foods.

We also discuss the surprising individual responses to various glycemic loads.

Even if you don't have diabetes, understanding the impact of each food on your blood sugar and insulin levels is a valuable tool for BIOptimization. First, good blood sugar control is important for longevity and health span.[1] Elevated blood sugar levels accelerate aging.

Because your brain is exquisitely sensitive to blood sugar fluctuations, stabilizing your blood sugar is essential for optimal cognitive performance and hormone balance. Also, improving your aesthetics is far easier with a higher level of insulin sensitivity.

Slow-carb followers eat more protein and fibers while reducing processed carbs. Overall, this combination increases the thermic effect of food. Also, the increased fiber composition can improve the microbiome toward the bacteria strains that favor metabolism.[2]

One of the advantages of this diet is that you can manage blood sugar without needing to go through keto adaptation. It can also be relatively easy to do and easier to adapt to different situations than ketogenic diets. For many, this diet is a gateway to keto.

Athletes or bodybuilders who are fueled by carbs need five or six meals a day to prevent energy crashing, or bonking. Wade calls this the "carb toilet," which refers to the extreme fatigue, irritability, and passing out when someone goes too long without eating. Focusing on carbs that don't spike blood sugar can help you feel steadier and prevent such crashes, which tend to happen more in leaner athletes.

Combining Slow-Carb with Other Diets

The slow-carb strategy can be easily combined with other diets, including paleo, veganism, and vegetarianism.

IS THIS DIET MAGICAL FOR WEIGHT LOSS?

Again, the answer to this question for every diet is always no. On the flip side, for some people who enjoy carbs and want a strategy to manage their blood sugar level, it's a great solution.

The premise of the slow-carb diet is to manage blood sugar by focusing on foods that have lower glycemic impact. As a result, many people experience increased satiety and fewer sugar-related cravings, so they end up eating less food, which can lead to fat loss.

Ultimately, to lose weight, you have to be in a calorie deficit. If you're just stabilizing your blood sugar and eating at maintenance, then your weight will remain the same. This is true for all diets.

However, I think most health experts would agree on one thing: keeping your blood sugar stable and within optimal range is important for health reasons.

The Original Slow-Carb Diet

The first slow-carb diet was a low-glycemic-impact diet popularized by Tim Ferriss in his book *The Four-Hour Body*. Ferriss made some modifications to make the diet easier to follow, which improved compliance and success rates, including:

- Eating the same few meals over and over again (one of our key principles also)
- Getting 30 grams of protein within 30 minutes of waking (protein for the win!)
- Avoiding all white, starchy carbohydrates, fruits, and dairy
- Avoiding drinking calories (a good strategy on any diet)
- One refeed day per week to enjoy your favorite foods as much as possible
- Using blood sugar support supplements (we suggest Blood Sugar Breakthrough)

This diet focuses on non-starchy vegetables, protein sources, legumes, nuts, and good fats. It tends to be low carb and high protein, with some variability in fats. Usually, legumes and pulses are the best types of carbs for this diet, because they have very low glycemic load, high protein, and high fiber. So, high-legume cuisines, like certain Mexican dishes, are good options.

Participants are advised to eat to their appetites instead of counting calories. While eating to your appetite usually works very well for beginners or obese people, we recommend eventually tracking calories and macro breakdowns as you progress with the diet. Remember the rule of thumb: you don't usually need to track or measure calories early on. Just shifting diets is usually enough to naturally create a calorie deficit.

However, to achieve elite levels of leanness, tracking is usually mandatory. That way, you can ensure consistent progress and troubleshoot when the progress stalls.

WHAT'S THE DIFFERENCE BETWEEN SLOW-CARB, PALEO, AND KETO?

- A slow-carb diet cuts out grains, refined sugar, and all fruits. It does include starchy vegetables, legumes, and beans.
- A paleo diet does not include grains, legumes, or any refined sugars. However, there's no real limitation on carbs, and you can consume fruits and starchy vegetables.
- A keto diet keeps a very tight control on carb consumption.

SLOW-CARB DIET 2.0: A DIET BASED ON PERSONALIZED BLOOD SUGAR RESPONSE

The glycemic index table gives lab measurements of one food at a time. However, that's not how we eat—we tend to eat a combination of foods at each meal, which has a massive impact on the glycemic response. Add some protein and fats to a meal, and the glycemic response will be blunted significantly.

There are also significant blood sugar variances from one person to another, even eating the exact same foods. The best approach is to get personalized data, which we cover in a moment. We suggest checking out the Glucose Goddess's page on Instagram for great examples.

Benefits of a Slow-Carb Diet

A 2019 meta-analysis of 54 studies shows that low-GI diets can improve blood sugar control and weight loss in people with diabetes and prediabetes.[3]

Glycemic Index vs. Glycemic Load

A high-glycemic-index food spikes blood sugar higher than a low-glycemic-index food. The glycemic index compares the blood sugar increase of a food that contains 50 grams of carbohydrates to the blood sugar increase from 50 grams of pure glucose.

However, to measure the glycemic index of any food, a research subject needs to consume enough of it to get 50 grams of carbohydrate.

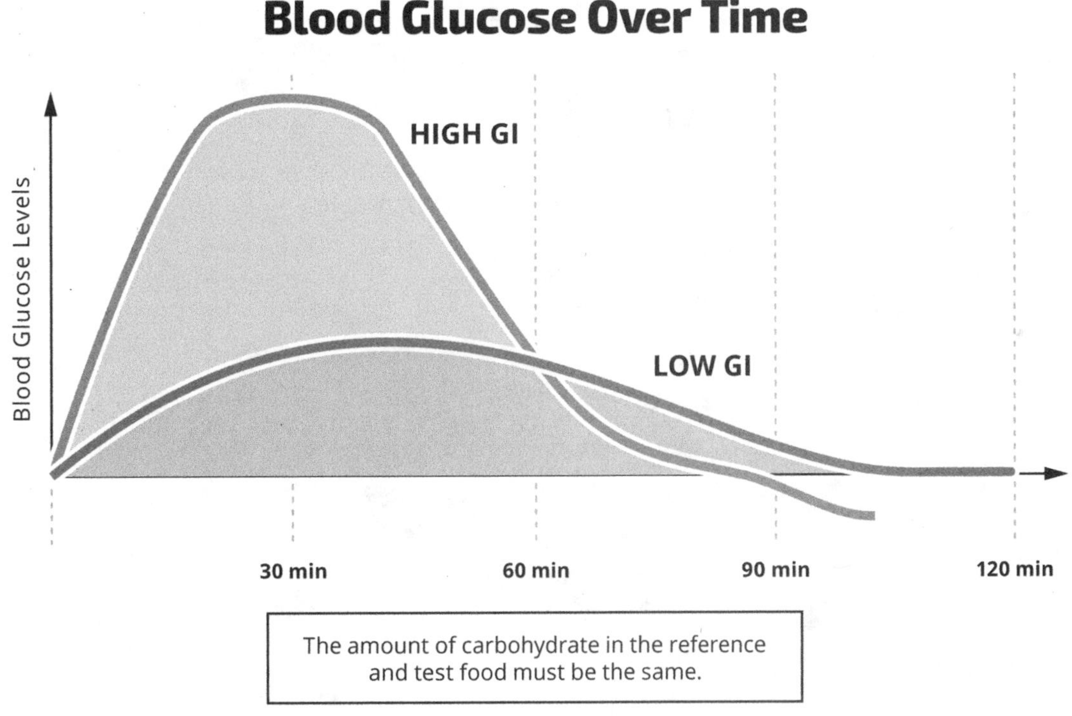

The amount of carbohydrate in the reference and test food must be the same.

The problem with this model is that many foods have fast (high-glycemic-index) carbs, while they have a low concentration of carbohydrates. In other words, the model takes into account only the *type* of carbs in a food, not the *amount* of carbs.

For example, carrots have a high glycemic index, but it takes a lot of carrots to get 50 grams of carbohydrates. Plus, carrots have a lot of fiber. As a result, carrots typically have a low impact on blood sugar.

That's why glycemic load is a far better measurement than glycemic index. Glycemic load is a more accurate measurement that takes into account both the type and the amount of carbs in each food. See the table on the next page.[4]

Glycemic Impact (GI) vs Glycemic Load (GL) of Different Foods

FOOD	GI	GL	FOOD	GI	GL	FOOD	GI	GL
Yogurt, plain, no sugar	14	2	Rye, grains	34	26	Pinapple juice	46	6
Peanuts	15	4	Soy milk	36	3	Grape	46	7
Soybeans	18	2	Chickpea	36	8	Linguini	46	12
Fructose	20	20	Tomato	38	2	Sponge-cake	46	27
Peas, dry	22	2	Tomato juice	38	3	Barley bread	46	30
Cherry	22	3	Apple	38	5	Lactose	46	46
Peanut butter	22	5	Pear	38	5	Peach, canned	47	4
cashew nuts	22	6	Plum	39	5	Macaroni	47	14
Chocolate milk, no sugar	24	2	Ravioli with meat	39	8	Fruit bread	47	23
Yogurt, lowfat with fruits	24	3	Strawberry	40	3	Grapefruit juice	48	5
Grapefruit	25	3	Carrot, cooked	40	4	Peas, fresh	48	7
Barley, grains	25	7	Apple juice	40	5	Grape juice	48	8
Milk, whole	27	2	Fettuccine	40	10	Spaghetti	48	14
Beans, Kidney	29	7	Chocolate cake	40	20	Bread, mixed grains	48	24
Plum, dry	29	16	Wheat germ	41	22	Oatmeal bread	48	25
Lentils	30	4	Peach	42	5	Chocolate bar	49	26
Beans, black	30	7	Pear, canned	43	4	Oatmeal	49	36
Apricot, dry	31	15	Orange	43	5	Orange Juice	50	5
Milk, lowfat	32	2	Lentils, soup	44	4	Tortellini with cheese	50	6
Beans, lima	32	7	Carrot juice	45	4	Ice cream, lowfat	50	10
Yogurt with fruits	33	6	Fermented milk	45	10	Pinapple	50	7
Chocolate milk with sugar	34	4	Capellini	45	11	Yam	50	12

Shockingly Individual Glycemic Responses

A 2015 study published in the prestigious journal *Cell* found that blood sugar responses to the same meal widely vary from person to person.[5] This was a surprising revelation. Researchers continuously monitored the blood sugar responses to 46,698 meals in 800 participants for a week.

Some of the findings were intriguingly counterintuitive and contradictory to the original glycemic load table. For some people, bananas are worse for their blood sugar than bread. For others, it's the opposite. While most participants experienced a significant spike in blood sugar after eating bread, a few of them maintained almost steady blood sugar responses to the same bread. Interestingly, the blood sugar responses to identical meals are very consistent.

The study found that the microbiome, along with genetics and other lifestyle factors, plays a role in determining the foods that are best for each person's blood sugar. The post-meal blood sugar response correlates with type 2 diabetes and other disease risks based on blood test results. Therefore, a personalized blood-sugar-control diet appears to be the healthiest option.

The study also used the meal content, physical activity, blood tests, blood sugar responses, and microbiome features from the 800 participants to create a computerized predictive model. It was found to correctly predict the blood sugar responses in another 100 participants. In a feeding experiment, it was found that the microbiome is better for metabolism, and blood sugar improves, when people eat the diet that is right for them based on this model.

That's why we suggest doing microbiome tests and optimizing your food selection even further using their insights.

As a general rule, the glycemic index and glycemic load predict the blood sugar response for many people. However, as this study finds, there are exceptions, and some of the theoretically high-glycemic-index foods could be the healthiest *for you*.

THE ULTIMATE STRATEGY: USE A CGM

To get out of the uncertain realm of dietary opinions and theories, you need your own personalized, high-quality data. Therefore, it's best to use a continuous glucose monitor (CGM) to understand your blood sugar responses to different meals and build your own personalized slow-carb diet. This is what we call the Slow-Carb Diet 2.0, which we'll refer to as the Slow-Carb diet going forward.

HOW TO DO OUR SLOW-CARB DIET

Step 1: Find Meals that Work for You with CGM and Microbiome Testing

Our Slow-Carb diet aims to keep your blood sugar as steady as possible by focusing your meals around protein and carbohydrate foods that won't spike your blood sugar.

Microbiome tests will suggest foods that your gut bacteria love. Incorporate them into your meals and observe the blood sugar response.

Use a continuous glucose monitoring device, such as a Nutrisense or Dexcom, and journal your food for at least a week with your typical meals. Also, write down your hunger levels and blood sugar response the next morning.

If certain foods or meals spike your blood sugar or result in extremely low blood sugar within a few hours, then they don't work for you, and you shouldn't be eating them on a regular basis. Keep eating meals and food items that stabilize your blood sugar.

Step 2: Find Your Individual Low-Glycemic-Impact Carbs

What we often find is that some people maintain blood sugar better with high-glycemic-impact carbs, such as rice and potatoes. You may want to test starchy foods individually to find out your personal responses to each of these. In real life, however, you'd almost always mix starchy foods with fat, fiber, and protein, so the actual impact on your blood sugar won't be as high.

Step 3: Plan Your Calorie and Meal Breakdowns Based on Your Goals

On a Slow-Carb diet, protein is still the king macro to focus on. Aim for 35 to 50 percent of your calories from proteins, 30 to 35 percent from carbohydrates, and the rest from fats. Some people may do better with fewer carbs and more fats, but you can't do high carb and high fat. You have to choose one dominant energy source and stick with it.

Refer to Chapter 7 to find out how many calories to start with. If you're working to lose body fat, you have to be in a caloric deficit. To maintain weight, simply stay at maintenance calories. If you want to lose fat, aim for a 500-calorie daily average deficit.

If you're trying to gain muscle, you should be getting at least a 500-calorie surplus. Some people may find better results with hypertrophy if they add a fast carb and protein around their training sessions.

Once you know how many calories you'll be eating, divide that number by the number of meals, which could be three to five per day, unless you're doing intermittent fasting.

Best Food for the Slow-Carb Diet

Protein	Legumes	Vegetables	Fats	Spices
Eggs	Lentils	Spinach	Butter	Salt
Chicken (breast or thigh)	Black beans	Cruciferous vegetables such as broccoli, Brussels sprouts, cauliflower, and kale	Olive oil or low-heat cooking	Garlic salt
Beef (preferably grass-fed)	Pinto beans	Sauerkraut and kimchi	Grapeseed or macadamia oil for high-heat cooking	White truffle sea salt
Fish	Red beans	Asparagus	Nuts like almonds, walnuts, and macadamias	Herbs
Pork	Soybeans	Peas	Ghee	
A good protein powder like Protein Breakthrough		Green beans	Creamer: dairy free, only 1–2 tsp (5–10 ml) per day	

THREE-DAY SLOW-CARB DIET SAMPLE MENU

You can find all of these delicious recipes in our *Primal Paleo Cookbook.*

Day 1

- Roasted Baby Kale (125 calories)
- Fish Tacos (590 calories)
- Pho-Flavored Brisket (732 calories)
- Marble Cake (364 calories)

Day 2

- Basic Cauliflower Rice (13 calories)
- Fish Sauce Chicken Thighs (449 calories)
- Korean Bibimbap (823 calories)
- Avocado Chocolate Mousse (573 calories)

Day 3

- Jicama Fries (253 calories)
- Cabbage Dumplings (614 calories)
- Vietnamese Chicken Wings (504 calories)
- Ice Cream Cake (445 calories)

Check out our YouTube channel at https://www.youtube.com/BIOptimizers to see some of the recipes from this cookbook in action.

SLOW-CARB TIPS

- *When you eat is important.* On the Slow-Carb diet, eat breakfast within an hour of waking up. Depending on your sleep schedule, space meals approximately four hours apart.
- *Don't overeat calorie-dense foods.* A lot of people tend to overeat certain foods included in the Slow-Carb diet (like nuts and hummus). This can easily add excess calories, so be mindful.
- *Get enough protein.* We recommend 30 grams of protein with breakfast and at least 20 grams per meal after that.
- *Continue protein-filled breakfasts even on refeed days.* Even though cheat days allow you to eat whatever you want, stick with 30 grams of protein at breakfast. This helps lower your blood sugar response to any carbs.
- *Take your time.* The diet suggests taking at least 30 minutes to eat each meal. This helps decrease your glycemic response.
- *Substitute veggies for starchy foods.* Choose vegetables or beans over carbohydrates like rice and pasta.

Lifestyle Recommendations

- *Start small.* If too many diet and lifestyle changes overwhelm you, start small. For example, commit to a protein-rich breakfast within 30 minutes of waking up, and then gradually build more rules into your routine.
- *Keep it simple.* Basic foods such as eggs, frozen veggies, or canned anchovies are easy, quick meals.
- *Prepare for traveling.* You can grab on-the-go meals like nuts or protein powder in water. Again, try to keep it simple.

Other Tools to Manage Your Blood sugar

Exercise

Exercise is one of the best ways to improve nutrient partitioning and ensure that the food you eat goes to your muscles. At the very least, try to walk for 10 minutes after eating a meal. Tim Ferriss also does some short resistance exercises around his cheat meals to increase muscle insulin sensitivity.

Supplements

Blood Sugar Breakthrough can help support your blood sugar levels, improve calorie partitioning, and potentially reduce cravings.

PROS AND CONS OF A SLOW-CARB DIET

Health

Pros

- Improved insulin sensitivity
- Reduced cravings
- Improved blood lipids and lower health risk
- Improved regularity due to increased fiber
- Good for gut bacteria

Aesthetics

Pros

- Easy to lose fat for people who have insulin resistance
- May minimize fat gain on an anabolic (muscle-gaining) phase

Performance

Pro

- Stable blood sugar improves mental performance

Con

- Power athletes may need higher-glycemic carbs during intense workouts and competition to maximize performance

Lifestyle

Pro

- Easy to adapt to on the road or eating out by substituting vegetables for starches; certain cuisines allow for easy substitutions

Con

- Must avoid cakes, cookies, pasta, and donuts except on refeed day (if applicable)

Psychological

Pro

- Stabilized blood sugar often stabilizes mood and cravings

Con

- The diet can still be restrictive in certain social situations

SUMMARY

Slow-carb (or low-glycemic-impact) diets focus on food that minimizes the impact on blood sugar. You eat more protein and fibers, and fewer processed carbs. This combination increases the thermic effect of food and decreases net calories.

Slow-carb diets are different from paleo or keto diets:

- Slow-carb diets cut out grains, refined sugar, and all fruits while including starchy vegetables, legumes, and beans.
- Paleo diets cut out grains, legumes, and any refined sugars. However, there is no limitation on carbs, fruits, or starchy vegetables.
- Keto diets keep a tight control on carb consumption.

To do the Slow-Carb 2.0 Diet, you must take these steps:

1. Find meals that work for you with CGM and microbiome tests.
2. Find your individual low-glycemic-impact carbs.
3. Plan your calorie and meal breakdowns based on your goals.

CHAPTER 25

IIFYM: THE MOST FLEXIBLE DIET OF THEM ALL

In this chapter, you're going to learn:

- What makes IIFYM the most flexible diet ever created
- What IIFYM means and what its advantages are
- How you can do an IIFYM diet in a three-step process
- How you can adjust your calorie intake based on your ultimate diet goals
- Two clear-cut examples of how to calculate your macros (proteins, fats, and carbohydrates) to align with your goals
- A thorough list of high-protein foods that should be foundational in an IIFYM diet
- How you can diet without having to give up your favorite foods
- How to select the fats to include in your diet
- How to select the carbs to include in your diet
- Four different times you can use the IIFYM diet in your life
- Three steps to target your calories and how to calculate BMR for men and for women using a simple equation
- The three macronutrients to track to have success on an IIFYM diet

The "If It Fits Your Macros" (IIFYM) style of diet is the default for most bodybuilders and physique athletes. It's effective for getting lean and for muscle building.

The structure of IIFYM is simple. You create the calorie and macro targets that will help you achieve your goals and *eat whatever you want* as long as you hit your targets.

IIFYM is also a good option for people who are repulsed by the concept of "diets" and giving up their favorite foods. You can keep eating your favorites—with some modifications in portions, of course.

IIFYM can be a good transition diet for people who want to achieve their aesthetic goals before moving on to another diet type. Both of us have gone through that process. When we were focused solely on bodybuilding, we concentrated mostly on protein and calories. It was effective for building muscle or getting lean. Over time, our personal nutritional strategies evolved. Wade moved to a plant-based lifestyle, and Matt has primarily followed a keto diet.

THE ADVANTAGE OF IIFYM

The primary advantage of IIFYM is that it's completely free of dieting dogma because of its wide-open flexibility. The only thing that matters is hitting your target macros and calories.

THE DISADVANTAGE (AND CONTROVERSY) OF IIFYM

The downsides of IIFYM are the potential health issues from eating inflammatory foods and a lack of mindfulness around micronutrients and other health benefits that can arise from eating healthier food options. However, there's a vital piece of data that most healthy food zealots don't want you to know: if someone's in a calorie deficit, their health markers usually improve.

On one side of the debate, nutritional experts attack foods that have seed oils, artificial sweeteners, GMOs, or anything unnatural. On the other side, IIFYM followers don't care about organic food or ingredient quality.

What's the truth? The truth is, there is *not* a lot of data showing damaging health effects from those "evil" foods. Now, that doesn't mean they don't negatively impact people's health.

What's our stance? That the truth is probably in the middle. There could be some negative consequences of eating unhealthy foods over time. Theoretically, it makes sense to eat food that has more nutrients and fewer toxins. We do believe that it's a smart insurance policy to eat organic food when possible. On the flip side, we don't believe in vilifying foods or those who eat them.

When it comes to food, the words *toxins* and *natural* get thrown around a lot. The reality is, when your body starts breaking food down, the components eventually all become chemicals. Arsenic is "natural," and it's certainly not good for you; it's a deadly toxin.

One of the potential long-term issues of IIFYM is micronutrient deficiencies. IIFYM does not focus on micronutrients, such as vitamins and minerals. According to the CDC, 2 billion people worldwide have micronutrient deficiencies.[1] We are big believers and proponents of giving your body all of the key nutrients it needs for optimal functioning. That's a foundational piece of being biologically optimized. We know that when the body has certain nutrient deficiencies over time, it leads to health problems.

HOW TO DO THE IIFYM DIET

People following the IIFYM diet keep track of these three macronutrients:

- Proteins
- Carbohydrates (including fiber)
- Fats

Start by using the calculator by downloading the Me Diet app:

- Step 1: Calculate your target calories.
- Step 2: Determine your target protein per day in grams.
- Step 3: Determine your target carbs per day.
- Step 4: Determine your target fats per day.

Step 1: Target Calories

We've covered this in previous chapters, but here's a brief overview:

1. **Calculate your BMR using the Mifflin-St. Jeor equation.**

- For men, BMR = 10 x weight (kg) + 6.25 x height (cm) – 5 x age (years) + 5
- For women, BMR = 10 x weight (kg) + 6.25 x height (cm) – 5 x age (years) – 161
- Add additional daily calorie expenditure
- Exercise (as a general rule, 500 calories per hour is a good number, but it obviously depends on intensity and difficulty)
- Brown fat activation
- Cold thermogenesis. If you get to the shiver zone, it can burn 800 to 2,000 calories a day.
- High-level anabolism. If you're in a rapid muscle-building phase, you can burn an extra 10 to 25 percent in calories per day.
- NEAT. If you move a lot throughout the day, you can burn an extra 300 to 700 calories.

If all of this is too complex, don't worry; just download the Me Diet app, and we will do all the calculations for you. Of course, we take out all of the guessing and use our formulas to design your personalized journey designed with the Me Diet app. Go to www.BIOptimizers.com/book/dietapp to download our app to make your Me Diet journey simple and easy to follow.

2. **Adjust your calories based on your goal.**

- For weight loss: as a starting point, subtract 500 calories
- For muscle building: as a starting point, add an extra 300 calories a day
- For maintenance: keep the calories the same

Step 2: Calculate Your Protein

Protein is the king macro and should be calculated first.

- Protein should be between 0.7–1.0 grams per pound of bodyweight

Step 3: Calculate Your Fats

- Fat intake should be between 0.25–0.4 grams per pound of bodyweight. (Note: most bodybuilders try to keep their fat intake on the lower side of the spectrum.)

Step 4: Calculate Your Carbs

All remaining calories are allocated for carbs.

Here are two examples of how this could look:

First, let's use Nicky. She's 40, weighs 200 pounds, and wants to lose 40 pounds. She trains three times per week.

- Her target calories are 2,254 per day.
- Her target protein is 154 grams per day.
- Her target fat is 86 grams per day.
- Her target carbs are 221 grams per day.

It's important to note that none of these calculations are perfect. However, it doesn't matter; these are all just starting points. The magic is in the ongoing adjustments. If Nicky doesn't lose weight in the first two weeks, then adjustments will be made. We'll either increase her calorie expenditure or decrease her calories by about 300, and then continue monitoring her progress.

Now, let's take a look at Uncle Tony, who wants to get huge. He's currently 200 pounds and wants to add 25 pounds of bodyweight (as mainly muscle).

- His target calories are 3,442 per day.
- His target protein is 219 grams per day.
- His target fat is 110 grams per day.
- His target carbs are 394 grams per day.

Again, we monitor Uncle Tony's results. If he's gaining too much body fat, then we pull back on the calories a bit. The goal is to have his weight gain be mostly lean muscle tissue.

Step 5: Track Your Macros

The last step is simply to track your calories and macros. The best way to do that is to use a food-tracking app.

Of course, we take out all of the guessing and use our formulas to design your personalized journey designed with the Me Diet app. Go to www.BIOptimizers.com/book/dietapp to download our app to make your Me Diet journey simple and easy to follow.

WHAT TYPES OF FOODS SHOULD YOU EAT ON IIFYM?

Even though you can technically eat anything on this plan, you won't be able to hit your macros unless you focus on high-protein foods.

Here's a list of high-protein foods that should be foundational:

Non-Vegetarian Options	Vegetarian/Vegan Options
Beef	Black beans
Salmon	Lima beans
Chicken	Broccoli
Eggs	Peas
Lamb	Pea protein
Cottage cheese	Pumpkin protein
Bison	Hempseed protein
Pork	Tempeh
Turkey	Spirulina
Milk	Chickpeas
Whey protein	Oats
Greek yogurt	Lentils
Shrimp	Chia seeds
Octopus	Edamame
Wild game	Tofu

As we discussed in previous chapters, protein is the key. Strive to have protein with each meal. Then you can add carbs and fats.

A Note on Animal Proteins

There are massive differences in the percentage of fats of various meats. This is important when you're building your meals and selecting your protein sources. It's okay to eat a fattier animal protein for one meal and then choose a leaner option for dinner. As long as your daily macros are met, you're fine. Strive to find the balance. If you're on a weight loss program, then you should progressively transition from fattier cuts to leaner cuts over time. See the Animal Protein and Fat Percentage Table in Chapter 20 for more insights.

How Should I Select My Fats?

We suggest that it's best to minimize inflammatory fats, including trans fats and vegetable oils. For vegans, focus on natural fats: olives, olive oil, avocados, and nuts. If you're not a vegetarian, then you'll probably be consuming enough fats from your protein sources. Simply track your total fat intake and make adjustments as needed.

How Should I Select My Carbs?

This is where there's the most flexibility. If you're dieting, read Chapter 10, Conquering Hunger, discussing hunger, and focus on satiating carbs such as potatoes, sweet potatoes, oatmeal, and high-fiber vegetables.

If you're trying to eat a lot of food to gain weight, then focus on faster-digesting carbs: some fruits, white rice, pasta, and so on.

To get an example of a three-day meal plan, go to www.BIOptimizers.com/book/resources to get all the extra content (and more meal plans).

COMBINING IIFYM WITH OTHER DIET STRATEGIES

IIFYM is just another tool in the toolbox. You don't need to go all in. You can use it strategically for:

- Vacations and holidays
- Refeed days
- Diet breaks
- Higher-carb days if you're on a cyclical keto diet

For example, Matt likes to use the IIFYM approach on refeed days and during vacations. He's keto from Monday to Saturday, and on Sunday, he eats whatever he wants within his target parameters.

Doing IIFYM can help give your brain a psychological break while still moving you toward your goals.

This is one of the simplest strategies there is. Most diet books would try to add another 100 pages of fluff to make it sound more complex and magical. It isn't. It's easy and straightforward. If you want to make it even easier, then download the Me Diet app and we'll provide the guidance for you.

Of course, we take out all of the guessing and use our formulas to design your personalized journey designed with the Me Diet app. Go to www.BIOptimizers.com/book/dietapp to download our app to make your Me Diet journey simple and easy to follow.

PROS AND CONS OF IIFYM

Health

Pros (if you're in a calorie deficit)

- Improved insulin sensitivity
- Reduced cravings
- Improved blood lipids and lower health risks

Con

- Potential health problems over time due to nutrient deficiencies

Aesthetics

Pros

- It's easy to lose fat and achieve your goals
- This is a great diet for gaining lean muscle

Con

- Some people may have increased food cravings due to blood sugar and insulin issues

Performance

Pro

- Diet macros can easily be adjusted for peak athletic performance

Con

- Power athletes may need higher glycemic carbs during intense workouts and competition to maximize performance

Lifestyle

Pro

- Easily one of the best "lifestyle" diets. Virtually any type of cuisine or food works, as long as you hit your macros

Con

- You have to count your calories and macros if you want this to work. If you start winging it, the odds are high you will go off track

Psychological

Pro

- It's the most psychologically flexible diet ever created

Cons

- None

SUMMARY

IIFYM stands for "if it fits your macros." Essentially, you can eat whatever you want, as long as it fits your target macros.

The primary advantage of IIFYM is that it's completely free of dieting dogma because of its wide-open flexibility. However, it's possible for the IIFYM diet to lead to nutrient deficiencies over time.

You can easily keep track of your macronutrients with these four simple steps:

- Step 1: Calculate your target calories.
- Step 2: Determine your target protein per day in grams.
- Step 3: Determine your target carbs per day.
- Step 4: Determine your target fats per day.

UNIVERSAL NUTRITIONAL OPTIMIZERS

This section is filled with strategies and tools that can be applied to every and any diet. They are powerful tools that will help you enhance your results and optimize your health.

CHAPTER 26

REDEFINING NUTRITION

This chapter is for everyone. You can apply these universal strategies and tactics to make any diet work better.

As we argued with each other for years about which diet was better (for example, keto vs. vegetarian), we eventually found core principles that helped both camps. These debates helped us discover universal truths about nutrition.

In this chapter you will learn:

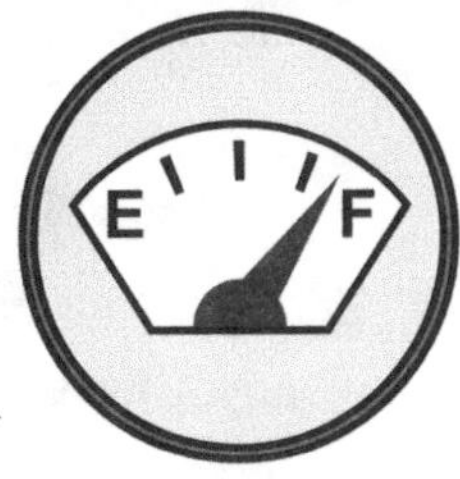

Nutrification

- What the definition of nutrition is, and what strategies you should use to optimize your consumption, conversion, and assimilation of nutrients
- Why reaching the optimal-dose zone is one of the most powerful things you can achieve
- The most important aspect to focus on is your macros, right? *Wrong!* Discover why focusing on your enzyme and probiotic levels plays a key role in nutrition.
- Why nutrition is more than simply eating good food
- The three phases of nutrification and how to optimize each properly to take your health, aesthetics, and performance to the next dimension
- What the primary bio-workers inside the body are, and how they work to help you build the ultimate dream body
- What BIOptimizing really means
- How much better you could feel and live if you moved into the optimal-dose zone
- How you can use your biofeedback, bloodwork, and other health analyses to optimize your nutritional choices and supplements even more precisely
- How to avoid entering the poison zone of nutrition
- Our redefinition of *nutrition* and how to enhance all of the most critical biological processes
- How to surpass the optimal zone of nutrition and achieve the world-class zone

We consider this one of the most important chapters in the book. It redefines what most people consider nutrition to be.

Most people think of *nutrition* as simply eating good food. Oxford's definition is "the process of providing or obtaining the food necessary for health and growth."

However, the accurate scientific definition is "the biochemical and physiological process by which an organism uses food to support its life. It includes ingestion, absorption, assimilation, biosynthesis, catabolism and excretion."[1] Our company, BIOptimizers, is devoted to enhancing all of these critical biological processes, and you'll find many powerful strategies for doing that in this book. This chapter gives you the big picture as we break down what we call our system of nutrification.

Nutrification is the consumption, conversion, and assimilation of food into nutrients. The system starts with consuming healthy, nutrient-rich foods, breaking them down into usable components, transporting them into your bloodstream, and then assimilating those nutrients into the body.

THE THREE PHASES OF NUTRIFICATION

Nutrification Phase 1: Consume

This one is simple. Eat the highest quality food possible—ideally, organic, nutrient-rich, toxin-free foods.

The ultimate objective is to grow and raise your own hyper-optimized food. Optimize your soil with nutrients and grow heirloom seeds. If you have the land, time, and inclination, raise your own animals. This is the best. However, most of us just can't do this.

Nutrification Phase 2: Convert

Most of the information in the dietary world is focused just on macros: "You need this many calories, this much protein, this many carbohydrates, and this many fats." What good are these materials if they're not bioavailable?

Bio-workers are just as important as the raw materials when it comes to nutrition. Inside the body, the primary bio-workers are enzymes and probiotics. They take apart macros into absorbable nutrients—carbs into glucose, proteins into amino acids, and fats into fatty acids. They're the construction crew working on your dream home. If they're not on site, you'll just have a bunch of building materials.

We'll dive much deeper into enzymes and probiotics in Chapters 8 and 9.

Nutrification Phase 3: Assimilate

Finally, nutrients move into the bloodstream and assimilate into building blocks or energy for the body. Glucose becomes energy. Amino acids morph into neurochemicals, muscle tissue, organ tissue, and much more. Fatty acids become energy, hormones, skin cells, brain tissue, and more.

Your health, aesthetics, and performance will go to the next dimension when you optimize all three phases.

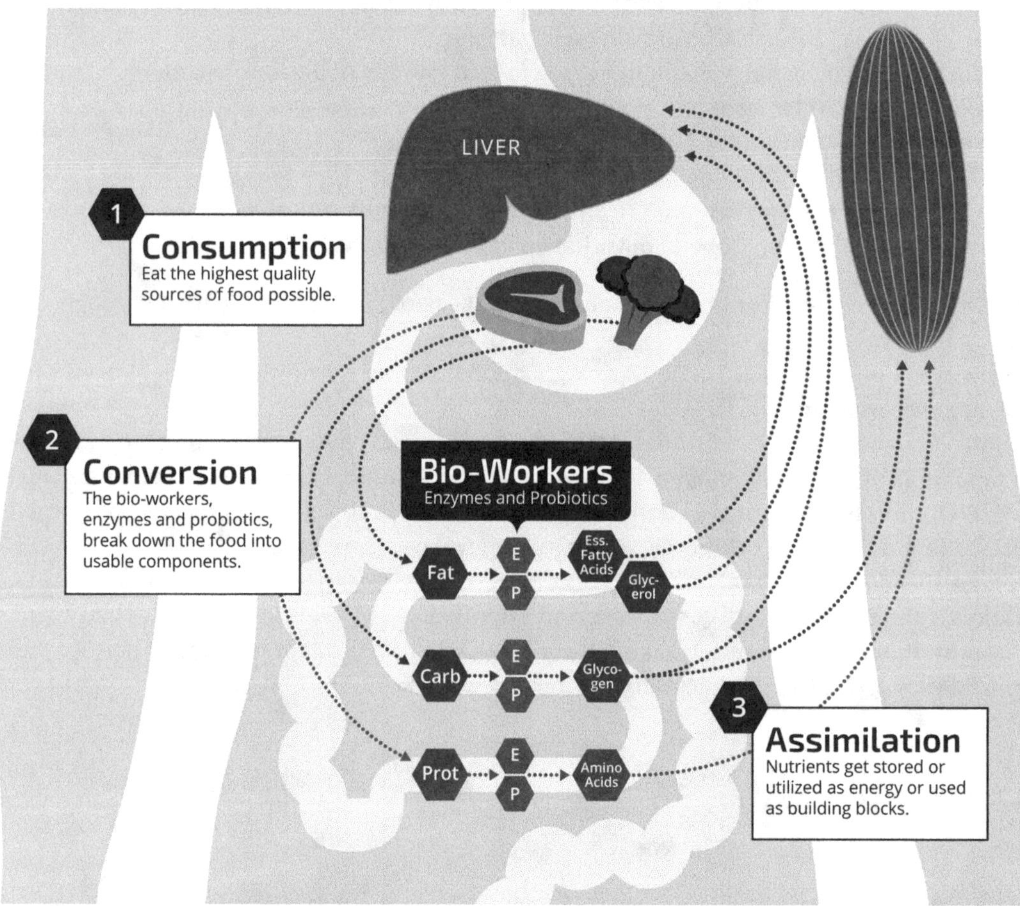

PHASE 1: CONSUME

In this phase, we flood your digestive system with the essential nutrients required for you to achieve your health and performance goals based on your genetics. Our goal is to give your nutritional system all the macronutrients and micronutrients it needs, including proteins, essential fatty acids, carbohydrates, and optimal levels of vitamins and minerals.

Phase 1 is aimed at giving your body all of the highest-quality nutrients it needs to be at its best. This is where buying the best real food possible matters. Buy organic vegetables and fruits if possible. Heirloom vegetables may even be better. When you buy meat, focus on grass-fed. Even better, eat wild game.

The real challenge here is modern food production systems. The food production world has focused solely on maximizing yield and profits at the cost of nutrients. Food today is calorie rich and nutrient poor. Nutrients in soil have dropped between 20 and 40 percent since 1975.[2, 3] And other data shows they were falling for decades before that.

Farmers focus on creating the biggest possible fruits and veggies, and most forgo the extra expense and effort of remineralizing their soils and rotating crops. We can expect commercialized mass farming to continue this trend, and for store-bought fruits and vegetables to keep declining in value and quality.

PHASE 2: CONVERT

The second phase is converting your food into usable nutrients. The stars of the show are enzymes and probiotics. These are the bio-workers who do all the hard labor of deconstructing your food into its bioavailable components.

Enzymes have more than 25,000 different functions in the body. They are involved in everything from thinking to blinking. They deconstruct protein into usable amino acids, fats into fatty acids, and carbs into glycogen. They enhance your body's ability to move toxins out, and more important, rebuild damaged tissues. They clean house.

This is why our company, BIOptimizers, has been obsessed with building the best digestive supplements. We've built the most powerful enzymes and probiotics on the market. We've been testing and optimizing all of our formulas in our BioLab with the University of Burch in Sarajevo (where we employ a team of Ph.D.s in microbiome, chemistry, and biology studies) for several years now, and we've beaten every competitor in effectiveness. Visit www.BIOptimizers.com to learn more.

Probiotics are organisms that break down food even further, help fight off bad bacteria and viruses, remove toxic garbage, and run an incredible array of biological functions for digestion. They also produce neurotransmitters, immune factors, vitamins, enzymes, and many other critical nutrients for the body.

They're among the best weapons to protect your immunity and maintain optimal digestive function.

Think of enzymes as a lawnmower and probiotics as a lawn mulcher. Together, they deconstruct food into the fuel and building blocks your body needs to be BIOptimized.

PHASE 3: ASSIMILATE

Assimilation is the final phase of nutrification. The amino acids, fatty acids, and glycogen cross the intestinal barrier and enter the bloodstream.

Nutrients are essentially inert substances, and they require workers to put them together. In this final phase, enzymes are the workers that do the assimilation as part of their more than 25,000 different functions. Enzymes help reassemble amino acids into peptides and proteins, which are assimilated as muscle, organs, neurotransmitters, and much more. Fatty acids become energy, brain matter, skin, hair, body fat, myelin sheath, hormones, and many other things.

Glycogen gets stored in the liver or muscle, or it turns into body fat via the gluconeogenesis process. Gluconeogenesis is a 25-cent word that means, "You didn't burn the excess carbs, so we're going to store it as fat." This is how most people become obese. They have an excess of energy. It's important to note that not just glucose causes this, but fat as well. The bottom line is that an excess of calories leads to body fat gain.

The key to optimizing assimilation is keeping your body's enzyme levels high. We do this by taking them as supplements with our foods, as well as on an empty stomach. There's more on this in Chapter 28.

Another important part of the assimilation team is the nutrient co-factors. They are the enzymes' teammates and vital parts of the process. That's why maintaining optimal levels of vitamins and minerals is important. For example, magnesium is a co-factor in more than 300 of the body's functions. We are discovering in our BioLab research that micro amounts of co-factors can multiply assimilation by 200 to 300 percent. This is why giving your cells all the micronutrients they need is so critical.

Now, let's move on to the next key part of the system.

FINDING YOUR OPTIMAL-DOSE ZONE

Our definition of *biological optimization* (aka *BIOptimization*) is: a state of existence where all of the body's and brain's functions exist in optimal quantities and operate in perfect harmony.

Most people are highly deficient in a wide variety of nutrients. They live in a suboptimal state that they see as normal because they're used to it. They have no clue how much better they could feel and live if they moved into the optimal-dose zone. Here's a nutritional axiom when it comes to all molecules: the dose creates the effect.

You can truly experience some life-changing benefits by going from suboptimal to optimal. When Matt took his testosterone from suboptimal to optimal, he went from living with a low drive to becoming highly driven. When Wade took his magnesium from minimum to optimal, he went from burnt out to rejuvenated. When Matt took his potassium from suboptimal to optimal, he improved his hydration levels and aesthetics. We could fill this chapter with examples like this.

When you move into the optimal zone with your nutrient levels, your health, aesthetics, and performance improve. *The dose creates the effect.*

There are two ways that nutrients in the wrong amounts can kill our progress:

1. With long-term deficiencies
2. With deadly overloads[4]

Our goal is to find that sweet spot in the middle.

For almost every nutrient there is a:

- Deficiency zone
- Minimum effective dose
- Optimal dose
- Maximum effective dose
- Deadly poison zone

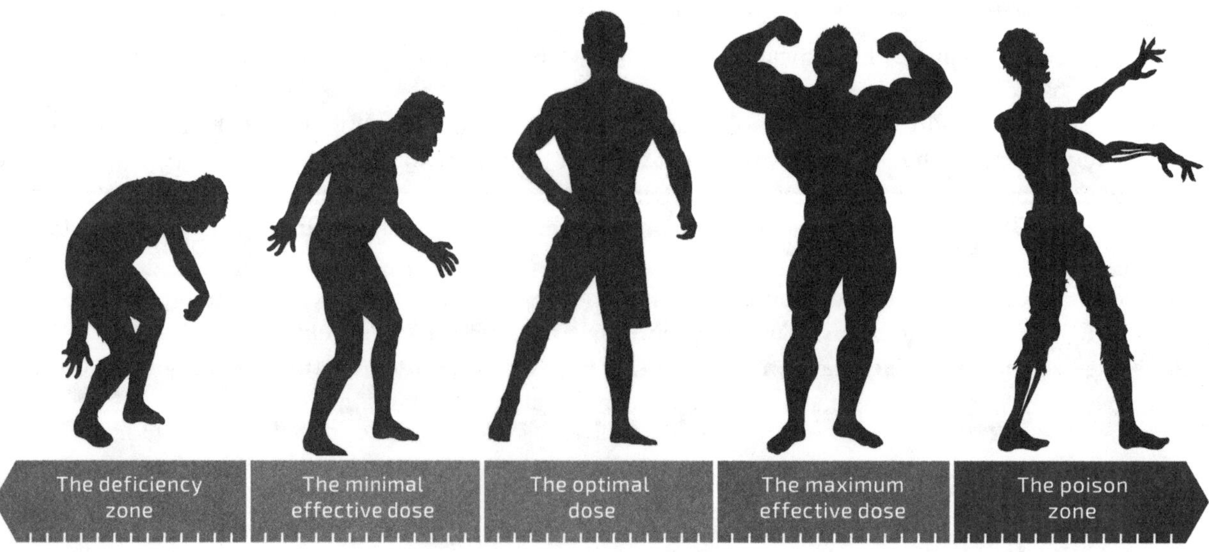

The Deficiency Zone

The deficiency zone is where there aren't enough nutrients for your body to operate at its peak, and diseases and other health problems occur.

This can create a cascade of secondary negative effects.

Here's an analogy to illustrate this point. When Matt was 16 years old, his father's car had transmission problems. His father said, "Don't go anywhere with the car, we need to fix the transmission. It could damage the engine."

Well, Matt being young, ignorant, and stubborn decided to go see his girlfriend, who lived 30 miles away. On the way back, the car was stuck in second gear and the RPMs were maxed out for the entire drive. By the time he got home, he had cooked the engine and it was completely destroyed. His father wasn't a happy camper.

The point of this story is that when one system in the body becomes compromised, it impacts other systems. This can create a dire chain of consequences.

The Minimum Effective Dose

Most people are in this zone with the majority of the body's critical nutrients. In this range, the body has some of the nutrients but not enough to operate at its best. Minimum effective doses eventually lead to suboptimal nutrient levels in your body.

One of the problems of being in this zone is that over time, it's easy to slip into the deficiency zone. As we age, a lot of our body's functions decline. We tend to absorb fewer nutrients and our ability to assimilate them gets weaker.

What are some of the consequences? Your body produces fewer neurotransmitters, which are vital for your brain to operate at its peak and feel happy. Your muscles lack amino acids, which leads to muscle loss. Loss of muscle leads to a slower metabolism and other negative issues.

The list goes on and on.

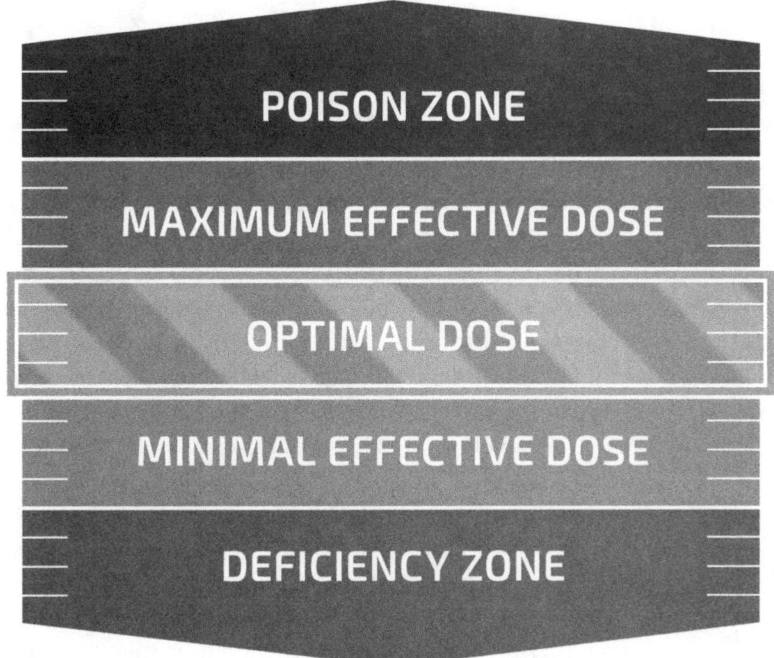

The Optimal Dose

There is an optimal zone at which you're giving your body the appropriate amount of nutrients for it to operate at its best. You will feel your best. Living in the optimal zone changes your energy levels. You feel like the best version of yourself.

The goal is to get each of your body's nutrients and hormones into the optimal zone. This is easier said than done. We're not just talking about macronutrients (carbs, proteins, and fats). We're talking about everything: micronutrients, enzymes, probiotics, phytonutrients, etc.

There are many considerations to help you figure this out:

- Your age: The older you get, the harder it is to absorb nutrients
- Your lean body mass: The more you have, the more you need
- Your metabolism: Some people utilize nutrients at a much faster rate
- Your genetics: This is one of the most significant ones because genetic mutations (which everyone has) can easily cause deficiencies. To learn about potential nutritional mutations, go to: www.BIOptimizers.com/book/genes.

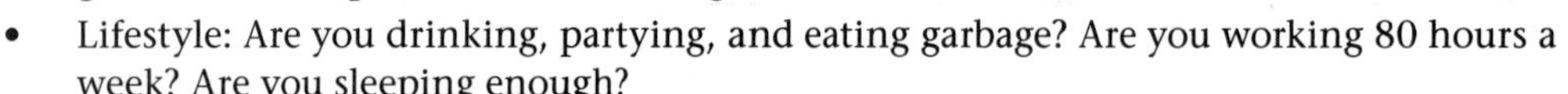

- Lifestyle: Are you drinking, partying, and eating garbage? Are you working 80 hours a week? Are you sleeping enough?

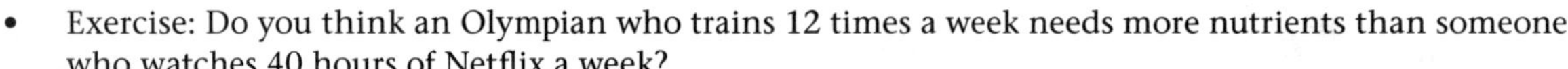

- Exercise: Do you think an Olympian who trains 12 times a week needs more nutrients than someone who watches 40 hours of Netflix a week?

The Maximum Effective Dose

Beyond biological optimization is maximization. The goal here is to achieve the most extreme results possible.

Professional athletes generally operate in the maximization zone. Their goal is maximum speed, maximum power, maximum endurance, or maximum performance.

They're willing to sacrifice the health side of the BIOptimization Triangle to achieve their goals.

Even many purpose-driven entrepreneurs fall into this category. They're on a mission and they're willing to sacrifice their health to get there.

First of all, we applaud the dedication and drive of these people. They're a special breed that are extremely driven to become the best at what they do.

Our message is that you can achieve even better levels of success by focusing on the health side of the BIOptimization Triangle. Longer careers and even better performance can be achieved by optimizing vs. maximizing.

The Poison Zone

Paracelsus, a Swiss physician from the 16th century, wrote, "*Sola dosis facit venenum.*" This translates to, "The dose makes the poison."

When the dose enters the poison zone, it becomes deadly. Virtually every substance has an LD_{50}, which means the median lethal dose. The lethal dose of a substance would kill at least 50 percent of the population.

On the extreme side, the deadliest toxin in the world, botulinum, kills a human at 1 nanogram per kilogram.

Everything at the right dose can kill us, including water. A lady who drank 10 liters of water later died. This is a bit misleading because it's a mineral deficiency that killed her. When you drink water, it pulls minerals out of your body. Some waters, like distilled water, aggressively eliminate crucial minerals and can create serious health issues, and even lead to death.

Our advice is to be mindful of the LD_{50} of supplements and other nutrients that you take.

HOW TO OPTIMIZE YOUR NUTRIENTS TO THE WORLD-CLASS ZONE

To become BIOptimized, you need data. Lack of good, convenient data can be solved for the most part with blood, urine, and saliva tests.

Then you use your biofeedback, bloodwork, and other health analysis to optimize your nutritional choices and supplements even more precisely. This is a core part of the Biological Optimization Process. Work with professionals that can help you interpret your data.

SUMMARY

In summary, nutrition is more than simply eating good food. We define nutrition as the consumption, conversion, and assimilation of nutrients. We call this process "nutrification."

1. Take your nutritional results to the next level by optimizing each of the three nutrification phases:
    - Phase 1: Consume. Eat the best food possible to feed your digestive system with high levels of micronutrients.
    - Phase 2: Convert. Break your food down into usable, absorbable components by using bio-workers (enzymes and probiotics).
    - Phase 3: Assimilate. Turn nutrients into energy, hormones, or tissue. Enhance the process with enzymes (on an empty stomach) and BIOptimizers supplements.
2. Seek to live in the optimal nutrient zone.
    - The deficiency zone. This zone is where there aren't enough nutrients for your body to operate at its peak, and diseases and other health problems occur.
    - The minimum effective dose. In this range, the body has some nutrients, but not enough to operate at its best. It's easy to slip into the deficiency zone from here. Your brain function goes down, you lose muscle, your metabolism is slower, and other negative issues arise.
    - The optimal dose. In this range, you give your body the appropriate amount of each nutrient for peak performance based on your age, lean muscle mass, metabolism, genetics, lifestyle, and more.
    - The maximum effective dose. Here, the goal is to achieve the most extreme results possible. However, by focusing on this range, you can compromise your health.
    - The deadly poison zone. Everything can kill us at the wrong dose. This can be either too little (long-term deficiencies) and too much (deadly overload).

Using the BIOptimization Process to Find the Sweet Spot

To become BIOptimized, you need a high-quality stream of data. Use your biofeedback, bloodwork, and other health analyses to optimize your nutritional choices and supplements even more precisely. Create a life-changing feedback loop by getting information, making adjustments, and then remembering. Embrace *kaizen* (the Japanese term for "continuous improvement").

CHAPTER 27

THE MAGIC OF MICRONUTRIENTS

This chapter is about optimizing your micro nutrition. In this chapter you will learn:

- Why the *dose* of each of your supplements is critical for taking you from a deficiency zone to your optimal levels of health, aesthetics, and performance
- The six key factors to take into consideration for bringing your body's nutrients and hormones into the optimal zone
- What we can learn from the "orthomolecular strategy" about using megadoses of vitamins and minerals to optimize health
- How to achieve your next level of success by focusing on the health side of your BIOptimization Triangle to cultivate longer careers and even better performance (hint: focus on optimizing rather than maximizing)
- Knowing the recommended dose of a vitamin or mineral is the most important thing, right? *Wrong!* Find out why you have to know *what's already in your system* first
- The seven master nutrients to pay attention to so you can become BIOptimized, including each nutrient's RDA, key benefits, top food sources, and extra insights
- Why salt *is not* your enemy, plus how to upgrade your salts to contain as many as 88 different trace minerals to keep your levels optimal
- What the SpectraCell Micronutrient Test is, and why frequent testing of your body's nutrient levels is important
- How to stack your fats and fat-soluble vitamins to increase absorption gains with many other key fat-soluble nutrients
- Eight critical micronutrients and the important roles they play in your body
- Why we believe that trace mineral deficiencies inevitably lead to compromised health

When most diet experts talk of nutrition, they focus on carbs, proteins, and fats. Those are the macronutrients. However, to fully optimize your health, you also need to focus on micronutrients, which include:

- Macrominerals
- Microminerals
- Trace minerals
- Vitamins

Nutrients are essential for life. Without them, your health would be compromised. Let's use minerals as an example. With extreme mineral depletion, you would die of a heart attack. In fact, many bodybuilders *have* died of heart attacks in competitions because they used diuretics, which pull out water *and* minerals. Going from suboptimal to optimal levels of various minerals (like magnesium) can have profound effects on health and performance.

One of the most important concepts in biological optimization is: the dose creates the effect. The following diagram illustrates our point.

The deficiency zone
The minimal effective dose
The optimal dose
The maximum effective dose
The poison zone

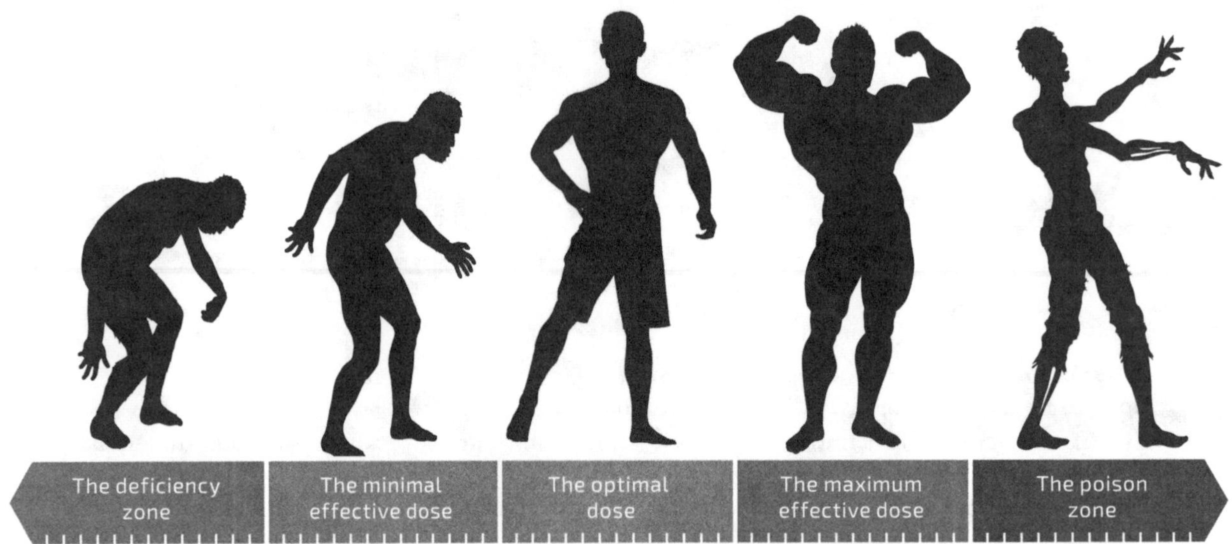

The truth is that the majority of people are at suboptimal levels of most minerals and vitamins. Let's take magnesium as an example. According to research, 61 percent of American adults are not consuming enough.[1]

When we increased our magnesium breakthrough dosage, we both experienced dramatic changes in our entire nervous systems and overall well-being. We went from feeling fried and stressed to calm and relaxed in just a month. This really revealed the power of going from suboptimal to optimal.

Every one of our clients has experienced new levels of cognitive performance and energy when they've optimized their body's nutrients.

THE DEFICIENCY ZONE

The deficiency zone is where you are when you don't have enough nutrients for your body to operate at its peak. Diseases and other health problems occur here, creating a cascade of secondary negative effects. When one system goes down, other systems are often impacted.

Your body is an intricate machine where all your organs and biological systems work in harmony.

As we learned from Matt's engine-blowing story in the previous chapter, when one system becomes comprised, it usually creates a domino effect of destructive health consequences. Cars don't run very long when they run out of oil. Similarly, the body doesn't work well when it's missing critical nutrients. This is how the body works.

THE MINIMUM EFFECTIVE DOSE

Most people are in the minimum effective zone with most of the body's critical nutrients. In this range, the body has some nutrients but not enough to operate at its best.

One of the problems of being in this zone is that over time, it's easy to slip down into the deficiency zone. As we age, a lot of our body's functions decline. We tend to absorb fewer nutrients; our ability to assimilate them gets weaker.

Take digestion, for example—as we age, our body's enzyme reserves get depleted. We produce less stomach acid, which means we absorb fewer nutrients, including critical amino acids.

What are some of the consequences? Your body produces fewer neurotransmitters, which are vital for your brain to operate at its peak and to feel happy. Your muscles lack amino acids, which leads to muscle loss. Loss of muscle leads to a slower metabolism and other negative issues.

THE OPTIMAL DOSE

There is an optimal zone where you're giving your body the appropriate amount of nutrients for it to operate at its best.

We're not just talking about macronutrients (carbs, proteins, and fats). We're talking about everything: micronutrients, enzymes, probiotics, phytonutrients, and so on.

The goal is to get each of your body's nutrients and hormones into the optimal zone. However, this is easier said than done.

There are many considerations when figuring this out:

- *Your age:* The older you get, the harder it is to absorb nutrients
- *Your lean body mass:* The more you have, the more you need
- *Your metabolism:* Some people use nutrients at a much faster rate
- *Your genetics:* This is one of the most significant factors, because genetic mutations (which everyone has) can cause deficiencies
- *Lifestyle:* Are you drinking, partying, and eating garbage? Are you working 80 hours a week? Are you not sleeping enough?
- *Exercise:* Do you think an Olympian who trains 12 times a week needs more nutrients than someone who watches 40 hours of Netflix a week?

Power Move: Get Regular Bloodwork and Other Tests

It's crucial, as a BIOptimizer, to get bloodwork done on a regular basis. We suggest every six months—or, if you can afford it, every three months.

Other valuable tests include genetic, gut health, and hormone tests. We're also big proponents of using biofeedback devices such as the Oura Ring and fitness trackers.

PROBLEMS WITH THE RDA

Here's one of the bigger challenges: we're still learning what the optimal dose is for most nutrients. And, in the United States, there are two standards for the recommended dietary allowance (RDA) of nutrients.

The first was produced by the U.S. Food and Drug Administration (FDA) and hasn't been updated since 1968. It gave the world a simplified estimation of nutrient needs based on a 2,000-calorie diet regardless of age, sex, or pregnancy status.

The second set was produced by the Institute of Medicine. Its numbers are reasonably precise because they're broken down by age and sex, and they're updated fairly often. Those numbers give us:

- An estimated RDA of how much of a nutrient you need based on your age, sex, and pregnancy status
- Adequate intake (AI)—how much of a nutrient you need to avoid an obvious deficiency disease
- Tolerable Upper Limit (UL)—how much of a nutrient you can safely take without overdose

The problems with such RDAs and daily recommended intakes (DRIs) are that they don't factor in your genetics, your goals, or other personal factors. Many people have genetic mutations that can easily lead them to become deficient in various vital nutrients.

There's a lot missing from following these recommendations if you want to become a biologically optimized human. That's why you should keep educating yourself and learning.

The field of health, fitness, and nutrition is evolving by the day. Hold all knowledge as provisional, because new knowledge makes old knowledge obsolete. This is also why you want to build a Jedi Council of health experts to guide you on your mission.

THE ORTHOMOLECULAR STRATEGY

Dr. Linus Pauling, Dr. Abram Hoffer, and Dr. David Hawkins published a book called *Orthomolecular Psychiatry* in the early 1970s. Orthomolecular medicine is the approach of using the optimal level of molecules (usually vitamins) to cure certain medical issues.

These doctors had developed megadose vitamin and mineral protocols to treat advanced states of medical illness, such as schizophrenia.

Although many traditional scientists and doctors refuted their work, thousands of people from around the world poured into their clinics for treatment. Many of these patients came from some of the most affluent families in the world who had tried everything with their ill family members.

Oftentimes, these clients were completely healed with mega doses of various nutrients and eliminating sugar and chemical toxins.

THE MAXIMUM EFFECTIVE DOSE

Beyond biological optimization is maximization. This is where the goal is to achieve the most extreme physical results you can.

Professional athletes in general operate in the maximization zone. Their goal is maximum speed, maximum power, maximum endurance, or maximum performance. Professional bodybuilders are the perfect example: their goal is to build as much muscle and lose as much body fat as humanly possible. They're going above and beyond any genetic limitation. That's why they use extreme doses of testosterone, selective androgen receptor modulator (SARMS), growth hormone (GH), and other drugs. All these pros are willing to sacrifice the health side of the BIOptimization Triangle to achieve their goals.

Sports researcher Robert Goldman polled 198 world-class athletes, asking, "Would you take a pill that would guarantee a gold medal, even if you knew that it would kill you in five years?" More than half said they'd do it. In other words, they want athletic success and a gold medal more than they want life itself.

Even many purpose-driven entrepreneurs fall into this category. They're on a mission, and they're willing to sacrifice their health to get there. We applaud the dedication and drive of these people. They're a special breed, extremely driven to become the best at what they do.

Our message, though, is that you can achieve even better levels of success by focusing on the health side of the BIOptimization Triangle. Longer careers and even better performance can be achieved by optimizing vs. maximizing.

The body can tolerate short bouts of maximization short term. The key is to cycle periods of recovery with these intense bursts. Similar to an engine, which can tolerate redlining its RPMs for short periods, if you redline your body for too long, you'll cook your engine (like Matt did).

THE POISON ZONE

Virtually every substance has an LD_{50}—a median lethal dose. This is the dose at which a substance would kill 50 percent of the population.

On the extreme side, the deadliest toxin in the world, botulinum, kills a human at a single nanogram per kilogram.

Everything can kill us at the right dose, including water. For example, one woman who drank 10 liters of water died. This is a bit misleading, because it was actually a mineral deficiency that killed her. When you drink water, it pulls minerals out of your body. Water of certain types, like distilled water, aggressively eliminate crucial minerals and can create serious health issues, and even lead to death.

Our advice is to be mindful of the LD_{50} of all supplements and other nutrients that you take. At a high level, macrominerals are the most important, then microminerals, then vitamins, and finally trace minerals.

Now let's review all of the key nutrients your body needs and the top food sources for each one.

THE MOST IMPORTANT THING

Yes, dosage is important. However, it's not the most important thing. What matters most is the amount of nutrients in your system and how well you are metabolizing them. You may need three times the dose. You may have a genetic mutation that makes it hard for you to absorb and use vitamin B. The only way to accurately figure out your optimal dose is by doing tests.

Power Move: Do the SpectraCell Micronutrient Test

This test checks for your micronutrient status over a three-to-six-month window. Your blood is split into 30 different sample tubes to test it for micronutrients like vitamin C, calcium, magnesium, chromium, and so on. The test also looks at your metabolism, oxidative stress, and immune response.

Once you have baseline data, you can keep track of whether you're heading in the right direction or not. If your markers are too high, lower the dose. If they're too low, increase the dose. It's that simple.

THE MASTER NUTRIENT LIST

Here's a list of all of the key minerals and vitamins you should focus on to become BIOptimized. We include each one's RDA, key benefits top food sources, and some extra insights.

MACROMINERAL	Recommended Daily Dose	Use/Function	Sources
Calcium	Age 19–50: 2,500 mg Age 51+: 2,000 mg	Healthy teeth and bones Nerve transmission Muscle contraction Blood pressure	1. Dairy 2. Sardines 3. Leafy green vegetables
Key Calcium Insights • Most people's calcium dosages are too high. Why? Because a lot of foods are "fortified" with calcium. High levels of calcium have been shown to increase risk of heart attacks by 30 percent. • A lot of age-related ailments are the result of overcalcification: heart attacks, arthritis, etc. • To maximize calcium absorption, you need enough vitamin D (see more on vitamin D below).			
Chloride	Age 15+: 2,300 mg	Heart health Nervous system health Production of stomach acid Assists in cellular nutrient absorption	1. Salt 2. Tomatoes 3. Seaweed 4. Olives 5. Rye
Key Chloride Insights • Unless you're avoiding salt, you probably don't have a chloride deficiency. Salt is 60 percent chloride.			
Magnesium	Age 19–30: 310–400 mg Age 31+: 320–420 mg In our opinion, optimal is between 1–2 grams.	Component of bones and teeth Nerve transmission and muscle contraction Over 600 different reactions	1. Leafy green vegetables 2. Nuts 3. Whole grains 4. Chocolate 5. Magnesium Breakthrough
Key Magnesium Insights • Magnesium is hard to absorb with food. We believe that almost everyone has suboptimal levels of magnesium in their bloodstream. • After looking at hundreds of research papers, our viewpoint is it's best to supplement with a variety of magnesium compounds. They seem to impact *different* systems in the body. That's why we've combined the top seven in one formula—Magnesium Breakthrough.			

Phosphorus	Age 19+: 700 mg	Structural component of: • Bones and teeth • DNA and RNA • Cell membranes	1. Chicken 2. Turkey 3. Organ meats 4. Seafood 5. Dairy 6. Nuts
Key Phosphorus Insights • This is a mineral that most people have in excess. • Vegans and vegetarians should be mindful of potential deficiencies.			
Potassium	Age 19+: 2,600–3,400 mg	Electrolyte balance Nerve conduction Muscle contraction Blood pressure	1. Bananas 2. Sweet potatoes 3. Cream of tartar (powder, not the sauce for fish) 4. Prunes 5. Oranges 6. Potatoes
Key Potassium Insights • Most people are potassium deficient, and their potassium-to-sodium ratio is out of whack. The average American consumes around 1,755 mg a day, and the optimal amount is around 4,700 mg. Hard-training athletes may even need more. • The ideal potassium-to-sodium ratio is 3 to 1 (that is, 3 parts potassium to 1 part sodium). Most people's ratios are inverted. • It's critical for athletic performance. • Many people report fixing blood pressure issues by simply increasing their potassium. • The easiest way to optimize this is by using potassium supplements and consuming with food to balance out the sodium.			
Sodium	2,300 mg	Electrolyte balance Nerve conduction Muscle contraction Blood pressure	1. Himalayan salt 2. Sea salt 3. Processed food
Key Sodium Insights • Even though the recommended dose is 2,300 mg a day, we know many people need much more than this, such as hard-training athletes, people who sweat a lot, etc. • Optimize your balance of potassium to sodium (see above). • Upgrade your salts so you get trace minerals with them (see Power Move on the next page).			
Sulfur	1,000 mg	Repairs DNA Joint health Skin Protein synthesis	1. Turkey 2. Beef 3. Eggs 4. Fish 5. Nuts/seeds 6. Chickpeas 7. Couscous 8. Lentils 9. Walnuts

Key Sulfur Insights

- Your body gets sulfur from proteins that contain it. Proteins contain between 3 and 6 percent sulfur amino acids. However, your body needs sulfur to break down certain proteins.
- Methylsulfonylmethane (MSM) is a good supplement source of sulfur.
- Chondroitin sulfate is another good option and great for joint health.

Power Move: Upgrade Your Salt

Fortunately, it's relatively easy to get the majority of trace minerals from certain salts. Traditional table salt is 97 to 99 percent sodium chloride (which is a combination of sodium and chloride).

Why not upgrade your salts to contain a massive array of trace minerals? A spectral analysis of pink Himalayan salt found that it contained 88 different minerals. According to Western Analysis, Inc., sea salt can contain as many as 75 minerals and trace elements.

From a cooking perspective, you will have to modify the amounts a bit. The saltiness of Himalayan salt is milder than that of traditional table salts.

Is salt the enemy? Absolutely not. High-quality salt is one of the most precious things you can consume.

Doesn't salt increase blood pressure and lead to more heart attacks? Let's take a look at the data from Japan. That country's heart attack rates are half those of the United States, and its people eat quite a few salty foods every day.

Does sodium increase blood pressure? Yes, it does. However, there are much healthier ways to lower blood pressure than avoiding salt. By lowering your body's overall carb levels and inflammation, your blood fluid volume will drop, and with that, your blood pressure. Lowering body fat is another effective way to lower blood pressure. Of course, consult your doctor before making these important decisions.

This Power Move leads us to our next section . . .

First let's review a list of key highly researched microminerals. We could compile an entire book of research on the impact that these minerals have on health.

Let's take bone health as an example. Microminerals and trace minerals, including boron, iron, zinc, copper, and selenium, in addition to macrominerals like calcium, phosphorus, and magnesium, play a part in bone metabolism. Most likely, the trace elements help regulate macromineral metabolism. They might also have direct effects by affecting osteoblast (a cell that secretes the matrix for bone formation) or osteoclast (a bone cell that absorbs bone tissue during growth and healing) proliferation, or by helping metabolize the bone mineral matrix.[2]

MICROMINERAL	Recommended Daily Dose	Use/Function	Sources
Chromium	Age 19–50: 25–35 mcg	Assists insulin action Heart health Cholesterol management Weight loss	1. Mussels 2. Broccoli 3. Grape juice 4. Brewer's yeast 5. Meat 6. Brazil nuts

<table>
<tr><td colspan="4">Key Chromium Insights
• Chromium is important for blood sugar management. This is why we included it in Blood Sugar Breakthrough.
• For people who struggle with blood sugar issues, dosages of 100 mcg may be advisable. Talk to your doctor.</td></tr>
<tr><td>Copper</td><td>Age 19+: 900 mcg</td><td>Frees iron for usage
Assists with antioxidant enzymes and formation of connective tissue</td><td>1. Liver
2. Shellfish
3. Spirulina
4. Shiitake mushrooms
5. Nuts
6. Legumes</td></tr>
<tr><td colspan="4">Key Copper Insights
• For copper and zinc, the optimal ratio 1:8, however, a 1:15 ratio is acceptable.
• If your home has copper water pipes, you may be consuming too much copper.</td></tr>
<tr><td>Iodine</td><td>Age 19+: 150 mcg</td><td>Structural component of thyroid hormones, metabolic rate, and cell growth</td><td>1. Seafood
2. Dairy
3. Iodized salt</td></tr>
<tr><td colspan="4">Key Iodine Insights
• The iodine patch test checks how quickly your body absorbs iodine. A doctor paints a patch of it on your skin and checks how it looks 24 hours later. If you're iodine deficient, the patch fades in less than 24 hours.</td></tr>
<tr><td>Iron</td><td>Age 19–50: 8–18 mg
Age 50+: 8 mg</td><td>Red blood cell formation
Immune function
Assists antioxidant enzymes
Energy</td><td>Heme:
1. Lean meat
2. Seafood
Nonheme:
3. Lentils
4. Fortified grain products
5. Beans
6. Nuts</td></tr>
<tr><td colspan="4">Key Iron Insights
• Most people are deficient in iron. It's extremely easy for vegans and vegetarians to become iron deficient.
• Vitamin C and vitamin A are iron co-factors for iron absorption.
• Iron deficiencies can take months to fix.</td></tr>
<tr><td>Manganese</td><td>Age 19+: 1.8–2.3 mg</td><td>Component of antioxidant enzymes
Bone development
Helps break down glucose
Hormones</td><td>1. Mussels
2. Brown rice
3. Hazelnuts
4. Pineapple
5. Spinach
6. Black tea</td></tr>
</table>

<table>
<tr><td colspan="4">Key Manganese Insights
• Manganese is a co-factor for magnesium absorption. That's why we included it in Magnesium Breakthrough. It's also a co-factor for calcium absorption.
• Manganese is a component of the antioxidant enzyme superoxide dismutase (SOD), which is one of your body's most significant antioxidants.</td></tr>
<tr><td>Molybdenum</td><td>Age 19+: 45 mcg</td><td>Assists in metabolism of: amino acids, nucleic acids, xenobiotics
Helps break down toxins
Enzyme cofactor</td><td>1. Organ meats
2. Beans
3. Lentils
4. Peas</td></tr>
<tr><td colspan="4">Key Molybdenum Insights
• Very few people are deficient in molybdenum. Average estimated daily intake is between 76 and 109 mcg/day.
• Some research suggests that in China, where molybdenum is low in the soil, there's a higher instance of esophageal cancer. Other research in Japan found similar trends with esophageal and rectal cancer in women.</td></tr>
<tr><td>Selenium</td><td>Age 14+: 55 mcg</td><td>Assists antioxidant enzymes
Thyroid hormone production
Immune function</td><td>1. Brazil nuts
2. Fish
3. Pork
4. Beef
5. Cottage cheese
6. Sunflower seeds</td></tr>
<tr><td colspan="4">Key Selenium Insights
• All you need is one Brazil nut a day. That's right, one. If you overconsume Brazil nuts, you could develop an excessive amount of selenium in your bloodstream.
• Selenium really showed its immune powers during the COVID spikes.</td></tr>
<tr><td>Zinc</td><td>RDA:
Age 9+:
Women: 8 mg
Men: 11 mg</td><td>Production of hemoglobin
Immune function
Component of hundreds of essential molecules</td><td>1. Oysters
2. Beef
3. Beans</td></tr>
<tr><td colspan="4">Key Zinc Insights
• Estimates are that about 25 percent of the population is deficient in zinc, and in our opinion, a far greater percentage is suboptimal in it.
• Zinc is especially vital for men's testosterone production.</td></tr>
</table>

TRACE MINERALS

We are big believers in the power of trace minerals because we believe that they are co-factors in hundreds—if not thousands—of biological processes. The term *co-factor* here means that something assists or synergizes certain metabolic processes.

The body has more than 102 minerals, and the majority are trace minerals. There's a reason they're in our bodies. Overall, there has been very little research on trace minerals and their impact on health. However, we know beyond the shadow of a doubt that nutrient deficiencies in general lead to health problems. A paper published by Castillo-Durán and Cassorla notes, "Trace mineral deficiencies may affect several biological functions in humans, including physical growth, psychomotor development and immunity."[3]

This is one of our key strategies with all BIOptimizers formulations. By adding certain co-factors, we've been able to improve the potency of particular products by more than 200 to 300 percent in our lab tests.

VITAMINS

We both grew up admiring Hulk Hogan, who had the famous saying: "To all my little Hulkamaniacs, say your prayers, take your vitamins, and you will never go wrong." Solid advice from the Hulkster. What's a vitamin? A vitamin is an organic molecule that is essential for the proper functioning of your metabolism.

A lot of people are vitamin and mineral deficient. They're running on fumes and unknowingly experiencing a performance deficit and suboptimal health. Going from nutrient deficient to nutrient optimal can have a massive impact on performance, especially with B vitamins. By ensuring your nutrient levels are optimized, you will experience better cognitive and physical performance.

Power Move: Stack Your Fats and Fat-Soluble Vitamins

Many vitamins, including A, D, E, and K, are fat soluble. In other words, they look for a source of fat to bond to, which helps the vitamins get absorbed into your bloodstream.

Stacking all your fat-soluble supplements with eating fats creates a major breakthrough in nutrient absorption. For example, research has shown you can boost cannabidiol (CBD) absorption in the bloodstream by 800 percent when taken with a high-fat meal. You can get similar absorption gains with many other key fat-soluble nutrients.

Matt has recently increased his vitamin D levels from 50 to 148 ng/ml using this approach, all while taking half of the vitamin D he had previously been consuming.

We suggest taking all your fat-soluble nootropics and fat-soluble supplements with fats in one shot. Your regimen can include such items as:

- Nootopia caps: Brain Flow, Upbeat, Ultimate Focus, and Apex
- Fish oil or krill oil
- Algae oil
- Buttered coffee (or with MCT oil)
- Vitamins: A, D, K, and E
- CBD/CBG/CBN (more on this in Chapter 3)
- Other high-quality fats: olive or macadamia nut oil

Taking the entire "fat stack" together will cause a powerful synergistic effect. It'll improve the uptake of your nootropics and moderate the uptake into the brain, which improves long-term performance. So, instead of a quick spike in performance, you'll get a long-term, controlled performance improvement.

We suggest doing blood tests every three months when making big shifts so you can track the changes in your biomarkers.

Let's look at the recommended RDA for fat-soluble vitamins:

<table>
<tr><th>Vitamin</th><th>Recommended Daily Dose</th><th>Use/Function</th><th>Sources</th></tr>
<tr><td>Vitamin A</td><td>Age 14+:
700–900 RAE</td><td>Immune function
Vision
Reproduction
Cellular communication</td><td>1. Dairy products
2. Fish
3. Meat</td></tr>
<tr><td colspan="4">Key Vitamin A Insights
• This vitamin is fat soluble, so add it to your daily fat stack regimen.
• Vitamin A deficiencies aren't common in high-income countries.</td></tr>
<tr><td>Vitamin D</td><td>Age 1–70: 15 mcg
Age 71+: 20 mcg</td><td>Helps your body absorb calcium
Helps your muscles move
Helps your nerves work
Hormone optimization
Immune system</td><td>1. The sun
2. Milk
3. Orange juice
4. Yogurt
5. Fatty fish
6. Beef liver
7. Egg yolks</td></tr>
<tr><td colspan="4">Key Vitamin D Insights
• Vitamin D is absolutely one of the most important nutrients to optimize.
• The majority of the population is highly deficient in vitamin D.
• Take vitamin D with your fat stack.
• Always stack with vitamin K to help absorption and minimize calcification. As a general rule, use 50 mcg of vitamin K for every 1,000 IU of vitamin D.
• Higher levels of vitamin D have correlated to much milder symptoms in cases of COVID.
• "Vitamin D" is actually a misnomer. It's really a master hormone that impacts multiple core systems in the body: other hormones, neurochemicals (adrenaline, noradrenaline, dopamine, and serotonin).</td></tr>
<tr><td>Vitamin E</td><td>Age 1–3: 6 mg
Age 4–8: 7 mg
Age 9–13: 11 mg
Age 14+: 15 mg</td><td>Antioxidant
Boosts immune system
Widens blood vessels
Heart health
Inflammation</td><td>1. Vegetable oils
2. Nuts
3. Green vegetables
4. Some breakfast cereals</td></tr>
<tr><td colspan="4">Key Vitamin E Insights
• We rarely recommend supplementing with vitamin E.
• Vitamin deficiencies and excess are rare.
• This is another vitamin that you can add to your daily fat stack if you want to.</td></tr>
</table>

Vitamin	Recommended Daily Dose	Use/Function	Sources
Vitamin K	Age 14–18: 75 mcg Age 19+: 90–120 mcg	Important for blood clotting Important for healthy bones Vitamin D co-factor	1. Leafy green vegetables 2. Natto 3. Broccoli 4. Liver 5. Prunes 6. Figs 7. Meat 8. Hard cheese

Key Vitamin K Insights

- We suggest using vitamin K_2. As a general rule, use 50 mcg of vitamin K for every 1,000 IU of vitamin D.
- This is another vitamin to add to your daily fat stack.
- Synergizes with vitamin D.

Now let's look at the water-soluble vitamins. As a general rule, most people can benefit from higher doses of B vitamins. Another rule is that vegans and vegetarians should monitor their B vitamin levels: a study done by the *American Journal of Clinical Nutrition* found that 92 percent of vegans had vitamin B_{12} deficiencies.[4]

Vitamin	Recommended Daily Dose	Use/Function	Sources
Vitamin C	RDA: Age 14–18: 65–75 mg Age 18+: 75–90 mg	Antioxidant Collagen Immune system Wound healing	1. Citrus fruits (oranges and grapefruits) 2. Broccoli 3. Strawberries 4. Potatoes 5. Tomatoes

Key Vitamin C Insights

- As a general daily recommendation, we suggest using 1 gram per day.
- When you feel your immune system needs extra support, you can take a megadose—1 gram every hour until you feel better (or you have diarrhea) is a popular protocol.

Vitamin	Recommended Daily Dose	Use/Function	Sources
Vitamin B_1: Thiamine	Age 14–18: 1–1.2 mg Age 19+: 1.1–1.2 mg	Helps turn food into energy Important for the growth, development, and function of cells Blood sugar management	1. Wheat germ 2. Whole grains 3. Meat 4. Fish 5. Legumes

Key Vitamin B_1 Insights

- When you go from vitamin B_1 deficiency to optimal levels, you will notice higher levels of energy and better brain function.
- Thiamine helps optimize food assimilation.

Vitamin B_2: Riboflavin	Age 14–18: 1–1.3 mg Age 19+: 1.1–1.3 mg	Important for the growth, development, and function of cells Helps turn food into energy	1. Eggs 2. Organ meats 3. Soybeans 4. Almonds 5. Fish and animal products
Key Vitamin B_2 Insights • B_2 helps optimize food assimilation. • Both deficiency and excess are rare for vitamin B_2. • This vitamin is another energy booster.			
Vitamin B_3: Niacin	Age 14+: 14–16 mg	Important for the growth, development, and function of cells Helps turn food into energy NAD co-factor Improves blood lipid profile	1. Poultry 2. Beef 3. Brown rice 4. Potatoes 5. Peanuts
Key Vitamin B_3 Insights • It's hard to overdose on B_3 because your body will shed the excess in urine. • Higher doses of niacin can create a "skin flush" that feels like a prickly, burning sensation. • Some people combine niacin with the sauna or intense exercise to maximize detoxing effects.			
Vitamin B_5: Pantothenic Acid	Age 14+: 5 mg	Important for making and breaking down fats Helps turn food into energy Healthy skin, hair, and eyes	1. Beef 2. Poultry 3. Seafood 4. Organ meats 5. Eggs 6. Milk 7. Mushrooms 8. Avocados 9. Whole grains 10. Peanuts
Key Vitamin B_5 Insights • Studies have shown that B_5 can help improve skin blemishes and wound healing.			
Vitamin B_6	Age 14–18: 1.2–1.3 mg Age 19–50: 1.3 mg Age 51+: 1.5–1.7 mg	Enzyme reactions involved in metabolism Enzyme reactions involved in brain development during pregnancy and infancy Immune function	1. Poultry 2. Meat 3. Fish 4. Potatoes 5. Non-citrus fruits
Key Vitamin B_6 Insights • B_6 is a mood enhancer because it's a critical co-factor for creating key neurotransmitters, including serotonin, dopamine, and GABA. This is why we use it in several of our Nootopia brain supplement formulas. • Vitamin B_6 deficiencies are more common in people who drink a lot of alcohol and are obese.			

<table>
<tr><td>Vitamin B_7: Biotin
Also known as
"Vitamin H"</td><td>Age 14–18: 25 mcg
Age 19+: 30 mcg</td><td>Helps turn the carbohydrates, fats, and proteins from food into energy
Important for healthy hair, skin, and nails</td><td>1. Meat
2. Eggs
3. Liver
4. Walnuts
5. Sweet potatoes
6. Spinach
7. Broccoli</td></tr>
<tr><td colspan="4">Key Vitamin B_7 Insights
• Biotin is critical for pregnant women. Vitamin B_7 deficiencies can lead to health issues for the baby.</td></tr>
<tr><td>Vitamin B_9: Folate</td><td>Age 14+: 400 mcg</td><td>Makes DNA and other genetic material
Helps our cells to divide
Brain health</td><td>1. Liver
2. Asparagus
3. Spinach
4. Oranges
5. Nuts
6. Beans
7. Peas</td></tr>
<tr><td colspan="4">Key Vitamin B_9 Insights
• B_9 deficiencies become more common as people get older.
• This is another critical nutrient for pregnant women.</td></tr>
<tr><td>Vitamin B_{12}</td><td>Age 14+: 2.4 mcg</td><td>Keeps the body's blood and nerve cells healthy
Helps make DNA
Helps serotonin production
Energy production</td><td>1. Fish
2. Eggs
3. Dairy products
4. Clams
5. Beef liver</td></tr>
<tr><td colspan="4">Key Vitamin B_{12} Insights
• If you're deficient in B_{12}, your energy will plummet.
• B_{12} deficiency is extremely common in vegans and vegetarians.
• Some people need to inject B_{12} to get their levels into the optimal zone.
• B_{12} is another critical nutrient for pregnant women.</td></tr>
</table>

SUMMARY

To fully optimize your health, you need to also focus on micronutrients:

- Macrominerals
- Microminerals
- Trace minerals
- Vitamins

The majority of people are at suboptimal levels of most vitamins and minerals.

The deficiency zone is where you are when your body lacks sufficient nutrients to function at its best, resulting in diseases and other health issues. This can lead to a chain reaction of undesirable consequences. When one system goes down, other systems are often impacted.

The goal is to get your body's nutrients into the Optimal Nutrient Zone and keep it there. Provide your body with the right quantity of these vital nutrients to help it function at its best. To ensure this, consistent, frequent testing is required.

Remember that our guidelines are general. Most people have genetic polymorphisms that affect their ability to metabolize various nutrients. This is why doing a nutritional genetic test is so important.

In summary, here are the key nutrients you should focus on the most, because the odds of being deficient in any of them are the highest:

- Vitamin A
- Vitamin B_6
- Vitamin B_{12}
- Vitamin B_9
- Vitamin C
- Vitamin D
- Vitamin E
- Vitamin K

We're still learning what the optimal dose is for most nutrients. And there are significant differences between people. To help you figure out what you need, consider your:

- Age
- Lean body mass
- Metabolism
- Genetics
- Lifestyle
- Exercise

Dosage is important; however, it's not the most important thing. What matters is the amount of essential nutrients in your system and how well you are metabolizing them.

CHAPTER 28

FROM FOOD TO POOP

Optimizing the Five Stages of Digestion

This chapter teaches you how to take your digestive health to the next level, and the principles here are universal. It doesn't matter if you're vegan or carnivore; an optimized digestive system is crucial to your health. We give you the essential Power Moves for superhuman digestive health.

In this chapter, you'll learn:

- How to optimize all five stages of digestion daily, why each of them matter, and why breakdowns in any stage can lead to health disasters
- How fewer bowel movements than meals per day is a sign of suboptimal digestion
- Sixteen signs that poor digestion is derailing your goals and killing you slowly
- What the bizarre story of the "gray man" teaches us about the surprising truth behind stomach acid and heartburn
- How to know if your stomach acid levels are low or high with a simple, at-home test
- How to select the right enzymes for your diet
- Six ways to strengthen your gut barrier to keep pathogens and bad bacteria *out* while supporting your good gut bacteria for healthier digestion
- Whether poor digestion is slowly killing you
- Heartburn and acid reflux are caused by too much stomach acid, right? *Wrong!* Find out the real cause
- Remarkable lessons from Dr. Michael O'Brien and how we used them to completely transform our digestion
- Vital mitigation strategies for achieving BIOptimized digestion

THE MAN WHO CHANGED OUR DESTINY

In 2005, we were invited to a health practitioner seminar held by a remarkable doctor named Michael O'Brien. Dr. O'Brien had reportedly healed himself and hundreds of patients from a variety of serious conditions—including cirrhosis of the liver and cancer—using some unconventional protocols.

The doctor was using a specialized protocol of high-dose proteolytic enzymes, proteolytic probiotics, and live amino acids. Intrigued yet skeptical, we decided to investigate the doctor and his so-called miracle protocols for ourselves.

He certainly looked the part. He had phenomenal skin, clear eyes, and a strong handshake that felt like that of a 28-year-old. We had never met a man in his 70s who looked like him, and neither have we since. Not only did he look the part, he proceeded to do an intense 10-hour lecture without eating any food. His mind was sharp and his focus unwavering. We were in awe.

After the impactful lecture was done, we looked at each other and said, "Bro, we need to try this." So, we did.

We spent $1,500 a month and megadosed therapeutic amounts of enzymes, probiotics, and other superfoods to kickstart one of the most amazing transformations of our lives. In three months, Matt got into the best shape of his life. In six months, Wade had completely healed his digestive system and renewed his energy and vitality levels. Wade decided to compete again using these new protocols.

A Record-Breaking Comeback, by Wade T. Lightheart

After optimizing my body from the inside out, I returned to the competition. I shocked the people around me by winning a national championship with only five weeks of preparation and consuming 85 grams of protein a day. The best part is, I felt amazing during the entire contest preparation with no rebound effects after the competition. I avoided the post-show weight gain and bingeing I had experienced before.

Dr. Michael O'Brien's protocols were so powerful that they inspired us to create MassZymes, the strongest protein-digesting enzyme on the market. These tools were too impactful not to share with the world. We learned the hard way how digestion affects all aspects of health. Also, most people suffer unnecessarily due to poor digestion.

Our experience with high-dose proteolytic enzymes and probiotics was so powerful that we looked at each other and said, "We've got to produce our own, make it even better, and sell it." And a few months later, that's what we did with MassZymes, which has been the strongest proteolytic enzyme formula on the market since 2005.

IS POOR DIGESTION DERAILING YOUR GOALS AND KILLING YOU SLOWLY?

Processed foods, fast food, mega portions, fast-paced lives, and eating on the go are all digestive stressors. As a result, suboptimal digestion has become normalized. If you experience even a few of the following symptoms on a weekly basis, you have both suboptimal digestion and nutrification:

- Bloating and/or belching after meals
- Excessive farting
- Fewer bowel movements than the number of meals you have in a day
- Feeling full or having a heavy stomach after a meal
- Easily upset stomach
- Constipation
- Diarrhea
- Nausea and vomiting
- Heartburn and acid reflux
- Stomach cramps or pain
- Poorly formed stool
- Very stinky stools
- Fatigue or brain fog, especially after eating
- Difficulty losing or gaining weight
- Nutrient deficiencies despite a well-rounded diet and supplementation
- Inflammatory health conditions, such as skin problems, autoimmune diseases, allergies, and high cholesterol

If some of these apply to you, it is critical to restore optimal digestion. The good news is that we've cracked the code on optimizing every stage of digestion, which we cover in this chapter.

OPTIMIZING THE FIVE STAGES OF DIGESTION

The five stages of digestion are:

1. Preparation and anticipation
2. Secretion
3. Breakdown
4. Absorption
5. Elimination

Stage 1: Preparation and Anticipation

This is the sensory response stage where the touch, taste, smell, and other senses trigger your body's conditioned response.

Your brain is as much a part of your digestion as your gut is. Digestion starts with your mind. The smell of food makes you salivate and prepares your body for the nutrients to come.

Power Move: Rest and Digest

One of the most powerful upgrades you can make to achieve BIOptimized health is learning how to manage your nervous system. This is crucial when it comes to digestion; to optimize it, you need to be fully relaxed in "rest and digest" mode. When your body is stressed, your digestive health is compromised.

Therefore, to maximize your digestive potency, don't eat dinner while watching action movies and scary flicks. Instead, be present with loved ones. Relax and enjoy the bonding experience of eating together. Relax your mind and body as much as possible before eating.

Chewing helps your brain know what kind of food you're eating, and then your body begins producing the right types of enzymes to digest that food.

Chewing grinds your food, mixes it with saliva, and lubricates it. It binds food into a bolus so you can safely swallow it.[1] Saliva also contains white blood cells, antibodies, and lysozyme (a bacteria-digesting enzyme), which kill pathogens that could be in your food.[2]

Power Move: 30 to 50 Mindful Chews

Mindful eating can aid in weight loss. Studies confirm some positive effects of mindful eating:

- Reduced food cravings[3,4]
- Eating less (portion control)[5]
- Making healthier food choices[6]
- Being able to recognize your body's hunger and satiety signs[7]

More chews = more weight loss? Yes, that's what the research indicates.[8] Research has shown that increasing chews and slowing down the meal reduced food intake by up to 14.8 percent.[9]

More chews help to create more mindful eating.

Two of the possible explanations are:

- Slowing down the meal allows the fullness signal to appear before the meal is done. Satiety signals take about 20 minutes to appear after your first bite.
- According to Japanese researchers, eating slower could help burn more calories (up to 2,000 extra calories per month, which could equal about seven pounds of fat per year).[10]

Stage 2: Secretion

In this stage, your digestive system secretes hydrochloric acid (HCl, aka stomach acid), enzymes, and bile to break down the food you just ate.

The Bizarre Story of the Gray Man and the Surprising Truth about Stomach Acid and Heartburn

Most people believe that heartburn and acid reflux–related issues are caused by too much acid. It's the opposite. Heartburn is caused by too little stomach acid.

Dr. Jonathan Wright, a holistic health practitioner from Lake Tahoe, has helped thousands of patients get relief from heartburn.[11] One client was a Caucasian man so devoid of pink hues in his skin that he looked gray. They called him the "gray man." The gray man's previous doctors had told him that he was producing too much stomach acid and gave him medications to lower it. His symptoms got worse, and he became grayer.

More than 90 percent of Dr. Wright's heartburn patients were never previously tested for stomach acid levels, had been misdiagnosed by their doctors, and were wrongfully prescribed proton pump inhibitors (PPIs) and antacids.

Without the proper test, patients suffering from heartburn are often assumed to have too much stomach acid and are wrongfully prescribed potentially dangerous drugs. Shocking fact alert: it's estimated that 20 percent of people's medical problems are misdiagnosed.[12]

The scientific literature says that heartburn and gastroesophageal reflux disease (GERD, aka acid reflux) are not considered to be diseases of excess stomach acid.

The Five-Minute Stomach Acid Home Test

You can determine if you need more HCl with a simple bicarb test at home.

Mix ¼ teaspoon of bicarbonate of soda (baking soda) in water (about 6 ounces) and drink on an empty stomach first thing in the morning, before eating or drinking. If you have sufficient levels of stomach acid, the bicarbonate will be converted into carbon dioxide gas, which should cause belching within two to three minutes. If you have not belched within five minutes, stop timing.

Early and repeated belches might be due to excessive stomach acid, but they also could be due to swallowing air when drinking the solution (this tends to show up as smaller belches). If "normal" belching doesn't occur until after three minutes, stomach acid is low.

To recap:

Low stomach acid → no belching

Sufficient stomach acid → belching

Experts now know that acid reflux is caused by excess gas forcing the lower esophageal valve (LES) to open and allow acid to flow up to your throat. Your esophageal valve is like a water dam. When you have too much gas inside your body, it opens the dam and forces acid up, causing heartburn pain and discomfort in your chest. That's when you taste that bitter stomach bile. The problem is the gas, not the acid, and insufficient acid is what creates excess gas.

Research has proven that low stomach acid leads to both poor digestion and reduced gut movement. Both of these lead to bacterial overgrowth, which can cause an overload of gas, especially when you eat carbohydrates or fermentable fibers.

Bad bacteria starts to party and feast when you eat the wrong foods for your body. This is another benefit to optimizing your food selection based on your gut biome, nutrigenomics, and other optimizers.

The point is that if you eat the wrong foods for your body and you don't have enough stomach acid, the result is intense fermentation . . . and too much gas.

The excess gas problem explains why PPIs and antacids often amplify acid reflux. By suppressing stomach acid with a PPI, the carb digestion can become worse. This increases bad bacteria and fermentation even more.

To wean the gray man off acid-blocking medication, Dr. Wright recommended three supplements: digestive enzymes, probiotics, and betaine hydrochloride. The enzymes were to help break down the food in his stomach (because with age, we naturally lose our ability to produce enough enzymes). The probiotics were to fight off the bad bacteria in his stomach and intestines and optimize food breakdown (see Stage 4).

The betaine HCl was the most important of all three supplements. It helped restore the gray man's stomach acid levels back to normal for a healthy, functioning stomach.

Power Move: Consume HCL Breakthrough with Each Meal

If you're in your 30s or older, it might be time to consider adding HCl to your digestive stack. Adding one or two capsules of HCL Breakthrough to each meal can make a night-and-day difference to your digestion.

It stacks wonderfully with enzymes and probiotics to create the ultimate digestive power.

Go to www.BIOptimizers.com/book/HCL and give HCL Breakthrough a shot.

Secretion #1: HCl (aka Stomach Acid)

After you swallow, food arrives in the stomach through a muscular ring (which opens and closes to keep acid from coming up into your esophagus).

Food in the stomach triggers the release of gastrin, a hormone that activates gastric acid secretion. After 30 minutes, your stomach releases hydrochloric acid, which activates stomach enzymes. These enzymes begin the nutrient breakdown. (We go into greater depth in Stage 3.)

The hydrochloric acid in your stomach plays many important roles, including:[13]

- Causing the muscular ring between the esophagus and stomach to close, preventing acid reflux
- Preventing infections by killing most pathological microorganisms and parasites
- Activating enzymes including pepsin, a key digester of protein in the stomach
- Partially breaking down foods, which helps maximize the effects of the enzymes
- Freeing up minerals such as calcium, magnesium, and iron into absorbable forms
- Freeing up vitamin B_{12} to mix with intrinsic factors to be absorbed in the large intestine
- When the food travels from the stomach to the small intestine, the acidity triggers gut movement, digestive juice secretion, and further stages of digestion

Low stomach acid creates an unhealthy ripple effect throughout the body, including reduced appetite, gut infections, and deficiencies in minerals, protein, and vitamin B_{12}.

These happen more frequently in the elderly, those under a lot of stress, and those with weak vagus nerves. Small-intestine bacterial overgrowth may also occur due to reduced peristalsis, resulting in gas, bloating, and potentially diarrhea or constipation.

Secretion #2: Bile and Your Health

The second digestive substance your body secretes is bile, which is critical for breaking down fats. It also helps us absorb fat-soluble vitamins like A, D, E, and K.

Bile is produced by the liver and concentrates in the gallbladder until it's needed to help digest food. When food enters the small intestine, bile travels through the common bile duct to reach the duodenum. The acidity of food that comes from your stomach triggers a healthy bile release, so taking betaine HCl also promotes healthy bile flow.

Also, your gut bacteria convert bile salts into metabolites for their own use. Some of these have health benefits, while others are toxic.[14, 15] Therefore, poor bile flow can lead to hormone imbalances, high cholesterol, and dysbiosis in addition to possible gallstones.

One of the natural herbs you can take to stimulate bile production is dandelion root, which is why we've included it in kApex, one of our digestive solutions.

Secretion #3: Enzymes

The next vital molecules your body needs for great digestion are its hardest workers: enzymes. Digestive enzymes are mostly produced in the pancreas, stomach, and small intestine.

Enzymes break down fats into fatty acids, proteins into amino acids, and carbohydrates into glycogen. This leads us to the next stage of digestion.

Stage 3: Breakdown

Digestive breakdown is when we deconstruct food into its basic elements and enzymes do their magic. According to Dr. Edward Howell, your enzymes determine how quickly, or how well, you're able to break down and absorb the nutrients you're consuming.

Nowadays, we eat a lot of cooked, processed, chemical-laden, and genetically modified foods. These interventions disrupt the natural digestive process by killing the enzymes naturally found in food. All other animal species eat their food in a live and raw state, with the bacteria and enzymes present in it.

Also, our enzyme reserves get lower and lower with age. We absorb fewer and fewer nutrients, leaving more undigested food for our gut bacteria, and this leads to other problems. It's a vicious cycle.

Therefore, we believe that using the right enzyme formulas has a massive impact on your digestive health and body overall.

Power Move: Take Enzymes with Every Meal

We always suggest taking three to five capsules of enzymes with every meal. Usually, one capsule per 200 calories is optimal.

- For high-protein meals, we suggest using MassZymes
- For high-fat meals, we suggest using kApex
- For high-plant meals, we suggest using VegZymes
- For refeed meals with gluten or dairy, we suggest using Gluten Guardian

How to Select the Right Enzymes for You

For high-protein diets, focus on full-spectrum proteases.

Protein is the king macro. It's vital for building and maintaining lean mass. It also increases satiety and requires more energy to digest and use, so most weight loss diets are high in protein. (See Chapter 25 for more insights on macros.) Protein can also be hard to break down for many people, meaning virtually everyone can optimize their protein breakdown.

However, high-protein diets can come with tradeoffs:

- High protein intake correlates with reduced life span, especially in middle-aged people[16]
- Protein tends to be expensive, and if you can't digest and absorb protein properly, you end up wasting money
- Incompletely digested proteins can lead to food allergies or food sensitivities, causing chronic inflammation[17, 18]
- Your gut bacteria ferment undigested proteins and unassimilated amino acids into unhealthy metabolites such as hydrogen sulfides, ammonia, and phenol.[19] These gases stink and may even cause colon cancers and ulcerative colitis.[20]

The key to get the most value from your protein is proteolytic enzymes, which break protein down into usable, absorbable amino acids.

Your food goes through a full range of pH in your gut, because different amino acids are assimilated at different pH levels. Therefore, it's important to find a proteolytic enzyme blend that's active across the pH range. That's why MassZymes contains not just one protease, but multiple proteases that work at various pH levels so you get maximum assimilation of amino acids.

If your digestive enzyme blend contains insufficient protease or only works within a narrow range of pH, you won't get the protein digestion you need. Most enzyme formulations are low on protease simply because it's very expensive to produce.

We suggest taking three to five capsules of a high-protease enzyme formulation with every meal to maximize your amino acid absorption, especially when you eat flesh protein such as fish or meat.

A Key to Living Longer?

Not only will proteolytic enzymes enhance your digestive powers, but we believe that taking them in high doses (especially on an empty stomach) can potentially extend life span. Here's our theory.

Kris Verburgh, in his book *The Longevity Code,* shares some mind-blowing data showing that the cause of death of supercentenarians (people who live to over 110) is often a disease we call amyloidosis. Some believe it accounts for at least 70 percent of supercentenarian deaths. Amyloidosis is the accumulation of protein everywhere in the body.[21]

You can potentially minimize amyloidosis and avoid some of its negative consequences by using proteolytic enzymes to maximize your protein digestion. More research will have to be done to prove or disprove this theory.

Plant-Based Diets

The challenge with plant-based diets can be digesting cellulose. The solution is pectinase, cellulase, and hemi-cellulase.

You also want an enzymatic formulation that is stable and plant-based. A lot of companies use animal-based enzymes because they're less expensive. We've found that they don't work nearly as well as plant-based enzymes, because they're less consistent in strength and function.

If you're consuming a lot of fruits and plants, we suggest using VegZymes, which is specifically designed to help break down cellulose (the cell walls of plants). Visit www.BIOptimizers.com to learn more.

Many people don't have enough enzymes to digest sugars and polysaccharides, so they get gas and bloating from foods that contain them. Plant-based enzymes are better at breaking these down so they don't cause gas and bloating. That's why MassZymes also contains a full spectrum of plant-based enzymes that break down sugars, polysaccharides, and fibers.

Gluten from wheat and casein from A1 dairy are highly allergenic proteins because they have chemical structures that are difficult to digest[22, 23] (see Chapter 31). A special fungal enzyme called dipeptidyl peptidase IV (DPP IV) can help break these down and prevent them from causing problems (although they don't make gluten safe for people with celiac disease). Gluten Guardian contains DPP IV and other enzymes to help with high-carbohydrate meals. In our lab tests, Gluten Guardian has also been shown to be the most effective formula for dairy proteins (casein).

For people first trying a ketogenic diet, the high-fat content of meals can cause digestive problems. kApex contains a lot of lipase to help you digest fat, along with dandelion root to stimulate bile flow. Check out www.BIOptimizers.com/book/kapex.

Stage 4: Absorption

Throughout your small and large intestine, the nutrients get absorbed through your gut barrier.

To increase the surface area for nutrient absorption, your small intestine has tissue folds, along with villi and microvilli. A healthy gut's small intestine has the surface area of a tennis court to absorb nutrients.

Sugars, amino acids, and peptides get absorbed through the gut lining into the bloodstream. On the other hand, fatty acids get packaged into chylomicrons and absorbed into the lymphatic system. Both the bloodstream and lymphatic flow from the intestine get screened by the liver before circulating throughout the body.

Your gut barrier is only one cell layer thick. It interfaces between the content inside the gut and your gut's immune system. A healthy gut barrier is permeable enough to absorb nutrients but is impermeable to pathogens and potential food allergens.

Some nutrient absorption requires energy (adenosine triphosphate, or ATP), so gut lining cells need to be able to generate ATP well. They are fueled mostly by the amino acid glutamine and small fatty acids, such as acetate, propionate, and butyrate (these are short-chain fatty acids, or SCFAs). Butyrate gives vomit its characteristic smell.

Inflammatory foods, stress, and infections can create an unhealthy gut that allows pathogens and food allergens through and does a poor job at absorbing nutrients. For example, celiac disease damages the villi, causes leaky gut, and leads to nutrient deficiencies. Inflammation also reduces ATP production.

Six Ways to Strengthen Your Gut Barrier

1. Eliminate inflammatory foods (see Chapter 31)
2. Work with a practitioner to ensure that you don't have gut infections or dysbiosis (Para Guardian and Biome Breakthrough can also help with these)
3. Ensure that your stomach acid and digestive enzyme levels are optimal at Stages 1 through 3
4. Take probiotics, prebiotics, and synbiotics (a mixture of prebiotics and probiotics)
5. Eat fermented foods
6. Use healthy biofilm builders like Biome Breakthrough to build a healthier intestinal tract

Go to www.BIOptimizers.com/book/biome to learn more.

Probiotics can help balance the immune response in the gut, which typically reduces inflammation. When you feed them with prebiotics or dietary fibers, they can ferment the prebiotics into SCFAs. SCFAs strengthen the gut barrier and help it heal from stress and inflammation. SCFAs also help prevent other infections and increase ATP in the gut lining.[24]

Some probiotic strains also have antimicrobial activities. They can eliminate bad bacteria, yeast, and viruses. See Chapter 9 to learn about the gut microbiome and different probiotic strains for your goals.

Stage 5: Elimination

After all that hard work, it's time to ship out the waste to the great sewer in the ground.

Whatever's left at this point enters the colon. Most of the water will be reabsorbed by the body. This is one of the reasons why consuming enough water, along with fiber-rich foods, can help digestion. Importantly, your colon is home to trillions of bacteria cells that make up most of your gut microbiome.

Probiotics continue to play a role in the colon, continuing the fermentation process. Also, SCFAs increase water and mineral absorption through the colon wall. Peristaltic movements continue to help move the semisolid waste through the colon.

At this stage, your rectum expands in response to the storage of fecal matter. Using peristaltic movements of the rectum, waste is ultimately eliminated through the anus, completing the digestive process.

The success of this process often has a lot to do with the stages before it. Otherwise, without adequate enzymes, hydrochloric acid, and digestion-enhancing probiotics, undigested food will make it to the colon.

World-renowned wellness and exercise physiology expert Paul Chek says that the shape of your poop is one of the best indicators of your health. Refer to the Bristol stool chart in Chapter 32. If your score is lower than three or more than four, you've got to work on your digestive health.

The following diet and lifestyle choices could be keeping your digestion suboptimal unless you actively implement mitigation strategies:

- Sitting and inactivity
- Stress
- Exposure to antibacterial chemicals in household products and antibiotic residues in food
- Eating late at night
- Inflammatory diets
- Lack of fiber and phytonutrients
- Eating too fast and while stressed
- Coffee, tea, and soda

OPTIMIZING ELIMINATION

Power Move: Use a Squatty Potty for Optimal Positioning

In 2010, Japanese researchers found that by optimizing your feet and body position, you could improve your bowel movements. The Squatty Potty does increase the rectal canal angle from 100 degrees to 120 degrees.

Thirty-three people took part in a 2017 research that confirmed similar results. Pedestal toilet bowel motions, when the user is seated on the toilet, took an average of 113.5 seconds, according to research. Using a footstool, however, reduced the average time to 55.5 seconds. Except for one person, everyone said it was easier to squat. [25]

SUMMARY

The five stages of digestion are:

Stage 1: Preparation and Anticipation

- Make sure you're in a relaxed state when you start eating
- Digestion starts with your mind; your brain is as much a part of your digestion as your gut is. The smell of food makes you salivate and prepares your body for the nutrients to come.
- Be mindful, chew slowly, and enjoy your food

Stage 2: Secretion

- Secretion #1: HCl (aka stomach acid)
- Secretion #2: Bile
- Secretion #3: Enzymes
- Use HCl, enzyme, and proteolytic supplements to maximize the value of every meal

Stage 3: Breakdown

- Next, you break down food into its basic elements as enzymes do their magic. Your enzyme pool determines how well you break down and absorb nutrients

Stage 4: Absorption

- Nutrients get absorbed through your gut barrier throughout the small and large intestine

Stage 5: Elimination

- After all that hard work, it's time to release waste

CHAPTER 29

BIOPTIMIZING YOUR GUT BIOME

by Matt Gallant, Monia Avdić, and Wade T. Lightheart

Regardless of which diet you choose, optimizing your gut health will make you healthier. We're excited to share the latest discoveries in probiotics. We co-wrote this chapter with our head of research and development, Monia Avdić.

In this chapter, you'll learn:

- Why your gut bacteria are a critical factor in your overall health, aesthetics, performance, and happiness
- The latest science behind improving your gut bacteria (it goes beyond probiotics)
- How to break the vicious cycle of dysbiosis and finally BIOptimize your microbiome
- How to choose the most powerful specific probiotic strains for digestion, cognitive function, and fat loss
- Why microbiome tests are not created equal and what you should do with them
- How you can have more bacteria in your body than cells
- What dysbiosis is and how it affects your health
- The amount of power your gut bacteria has over your diet and food cravings
- Critical signs that you may have gut dysbiosis and how to mitigate it
- The role probiotics play in your gut health
- About various microbiome tests you can take and the benefits of testing
- The difference between micro and microbiome

YOU'RE MORE BACTERIA THAN HUMAN

For the first half of geological time, the world was inhabited only by bacteria, and these bacteria exist still today. They are very plastic. They can evolve, they can adapt, and they're all around us. Most of us is still bacteria.

— Monia Avdić, Ph.D., microbiology/genetics and bioengineering

When the Human Genome Project was underway in the early 2000s, scientists overestimated the number of human genes by up to fivefold. After all, we're a lot more complex than roundworms, which have about 20,000 genes, right?[1]

To their surprise, once the genome project was complete, our gene numbers were also in the 20,000s.[2] It turns out that humans have a "back pocket" of genes (pun intended) called our microbiome.

> **Microbiota** = The composition of *microorganisms* in an ecosystem, including bacteria, fungi, and viruses
>
> **Microbiome** = The composition of *genes* of all the microorganisms in an ecosystem, which is more reflective of your gut microbes' collective metabolic capacity

According to the latest estimate, you have about 30 percent more bacterial cells than your own cells.[3] Your gut bacteria possess over a million genes.[4]

In your skin, your nose, your gut, you're filled with bacteria. And we can literally see that we are 10 percent human and 90 percent bacteria. The bacteria that inhabit us inside and outside are the key to sustaining our health. And you can see in the newspaper from Good Health, that it's thanks to 100 trillion bacteria that are in us, on us, and around us.

— Monia Avdić, Ph.D., microbiology/genetics and bioengineering

The bacteria in your gut, mouth, skin, nostrils, and even genitals form the interconnected micro ecosystems that give you a dynamic, ever-changing gene pool, which allows you and your bacteria to adapt to your diet and environment.

While the latest research has barely scratched the surface of what your microbiome can do, we know for sure that:

- Dysbiosis leads to poor health and reduced resilience[5]
- The gut biome works almost like a separate organ that interacts with your gut and your brain[6]
- Your gut bacteria can control your cravings and food preferences[7]
- Humans don't have all the enzymes to digest our foods. Your collection of gut bacteria is your digestive powerhouse[8]
- Your supplements and medications work with your gut bacteria, and the microbiome controls how effective your drugs and supplements are[9]

A BEAUTIFUL SYMBIOSIS

In your gut, you have huge biofilms where the bacteria inside are acting as one, and you can affect it by the food that you're taking, by the supplements you're taking, because what you're actually inserting are signals. The chemical language of bacteria. We have to be really careful in how to use them to enhance the bacteria that we have. This is scientifically known as quorum sensing. They talk to one another with this chemical language. They produce a signal and they have a receptor for the signal where it turns on group behavior genes.

— Monia Avdić, Ph.D., microbiology/genetics and bioengineering

Bacteria and humans have been evolving together for eons. When you acquire and feed the right probiotics, the benefits for you are massive: better immunity, better digestion, more enzymes, more vitamins, protection against destructive pathogens, and much more. Just like with people, the key is building a healthy relationship with the *right* ones. However, the opposite is true also: if you have a relationship with the "bad guys," your health will be compromised.

There's no question that you must optimize your gut microbiome to expand all three sides of the BIOptimization Triangle: health, performance, and aesthetics. But remember that it takes two to tango; you have a two-way relationship with your gut bacteria. Every bite you eat, every thought you think, and every action you take changes your microbiome.

Fortunately, thanks to the latest research and this book, you can now take charge of this relationship.

This chapter is divided into four sections:

- Part 1: Hippocrates' Profound Wisdom
- Part 2: What's a Healthy Gut?
- Part 3: How to BIOptimize Your Gut Biome
- Part 4: The Biological Optimization Process (Assess, Test, Optimize) for Improving Your Gut Health

PART 1: HIPPOCRATES' PROFOUND WISDOM

Hippocrates, the ancient Greek physician, said 2,500 years ago, "All disease begins in the gut." He was certainly downloading some deep codes from the universe when he realized this, because he was pretty accurate.

Do You Have Gut Dysbiosis?

If you have suboptimal health or a disease state, you have dysbiosis. Here are a few common symptoms of gut dysbiosis:

- Brain fog and a lack of mental clarity and focus
- Bloating and gas
- Indigestion
- Food intolerances and sensitivities
- Allergies
- Chronic inflammation
- Cravings and excessive hunger
- Poor sleep
- Anxiety and depression
- Fatigue and sluggishness
- Chronic pain
- Lack of motivation

What Is Dysbiosis?

Dysbiosis is when you have imbalanced gut bacteria. There are a few ways this can happen:[10]

- Pathogenic bacteria take over and start to promote a disease state
- Loss of health-protective bacteria
- Increase in bacteria that degrade the mucus that protects your gut lining, which may inflame the gut lining and cause leaky gut[11]
- A combination of the above

It's unclear whether dysbiosis is the consequence, the cause, or both for changes in your gut lining and overall health. You've heard the expression, "Which came first, the chicken or the egg?" A healthy gut microbiome is like this.

If you take care of your health and follow other lessons in this book, your microbiome improves. Yet you must also proactively work on your gut microbiome to optimize your health. This means disrupting the vicious cycle of dysbiosis (more on this later in the chapter).

How Dysbiosis Can Cause Weight Gain

An unhealthy state due to bacterial toxins in the blood can cause obesity, along with many other ailments.[12] In this state, there's enough toxin in the blood to cause chronic low-grade inflammation, but not enough to cause sepsis (a life-threatening inflammatory shock).

Metabolic endotoxemia can cause leptin resistance, which makes people lethargic and perpetually hungry, setting them up for weight gain.[13]

Probiotics, prebiotics, and other interventions that support the microbiome and repair the gut can reverse metabolic endotoxemia.[14] Low gut microbial richness correlates with body fat, insulin resistance, and inflammation.[15] However, once you fix your gut microbiome, you'd still need to create a caloric deficit to achieve your weight loss goals.

A strong driver of cravings is neurochemical deficiencies. Neurotransmitters like serotonin are almost exclusively manufactured in the gut by your bacteria. Serotonin is responsible for a feeling of stability, and when we eat sugar, we get a quick boost in serotonin. Many people use sugary foods as a way to give them fast serotonin jolts.

Dopamine is another key neurochemical that certain probiotics produce. When people are low in dopamine, they find other ways of boosting it, including watching violent, intense shows; attending sporting events; or bingeing. Eating hyper-palatable food jacks up your dopamine levels, especially if it's something you've been anticipating.

One of our core goals at BIOptimizers is to create a superhuman gut biome. That's why we decided to create a BioLab with the University of Burch in Sarajevo, Bosnia and Herzegovina, where we employ a team of Ph.D.s in microbiome, chemistry, and biology studies. They conduct research to see which probiotics can help address neurotransmitter deficiencies that lead to bingeing, yo-yo dieting, leaky gut, and other conditions that compromise the immune system. One of our formulas, Cognibiotics, focuses on that. In our lab tests, it was the most powerful dopamine-producing probiotic blend we've ever tested.

The mood-elevating effects of the products we develop are very helpful for people who are prone to low mood, yo-yo dieting, and sudden changes in weight.

This story from Krista, one of Wade's clients, perfectly illustrates the power of optimizing one's gut microbiome:

> After three years as a bikini competitor, having earned two championship titles, I hit rock bottom when my sister passed away in a car accident.
>
> On the outside, I had never looked better; yet on the inside, I was really sick. The stress from competition preps and trauma had thrown my body off balance.
>
> Prior to all of that, I'd had 10 years of a chronic yeast infection that just wouldn't go away. It turned out to be systemic candida overgrowth. I also suffered from chronic allergies, frequent hives, depression, and hypoglycemia. Doctors couldn't help me and only recommended Canesten [a topical antifungal].
>
> I tried every brand of probiotics at Whole Foods, sometimes eating a whole bottle at a time. None of them made any difference.
>
> Then, I met Wade T. Lightheart, who introduced me to the BIOptimizers' probiotics. I started making coconut yogurt with P3-OM, which immediately cured my yeast infection.
>
> It started my journey with natural health and gut healing. Over the next 12 months, I healed my gut with MassZymes and P3-OM, and after clearing other infections and leaky gut, removing mercury amalgam, and a detox protocol, I'm now healthier than ever.

Krista's story goes to show that just because someone looks incredibly fit and beautiful, it does *not* mean they are healthy on the inside.

Obesity Is Transmissible via the Gut Microbiome?

A study in *Science* magazine examined the microbiomes of one identical and three fraternal twin pairs who had discordant obesity phenotypes. Despite being genetically very similar or identical, one of each pair was lean, whereas the other was obese. When their fecal matters were transplanted into mice, the recipient mice adopted the obesity or lean phenotype of the fecal donors.

Interestingly, when the newly transplanted mice were housed together and shared food, the mice with the obese fecal transplant did not develop obesity. They found that this is because some Bacteroidetes bacteria species from the lean fecal transplant recipients invaded the microbiome of the obese fecal transplant recipients.[16]

In agreement with the twin study, most microbiome-profiling studies have shown that the Firmicutes bacterium correlates with obesity. However, a few studies also showed no significant correlation, or even inverse correlation.[17] The conundrum suggests that Firmicutes could be both a contributor and a symptom of weight gain.

Weight loss also reduces the ratio of Firmicutes to Bacteroidetes, whether it's from a diet or gastric bypass.[18]

In a clinical study that precisely measured calorie intake and stool calories, lean subjects overeating about 3,400 calories per day had more Firmicutes compared to when they ate 2,400 calories. Also, the 20 percent increase in Firmicutes was associated with an extra 150 calories in energy harvest. However, the stool of lean individuals contained significantly more energy when they consumed 3,400 calories, while the stool of obese individuals contained the same number of calories whether they ate 3,400 or 2,400.[19]

Western-style diets, which are high in meat, fat, and sugar, increase Firmicutes at the expense of Bacteroidetes in both humans and mice.[20] On the other hand, a plant-based, low-fat diet has the opposite effect on the microbiome.

Time-restricted feeding increases the bile acid metabolites that promote the lean microbiome, even when caloric intake hasn't changed. Also, around-the-clock eating can throw off the microbiome because the microbiome also has its own circadian rhythm.[21]

Stress, Relationships, and Circadian Rhythm Affect Your Gut Bacteria

A study examined Lactobacillus levels in the stool, along with subjective stress and cortisol levels. They found that the longer participants were exposed to exam stress, the less Lactobacilli they had.[22]

The quality of your relationships shapes your microbiota, according to a study published in *Nature Scientific Reports*. It looked at the microbiota of 94 couples and 83 sibling pairs and found that spouses had more similar microbiomes, even when their shared diet was accounted for. Married individuals had better bacteria diversity and richness than those living alone. Also, couples who reported having close relationships had the greatest gut bacteria diversity.[23]

A chimpanzee study published in *Science* magazine found that frequent social interactions among the chimps created more microbial diversity and richness.[24]

The gut microbiota has day/night rhythms that respond to our fasting and feeding cycles. Therefore, circadian rhythm and sleep disruptions can change gut bacteria.[25] For example, healthy young men with 4.25 hours of sleep for two nights have increased Firmicutes relative to Bacteroidetes, among other changes.[26] In mice, sleep deprivation increases bacteria strains that feed on undigested foods.[27] These bacteria changes may be one factor in why sleep deprivation and thrown-off circadian rhythm can cause weight gain.

Firmicutes and Bacteroidetes are phyla (groups) of bacteria that together make up ~97 percent of your gut biome. Neither group is inherently bad by default.

Firmicutes are mostly gram-positive and spore-forming bacteria. These are associated with weight gain.

Bacteroidetes are mostly gram-negative, non-spore forming, rod-shaped bacteria. These are associated with leanness.

An Inflamed Gut Lining Causes Dysbiosis

Friendly bacteria, such as Lactobacilli and Bifidobacteria, are anaerobic. They are more comfortable with no oxygen around. The bad bacteria, such as Streptococci, tend to like oxygen.

Healthy gut linings have well-functioning mitochondria, which use up all the oxygen and create a zero-oxygen environment for friendly bacteria. On the other hand, unhealthy gut cells have poorly functioning mitochondria, leaving oxygen available for bad bacteria.[28] While dysbiosis causes inflammation, gut inflammation also allows dysbiosis and makes your gut less hospitable to friendly bacteria.[29]

How Gut Dysbiosis Impacts Your Mind

In order for you to be happy, in order for you to function optimally, you have to get good bacteria in your stomach. The gut-brain connection is amazing. The bacteria actually produce neurotransmitters that make your brain function. This is very important for different disorders and different diseases. For autistic spectrum disorder, the side effects can be lowered by applying the right probiotics. On the other hand, if you're a human with no disorders, you can enhance your health. You can get rid of brain fog and other ailments.

— Monia Avdić, Ph.D., microbiology/genetics and bioengineering

Depression Is Transmissible via Stool Microbiome

Depression patients have major changes in their gut biome compared to people without depression. When fecal bacteria from unmedicated depression patients were transplanted into mice without gut bacteria, they developed more depression-like behaviors.[30]

Transplanted Microbiome Can Change Your Personality

When a shy strain of mice was treated with antibiotics, they became more exploratory and had more brain-derived neurotrophic factor (BDNF) in the brain. Also, taking the gut microbiota from a more outgoing strain and transplanting it into the shy mice caused the mice to become more outgoing, and vice versa.[31]

Dysbiosis and Yeast Overgrowth Can Worsen Anxiety and Depression

Scientists still don't fully understand what causes mood disorders, which is why there isn't a lab test for any psychiatric condition. The microbiome is definitely one piece of the puzzle.

Mood disorders are associated with dysbiosis and digestive problems. The bad bacteria and yeast overgrowth increase inflammation by causing leaky gut and increasing blood bacterial toxins.[32]

In caveman times, inflammation meant you were healing from an infection, so it was best for you to rest and stay away from your group. Scientists call this "sickness behavior," which is when inflammation causes fatigue, malaise, withdrawal, reduction in appetite, and unhealthy sleep patterns.[33] It's one of the most likely explanations of depression.

Inflammation stimulates the stress response, which is typically overstimulated in mood disorders.[34] It also increases the production of neurotoxic tryptophan metabolites, which induce serotonin and melatonin deficiency, which in turn can cause anxiety and depression.[35, 36]

Fortunately, we now know how to fix the abnormal gut-brain axis. In mice, probiotics have been shown to relieve this sickness behavior.[37]

PART 2: WHAT CREATES A HEALTHY GUT BIOME?

Scientists are still working to completely understand what makes a healthy (or unhealthy) microbiota.

It seems that the more diverse your gut microbiota is, the better. The diversity and richness make the microbiota more resilient to invasion, bad bacteria overgrowth, antimicrobials, and antibiotics.[38] It also allows you to adapt to changes in your diet, lifestyle, and environment.

Gut bacteria diversity has been associated with health and happiness. You want your gut to resemble the Amazon's lush jungle, not a barren desert.

Richness = total number of bacterial species in your gut microbiota
Diversity = the number of individual bacteria from each species that is present in your gut biome
Postbiotics = substances produced by your gut bacteria when they consume or ferment the food or prebiotics that you eat

A healthy microbiome should also have healthy metabolic capacity and flexibility. It can produce more beneficial postbiotics and less harmful ones.

How Your Gut Microbes Mastermind Your Metabolism and Cravings

A scientific principle that I always return to is "everything depends on everything." And this is what happens when you come to the molecular realm. When you study these tiny microorganisms, the conclusion that you get is, you wouldn't be able to digest your food the way that you digest it, if you didn't have the microbes in your gut. They're the key to enhancing your ability to digest food, to drain the marrow out of the building blocks that you get when you break the chemical bonds of molecules of food. They allow you to get so much out of food and to enhance your body. If you take the right substances, you will enhance their properties even more.

— Monia Avdić, Ph.D., microbiology/genetics and bioengineering

Your gut microbes help you digest food, and then they get to eat whatever is left from the first few stages of digestion. Importantly, they extract calories from your foods and influence your nutrification.[39] Studies have confirmed that a disrupted microbiome is partly to blame for obesity and any modern chronic diseases.

Your Cravings Are Your Gut Bacteria's Cry for Their Favorite Foods?

We've come to believe that a lot of food cravings and bingeing are driven by the bacteria in our bodies. We believe that they send signals to our brains to feed them.

Every time we switch diets, we've noticed food cravings for the things we used to eat, but they stop. For Matt, a craving lasts about a week. Your body starts craving the new things you're eating. Wade notices that when his clients switch to a new diet, they may experience about two or three weeks of appetite changes in their bodies.

Back in the day when Wade and Matt used to argue about which was the best diet, Matt decided to follow Wade's advice. Wade brought Matt to the best salad bar in downtown Vancouver. Matt has always been a keto-carnivore guy and not so much a salad person. He didn't like it at first, but after about six days, he became excited for huge salads and started craving them. He was shocked at the shift.

Eating the foods that you have fewer bacteria to digest can eventually create a preference for the food. For example, the gut bacteria in Japanese people who regularly eat seaweed adopt the genes for the enzymes that digest the seaweed's carbohydrates.[40, 41]

We believe most of the symptoms that occur when we change diets are due to such microbiome changeovers. Some bacteria prefer fats because they do better with more bile, while others prefer sugars or fermentable carbohydrates. When you go from a high-carb, low-fat diet to a low-carb one, you starve your carb-eating bacteria—and they will make you crave carbs before dying off.

All of these hypotheses have a lot of circumstantial evidence, but we can't say they've been proven.[42] However, scientists have found that your gut bacteria can influence your behavior and mood, including ones that cause you to reach for ice cream and cookies.[43] The bacteria can also cause pain or manipulate your neurotransmitters when certain nutrients are missing.[44]

Your Gut Microbiome Is Its Own Ever-Evolving Organ

The gut microbiome is like a distinct organ that adjusts to your diet, lifestyle, and even health status. All of these factors decide if you have a healthy microbiome—or dysbiosis. Every meal impacts your gut biome.

Your Microbiome Adapts to Your Diet Overnight

A 2013 study published in *Nature* found that people fed with animal-based diets have distinctive microbiome patterns compared to those with plant-based diets. The gene activities in these microbiomes are similar to those of carnivorous and herbivorous mammals, respectively. Also, when people on one of these diets switched to the other, their gut microbiome adopted the diet's respective patterns within 24 to 48 hours.[45]

That's great news, because it means you can make radical improvements quickly. Your microbiome is constantly changing—in fact, it does this with *every meal*. When you feed certain strains, they proliferate. When you starve certain strains, they begin to die within 48 hours.

What Do Probiotics Do?

We're approaching an era that's called the post-antibiotic era, where we're thinking we are losing all the antibiotics. They're all becoming resistant. This is the era where antibiotics don't have an effect. This means that we're approaching an era where we will not have any more antibiotics to fight the pathogens with. So what's the solution? Well, in my opinion, the solution is fighting the pathogens with live organisms, with probiotics.

— Monia Avdić, Ph.D., microbiology/genetics and bioengineering

Your healthy gut bacteria and probiotics support your health by:[46, 47]

- Strengthening your gut barrier by secreting postbiotics, stimulating protective mucus, or preventing pathogenic bacteria from adhering to the mucus layer
- Competing with pathogenic bacteria for space and resources. The probiotic strains that can pitch a biofilm "tent" to adhere to your gut are more capable of this.
- Producing antimicrobial substances to inhibit the growth of bad bacteria, which can sometimes initiate a shift in the microbiome without themselves making your gut a permanent home
- Balancing the immune system so it can fight off pathogens, but not so overactively that it leads to allergic or autoimmune diseases
- Producing enzymes to digest food and food substances we can't digest
- Metabolizing (activating or degrading) supplements, drugs, hormones, nutrients, and neurotransmitters
- Communicating with your brain through neurotransmitter metabolites and the vagus nerve
- Producing and activating vitamins, such as vitamin K and some B vitamins

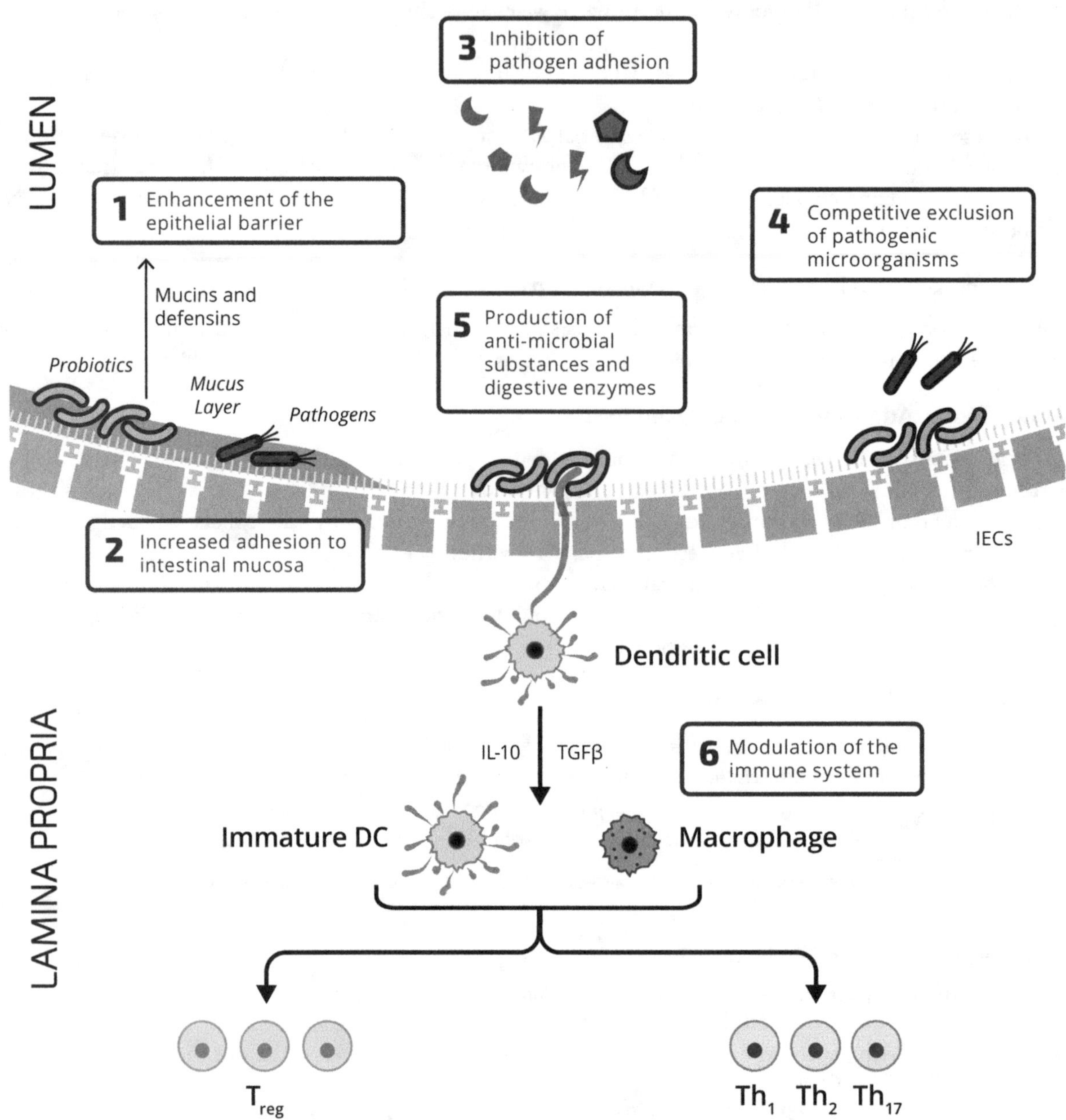

Most supplemental probiotics share their genes and metabolites that provide these benefits without making your gut a permanent home. These are called *transient bacteria.*

Now, let's talk about what it takes to optimize the gut microbiome.

PART 3: THE SCIENCE OF THE HEALTHY GUT

The key to getting BIOptimized is actually by optimizing the part of you that you can alter by taking the right probiotic and the right bacteria.

— Monia Avdić, Ph.D., microbiology/genetics and bioengineering

The Science of Microbiome BIOptimization: How to Break the Vicious Cycle of Dysbiosis

Most probiotic foods and supplements on the market do nothing at all, because your gut microbiome has a mind of its own. Microbiologists have been racing to find magic weight loss and disease-curing strains, mostly to no avail.

It turns out that the microbiome is more complex than previously thought, which is why probiotics don't have the same effect as fecal microbiota transplants. Any microbiome therapy has to take into account these complexities to be safe and effective at improving your health.

Eliminate the Bad and Reseed the Good

Studies have confirmed that diet composition can change your microbiome more than probiotic supplements. With every bite you eat, you're selecting your own gut bacteria. Therefore, you need to feed them the right foods. A gut health test can tell which foods your bacteria prefer or dislike by combining stool sample tests with DNA blood testing.

Also, many studies have shown that prebiotics and synbiotics (prebiotics plus probiotics) can often have a bigger impact on the gut microbiota than probiotics alone.[48, 49] The added prebiotics provide food for the probiotics, which enhance their survival and growth. Also, the fermentation of prebiotics produces postbiotics that are beneficial for your health and help improve your microbiota.[50]

Remove Sources of Inflammation

An inflamed gut makes a great breeding ground for dysbiosis.[51] Therefore, to rebalance your microbiome, you have to remove any gut irritants, including foods currently causing inflammation and infection.

To learn more about food allergies and sensitivities, refer to Chapter 31.

Weed and Reseed

Gut infections can cause dysbiosis by causing gut inflammation and inhibiting the growth of good bacteria.[52] Para Guardian can help with killing parasites and pathogenic yeasts. On the other hand, P3-OM specifically kills bad bacteria and yeast to make room for the good ones, which can improve the overall microbiota composition.

Biome Breakthrough contains IgYmax, a mixture of egg-based antibodies that can target and remove 26 strains of bad bacteria. IgYmax has been clinically shown to reduce gut lining inflammation and improve the overall gut bacteria composition.[53] Biome Breakthrough also contains beneficial bacteria that can form biofilm to replace the bad bacteria, along with prebiotics that improve probiotics survival and overall microbiota.

Optimize Your Digestion

Optimal digestive function is also crucial, because partially digested food particles can trigger the immune system and cause gut inflammation. Also, leftover amino acids and fats tend to favor dysbiosis, so be sure to practice good eating hygiene and take your digestive enzymes and HCL Breakthrough.

Live a Microbiome-Friendly Lifestyle

Your gut microbiota will reflect if you're unhappy, inflamed, stressed out, lonely, or not sleeping properly. If you want a healthy microbiome, manage your stress, optimize your sleep, and address sources of unhappiness in your life.

Eat Ferments Every Day

One of the easiest ways to upgrade your digestive health is to eat ferments every day. Even better is to eat them at every meal. Here are the top 10 fermented foods that you should integrate into your diet:

1. **Real yogurt.** Most commercial yogurts are filled with dead probiotics and an overload of sugar. Real yogurt is incredibly sour to the taste because its live probiotics have consumed the sugar and produced beneficial acids.
2. **Kefir.** Closely resembles yogurt. It provides a good dose of calcium as well as healthy bacteria. Choose unflavored kefir, since any added sugar may prevent your healthy bacteria from thriving.

3. **Sauerkraut.** The primary bacteria found in this type of food is *Lactobacillus*, which is found in even higher concentrations than in yogurt. Prepare sauerkraut yourself rather than purchasing it, because store-bought versions are typically prepared using vinegar, killing off much of the beneficial bacteria.
4. **Tempeh.** Tempeh is a type of fermented tofu. It not only provides a good dose of protein but is also an excellent way to boost your probiotic intake. It's a great source of calcium too.
5. **Kimchi.** Kimchi is prepared using cabbage, radishes, and scallions and may also contain red pepper or salted shrimp. The probiotic strain found in kimchi is called *Lactobacillus brevis*, which may help promote greater weight loss.
6. **Miso.** Miso soup is made from fermented soybeans along with salt and koji, an edible fungus. Taking miso helps to boost your digestive system and enhance your immune system, and it may also help to lower your overall risk for cancer.[54, 55]
7. **Kombucha.** Kombucha is a fermented probiotic drink made with black or green tea along with yeast.
8. **Pickles.** Just as with sauerkraut, you want fermented pickles, which are usually best made yourself. You need only cucumbers (or any other vegetable you desire), salt, and water. And if you make your own, you sidestep the additives in supermarket pickles.
9. **Natto.** This is a Japanese dish made from fermented soybeans and has a sticky sort of texture. Very rich in vitamin K, it can help with skin health as well, preventing wrinkles and boosting skin elasticity.[56]
10. **Fermented raw fruits and vegetables.** These are a great natural source of probiotics and have a very diverse range of live bacteria.

Almost all fermented foods are upgrades to *every* diet, including keto and even carnivore diets. They're almost all low-carb, raw, low-calorie foods and high in probiotics. They contain many acids beneficial for your body.

High Fiber Diet

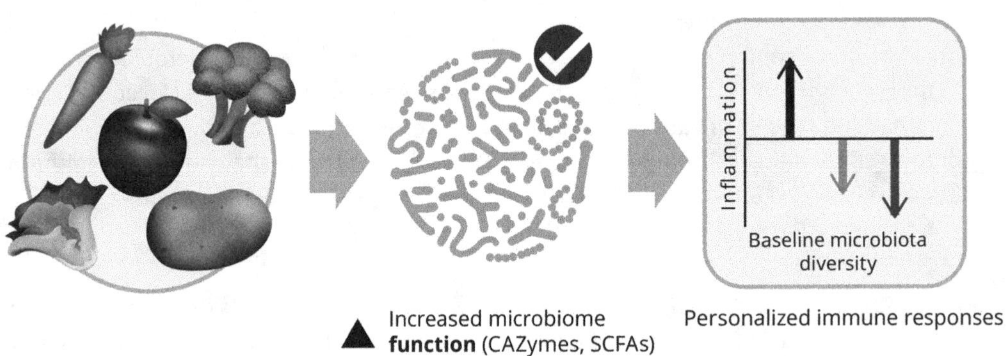

High Fermented Food Diet

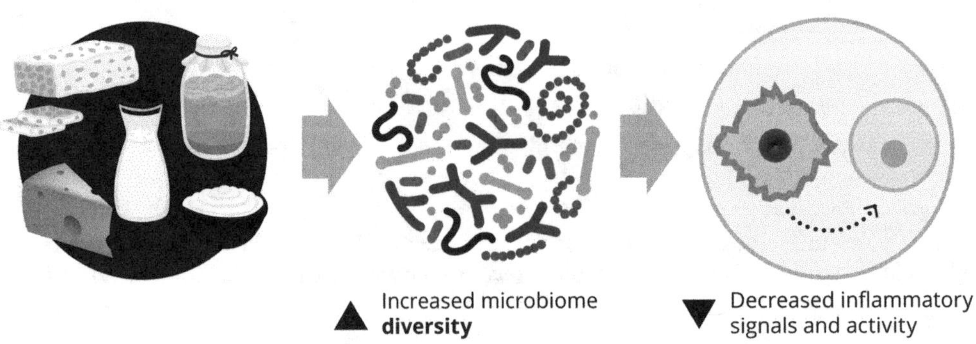

Healthy adults did a 17-week study in which they were given either a high-fiber diet or a high-fermented-food diet. The study measured their microbiomes and hosts, including extensive immune profiling.[57] What was the result?

- The high-fiber diet increased microbiome function; however, it did not increase microbiota diversity. It also increased markers of inflammation.
- The high-fermented-food diet steadily increased microbiota diversity and decreased inflammatory markers.

Now that you understand how to cultivate a healthy microbiota, we will cover what probiotics and the friendly bacteria do.

Probiotics for Optimal Digestion

Suboptimal digestion can leave a lot of undigested foods unsuitable for your bacteria. Poor fat digestion may drive dysbiosis and leaky gut,[58,59] whereas on a high-protein diet, leftover amino acids can get converted into harmful metabolites.[60]

P3-OM contains *Lactobacillus plantarum OM,* the patented probiotic strain with potent protein-digesting ability. It is the most proteolytic probiotic we have ever tested. This means it's the best at breaking down protein. It also helps digest gluten, casein, and even big chunks of red meat.[61] Therefore, if your goal is to maximize the proteins that you eat and optimize digestive health, P3-OM is the strain for you.

L. plantarum OM also secretes substances that kill bad bacteria, yeast, and retroviruses, which explains why it's particularly helpful to prevent or treat food poisoning.

The Gut-Brain Connection

The aim will be to get new environmental species that are beneficial to humans and give you a lot of neurotransmitters that make your brain function optimally, that will make your body function optimally, and provide you with health. Because, how I see it, you have what you have. Your genome is your genome. But you can enhance your body by inserting an organism that co-exists with you in your gut, and in your gut, it can do the digestion for you. Then you'll just get the benefits. This is what probiotics are. Because when we think of it, we are 90 percent bacteria, 10 percent human.

— Monia Avdić, Ph.D., microbiology/genetics and bioengineering

How Psychobiotics Improve Mood and Brain Function

Psychobiotics aren't the latest creatures from a Hollywood movie. They are specific strains of bacteria that have been shown to produce significant impacts on mind and mood. Those are the types of strains we use in Cognibiotics—the first brain-enhancing probiotic formula that works by improving your gut-brain-microbiome axis.

Given how intertwined your gut microbes are with your brain and mental health, it is not possible to fully restore healthy brain function without improving your gut bacteria. In our experience, very few people successfully improve their mood or cognitive function with probiotics alone. This led us to formulate Cognibiotics.

Cognibiotics contains the synergistic (combined effect greater than the sum of their separate effects) mix of bacteria strains and Chinese herbs that have been shown to improve brain health, especially in stressful environments. This combination provides greater benefits than the effects of each individual strain.[62, 63] The Chinese herb formula *chaihu shugan san* has also been shown to reverse dysbiosis and reduce inflammation.[64, 65] Our lab tests have shown that it's a dopamine-producing powerhouse.

The Science behind "Gut Feelings"

For generations, people have told us to trust our guts when something feels off. And now, studies have confirmed the intertwined connections between the brain, the gut, the microbiome, and all aspects of health. Here are a few mind-blowing studies that demonstrate these connections.

Gut Bacteria Control Brain Development, Mood, and Intelligence

Rodents without gut microbiomes have abnormal brain and gut-brain development.[66] They have less anxiety and fewer depressive behaviors, but they are also less intelligent.[67]

Maximum Mental Performance: Seven Ways to Boost Your Gut Biome

1. Short-Chain Fatty Acids (SCFAs)

Short-chain fatty acids, such as acetate, propionate, and butyrate, are very beneficial postbiotics that our friendly gut bacteria produce by fermenting prebiotic fibers.

Neurons that can't get enough energy (ATP)—because excess oxidative stress jams their mitochondria—become sluggish, causing low mood, brain fog, and fatigue.[68, 69, 70] SCFAs can get absorbed in the blood and easily enter the brain to neutralize the oxidative stress and jump-start the mitochondria. They also work as a source of clean-burning fuel for your neurons without generating more oxidative stress.[71]

Chronic inflammation, leaky gut, and leaky brain can cause brain fog and mental health problems. SCFAs counteract such lifestyle-related chronic inflammation and strengthen the gut- and blood-brain barriers.[72] The chronic inflammation, leaky gut, and leaky brain can cause brain fog and mental health problems.[73, 74]

Butyrate also increases proteins, such as brain-derived neurotrophic factor (BDNF), that boost neuronal growth and regeneration. Therefore, it boosts mood and improves memory, learning, and neuronal repair.[75]

2. Balancing Your Stress Response and Improving Stress Resilience

Both the Chinese adaptogens and friendly bacteria in Cognibiotics help balance the stress response. *L. plantarum, L. helveticus, L. fermentum, L. rhamnosus,* and *L. casei* supplementation reduces the stress hormone cortisol and mitigates some stress-related symptoms in rodents.[76, 77, 78, 79, 80]

Many herbs in Cognibiotics are adaptogens that help the body better adapt to stress, such as by mitigating stress-induced fatigue, irritability, and cognitive dysfunction.[81, 82] They promote calmness and focus.

3. Improving Neurotransmitter Balance

A balanced neurotransmitter profile is key to a well-functioning brain. For example, serotonin imbalance may cause depression, while acetylcholine is important for memory.

Several herbs in Cognibiotics, including *P. multiflorum, S. miltiorrhiza,* and *R. glutinosa* may increase acetylcholine levels.[83]

L. plantarum, L. helveticus, L. fermentum, L. rhamnosus, and *B. infantis* change animal behaviors partly by influencing levels of the neurotransmitters serotonin, dopamine, and GABA in the brain.[84, 85] These good bacteria also crowd out the bad bacteria and reduce the enzymes that may convert healthy neurotransmitters into anxiety-causing metabolites.[86]

4. Promoting Neuroregeneration and Neuroplasticity

The good bacteria and herbs in Cognibiotics work together to stimulate the production of proteins that help the brain grow, reorganize, and adapt.[87, 88] These proteins include brain-derived neurotrophic factor and neural growth factor (NGF). Increasing these proteins helps with learning and memory, while low BDNF is also implicated in depression.[89]

5. Protecting the Brain against Oxidative Stress

Many modern lifestyle factors are unhealthy for the brain because they increase oxidative stress and inflammation. Some scientists also believe that infections, together with chronic inflammation and high blood sugar, increase amyloid beta, the abnormal protein in Alzheimer's disease.[90, 91]

L. acidophilus, B. lactis, and *L. fermentum* increase antioxidant enzymes and improve cognitive function in diabetic rats.[92] All herbs in Cognibiotics have some antioxidant activities, including several compounds that can easily enter the brain and protect neurons from oxidative stress.[93, 94]

6. Increasing Blood Flow to the Brain

Oxygen and vital nutrients are very important for brain function, but the brain is located at the highest point in the body with numerous tiny blood vessels. Stress, poor cardiovascular health, and low blood pressure can reduce blood flow to the brain, causing the brain to be starved of oxygen and vital nutrients. This can contribute to fatigue, brain fog, poor cognitive function, and depression.

The *chaihu shugan san* herb formula in Cognibiotics may help increase blood flow to the brain in people experiencing depression.[95]

7. Stimulating the Vagus Nerve

The vagus nerve is an important nerve bundle within the rest-and-digest (parasympathetic) branch of the nervous system. It links the gut and the brain, and scientists believe that it is one pathway that our gut bacteria use to control our minds within the gut-brain axis.

B. longum and *L. rhamnosus* stimulate the vagus nerve,[96, 97] which can potentially improve mood, reduce inflammation, and improve well-being.[98]

Therefore, Cognibiotics is the most potent probiotics and brain-enhancing formula that works with the gut-brain-microbiome axis.

Power Moves to Promote the Lean Microbiome

- Feed your microbiome with fiber and the right probiotic strains
- Entrain a healthy circadian rhythm and work on optimal sleep (see Chapter 8)
- Heal your gut

Probiotics for Weight Loss

To maximize your weight loss success and improve your metabolic health, it's a wise move to improve your gut microbiome and seal leaky gut in addition to optimizing your diet and exercise.

Probiotics can help improve the gut barrier function and reduce metabolic endotoxemia. They ferment prebiotics and produce SCFAs that help seal the gut and reduce chronic, low-grade inflammation.[99] In addition, some specific strains have been shown to help reduce body fat, potentially by improving the overall gut microbiome.

Lactobacillus gasseri

A Japanese study published in the *British Journal of Nutrition* gave subjects *L. gasseri* in fermented milk for 12 weeks. By the end of the study, their abdominal fat decreased by 8.5 percent, along with their BMI, waist and hip circumferences, and body fat mass.[100] A Korean study also found that *L. gasseri* reduced visceral fat and waist circumference in obese adults.[101]

In mice, *L. gasseri* reduced inflammation from fat cells and sealed the leaky gut that can cause metabolic endotoxemia. As a result, the mice had less bacterial toxin in their blood.

Lactobacillus rhamnosus

A clinical study tested the effect of synbiotic containing *L. rhamnosus* in dieting obese men and women. The women in this study lost 50 percent more weight and had lower leptin than other groups. The prebiotics in the synbiotic formula improved the survival of *L. rhamnosus* in the gut.[102]

Biome Breakthrough is a symbiotic product that's rich in *L. gasseri* and *L. rhamnosus*, with a powerful prebiotics blend. It also contains IgYmax, which helps reduce harmful bacteria, especially gram-negative ones, which are sources of harmful bacterial toxins. Together, these ingredients can support weight loss by reducing inflammation, fixing leaky gut, and improving the overall microbiome.

Lactobacillus plantarum

In mice, *L. plantarum* reduced low-grade inflammation and suppressed weight gain from the inflammation. The bacteria also helped normalize lipid profiles.[103]

P3-OM contains *L. plantarum OM,* which is a powerful patented strain of *L. plantarum.* Not only does it kill bad bacteria, but it also improves digestive function and supports gut barrier function.

PART 4: ASSESS, TEST, AND OPTIMIZE

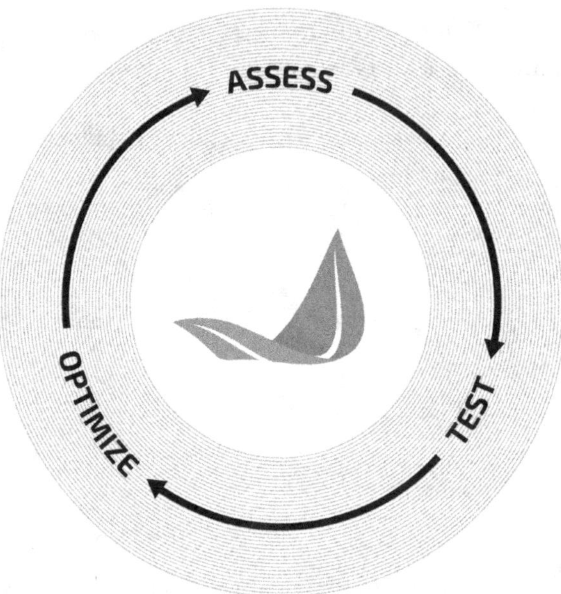

You can stop the bacteria from seeing the molecule. If you want to stop some traits that you don't want, then you go into the realm of "see no molecules, hear no molecules, speak no molecules." But if you want to enhance some behaviors, you just add the right signal.

— Monia Avdić, Ph.D., microbiology/genetics and bioengineering

For people who want to go to the ultimate level of health, we recommend following the Biological Optimization (BIOptimization) Process. This is an ever-evolving cycle of assessing, testing, and optimizing. You can use this process to upgrade any part of your health, including your gut biome. This section will discuss how you can test your gut biome and use the data to make smart upgrades.

Testing Your Microbiome

You can only manage what you can measure, and we're all about data-oriented strategies. With next-generation sequencing technologies, it is now possible to profile your gut microbiome by taking a "snapshot" with a direct-to-consumer test. The bad news is that these tests are still in their infancy, and you need to take the results with a grain of salt (see our caveats below).

What Is Next-Gen Sequencing?

Next-gen sequencing (NGS), also called *massive parallel sequencing,* refers to technologies that make it possible to sequence the DNA for millions of DNA fragments at a time. Previous technology could determine only one fragment of DNA at a time.

Because we can now sequence millions of fragments in parallel, we can count the number that have the same sequence. This means that we can count the number of bacteria or copies of genes within a sample.

Previously, to identify the bacteria species in a stool sample, they had to be isolated in a petri dish. But gut bacteria are mostly anaerobic—they dislike oxygen, or it's toxic to them. However, lab culture environments contain oxygen. Also, many strains of gut bacteria are not yet possible to grow in a lab.

NGS provides a massive breakthrough because we only need DNA samples, not live bacteria—so we don't need to grow it. The process of identifying, counting, and studying the genomes of microbes in an environment using NGS is called *metagenomics*.

Microbiome Tests Look at Different Parts of the Genome

When we talk about how to modify these bacteria, you get to know that the bacteria genome works like a babushka doll, where you have a core part of the genome, and this core part of the genome stays the same. But the accessory parts of the genome can change due to stress. And you can expose the bacteria to different levels of stress in order to change these accessory parts of the genome. You're creating novel environmental species like this and in doing so, you're activating other genes. You're making mutations and you can monitor in the lab the new molecules that you're gaining through this process.

— Monia Avdić, Ph.D., microbiology/genetics and bioengineering

Not all microbiome tests are created equal, and if you sent the same stool sample to all the different test companies, you might very well get different results.

While the cost per base pair of DNA sequence has decreased significantly, prices still depend on how long the total DNA sequence is. Therefore, 16S rRNA (part of the synthesizing organelle ribosome that's exported to help translate information to mRNA) is less expensive than full-genome and transcriptome sequencing, respectively.

16S rRNA

16S rRNA is a small portion (~1,550 base pairs) of bacterial genomes that has a unique signature for each species. This is the least expensive and most reliable way to profile the bacteria composition of a sample, although it doesn't determine the genes. Most microbiome profiling studies use this test.

It may be possible to project the genome composition by querying the database of full bacterial genomes. However, bacteria can gain or lose genes, or transfer them to each other, so this approach will provide only an estimate of your biome's metabolic capacity.

Whole-Genome Bacteria Sequencing

Instead of sequencing only the 16S rRNA, whole-genome sequencing determines all the DNA sequences present in your stool sample and therefore all the genes present in your microbiome. Genetic data can be deduced for biochemical activities.

Transcriptome

Simply because a gene is present doesn't mean it's being read from. The transcriptome test measures the degree from which a gene is read. So far, it's the most direct measurement of the metabolic and biochemical activities in your sample, although it's less reliable at detecting all the species present. Go to www.BIOptimizers.com/book/guthealth to do a gut health test; this will help you choose better foods for your gut biome.

Matt's Gut Biome Testing Experience

Matt has undergone many gut biome tests. Here's what he says about them.

I think doing gut biome tests is a great way to upgrade your diet. First of all, it confirmed some of my biofeedback with certain foods. I never liked chicken and felt I didn't digest it well. I always loved beef and felt great afterward. The test told me to minimize chicken and that beef is a superfood.

The other benefit was being shown "personal superfoods" that I wasn't aware of. Foods like watercress, Jerusalem artichoke, pumpkin, and spirulina are all suggestions that I wasn't eating. So now when I want to make a big-ass salad, everything I put in is considered a "superfood," and I feel amazing. My digestion operates at its peak when I eat based on my gut biome.

Caveats of Direct-to-Consumer Microbiome Tests

- Next-gen sequencing technologies are relatively new, error prone, and still rapidly evolving.
- Most direct-to-consumer microbiome tests only test the stool microbiome, which is only what passes through your system. However, your gut is not a uniform fermentation chamber. Rather, there are micro-communities of microbes, which can be very different from spot to spot. Colonoscopy biopsy microbiomes can be very different from stool microbiomes.[104] The colonoscopy microbiome tests won't be easily available direct-to-consumer any time soon.
- Stool microbiome only gives a snapshot, but we know that the microbiome can change quite quickly. So far, there isn't a specific protocol on how often to test or what to do with the results. Therefore, you should see a practitioner who can help you decode it and decide how to address this.
- Scientists are still discovering how individual microbiome components affect our health.
- In our experience, the tests provide useful insights that will help you upgrade your diet. However, the suggestions shouldn't be seen from a dogmatic lens (which is true for all diet advice, including this book).
- Go to www.BIOptimizers.com/book/guthealth to do a gut health test, this will help you choose better foods for your gut biome.

It is also important to keep in mind that so many factors affect our gut biome, whereas the current scientific framework favors studying one factor at a time for the same effects in large populations. This also explains why metagenomic microbiome studies have been producing mixed results or failing to establish a scientific consensus.

SUMMARY

Part 1: The Profound Wisdom of Hippocrates

"All disease begins in the gut."

- Dysbiosis is when you have imbalanced gut bacteria
- Dysbiosis can cause weight gain and decrease mood
- An inflamed gut lining causes dysbiosis
- Fortunately, we now know how to fix the abnormal gut-brain axis. In mice, probiotics have been shown to relieve this sickness behavior.

Part 2: What Creates a Healthy Gut Biome?

- The richer and more diverse your gut microbiota are, the better
- Diversity and richness make the microbiota more resilient to invasion, bad bacteria overgrowth, antimicrobials, and antibiotics
- This also allows you to adapt better to changes in your diet, lifestyle, and environment

Part 3: The Science of Healthy Gut

- It turns out that the microbiome is more complex than previously thought. Probiotics don't have the same effect as fecal microbiota transplants.
- To be safe and effective at improving your health, any microbiome therapy has to take into account these complexities
- With every bite you eat, you're selecting your gut bacteria. Therefore, you need to feed them the right foods.
- Remove sources of inflammation, weed out any bad bacteria, and reseed the good bacteria

Part 4: Assess, Test, Optimize

It's important to use high quality data to take your results even further. Do a gut biome test and start experimenting with eating different foods in order to optimize your gut health to the next level.

CHAPTER 30

HOW TO INTEGRATE FASTING INTO YOUR LIFE

This chapter is going to open your eyes to the unparalleled power of fasting to help support your overall biological optimization and body transformation.

In this chapter you will learn:

- How you already fast every single day, driving a process called autophagy
- The five key benefits of implementing fasting in your life
- The five different types of fasting, how to do each one, and the various benefits each type has on your body
- How shifting your ghrelin is advantageous
- When and how you should do multiple-day fasts
- How you can integrate fasting into your life to support weight loss
- Eleven ways you can optimize your fasting results
- Potential risks that may come with fasting
- The appropriate way to safely end an extended fast and get back into your normal diet comfortably

Fasting is one of the human body's great marvels. It allowed our ancestors to function during times of famine and not perish.

And guess what? You're already fasting every day. That's right—when you're sleeping, your body is in a fasted state for 8 to 12 hours. During that time, an important process called *autophagy* ramps up. *Auto* means "self," and *phagy* means "eating." So, the literal meaning of *autophagy* is "self-eating."

THE POWER OF AUTOPHAGY

Autophagy is the body's way of cleaning house—getting rid of damaged cells and creating healthier ones, according to Priya Khorana, who has a Ph.D. in nutrition education from Columbia University.

Autophagy is always happening, to a certain degree. However, it ramps up higher the longer we go without food.

Getting Back into Alignment with Nature

Historically, almost every culture has used fasting to accelerate healing. Many animals won't eat when they get hurt or injured. Oftentimes they will not eat for days. Humans also do this. When people get sick, they often lose their appetites and reduce their food consumption.

Periods of fasting are actually more in alignment with our biological natures than our current constant overabundance of foods.

KEY BENEFITS OF FASTING

The health benefits from fasting are numerous. That being said, despite what many intermittent fasting (IF) zealots claim, it's not a magical bullet for weight loss. However, it is a powerful tool when used properly. Let's look at some of the key benefits you get from fasting.

The Brain Benefits of Fasting

On the brain level, we know that fasting can boost brain-derived neurotrophic factors (BDNF), which is kind of a fertilizer for your brain. Boosting BDNF helps keep your brain young and healthy.

Fasting Is a Huge Time-Saver

The time you save by fasting is massive. How much time do you spend thinking about food every day? *What am I going to eat for lunch? Dinner?* Then there's prepping the food, eating the food, and cleaning the plates and the kitchen. Fasting saves a massive amount of time.

Fasting Transforms Your Emotional Relationship with Food

One of the biggest benefits that almost everybody reports is that their emotional relationship with food changes. Our brains are hardwired to always be thinking about food because it's a key to survival. We've been conditioned to eat multiple times a day since we were kids.

Most people have never consciously gone a long period without feeding themselves. The majority of the world has an "I must eat at least three times a day" mental programming, and fasting helps change that.

Fasting helps reduce the fear of, "If I don't eat, I'm going to die." When we suggest people try fasting, oftentimes their initial reaction is, "I'll die." This is obviously not true, but the only way to realize this is to go through a fasting experience.

Wade shares his initial fasting experience:

> The first time I can remember fasting, there were struggles. I can recall when I first started fasting. The first three days really sucked. I was a guy that ate five or six meals a day for probably 10 to 15 years before I started fasting. Once I got through the first three days, I felt great.

ACCELERATED KETOSIS AND FAT BURNING

There is significant synergy between following a ketogenic diet and fasting. Why? Because you're already using fat for fuel, it's easy for the body to keep doing that when there's no food present.

Fasting strengthens your fat adaptation. The longer you fast, the more ketones your body produces and the better you use them. That's why the first fast is the most challenging for people. They haven't built that biological adaptation to be able to convert fats into ketones easily.

Improved Neurochemistry

Also, Western physicians have used fasting as a treatment for mood disorders and chronic pain.[1] Between days two and seven, fasters can experience improved mood, alertness, and a sense of tranquility.

Researchers have hypothesized that the ketone body beta-hydroxybutyrate (BHB) is sufficiently similar to gamma-hydroxybutyrate (GHB),[2] and based on this hypothesis, BHB may partially bind to GABA receptors, which has a calming effect and overall slows down the activity of the brain.

Fasting may also boost dopamine to drive your motivation to find food.[3]

FASTING ISN'T FOR EVERYONE

There's a small group of people who should not fast. Why? Because they don't have great genetics for it.

Many people with Mediterranean genes are not built for fasting, because that area of the world has had a perpetual abundance of food. The epigenetics of Mediterranean people evolved differently than those of Caucasians who survived long, brutal winters.

We've seen this with many of our clients. When they fast, their bodies have stressful responses like the ones listed below:

- Their cortisol goes up
- Their HRV goes down
- Their heart rate goes up
- They don't feel well
- Their sleep quality usually goes down the drain

Matt shares his experience of multi-day fasting:

> When I fast, I feel great. My HRV goes up, my heart rate hits new lows, and by the third day of fasting, my heart rate is dropping even more. However, I've seen the opposite with several clients who have Mediterranean genes.

TYPES OF FASTING

1. Intermittent fasting
   - 16 hours fasting–8 hours not
   - 20 hours fasting–4 hours not
   - One meal a day
2. Alternate-day fasting
3. 3-day fasts
4. 5-to-10-day fasts
5. 40-day fasts and beyond

Intermittent Fasting

If you've never fasted before, intermittent fasting is a good place to get started.

First, you can start with 12 hours of fasting. This means if you start eating at 8 A.M., your last bite would be at 8 P.M. If you're someone who is snacking until you go to bed, this is a big improvement. First of all, your sleep quality will improve. Second, you will probably lower your overall calories.

From there, you can go 14–10, meaning 14 hours of fasting and 10 hours of eating. This means if you start eating at 8 A.M., you stop at 6 P.M.

Many people promote the 16–8, meaning 16 hours of fasting and 8 hours of eating. In general, the longer you fast, the more autophagy ramps up in the body. These smaller eating windows may make it easier for you to eat less food. However, to reiterate: there's no magic metabolic weight loss advantage to intermittent fasting. It does not ramp up your metabolism. Your weight loss still comes down to calories in and calories out.

Remember: if you consume more than you expend, you will still gain weight.

The Biggest Advantage to IF Dieting: Ghrelin Shifting

There's one key advantage that is unique to IF: ghrelin shifting.

Our bodies typically release a ghrelin spike an hour before our usual eating times. For example, if you typically eat breakfast at 9 A.M., you'll start to feel hungry around 8 A.M. Your body pings your brain and says, "Hey, get ready. I want to eat soon."

However, when you do IF for a few days, there's a powerful adaptation that occurs; the ghrelin response changes. You lose that one-hour ghrelin spike before the meal, and that can be a game changer for managing hunger and lowering calories. Eliminating hunger a few hours per day can make it easier to eat less.

Some dieters find themselves living in a perpetual state of hunger when they eat four to six small meals a day. IF dieting can lower the amount of time that you experience hunger.

Some people will push their fasting window to 18–6 (18 hours of fasting and 6 hours of eating). That usually means you're eating maybe two meals and a snack.

Some do 20–4 (20 hours of fasting and 4 hours of eating). Then, some people do just one meal a day. If you can manage the hunger, it's hard to overeat in an hour if your meal is vegetables and good quality protein sources. However, if you're going to pound a 14-inch pizza, it's easy to go over your daily calorie target.

Alternate-Day Fasting

Alternate-day fasting is when you eat normally one day and then don't eat the next. Basically, you're eating for 12 hours out of every 48. You're doing a 36-hour fast, and you're eating during a 12-hour window. This does allow the body to go pretty deep into autophagy.

We decided to try this a couple of years ago. We both got good results . . . however, we found two big downsides:

1. Our hunger was way higher than usual, probably because there wasn't enough consistency to create the ghrelin shift. We would eat all day one day, and not eat the next.
2. We found it catabolic. And this seems to be the consensus for a lot of people who fast for long periods. Dr. Peter Attia and Tim Ferriss shared this on their podcast. Their weight stayed the same, and their body fat increased. Wade also noticed that most of the fat loss benefits stopped after 14 days. There was significant muscle loss.

Bottom line is, it's another potential calorie-management strategy. However, because they don't get the benefits of the ghrelin shift, we don't advise our clients to follow this strategy.

Psychologically, the plus side is, you wake up one day and say, "Okay, I'm going to eat normally today." Then, the next day, you say, "Okay, I'm not eating today." The biggest downside is hunger. It's also normal to overeat when you're ravenous on the days that you can eat.

We also noticed one more downside: there was an increased desire for calories for an extended period after the fast. We had activated our body's starvation self-defense mechanisms.

Three-Day Fasts

Once you've done a full day of fasting and you feel comfortable with it, you may want to consider doing a three-day fast.

There's limited clinical data on this, but an animal study found that autophagy kicks into full gear 24 to 48 hours into a fast.[4] So, if you want full autophagy benefits, consider a three-day fast after you've tried shorter fasts.

Benefits of a three-day fast:

The extended phase of autophagy produces several interesting benefits in the body:

1. You'll be in deep ketosis and burning mostly fat. You may become fat adapted.[5]
2. Significant amount of weight and fat loss[6]
3. You reboot your neurons as autophagy prunes away gummed-up proteins that can cause neurodegenerative diseases[7]
4. Reduced chronic inflammation[8]

Psychologically, a three-day fast is a very different experience. This is when you really get to change your relationship with food.

Most other studies about fasting and the gut say the microbiome changes positively, improving metabolic conditions and so forth. One study actually profiled the microbiome and found that when mammals go through long fasts (such as during hibernation), their villi temporarily atrophy and their fiber-eating microbes decrease.[9] Meanwhile, mucus-eating bacteria increase. But these changes go away quickly when the animals go back to feeding.

In one study, a 10-day fast did increase gut permeability and inflammation markers, but it wasn't a problem for the healthy subjects. Other studies it cited found that fasting reduced gut permeability and blood bacterial toxins.[10,11,12] Fasting reduces blood lipopolysaccharides (LPS), because eating usually increases bacterial toxin translocation into the blood.

How often should you do a three-day fast?

- Every quarter is a good idea. We believe that there could be some powerful longevity benefits in doing three-day fasts on a regular basis.
- At the end of a dieting phase, before going on a diet break. This is a good strategy to cut calories. However, be mindful of the hunger that can occur when you start eating.

5-to-10-Day Fasts

Some people choose to do longer fasting to truly maximize detoxification or to help their body heal itself.

Wade shares his experience of his first 10-day fast:

> My first 10-day fast was a major transformer. I can remember still crapping 10 days into the fast, and the stuff that came out of me looked like recycled tires.
>
> I also combined it with colonics to accelerate the cleansing process. But with colonics, you have to be very mindful not to overdo it. Once every couple of days, starting around day four, is probably enough.
>
> One major upgrade I did was using massive doses of MassZymes with my fasts. I truly believe this accelerated the detox.
>
> Then, I started doing a 10-day fast twice a year. However, after a few years, it got to the point where somewhere between five and seven days, I would just start going catabolic. In other words, I would start losing so much muscle mass that I would have to abandon the fast. Matt also reports the same thing.

There's a moment, usually between days five and seven, in which you feel your body go catabolic. This is when we end the fast.

One more benefit that we see during extended fasting is on a brain wave level. If you pay attention, you'll see your body move less day by day. Your NEAT lowers significantly. The body starts making it harder for you to move. Research with fasting and NEAT has proven this.[13] One of the things you'll notice is your brain waves slowing down. We have not seen data on that, but having done a lot of neurofeedback, we definitely think beta brain waves go down quite a bit and alpha and theta brain wave activity become more dominant. You just feel chill.

During extended fasts, it's not a time to be pushing your body, competing in athletic events, being in a period of emotional stress, or needing to be in peak cognitive state. Choose a time when you can do a lot of resting and relaxing.

40-Day Fast

Throughout history, usually associated with spiritual practices, some people have done 40-day fasts. Buddha, Jesus, and Muhammad reportedly all did them as part of their spiritual practices.

Our mentor Dr. Michael O'Brien shared that he overcame cirrhosis of the liver and colon cancer using a combination of 40-day fasts and the massive intake of enzymes and proteolytic probiotics.

He also did a similar process with Bernard Jensen, who wrote 65 books on health and was the master of iridology. In one such book, Jensen details how he overcame paralysis and death, which was Bernard Jensen's story of how Michael supervised him through a fast and then a massive intake of proteolytic enzymes and proteolytic probiotics in specific tocotrienol-based amino acids.

Health expert Lou Corona has shared his story with us. He had a very large tumor. His health mentor at the time said, "Let's fast for 40 days." He did, and he said the tumor was gone.

That being said, we do not advise any healthy individual to do a 40-day fast. Magician David Blaine, who has done many of the craziest stunts ever performed, has said in multiple interviews that he felt he never fully recovered from his 44-day fast. He:

- Lost 10.4 kg of muscle
- Developed some nutritional deficiencies (B vitamins, low potassium, low vitamin A, and others)
- Experienced faintness and dizziness upon standing up quickly (at two weeks in)

- Developed sharp, shooting pains in his trunk and limbs
- Experienced nausea and abdominal discomfort
- Has stated that the negative effects have lingered for many years

Never attempt to do an extended fast without medical supervision.

180-Day Fast

There have been a few experiments with extremely long fasts.

Angus Barbieri's 382-Day Fast Experiment

A man named Angus Barbieri fasted for 382 days between June 1965 and July 1966. This may be the world's longest medically documented fast He weighed 456 pounds when he checked into a hospital in Dundee, Scotland.

Angus had shed 276 pounds throughout his fast. He dropped all of his additional body fat and weighed roughly 180 pounds at the end. Once he achieved this healthy weight, he kept it for the duration of his experiment's five-year follow-up period.

During his fast, he simply drank water, coffee, and tea, and he took a few supplements. Blood and urine samples were taken, as well as notes and observations on his progress. Not that it matters, but his fecal evacuations were quite impressive. The typical interval between stools was 37 to 48 days. A fast this long is only advisable for people who really have extremely high levels of body fat.

- This is not something you want to do if you have only 10 pounds to lose. But very obese individuals may see incredible results for fat loss. You absolutely must be supervised by medical professionals.
- It's critical to give your body the vital nutrients it needs: water, minerals, and vitamins.

HOW TO END AN EXTENDED FAST

The following key points are important for any fast past 48 hours. When you fast for several days, the bacteria in your intestinal tract will begin to die. Bacteria have around a 48-hour life span, and if you stop feeding them, they stop reproducing.

Prolonged fasting can temporarily put your gut lining cells into a resting, atrophic state, which can cause leaky gut and gut inflammation. You'll also lose some bacteria that eat fibers from your food, while gaining the bacteria that eat the mucus your gut cells produce.

However, while you're fasting, you're not getting any inflammation from food, so you may feel less of it.[14] However, once you get back to eating, you have to provide your gut lining with what it needs to grow back, so make sure to eat gentle foods.

Your first few meals are really important.

- Biome Breakthrough is a phenomenal option for your first meal. It helps rebuild a strong, healthy biofilm.
- Bone broth also helps rebuild the biofilm.
- Drinking a healthy protein shake (we suggest Protein Breakthrough) with fruits is a good option.
- Easily digestible carbs like white rice are good later in the day.
- Add fermented foods every meal: real yogurt, kimchi, and sauerkraut.

For your second and third meal, make sure to include some fibrous food to help feed your bacteria. Fish is a good option as well. And then the following day, start to eat your normal diet.

One of the most difficult things we can surely attest to is that when you start eating, your body wants to make up for the last few days of calorie deficit. It may be psychologically challenging because your body can ramp up hunger to recoup those lost calories. If you're not conscious of that and don't have a game plan for it, you can easily overeat.

If you do an extended fast for fat loss (more than seven days), we suggest you reverse-diet your way out of it for a couple of weeks.

Let's say your normal maintenance is 2,500 calories. Then, we suggest you eat 1,800 calories for week one after the fast. Week two, eat 2,000, and week three, have 2,250. This will help prevent fat regain and may in fact lead to further fat loss post fast. This all requires planning, mental vigilance, and mindfulness.

USING FASTING FOR WEIGHT LOSS

We see fasting as a simple tool in the toolbox that can help you cut calories in the later part of your journey. Save it for the last half or last third of your weight loss program. We don't recommend using it as your primary weight loss method.

Here are some tips to using fasting as a part of your weight loss program:

Do IF infrequently. Your body will adapt if you do it constantly. Here are some strategies:

- Do IF two days a week to cut an extra 20 to 40 calories (assuming you don't overeat the rest of the day).
- Fast an entire day every week. This will cut your weekly calories by 15 percent.
- Do a three-day fast every three months before doing a diet break. You can lose one or two pounds of body fat during those three days.

HOW TO OPTIMIZE YOUR FASTING RESULTS

- Get sunlight exposure. It's much easier if you're in a warm climate or you're exposing yourself to full-spectrum light for as much as you can while keeping UV safety in mind. Your body temperature will drop during extended fasts, so sunlight can help.
- Do saunas. However, make sure to consume a lot of electrolytes and water to compensate for sweating.
- Consume 5 to 10 grams of high-quality salt a day. We suggest mixing it with your water. Running out of electrolytes can be deadly.
- Consume 4 to 6 liters of water a day.
- Consume 20 to 50 MassZymes a day. The proteolytic activity will help your body clean house.
- Consider doing colonics starting on day three and beyond.
- Move every day. We recommend walking, rebounding, or yoga. After a couple of days, you'll have to fight your body's desire *not* to move.
- Get massages.
- Get acupuncture.
- Use hyperbaric chambers.
- Do skin brushing.

THE RISKS OF FASTING

Some people experience euphoria, mental clarity, and increased subjective well-being on fasting, which may explain why many spiritual practices incorporate it.

Ramadan fasting studies find that participants increase endorphins and endocannabinoids.[15] Importantly, it activates stress hormones, including adrenaline, noradrenaline, and cortisol, which suppress pain and increase energy.

The Risk of Addiction

For certain people, neurochemical changes can be addictive. We've seen people fast themselves into illness because they become addicted to it. Their extended catabolism and nutritional deficiencies compromise their health.

People with disordered eating tendencies may use the high from fasting to cope with their anxiety.[16] So, if you have a history of disordered eating, that's a contraindication for fasting. If you have a history of addiction, you should be extra mindful.

Some people become addicted to cycles of fasting and binging. They do extended fasts and then go on massive binges. Matt went through this stage for a few years. He would do a couple of days of fasting during the week and then eat 6,000 to 10,000 calories in a day. He was using food as a drug.

Metabolic Risks

Metabolic effects of fasting are both positive and negative. In a fasting and feeding study, leptin drops 12 hours into the fast and bottoms out at 36 hours.[17] However, studies in lean young men found that resting energy expenditure increased from the higher norepinephrine during the first four days of the fast.[18, 19]

A study in obese people detected about a 400-calorie drop in adaptive thermogenesis and resting energy expenditure at about two weeks on a very low-calorie diet. At the time, the subjects lost about 5 percent of their bodyweight.[20] A 400-calorie drop in two weeks is a massive amount.

An interesting observation across multiple weight loss trials is that fasting tended to preserve muscle mass more than the same caloric deficits created by steady low-calorie diets. This is because fasting increases growth hormone and insulin growth factor while inhibiting somatostatin.[21] IF participants also tend to regain less weight, and they regain more muscles than fat.[22]

Your metabolism doesn't drop, but you'll move less (aka have a drop in NEAT). Over time, your body will start downregulating, especially with longer fasts.[23]

Two Metabolic Types

A small clinical study suggested that there could be two metabolic phenotypes—spendthrift and normal. The thrifty phenotype could be epigenetic, such as from their mothers being nutritionally stressed during pregnancy. After the 24-hour fast, the researchers made their subjects eat twice their maintenance calories.

During 24-hour fasting, energy expenditures dropped by 158 ± 81 calories per day. Those with a lower drop in energy expenditure during fasting gained less weight and fat mass, and they also stored fewer calories during the overfeeding. Therefore, if you have a history of spendthrift phenotypes (i.e., you get fat easily) in your family, you need to watch out for overeating post fast.[24]

CREATING A FASTING GAME PLAN THAT WORKS FOR YOU

We always suggest following a gradual process with fasting.

Start with intermittent fasting: a 12–12 fasting-to-feeding window. Then move to 16–8.

Once you feel confident, shoot for a one-day fast.

Then try doing a one-day fast every two weeks for three months.

After three months, do a two-day fast. You can break that up either as two full days (which ends up being around 60 hours), or you could eat lunch on a Friday and then restart eating on Sunday around noon. This would be a 48-hour fast.

Once you feel ready, graduate to a 72-hour fast. Once a month is a good interval for 72-hour fasts.

Once you've mastered that, your body has adapted to fasting, and it becomes easy for you, then you can go for a 5-to-10-day fast.

SUMMARY

- From a psychological standpoint, are you built for fasting? Usually, people with extreme personalities enjoy fasting.
- Key benefits of fasting include:
    - Boosts brain-derived neurotrophic factors (BDNF)
    - Saves a ton of time
    - Improves your emotional relationship with food
    - Improves mood and alertness, and provides a sense of tranquility
    - The longer you fast, the more ketones your body produces, and the more it learns to utilize them

Do you have the genetics for fasting? If your ancestors lived in brutal winters, you probably do.

- Types of fasting include:
    - Intermittent fasting

        16 hours fasting, 8 hours eating

        20 hours fasting, 4 hours eating

        One meal a day
    - Alternate-day fasting
    - 3-day fasts
    - 5-to-10-day fasts
    - 40-day fasts and beyond
- When ending an extended fast, your first few meals are really important. Start slow with Biome Breakthrough, bone broth, a healthy protein shake, easily digestible carbs, and fermented foods. Then you can start to eat your normal diet the following days.
- While we don't recommend using fasting as your primary weight loss method, here are some tips to using fasting as *part* of your weight loss program:
    - Do a two-day-per-week IF, infrequently
    - Fast an entire day every week
    - Do a three-day fast every three months
- Finally, create a fasting game plan. Gradual integration is always better. Start with IF, then go to a one-day fast and work your way up from there.

CHAPTER 31

ELIMINATING FOOD TOXINS

In this chapter, you will learn:

- How hidden food allergies and intolerances keep you from optimal health, performance, and aesthetics
- How to uncover and manage food sources of inflammation and pesky symptoms
- Why foods are the scapegoat (and not the culprit) in food reactions
- How to heal your gut and maximize your resilience so you can thrive despite any existing food-related inflammation
- How to optimize your digestion, strengthen your gut lining, and balance your immune system so you can avoid developing more food sensitivities
- Why healing your gut lining, restoring your digestion, and optimizing your gut flora are the three key areas to focus on for long-term avoidance of symptoms caused by allergic inflammation
- How to discover the tools and resources that can help you expand your food options over time and thrive despite your food allergies, intolerances, and sensitivities.
- What Dr. Nattha Wannissorn's story about allergic reactions and eczema can teach us about how food sensitivity is often a symptom and not a root cause
- What your biofilm is and why it's important to build a strong one
- Food allergies and sensitivities are determined only by genetics, right? *Wrong!* Find out how even stress, past traumas, and recent traumatic experiences can be a multiple whammy that leads to food sensitivities
- What Matt's story with digesting A1 dairy and Wade's story with a plant-based protein powder can teach us about how to discover what ingredients affect your gut health
- The pros and cons of following an elimination diet to discover your food sensitivities, and what other options there are to determine your sensitivities successfully

Removing foods that stress and harm your body is another important layer to the hierarchy of nutrition. In the short term, such foods stress your nervous system. Long term, the situation could lead to more serious health issues. This chapter will discuss virtually every known possible food stressor.

KEY NUTRITIONAL PRINCIPLE: ONE PERSON'S FUEL MAY BE ANOTHER'S POISON

Nutrigenomics are so important because your genes can help you eliminate foods that are harmful to you.

However, foods can become harmful for other reasons than incompatibility with your genetics:

- Leaky gut is a primary cause of food allergens as undigested food particles enter the bloodstream
- Food allergies may develop over time due to eating them too often, or for other reasons

As you read this chapter, remember another key principle: the dose creates the effect. This is true for most of the things in this chapter. This means that if you eat a little bit of the wrong things, you're fine, but if you eat too much of them, it will affect your health.

However, for some people, certain foods are simply binary: there is either zero response or a significant response—even small amounts can have detrimental impact. This means they must avoid that food completely. For example, those with celiac disease and severe food allergies need to avoid the foods that they react to altogether.

Now, let's get into it.

Do you suffer from any of the following symptoms?

Digestive Problems	Mental Health Issues	Metabolic and Energy Production	Pain Disorders
• Gas • Bloating • Belching • Constipation • Diarrhea • Irritable bowel syndrome	• Brain fog • Anxiety • Depression • Mood swings • Psychosis • Insomnia and poor sleep quality	• Fatigue • Inability to regulate blood sugar • Inability to lose excess fat or gain muscle mass	• Headaches and migraines • Fibromyalgia • Joint and muscle pain • Arthritis
Nutrient Deficiencies	**Allergy and Autoimmunity**	**Skin Problems**	**Hormonal and Reproductive Health**
• Stubborn iron-deficiency anemia that doesn't respond to iron supplements • Inability to increase vitamin D • Loss of bone mass, leading to osteopenia and osteoporosis	• Allergic rhinitis • Asthma • Inflammatory bowel disease • Hashimoto's disease • Multiple sclerosis • Lupus • Type 1 diabetes	• Eczema • Hives • Psoriasis • Acne	• Infertility • Painful menstrual symptoms

This list is not exhaustive. But if you're suffering from any of these health issues, it's possible that what you're eating is causing inflammation. And while food might not be the only cause of your inflammation, it can be a key contributor.

To maximize all three sides of your BIOptimization Triangle, you need to lower the inflammation in your body as much as possible. This starts with knowing which types of food reaction you have and to which foods. In the short term, you need to avoid or minimize problematic foods. In the long term, you need to heal your gut lining, restore your digestion, and optimize your gut flora.

Many common inflammatory foods are staples that make up your favorite comfort foods, such as cakes, pastries, ice cream, and bread.

At BIOptimizers, we're about optimizing health, performance, and aesthetics while living an awesome life—which includes being able to enjoy your favorite foods and food-related occasions. The key is to counter the negative effects of problem foods with enzymes like Gluten Guardian.

Later in this chapter we'll cover tools and resources that can help you expand your food options over time and to thrive despite your food allergies, intolerances, and sensitivities.

And on the occasion that you do get exposed to these inflammatory foods, there are ways to manage inflammation and quickly recover from the symptoms.

Dr. Nattha's Story

During the fourth year of my Ph.D., after one and a half years of failed experiments, I fell into depression and orthorexia as my academic hopes and dreams fell apart. I was doing bodybuilding workouts and HIIT for two to three hours a day, and aggressively cutting calories. At the same time, I was working long hours in the lab, studying fitness and nutrition.

As my naturopathic intern friend put it, my "adrenals were tanked." Instead of listening to her, I used four different types of stimulants to burn fat and stay awake. Eventually, I decided to introduce intermittent fasting. I started to fast for 24 hours once a week, despite the contraindications with my history of disordered eating.

The fasting was the last straw on my stress response system. A few weeks later, I woke up with my entire upper body covered in eczema.

Having watched my brother have to lather himself with very strong steroid creams to (ineffectively) control his severe eczema his entire life, I decided to opt out from steroids altogether. The itching was so bad I had to take a semester off from graduate school to recover both physically and emotionally.

My naturopathic intern friend suggested an elimination diet.

I met with an allergist, and he diagnosed me with a ragweed (dandelion) allergy from the skin test and told me to avoid chamomile tea. I then discovered that my vegan protein powder contained dandelion. I had also been enjoying spoonfuls of sunflower butter. Within a week after I stopped ingesting these, my neck (which was entirely covered in red and raw eczema) had completely cleared up.

I also realized that the generic elimination diet handout might not have been restrictive enough. So, I came up with my own diet version that consisted of poultry, rice, apples, and leafy greens.

I stuck to the diet, and within a month, not only did I clear the eczema, my overall outlook on life was better. I was able to return to graduate school and finish my Ph.D.

While I wouldn't wish this experience on anyone, I now recognize that my journey was a blessing. Eczema often plagues people for years—or even a lifetime. But I was able to put an end to it within a month, while managing to avoid antidepressants and many other drugs.

WHY FOODS ARE NOT THE REAL CULPRIT IN FOOD ALLERGIES, INTOLERANCES, AND SENSITIVITIES

Many people suffer from inflammation due to foods, especially if they're on the standard American diet. However, they may not have connected their symptoms to their foods. These reactions can be very individual, depending on where the weakest links are in someone's body.

Keep in mind that food allergies, intolerances, and sensitivities are typically symptoms of deeper underlying problems. These are neither normal nor healthy. And in many cases, simply avoiding the inflammatory foods may not fix the root causes.

Here are a few common dysfunctions that contribute to food allergies, intolerances, and sensitivities:

1. Intestinal Permeability (aka Leaky Gut)

You have a leaky gut when undigested food particles can pass your intestinal tract and enter your bloodstream. Basically, it means you've got holes in your gut. The gut lining (mucosal barrier) consists of a single-cell layer and the mucus covering it. The barrier separates the gut immune system and the gut contents. Between the cells of the gut lining are proteins that zip the cells together, such as tight junctions, desmosomes, and adherens junctions.

Your gut lining is naturally permeable to allow the absorption of some nutrients. Substances and nutrients can get transported between the cells or across the cells.

How to Know if You Have Intestinal Permeability

- You have some symptoms or health issues listed at the beginning of this chapter
- You get one of the following lab test results indicating intestinal permeability:[1, 2]
  - Elevated or low secretory IgA (sIgA), an important gut antibody, in the saliva or stool
  - Elevated IgG (the most common antibody found in blood circulation) in response to many foods
  - Elevated ratios of lactulose to mannitol in the lactulose-mannitol test

    Mannitol is a smaller sugar molecule that is readily absorbed, whereas lactulose is a larger molecule, so the presence of it in the bloodstream means that the gut is leaky[3]

- Elevated blood lipopolysaccharides (LPS)
- Elevated zonulin shows that the tight junctions may be opening up through the zonulin pathway.
  - Zonulin can be a marker of celiac disease and non-celiac gluten sensitivity, especially when they're actively consuming gluten. We suggest getting a Zonulin test to get a baseline.[4, 5]

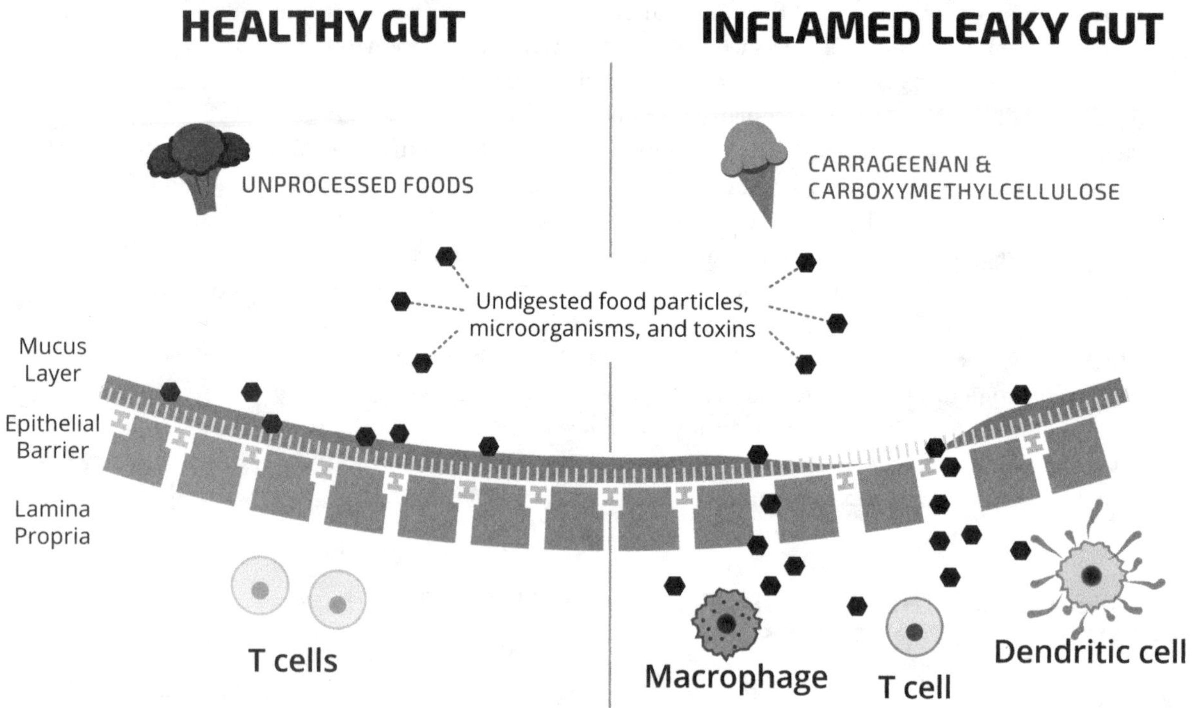

HEALTHY GUT | **INFLAMED LEAKY GUT**

UNPROCESSED FOODS

CARRAGEENAN & CARBOXYMETHYLCELLULOSE

Undigested food particles, microorganisms, and toxins

Mucus Layer

Epithelial Barrier

Lamina Propria

T cells

Macrophage

T cell

Dendritic cell

Healthy and strong gut barrier:

- Healthy anti-inflammatory gut microbiome
- Healthy level of protective mucus
- Balanced immune function
- Better food tolerance
- Strong immune system to fight off infection
- Minimal food exposure to the immune system
- Healthy enzyme production and nutrient absorption

Leaky gut and pro-inflammatory gut barrier can expose food particles to the bloodstream, which can create:

- Increased pro-inflammatory gut microbiome
- Reduced protective mucus
- Food sensitivities
- Gut and whole-body inflammation
- Allergies or autoimmunity
- Weak immune function
- Reduced enzyme production and nutrient absorption

Causes of Leaky Gut

There are many different ways people can get a leaky gut, including:[6, 7]

- Disruption of tight junctions from inflammatory foods such as gluten
- Cellular death (apoptosis) and ulcers, such as in IBD and celiac disease
- By translocation of bacteria or bacteria toxins, such as lipopolysaccharides (LPS)
- Extended fasting and then not properly rebuilding a healthy biofilm post fast
- Major illnesses, injuries, and surgeries
- Medications, including nonsteroidal anti-inflammatory drugs and proton-pump inhibitors
- High-fat and high-sugar meals

- Lack of dietary fibers and polyphenols
- Deficiencies in nutrients that are important for mucosal barrier function, such as vitamins A and D, and zinc
- Dysbiosis and gut infections

Gut Leaks

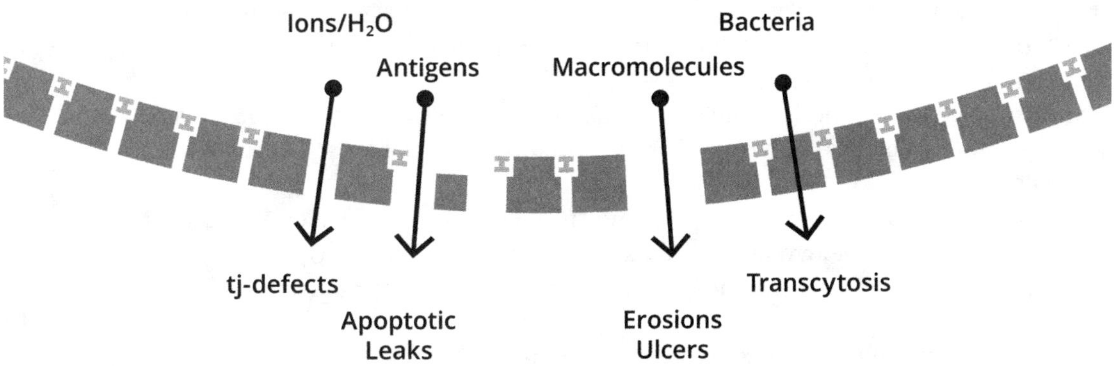

Leaky gut alone is not a disease. Most people's gut linings open up multiple times a day before resealing and bouncing back with no problem. It only becomes problematic when the gut lining fails to heal itself and the immune system sustains the inflammation. Our answer to leaky gut is called Biome Breakthrough.

Power Move: Add Biome Breakthrough to Your Diet

Biome Breakthrough is a delicious probiotic/biofilm stack that will help boost your immunity and increase the health of your biofilm. We've proven in our BioLab that it's one of few probiotic stacks that actually increases biofilm formation. Biofilm is the layer that, if built of the proper cultures of bacteria, will create a powerful line of defense against inflammation. Healthy biofilm formation is also the solution to leaky gut.

Biome Breakthrough is synergistically designed to eliminate bad bacteria, implant the good ones, and repair your gut lining. It will also:

- Promote overall gastrointestinal (GI) health
- Possibly reduce intestinal permeability
- Eliminate bloating and gas
- Promote healthy immune response
- Possibly reduce gut inflammation
- Increase nutrient absorption
- Raise your energy levels

2. Reduced Immune Tolerance and Increased Inflammatory Tendency

A healthy immune system should be able to ignore harmless antigens such as foods, dusts, pollens, and your own proteins. This is why most people tolerate many foods and environmental allergens without developing allergies, autoimmune issues, or food-related inflammation. However, those with weaker immune systems find their bodies reacting.

Your immune system has many checks and balances to ensure you tolerate your foods and don't develop autoimmune diseases. Food-related inflammation is a sign that some of these defenses are breaking down. Here are three variables you should keep a close eye on.

Check & Balance #1: Killing and Deactivating Budding Autoimmune Cells

As your white blood cells develop in your thymus and bone marrow, your immune system eliminates the young white blood cells that attack your own tissues.[8] Even when you have antibodies against your own tissues or foods, it rarely becomes a problem.

Check & Balance #2: Not Mounting an Immune Response Even Though You Have Antibodies

Having antibodies against foods or your own tissues rarely leads to autoimmune diseases.

For example, about 8.5 percent of men and 16 percent of women have thyroid peroxidase (TPO) antibodies.[9] This suggests that most TPO antibodies don't interfere with thyroid function or trigger the immune system to destroy the thyroid tissues.

Similarly, in a study of 500 healthy subjects without autoimmune diseases, 8 to 15 percent of them have antibodies against common food lectins. Test tube assays found that some of these antibodies can bind to proteins of human tissues.[10]

Now, this doesn't mean you don't have to be concerned if you have antibodies. You're at a higher risk, and you should proactively monitor your autoimmune markers, but keep in mind that you also have the power to improve your immune balance through your epigenetic activation and boosting your microbiome health.

Check & Balance #3: Your Immune System's Zen Master, Regulatory T Cells

Regulatory T cells (Treg) are present in your bloodstream and tissues. They ensure that your immune system ignores the harmless antigens, preventing allergies and autoimmunity. Also, Treg ensures that inflammation resolves after an infection or episode of inflammation.[11]

Treg cells help make sure you don't react to all your foods and bacteria in your gut.[12]

Even if you have a leaky gut, Treg cells calm the immune response and make sure you don't react to the foods. This allows your gut lining to reseal itself.

If you're suffering from symptoms of chronic inflammation or getting inflammation from foods, you have Treg dysfunction.

Also, you can't just increase Treg so that you can eat whatever you want. Excessive Treg activity can suppress immune responses that prevent cancers, possibly allowing cancers to develop.[13]

Power Moves to Promote Healthy Treg Levels and Overall Immune Balance

- Ensure that your vitamin A and D levels are optimal by testing and supplementing accordingly.[14]
- Use synbiotics, such as Biome Breakthrough, to increase short-chain fatty acids that promote gut Tregs.
- Optimize your sleep.[15] We have three highly effective sleep formulas: Magnesium Breakthrough, Sleep Breakthrough, and Dream Optimizer. To learn more, go to www.BIOptimizers.com/book/sleep.

3. Stress and Traumas

Stress, past traumas, and recent traumatic experiences can cause a multiple whammy that all lead to food sensitivities. Chronically elevated levels of stress can wreak havoc on the digestive system. One of Matt's clients, Juan B., shares his story:

> I was going through some extremely difficult times in my life and I was struggling to digest food. My gut biome was turned upside down. Sometimes I had diarrhea and other times I was constipated. It was amazing to see all of these symptoms disappear once the stress was gone.

Stress can cause a leaky gut and keep your body in a state that cannot effectively repair one.[16] For your body to heal, you need to be in a parasympathetic state. If you're constantly in "fight, flight, or freeze," your body's natural abilities to repair itself become compromised.

Chronic stress also increases corticotropin releasing hormone (CRH), which is the highly inflammatory stress hormone that also increases leaky gut and immune reactivity. Elevated CRH also disrupts the gut bacteria.[17]

Many people with food-related inflammation also benefit from neuronal rewiring practices such as the Dynamic Neural Retraining System, meditation, and neurofeedback. You can learn more about that here: www.BIOptimizers.com/book/neurofeedback.

Power Move: Include Cognibiotics in Your Daily Routine

Cognibiotics contains powerful stress adaptogenic herbs and bacteria strains. It can help with normalizing both the stress response and the gut lining.

It supports your brain-gut connection and improves brain health, mental clarity, learning, memory, and focus. Cognibiotics also boosts your cognitive function, mood, and stress resilience by improving your gut flora. It will even improve the balance of your neurotransmitters, including acetylcholine, serotonin, GABA, and dopamine in the brain.

4. Molecular Mimicry

Molecular mimicry is when an outside protein has sections that are very similar to your own proteins. When the immune system develops antibodies or immune cells against these sections of proteins, it can lead to autoimmune diseases.[18]

These outside proteins can come from foods or infections. However, very rarely does eating foods that contain molecular mimics or having antibodies against them lead to autoimmune diseases.[19] For an autoimmune disease to occur due to molecular mimicry, four conditions need to be in place:

1. Low stomach acid and poor digestion, especially incomplete protein digestion.[20] This often happens with proteins that are hard to digest, such as lectins, gluten, and casein.[21, 22]
2. Leaky gut, which allows the gut content to meet the immune cells.[23]
3. Environmental triggers causing the immune system to be on high alert, such as infections, stress, or toxin exposures.[24]
4. Loss of immune tolerance, or the breakdown of the immune system's ability to ignore self-attacking immune responses.[25]

You can have genetic predispositions for leaky gut, overactive immune system, and loss of immune tolerance. However, keep in mind that your epigenetics, gut flora, and lifestyle can contribute to any of the four factors. Having healthy gut flora protects against all of them.

If you already have an autoimmune diagnosis, it's worth working with a practitioner to find out if you have ongoing molecular mimicry in your body. Get a blood test—such as from Cyrex—to find these antibodies against common foods. Then, eliminate the foods to see if your symptoms or autoimmune markers improve.

Power Moves

If you don't have an autoimmune condition, optimizing your gut health allows you to enjoy all foods without developing abnormal immune responses.

If you have an autoimmune condition, it becomes even more important to optimize your gut and your gut microbiome health. You can use:

- HCL Breakthrough to support healthy stomach acid levels
- MassZymes to ensure optimal protein digestion
- Gluten Guardian to ensure digestion of gluten and casein
- Biome Breakthrough to support and heal the gut lining

In conclusion, the combination of leaky gut, loss of immune tolerance, stress, and traumas can cause you to develop inflammatory reactions to food.

THREE WAYS YOU CAN REACT NEGATIVELY TO FOODS

1. Food Allergies

Food allergies are medically recognized food reactions; you can be diagnosed with a blood or skin-prick test. If you have a food allergy, you will have IgE (the antibody that plays a role in allergic reactions) antibodies that recognize the protein from the food.

Once the IgE detects the food in your system, even a tiny amount, it can quickly activate mast cells and other types of immune cells. This can lead to severe and immediate allergic symptoms, such as:[26]

- Hives and skin itchiness
- Swelling (edema) of the tongue, mouth, or face
- Mucus in the nose, throat, and ears
- Vomiting and diarrhea
- Anaphylaxis, which can cause a life-threatening drop in blood pressure and cardiac arrest
- Breathing difficulty due to airway constriction

Most people know they have food allergies because they have immediate symptoms, and the symptoms tend to be severe. In some cases, they may even have reactions if they inhale the dust of the foods to which they're allergic.

However, some people do develop milder allergic conditions, such as eczema or ear problems, due to IgE-mediated food allergies. They may not even be aware that their conditions come from food allergies.

The most common food allergies are reactions to:

- Dairy proteins
- Tree nuts
- Eggs
- Peanuts
- Shellfish
- Wheat
- Soy
- Fish

Oral Allergy Syndrome: Can Environmental Allergies Make You Allergic to Foods?

Oral allergy syndrome is a type of food allergy that relates to environmental allergies. Many environmental allergens have proteins that are similar to some in foods. As a result, the IgE that reacts against these environmental allergens may also recognize similar foods. This is called *cross-reaction.*

Dust mites and cockroaches vs. shellfish. Dust mites and cockroaches have parts that are similar to some in shellfish. So, if you're allergic to these environmental allergens, you are more likely to be allergic to shellfish.[27]

Fungus allergies vs. moldy foods. Many people exposed to mold develop IgE, IgA, and IgG antibodies against mold and mycotoxins.[28, 29] These antibodies can cause you to react to any foods that contain fungus parts or metabolites, including:

- Moldy foods
- Foods that are made or fermented with fungi
- Fungal proteins such as Quorn
- Nutritional yeasts
- Moldy cheeses
- Cured meats
- Moldy fruits and vegetables
- Moldy grains, legumes, and flour
- Baker's and brewer's yeasts, along with beers and wines
- Mushrooms

Cat dander allergy vs pork. About 1 to 3 percent of cat-allergic people are at risk of allergy to pork meat.[30]

Pollen vs. certain fruits, vegetables, and spices. Allergies to common pollens also produce IgE that recognizes certain fruits, vegetables, and spices. Oral allergy syndrome due to pollen can be worse during pollen season.

Symptoms of pollen oral allergy syndrome tend to be limited to the mouth, nose, and throat, such as itchiness, tingling, and nasal congestion. However, in rare cases, the reactions can be systemic or life-threatening.[31]

Alder Pollen	Birch Pollen	Grass Pollen	Mugwort Pollen	Ragweed Pollen
• Celery • Pears • Apples • Almonds • Cherries • Hazelnuts • Peaches • Parsley	• Apples • Peaches • Apricots • Cherries • Plums • Pears • Almonds • Hazelnuts • Carrots • Celery • Parsley • Caraway • Fennel • Coriander • Aniseed • Nectarines • Soybeans • Peanuts • Kiwi • Parsnips • Peppers • Potatoes	• Melons • Tomatoes • Oranges • Swiss chard • Peanuts • Raw white potatoes	• Celery • Carrots • Parsley • Caraway • Fennel • Coriander • Sunflower • Peppers • Aniseed • Bell pepper • Black pepper • Mustard • Cauliflower • Cabbage • Broccoli • Garlic • Onion • Peach	• Cantaloupe • Honeydew melon • Watermelon • Cucumber • Kiwi • Banana • Zucchini • Chamomile tea • Sunflower seeds

Source: https://www.chkd.org/patients-and-families/health-library/way-to-grow/oral-allergy-syndrome/

Keep in mind, however, that if you're diagnosed with a pollen allergy, it doesn't mean the entire cross-reacting food list is off limits for you. Having these allergies means you're more likely to develop an allergy to cross-reacting foods, but it doesn't mean you will. The best way to find out is to eliminate them and bring them back to confirm whether you're allergic to the foods.

Responses to potential allergens can be highly individual. Testing for and challenging food allergens should be done under medical supervision, especially since it can lead to life-threatening anaphylactic reactions.

2. Food Intolerances

Food intolerances happen when your body lacks the enzymes to digest certain substances in foods, such as lactose, histamine, and fermentable oligosaccharides, disaccharides, monosaccharides, and polyols (FODMAPs).

People with food intolerances may be able to handle problematic foods in small doses. Some people can fully tolerate such foods by supplementing with enzymes they lack, while others need to completely avoid them.

Histamine Intolerance

Histamine intolerance refers to the inability to break down biogenic amines. Bacteria in foods convert amino acids into amines, such as histidine to histamine, tyrosine to tyramine, and tryptophan to tryptamine.[32] These are found in spoiled foods and fermented foods.

One of our VIP clients, Todd, activated a multi-month histamine response when he overloaded his system with toxins. It seems that the off-gassing of plastics and rubbers in his new home was the culprit. The incessant need to scratch destroyed his sleep, and the itching drove him mad. If he ate the wrong thing, the itching went out of control. We had to put him on an antihistamine diet to help manage the symptoms.

People with histamine intolerance have allergy-like symptoms in response to lower doses of biogenic amines than people without histamine intolerance. These symptoms may include:[33]

- Diarrhea and vomiting
- Brain fog
- Headache or migraines
- Asthma-like symptoms or asthmatoid coughs
- Acid reflux
- Dizziness, fainting, and drops in blood pressure
- Rapid heartbeat
- Hives and skin itchiness
- Flushing
- Muscle and joint pain
- Anxiety and depression
- Insomnia

In the short term, you can manage histamine intolerance by eating a low-histamine diet and supplementing with diamine oxidase (DAO) enzymes. Many people with histamine intolerance also feel better eating fewer lectins and other types of dietary gut irritants. Such irritants often trigger more histamine release and increase inflammation, especially in people with histamine intolerance.[34]

IgYmax is a type of antibody produced in chicken eggs targeted against 26 species of bad bacteria. It works by escorting out bad bacteria, making room for the good ones. An open-label clinical study showed that two grams per day of IgYmax for eight weeks significantly increased DAO production and the ratio of DAO to histamine. It also reduced zonulin, a marker of leaky gut, while increasing good bacteria.[35]

This is why we included IgYMax with synbiotics in Biome Breakthrough. Synbiotics also increase the production of postbiotics, which reduces gut lining inflammation and helps reseal a leaky gut.[36]

FODMAP Intolerance

FODMAP stands for fermentable oligo-, di-, and monosaccharides, plus polyols. These are carbohydrates that your gut bacteria can ferment. High-FODMAP foods include:

- Onions and garlic
- Beans
- Cruciferous vegetables
- Asparagus
- Chicory root
- Grains
- Some fruits, such as apples, stone fruits, and figs

For people who tolerate FODMAPs, the FODMAPs feed their good gut bacteria in the large intestine. It's healthy to consume FODMAP-containing foods.[37]

However, FODMAPs can cause bloating, gas, diarrhea, or even alternating constipation and diarrhea in those who are intolerant to them. Up to 80 percent of people with irritable bowel syndrome may have small-intestinal bacterial overgrowth (SIBO), although this number is also controversial.[38]

As we always say, the dose creates the effect. Many bodybuilders and athletes who consume massive amounts of calories run into digestive troubles when they eat too much of the FODMAP foods. That's why Stan Efferding eliminates all FODMAP foods in his Vertical Diet.

VegZymes is a full-spectrum, plant-based digestive enzyme blend that can break down most FODMAPs. We've found it to be very helpful with digestive symptoms related to FODMAPs.

FODMAP intolerance and IBS are linked to fibromyalgia, anxiety/depression, and chronic fatigue syndrome.[39,40,41] If FODMAP foods cause body pain, mood changes, or crippling fatigue, you should see a qualified practitioner to investigate.

3. Food Sensitivity

Matt's Food Sensitivity Story

I used to have trouble digesting A1 dairy (the A1 protein molecule is in the milk from most cows, and it can be problematic for certain people). It sits in my stomach and increases inflammation, causing bloating, gas, heaviness, and water retention. Whenever I was on a fat loss program, the dairy, specifically casein, would halt my progress no matter how I changed things from a caloric perspective. However, I didn't have the same problem with A2 dairy.

Some people can tolerate dairy just fine if they don't have a leaky gut. Now, when I supplement with Biome Breakthrough and Gluten Guardian to ensure that the A1 dairy is completely digested, it's no longer a problem.

Whenever I eat pork, my heart rate and body temperature go up, while my heart rate variability goes down. So clearly, there is some sort of reaction there, especially if I eat too much of it.

Power Move: Consume A2 Dairy Sources

If you find you have digestive issues with cow's milk, there is another option. Dairy that comes from animals other than cows contains A2 protein. These include goats, sheep, and buffalo. There are also new brands of cow milk products focused on A2 protein. All cows produce at least some A2 β-casein, but certain breeds have predominantly A2 in their milk. This includes the Guernsey, Jersey, Charolais, and Limousin breeds.

Casein Can Act Like Opiates

Like gluten, casein is high in glutamine and proline, making it difficult to digest with your body's natural digestive enzymes. Therefore, casein tends to be partially digested, leaving casein peptides, which can be inflammatory for some people.

A1 beta-casein, which is found in A1 milk, has the substitution of proline to histidine at position 67. This makes it possible for a proteolytic enzyme to cut out a peptide, generating an opiate-like peptide called beta-casomorphin-7 (BCM-7).

In adults, BCM-7 tends to be more problematic in those with a leaky gut and those who have limited production of peptidase DPP4, the only enzyme that can digest casein.[42]

Other Food Substances That May Cause Inflammation and Other Health Problems

You can develop a sensitivity to any protein or substance in foods. The most common food sensitivities include those to gluten, eggs, grains, dairy, chocolate, coffee, and nightshades (potatoes, tomatoes, eggplant, and peppers).

Some people are sensitive to specific food substances such as oxalates, salicylates, and lectins. Let's go through a variety of food types and discuss potential problems.

Lectins

If grains, nightshades, and legumes cause inflammation for you, it is likely you're sensitive to lectins.

Symptoms of lectin sensitivity may include:

- Post-meal brain fog or fatigue
- Pain
- Mood problems
- Digestive issues
- Autoimmune conditions

Lectins are proteins that help cells recognize or correctly "select" each other, and it's present in all species.[43] A few properties make lectins potentially an inflammatory gut irritant.

- They are very difficult to digest. They're poorly digested by human digestive enzymes, so scientists have found intact lectins in human stool samples.[44]
- Some plant lectins are recognized by lectin receptors in your gut, so they tend to irritate the gut lining.
- They can be potent immune activators—so much so that they're tested as adjuvants in vaccines.[45] In fact, everyone has some antibodies against dietary lectins in the blood.[46]
- They can throw off the gut microbes and increase bacteria strains that are linked to autoimmune diseases.[47]

Therefore, many dietary lectins are more likely to cause leaky gut and autoimmune diseases than others—such as lectins in grains, legumes, nuts, seeds, nightshade plants, and plants in the cucumber family. Pesticidal proteins engineered into genetically modified corns and soybeans may also cause leaky gut.

For people who are not sensitive to lectins, natural lectin-containing foods are perfectly healthy, especially if they're prepared properly.

However, for people with the preexisting genes and epigenetics for autoimmune diseases, lectins can contribute to the development of autoimmunity.

According to Alessio Fasano, M.D., autoimmunity requires three things:[48]

1. Genetic predisposition
2. A leaky gut, which can be caused by zonulin or lectins
3. A trigger that tips over the immune system, such as very stressful life event, an infection, or a pregnancy

A few lectins are just outright toxic whether you're sensitive or not. For example, raw white kidney bean lectin causes food poisoning in everyone.[49] Ricin, the castor bean lectin, has been used as a toxic weapon (and was used in the TV series *Breaking Bad*).[50] Gluten and wheat germ agglutinin, both found in wheat, can be harmful to people who are sensitive, celiac, or allergic to those proteins.

You can degrade legume lectins by cooking or sprouting, whereas grain lectins don't fully degrade through these processes.

Gluten Sensitivity

Gluten is a family of proteins including gliadins and glutenins. These are found in wheat, rye, and barley. However, gluten-sensitive people and celiacs may react to only a few parts per million of gluten, such as from foods processed in the same facility or particles in a restaurant kitchen.

Celiac Disease

Celiac disease is a serious autoimmune disease where the immune system attacks the small intestine lining when someone is exposed to gluten. The inflammation can destroy the nutrient-absorbing, finger-like structures (villi) in their gut and cause major gut leakage.

People with celiac disease may experience symptoms including bloating, gas, diarrhea, vomiting, bloody stool, and nutrient deficiencies. Untreated celiac disease can lead to other serious conditions, such as other autoimmune diseases, osteoporosis, anemia, and cancers.

Celiac disease is diagnosed with the following steps:[51]

- Blood testing for specific antibodies against gluten, including anti-transglutaminase and anti-endomysium antibodies
- Genetic testing for the presence of HLA-DQ2 and HLA-DQ8 genes
- Endoscopy and gut tissue biopsy to observe for visible damage to the villi

People with celiac disease need to completely avoid gluten. Even parts per million of it can make them very sick. This is why certified gluten-free foods have to be made in a facility that doesn't handle any gluten.

Once people with celiac disease completely eliminate gluten, the autoimmune destruction of the gut lining is so extensive that it can take three to six months for the gut to fully heal. For older patients, it may take up to two years.[52]

Some people with celiac disease also react to nongluten grains if their antibodies cross-react between gluten and those grains. In these cases, they may do better to avoid grains altogether.

It's typically very hard to be 100 percent sure that restaurant food is completely free of gluten. There can be cross-contamination in your food even if you order gluten free. That's why many people with celiac disease protect themselves with Gluten Guardian when they eat out, unless it's a 100 percent gluten-free restaurant.

However, Gluten Guardian is not a treatment for celiac disease; neither does it make it possible for people with celiac disease to enjoy gluten-containing foods.

Non-Celiac Gluten Sensitivity (NCGS)

NCGS refers to inflammatory reactions against gluten that are not from celiac disease, FODMAP intolerance, or gluten allergy.

Symptoms of NCGS have a wide range that can include digestive problems, fatigue, headaches, joint or muscle pain, numbness, brain fog, skin problems, depression, anxiety, and more.[53]

People with NCGS may experience these symptoms within a few hours of eating gluten. Once they stop eating it, the symptoms may resolve within a few hours to a few days.

Gluten can open the gut lining through the zonulin pathway. People with non-celiac gluten sensitivity also have elevated blood zonulin levels. Some also have the HLA-DQ2 and DQ8 genes.[54]

Eggs

Eggs contain many different proteins, and some of them can trigger food sensitivities that are not mediated by IgE but rather by other types of immune responses.[55] This type of inflammatory reaction to eggs can cause skin problems like eczema as well as gut issues.

Egg white proteins in particular are strong immune system sensitizers, so they may worsen other food sensitivities or allergies.[56] Eggs are commonly tested in food sensitivity tests and excluded in elimination diets.

Is Dairy a Problem for You?

Dairy sensitivity can be highly individual. It can range from fully tolerating all dairy to only tolerating A2 or non-cow dairy to not tolerating any dairy at all. The best way to find out is to eliminate and reintroduce it.

Given that partially digested casein from all types of dairy can be a problem, it is a good idea to ensure that all casein and milk proteins are fully digested. Gluten Guardian contains the enzyme that can digest casein and lactase, which can minimize any digestive problem or inflammation you may get from dairy.

Milk has a mixture of many different proteins; about 80 percent is casein and 20 percent is whey. Casein is a large protein and can be difficult for some people to break down.

By nature, milk is a mammalian newborn's first food, so it may also contain antibodies and other immune signals from the mother.[57] Milk components also keep an infant's gut leaky so they can absorb the antibodies and immune signals.

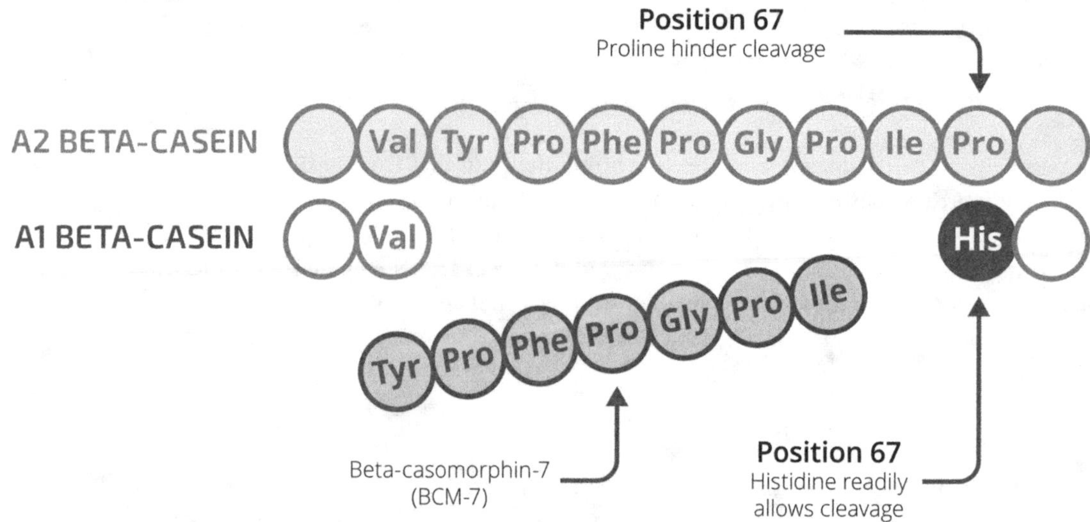

Region of A1 casein that generates beta-casomorphin, compared to the same region by A2.

Gut Issues and Brain Function

Your gut and entire body have opioid receptors. The opioid also naturally controls gut motility. So, dairy can generate pleasurable responses, especially when combined with sugar.[58] It's no wonder people use ice cream to numb emotional pain.

Problems with Insulin and Blood Sugar

Both whey and casein stimulate a high insulin response.[59] High proline proteins like casein and gluten stimulate the production of dipeptidyl peptidase 4 (DPP4) in the gut.

Aside from digesting casein and gluten, DPP4 also degrades GLP-1 and GIP, which work like insulin or stimulate insulin actions.[60] Some people who struggle with blood sugar and insulin sensitivity may be better off avoiding dairy. However, Gluten Guardian is loaded with DPP4, which makes it the best enzyme stack for dairy.

This is especially the case for type 1 diabetics, as some evidence also suggests that A1 casein may trigger the autoimmunity that leads to type 1 diabetes.[61]

Lactose Intolerance

Lactose intolerance is caused by a lack of the enzyme lactase, which digests the milk sugar lactose. It can cause digestive symptoms such as gas, bloating, diarrhea, nausea, vomiting, and gut cramps. Up to 65 percent of the population has lactose intolerance. Some develop it after an episode of gut infections, food poisoning, or due to other factors that affect the gut lining.[62]

Most lactose-intolerant people can have some dairy with supplemental lactase, or a digestive enzyme blend that contains lactase, such as Gluten Guardian.

Protease Inhibitors

Protease inhibitors are substances that block the function of protease enzymes. Many plants naturally propagate through animals eating and defecating seeds intact, so they produce protease inhibitors to keep their seeds from being digested. Therefore, grains, legumes, nuts, and seeds tend to be higher in protease inhibitors. Most of these can be reduced by soaking, sprouting, fermenting, and cooking.

Dairy also contains proteins that inhibit the function of digestive proteases.[63] Having protease inhibitors in the gut can reduce digestion of all proteins, which tells the pancreas to release more enzymes. It also throws off the balance between proteases, which allows trypsin to chew up the tight junctions and cause leaky gut.[64, 65, 66]

Oxalates

Oxalates can be found in leafy greens, cruciferous vegetables, rhubarb, black peppers, chocolate, tea, nuts, and berries. These can cause kidney stones and pain in people with oxalate intolerance. In healthy people, they can bind minerals in the gut and prevent absorption. Boiling vegetables and discarding the water may reduce oxalates by 30 to 87 percent.[67]

If you have severe oxalate sensitivity that causes excruciating pain, you may have to be very careful with vegetables.

Goitrogens

Goitrogens are substances that prevent healthy thyroid function by blocking iodine entry, interfering with thyroid peroxidase, or interfering with thyroid-stimulating hormone. These are found in unfermented soy products such as tofu, soy milk, and edamame, as well as fresh or fermented cruciferous vegetables. Therefore, you should limit your soy consumption and avoid relying on it for protein.

Salicylates

Salicylate sensitivity (also called salicylate intolerance) can trigger pseudoallergic reactions. These aren't true allergic reactions, because they're not mediated by IgE antibodies.

However, symptoms of salicylate sensitivity are similar to those in allergies, such as asthma, congestion, nasal polyps, hives, and gut inflammation. In children, salicylates can cause migraines and hyperactivity. In rare cases, anaphylactoid reactions can occur.[68]

People who are sensitive to salicylates will also react to medications and cosmetics that contain salicylate-like molecules. Aspirin, acne medications, and nonsteroidal anti-inflammatory drugs are examples of salicylates. Many herbs and essential oils also tend to be high in salicylates.

Salicylate Content of Foods

FRUITS					
VERY LOW SALICYLATE	LOW SALICYLATE		MEDIUM SALICYLATE	HIGH SALICYLATE	VERY HIGH SALICYLATE
mango passion fruit pears pomegranate rhubarb	bread fruit casaba melon coconut Crenshaw melon figs honeydew kiwi	kumquat lemons limes loquats papaya persimmon watermelon	avocado banana cantaloupe grapefruit pineapple (cooked or canned)	raw pineapple	dates guava

HERBS, SPICES AND CONDIMENTS					
VERY LOW SALICYLATE		LOW SALICYLATE	MEDIUM SALICYLATE	HIGH SALICYLATE	
allspice basil bay leaf black pepper caraway cardamom	fennel garlic malt vinegar nutmeg saffron white pepper	coriander soy sauce (MSG)	aniseed cinnamon cloves cream of tartar cumin garam marsala oregano sage tarragon sweet paprika white vinegar	cayenne chilli powder Chinese five spice curry dill ginger	hot paprika mint olives pimiento rosemary turmeric

SUGARS		
NO SALICYLATE CONTENT	MEDIUM SALICYLATE CONTENT	HIGH SALICYLATE CONTENT
granulated sugar maple syrup	honey (wide variety of salicylate content)	clover honey molasses

NUTS AND SEEDS				
VERY LOW SALICYLATE	LOW SALICYLATE	MEDIUM SALICYLATE	HIGH SALICYLATE	VERY HIGH SALICYLATE
cashews hazelnuts pecans sunflower seeds	Brazil nuts poppy seeds sesame seeds walnuts	macadamia nuts pine nuts pistachio nuts pumpkin seeds	peanuts	

VEGETABLES					
VERY LOW SALICYLATE	LOW SALICYLATE		MEDIUM SALICYLATE	HIGH SALICYLATE	VERY HIGH SALICYLATE
bamboo shoots cabbage (green/red) celery lettuce lentils	artichokes asparagus bean sprouts beans (all dried) beets Brussel sprouts broccoli carrots cauliflower chives chard collard greens corn green beans kale	kohlrabi leek mushrooms mustard greens onion parsley parsnips pumpkin peas rutabaga sorrel sweet potato turnip greens water chestnuts yams	alfalfa sprouts sweet corn baby squash white potato okra spinach	broad beams chicory eggplant radish zucchini	endive

Glycoalkaloids and Saponins

Glycoalkaloids are nitrogen-containing toxins found in nightshade plants. Plants in this family include:

- Tomato
- Tomatillo
- Potato
- Tobacco
- Eggplant
- Pepper (hot and bell peppers, and their products—such as cayenne, chili pepper, paprika, and dried peppers)

Saponins are soap-like glycoalkaloids that can poke holes in cell membranes, causing the cell to burst. They're found in legumes, quinoa, onions, garlic, asparagus, oats, spinach, sugar beet, tea, and yams.[69] Saponins may also inhibit digestive enzymes.[70] This is another example of something that can be tested using the BIOptimized Gene Testing Kit.

Toxic Exposures and Contaminated Toxins in Foods

Mycotoxins

A 1994 study by the Lawrence Berkeley National Laboratory found that about 47 percent of homes and 85 percent of commercial buildings have water damage and mold.[71] Therefore, mold toxicity has become much more common.

Mold toxins (mycotoxins) can activate mast cells and make your immune system more reactive to many things.[72] It can also tip the immune system toward allergies and intestinal permeability.[73] If you start developing symptoms or become sensitive to many foods after being in a new environment, you should see a practitioner to investigate mold toxicity.

Aside from environmental mold exposure, foods can also be a source of mold toxins. The following crops can get contaminated with mycotoxins:[74]

- Cereals
- Grains
- Nuts
- Seed oils
- Fruits and dried fruits
- Vegetables
- Cacao
- Coffee
- Wine
- Beer
- Herbs and spices
- Meats of animals fed with mycotoxin-contaminated crops

Food Emulsifiers and Texturizers

Wade's Rice Story

Years ago, Wade was associated with a top protein powder company that promoted a product containing rice bran protein. It was one of the best-tasting plant-based protein powders in the world. When Wade first tried it, he liked the texture and the taste.

As the company grew, it ran into some trouble with production and the supply chain, so it substituted the fermented rice bran with cheaper ingredients. Wade started to notice some bloating and stomach discomfort. He couldn't digest the product anymore—the new version had caused him to develop a new food sensitivity.

He believes the additives in the new version were the likely culprit. Emulsifiers, excipients, preservatives, coloring, and flavoring are commonly problematic ingredients in protein powder.

Many legal food emulsifiers (soaplike substances) such as xanthan gum, carrageenan, and other texturizers can cause leaky gut and digestive problems. However, natural emulsifiers such as lecithin and egg yolk are typically safe to eat.

Carboxymethylcellulose, carrageenan, and propylene glycol can cause the gut inflammation that contributes to the development of inflammatory bowel disease.[75]

Watch out for these chemical ingredients on food labels:[76]

- Monoglycerides, diglycerides, sucrose esters, polyglycerol esters, and sorbitan esters of fatty acids
- Fatty alcohols
- Saponins
- Stearoyl lactylates
- Propylene and ethylene glycol
- Polyglycerol esters
- Polysorbate 80
- Polyglycerol polyricinoleate

Foods that often contain these emulsifiers and texturizers include:

- Bakery products
- Confectionery
- Dairy
- Fat and oil
- Sauces
- Butter and margarine
- Nut and peanut butters
- Ice cream and ice milk products
- Cream liqueurs
- Milk-based beverages
- Gum
- Soy, nut, oat, and other plant-based milks
- Chocolate
- Convenience foods

Fortunately, many new food brands that avoid harmful ingredients have emerged in the last few years, so we can now enjoy similar items without the dangerous emulsifiers. Learn to read labels. The easiest way to go about eating is to focus on whole and unprocessed foods, and ingredients that don't require a chemistry degree to understand.

Food Coloring

Many food dyes can stimulate the immune system, causing allergic reactions and ADHD. You may find them in any colored foods such as burgers, sausages, drinks, candies, yogurts, condiments, cereals, and even cosmetics.

These colors include:

- Carmine, also called Red #4, FD&C 4, or E120
- Allura red, also called Red #40, FD&C #40, or E129
- Tartrazine, also called Yellow #5, FD&C #5, or E102
- Brilliant blue, also called Blue #1, FD&C #1, or E133

Pesticides and Fungicides

High levels of pesticides, such as dichlorophenols, are associated with sensitization to food allergens.[77] These pesticides in general are hormone disruptors that damage your DNA and nervous system.

THE SOLUTIONS

Elimination Diets

The gold standard to identifying food sensitivities is to do an elimination diet for at least 21 days or long enough for symptoms to subside. During these 21 days, you eliminate food groups that are most likely to be problematic.

After that, you bring back these foods one at a time in increasing doses, for three days each. Monitor for any changes in symptoms.

What to exclude on an elimination diet:

- All sources of gluten, such as wheat, rye, barley, and sauces (which may contain hidden glutens)
- All sources of dairy
- Nuts and seeds*
- Peanuts
- Soy and its derivatives
- Corn and its derivatives
- Sugar and all sweeteners (both natural and synthetic)
- Eggs*
- Fish
- Shellfish
- Coffee, tea, and cacao or chocolate
- Alcohol
- Nightshade plants, including tomatoes, potatoes, tomatillos, peppers, and ground-cherries
- Processed foods that may contain artificial additives
- Citrus fruits
- Vegetable seed oils

What to include:

- Non-nightshade vegetables
- Fruits*
- Gluten-free grains*
- Legumes*
- Coconut and avocados, and their products*
- Herbal teas*
- Animal fats
- Tubers
- Animal proteins

*Some practitioners may suggest excluding or including these depending on your circumstances.

Pros of elimination diets:

- They cover all possible mechanisms through which you could be reacting to foods
- They work well if you have only a few food sensitivities

Cons of elimination diets:

- They require being in tune with and observant of your body to notice changes in symptoms
- They can be difficult to do and take a lot of preparation
- They can be triggering for people with a history of disordered eating and orthorexia
- They may not work well if you happen to include the foods you're sensitive to during your elimination diet
- They may not work well if you're sensitive to food substances that are present in most plants, such as oxalates or salicylates
- The diets can be very restrictive, so following them for a long time can increase the risk of nutrient deficiencies and not eating enough
- Food reintroduction can be confounded by placebo and nocebo effects. In other words, your mindset, perception, and fear of certain foods can create symptoms and give you the false idea that you're sensitive to the food

Food-and-Symptoms Journaling

One of the best ways to notice if your symptoms follow a pattern that could be linked to certain foods is to keep track of your foods and symptoms.

Pro of food journaling:

- Doesn't require you to eat differently

Cons of food journaling:[78]

- Hard to follow through
- You may be reluctant to record your foods in social situations
- Journaling may not capture all the ingredients, especially in food from restaurants

Tests to Optimize Your Diet

How to Test for Food Sensitivities

Most people who are allergic to certain foods know they are, because their symptoms are fairly immediate. However, food sensitivity reactions can be delayed up to 48 hours after ingestion. Sometimes, people can tolerate small amounts of foods they're sensitive to and only react to at higher doses. As a result, many people don't even piece together that foods could be causing their conditions.[79]

While some studies have linked the presence of IgG, IgA, and IgM to foods that cause sensitivity responses, it's totally possible to react to foods without having antibodies to them.

Also, the presence of IgG induces immune tolerance, preventing IgE-mediated food allergies.[80, 81] Therefore, the gold standard for identifying food sensitivities is to do an elimination diet.

There are also other tools, such as food journaling, food sensitivity tests, monitoring heart rates and HRV, and blood tests.

Testing Food Sensitivity via Blood Tests

A few studies have shown that elimination diets based on the presence of IgG improve the symptoms of Crohn's, migraine, and IBS.[82, 83, 84, 85]

However, many studies have found that the presence of IgG antibodies simply indicates the exposure of the immune system to the food. Most people have some IgG antibodies against foods that they eat on a regular basis. If the foods are not causing any symptoms, the presence of IgG antibodies shouldn't be a concern.[86]

Among people with food allergies, the presence of IgG appears to facilitate tolerance and reduce reactions. Therefore, many allergists believe that IgG testing has no clinical value.[87]

If you already have symptoms that may be related to food, testing for antibodies may uncover some sensitivities. Also, if you already have an autoimmune disease, it's possible that eliminating foods for which you have molecular mimicry antibodies may improve your prognosis.[88] These tests can be especially helpful if you are sensitive to foods that are not typically excluded on elimination diets.

Be aware that food sensitivity tests commonly turn up so many positive hits that you're left with no idea what to eat next, but remember that the presence of IgG may not indicate that those foods are problematic. Your body has numerous checks and balances to prevent these immune responses from becoming a problem.

The best way to use test results is to confirm them by temporarily eliminating the foods in question to see if your symptoms resolve, and then bringing them back to see if the symptoms also return.

The food sensitivity testing industry is unregulated, so the tests' quality and results can vary widely. In a study published in *Alternative Medicine Review*, a naturopathic doctor had her blood tested at several different labs, whose resulting lists of food sensitivities disagreed by 79 to 83 percent.[89]

Another issue is that the same foods can trigger immune responses differently in raw and cooked states, and most labs don't test foods in both forms. If you want to run a food sensitivity panel, we recommend Cyrex because of its excellent quality control and ongoing research, and the fact that it tests foods in all the forms that people typically eat.

Also, it is possible to react to foods without having any antibodies to them. So, if some foods are causing you trouble, they are still problematic foods for you even if they turn up negative on tests.

Heart Rate and Heart Rate Variability

Inflammation can increase heart rate while reducing heart rate variability.[90] A Korean study found that elevated C-reactive protein correlates with increased heart rate.[91]

Your autonomic nervous system (that is, your sympathetic and parasympathetic nervous systems) controls how fast your heart beats. Heart rate variability (HRV) refers to the variability of the length of time between your heartbeats.

Power Move: Use HRV to Monitor Your Body's Response to Food

HRV is a very good tool to measure your body's stress response. HRV is a powerful measure of well-being and stress in real time.[92] In the long term, people with persistently lower HRV have a 112 percent higher risk of all-cause mortality.[93] Ideally, you should combine food-and-symptoms journaling with monitoring your HR and HRV, so you can observe the patterns. If drops in your HRV or surges in your heart rate correspond with certain foods, then it's likely the foods aren't good for you.

If you are getting inflammation from any source, your heart rate will temporarily increase, while your HRV may decrease.

Keep in mind, however, that your nervous system reacts to *everything* in real time, so these changes may not be from food-related inflammation. Any changes in diet that your body perceives as stressful, such as cutting carbs or going on a juice cleanse, can tank your HRV.[94]

SUMMARY

Hopefully, this chapter didn't scare you. We're not here to create food fears. If you eat unprocessed foods, the chances are low that you will have problems. It's not about being a health food purist who never touches inflammatory foods; it's more about healing the gut and maximizing your resilience so that you may enjoy these foods occasionally. Never forget: the dose creates the effect.

However, for those who are experiencing any of these issues, solving them can be a lifesaver.

To maximize all three sides of your BIOptimization Triangle, you must lower inflammation in your body. This begins with understanding which types of food reactions you have and to which foods.

Many people suffer from inflammation from food; however, they may not have connected their symptoms with what they eat.

Here are a few common dysfunctions that contribute to food allergies, intolerances, and sensitivities:

- Intestinal permeability (aka leaky gut)
- Reduced immune tolerance and increased inflammatory tendency
- Stress and traumas
- Molecular mimicry

Leaky gut, loss of immune tolerance, and stress and traumas in combination can cause you to develop inflammatory reactions to food.

THREE WAYS YOU CAN HAVE NEGATIVE REACTIONS FROM FOODS:

Food Allergies

The most common food allergies include those to:

- Dairy proteins
- Tree nuts
- Eggs
- Peanuts
- Shellfish
- Wheat
- Soy
- Fish

Food Intolerances

- Lactose intolerance
- Histamine intolerance
- FODMAP intolerance

Food Sensitivities

Other substances in food that may cause inflammation and other health problems (such as gut issues, brain dysfunction, and problems with insulin and blood sugar) include:

- Lectins
- Gluten (whether in a case of celiac disease or not)
- Eggs
- Dairy

Food Toxins and Contaminations

The most common food toxins and contaminations include:

- Mycotoxins
- Food emulsifiers and texturizers
- Organic solvents
- Microbial transglutaminase (mTG)
- Food coloring
- Pesticides and fungicides

There are various ways to test for food sensitivities:

- Elimination diets
- Food-and-symptoms journaling
- Heart rate and heart rate variability
- Blood tests for food sensitivities

CHAPTER 32

DATA SHAPES DESTINIES

Accurate, high-quality, data-driven feedback loops make the difference in the world. Feedback loops will multiply your learning speed and help you maximize your results.

In this chapter, you'll learn:

- How to know if a diet, supplement, or biohack will bring you toward your biological optimization goals
- Our tried-and-true three-step framework that has helped thousands of people achieve biological optimization against all odds
- Critical biofeedback measurements you can take daily for free (or for less than $50)
- Five key tests that provide the most leverage when it comes to improving your health
- The five most powerful health-tracking technologies you need in your BIOptimization journey
- Subjective assessments vs. objective assessments and how to use each to understand what's going on in your body
- The meta-feedback-loop process and how to use it to achieve BIOptimization
- A variety of ways that your personal feeling aligns strongly with data measurements
- What bioimpedance is and why we strongly advise against it
- The importance of capturing good baseline measurements before you start your Biological Optimization Process
- The *most* effective methods for tracking body fat changes that won't cost you a dime
- Why you need to monitor your blood sugar levels and the two different ways you can do so

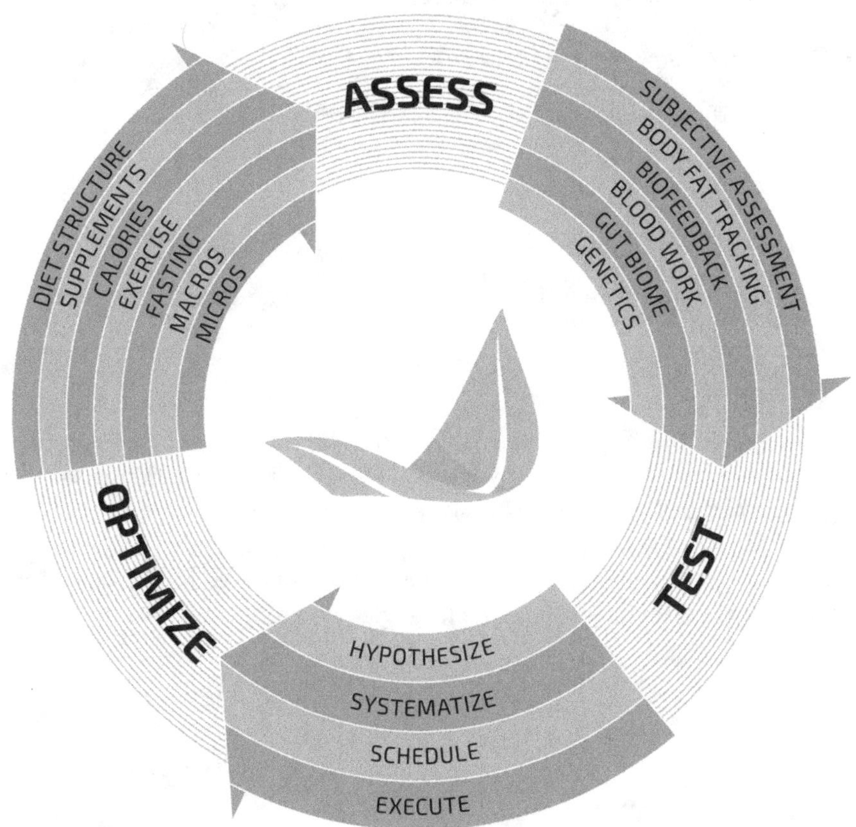

THE BIOLOGICAL OPTIMIZATION PROCESS

As we've shown, there is not one universal diet that works for everyone. You're biologically unique, with your own genetics, life experiences, and personal preferences. Even the best clinical studies cannot predetermine the right combination of nutritional strategies, supplements, exercise, or biohacks that will instantly put you in an optimal metabolic state.

Some of these actions can add incremental gains toward your goals, while others subtract. Make random changes without a system or understanding of biology, and you might end up going nowhere fast (or worse, going backward).

This chapter will give a more scientific, data-driven framework for things that bring you toward your goals while preventing you from wasting time and money on things that set you back.

THE LIFE-CHANGING POWER OF FEEDBACK LOOPS

We've all experienced the power of feedback loops. Your parents telling you, "Don't touch the stove" created a feedback loop. Every test at school was part of a feedback loop that helped you gauge your understanding and memorization of a topic. Every coach you've ever worked with was part of a feedback loop that helped you maximize your performance. Every form of pain creates a feedback loop.

Thanks to exponential biotechnical advances, we can now use technology to give us far more insight than humans could ever gather without it. For example, sleep and fitness trackers offer data that was never available before. This chapter outlines what we feel is a meta-feedback-loop process.

Matt's Shocking Sleep Quality Story

I remember looking at my Oura sleep score that said: zero deep sleep. I kept tracking for a couple of weeks, and the best I would get was 15 minutes. The shocking data didn't stop there.

A DEXA scan showed my body fat at 33 percent. My testosterone had dropped to the 200s. At the time, I wasn't as knowledgeable about sleep and hadn't yet discovered how critical it was for hormone health.

I had a "Eureka!" moment and realized that improving my sleep was the number one thing I could do to improve every part of my life. So, I started investing heavily into mattresses, Faraday cages, cooling mats, pulsed electromagnetic field therapy (PEMF) sleeping tech, air optimizers, and supplements.

Using data from the Oura Ring and DREEM, I've been able to take my deep sleep from 1 hour to 90 minutes with 2 hours of REM per night. The changes to my brain function and overall health have been life changing. This is also why we created the Sleep Potion formula. It took us years of experiments to find the synergistic stack that really moves the needle on sleep quality. Magnesium Breakthrough has been another game changer.

HOW TO GET GOOD MEASUREMENTS AND NOT GET STRESSED OUT

It's important to not get overly obsessed with health data. As Saint Francis of Assisi said, "Wear the world like a loose garment."

1. Compare Apples to Apples

The human body changes from minute to minute. Despite zero change in body composition, you can gain five pounds of pure water and food mass in one hour by just pounding a pizza and drinking soda. In pictures, it's possible to go from looking out of shape to having the physique of a cover model in minutes just by using the right poses and the right lighting.

For data that's usable, always compare apples with apples. Always take your measurements at roughly the same time of day. Use the same devices, the same photography angles, and so on.

2. Understand the Limitations of Each Measurement Technology

There's no such thing as a perfectly objective measurement. For example, all body fat measurements are only estimates and have a lot of room for user variability. You can have perfectly healthy blood tests and still feel awful. Every measurement introduces some errors.

Compared to a full-on clinical sleep study, the Oura Ring has:[1]

- 65 percent agreement in detecting light sleep
- 51 percent agreement in detecting deep sleep
- 61 percent agreement in detecting REM sleep

Therefore, it's important to develop the skills to correlate your subjective measurements and symptoms with the objective test results. The most important thing to know is, are you heading in the right direction?

3. Stay Objective and Patient

After his weekly refeed weekends, Matt's weight might go up by 10 pounds. There's zero worry when he sees this. He knows his weight will be back to normal by Wednesday, and lower still by the following week if he's in a calorie deficit on the weekly window.

It takes time for your body to adapt to nutritional strategies and training. The results often become evident only after a few weeks.

4. The Right Frequency for Data Collection

For fat loss and muscle gain, we suggest measuring by week. However, two to four weeks is the typical amount of time to see any significant change in appearance and body fat measurements if you're starting off with healthy body fat levels.

Biological processes have various cadences. Health markers can take a few months to move in the right direction sometimes. For blood tests, we suggest every three months unless your medical practitioner advises more frequently.

5. Keep an Accurate Journal

Wade would have clients write down their diet, sleep, workout, and every other habit for two weeks before they started his program.

Wade found that most people would say their diet was "pretty good." Yet, after two weeks, they would come back with their heads hanging and say, "Well, I guess it wasn't as good as I thought." Seeing it on paper gave them an objective view.

You're not going to remember your measurements from even yesterday, so journaling will provide you with the data you need to learn about your body and make decisions. For your data to be usable, you need to be disciplined and organized about it, and also document potential sources of variability in your measurements. That's one of the reasons why we created the Me Diet app. We've made it super easy to track all your diet data.

Of course, we take out all of the guessing and use our formulas to design your personalized journey designed with the Me Diet app. Go to www.BIOptimizers.com/book/dietapp to download our app to make your Me Diet journey simple and easy to follow.

6. Work with an Expert

With all of this data, it's easy to do the dance of delusion in the land of confusion. An expert coach will have the wisdom to help you prioritize and maximize. They will keep you on track, minimize distractions, and avoid common pitfalls. We'll talk more about this in the next chapter.

The Kaizen of Becoming a Superhuman

Kaizen is the Japanese term for continuous improvement. Rather than a "one and done" process, Biological Optimization is a never-ending process that consistently leads to improvements.

In the past 20 years, we've coached thousands of clients from all walks of life to achieve Biological Optimization. They were often looking at an uphill battle, against all odds. Thanks to the genius mentors and coaches on our team and the kaizen approach, we've watched client after client enjoy world-class results. And now it's *your* turn.

THE BIOLOGICAL OPTIMIZATION PROCESS IS A THREE-PHASE FEEDBACK LOOP

- Assess the relevant data to get an accurate picture of where you are
- Test by formulating a hypothesis (game plan) before testing new strategies, diets, exercise programs, and more
- Optimize your results by tweaking parameters (diet, supplementation, exercise, technology, and sleep)

The lifelong journey of Biological Optimization will help you continuously improve the three sides of the BIOptimization Triangle: aesthetics, performance, and health.

THE ASSESSMENT PHASE

As legendary CEO Peter Drucker said, "What gets measured gets managed." In other words, if you can't measure it, you can't improve it. To optimize your health, you must assess, measure, and track its subjective and objective data.

There are multiple data sources that must be assessed in this phase to get the most complete possible picture. Remember: the more accurate the data is, the more you can improve. Bad data can lead to bad decisions.

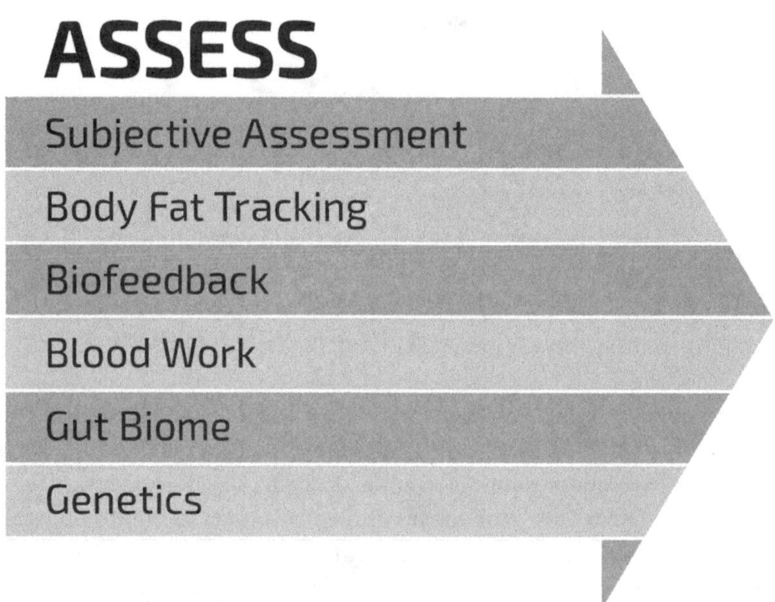

Assessment Factor #1: Subjective Assessments

Subjective assessments are your own qualitative, personal assessment of your:

- Psychological health
- Energy levels
- Mood
- Appearance in the mirror
- Appetite and cravings
- Pain and any other symptoms

Objective Assessments

The next five measurements are all objective. Objective assessment involves measurable data of what's going on in your body, including measurable biofeedback, such as:

- Data from your Oura Ring or fitness trackers
- Biomarker tests
- Body composition measurements

Synching Subjective Biofeedback with Objective Data

We're big believers in synching biofeedback to hard data. One should validate another. This is because neither subjective feelings nor measurements are perfect.

Understanding how your subjective measurements correlate with data can help you understand why you're experiencing symptoms or seeing improvement. Learning to read your body will teach you about the biggest needle-movers for yourself. Sometimes the patterns that keep coming up will give you the biggest insights.

Pay attention to how your personal feeling aligns strongly with data measurements. Some examples include:

- Feeling refreshed after a night of quality sleep. This correlates with high deep sleep scores, high HRV, and low resting heart rate
- Sensations in your body (fatigue or feeling cold) that indicate your body temperature's dropping when you're in an aggressive caloric deficit—such as your feet getting cold easily
- Feeling excessively sore and tired when your HRV is low the day after hard training
- Having a better mood and cognitive function once your HRV improves
- Feeling fewer cravings once your sleep and nutrition status become optimized
- Satiety and soreness responses to different macros, fiber intake, training intensity, and sleep quality

As you become more experienced in your BIOptimization journey, you will become more in tune with your body. Your subjective assessments will dramatically improve when you connect the body's sensations to hard data. As a result, you may need fewer measurements over time.

Throughout this chapter, we'll share our experience on these correlations that we observe with ourselves or our clients.

The Importance of Getting a Good Baseline

It's crucial to capture your baseline data as early as possible. You'll regret not doing this later if you don't. We understand the natural aversion to capturing your baseline when you're at your worst, but it's the best time. This is the baseline that helps create all of the dopamine loops that will empower you later.

Capture as much data as you can: pictures, tape measurement, full blood panel, body fat percentage, fitness levels, sleep quality, and so on.

Keep in mind that wearables (such as the Oura Ring or a fitness tracker) don't come with standard normal values, because everyone is different. To optimize your biology, first collect and assess your data at baseline. Then compare your progress to your baseline starting point as you go through the Biological Optimization Cycles.

Assessment Factor #2: Aesthetics (Body Fat and Lean Muscle)

Lowering your body fat is one of the most powerful things you can do to improve your health and aesthetics and—in many cases—athletic performance.

Measuring body fat isn't an exact science, and that doesn't matter. What we are tracking is the overall direction of progress. Are we losing body fat or not? If we are, we're winning. If not, let's make some modifications.

The Gold Standard for Body Composition Measurement

Out of all available body fat assessment techs, we believe that the dual-energy X-ray absorptiometry (DEXA) scan is the most reliable. DEXA scans will give you both body composition and bone density assessment, which is important for health span and longevity. It also helps track whether or not you're gaining fat. We recommend against other methods of body fat testing other than body fat calipers and hydrostatic weighing.

Your glycogen and hydration levels can increase lean body mass on your DEXA scan results. So, whatever condition you're in when you go, make sure it's the same every time. If you go carb loaded, always be carb loaded at every rescan. Aim to go the same time of day, the same day of the week every time (especially if you're doing refeeds). Otherwise, you'll see massive fluctuations in lean body mass that aren't accurate. Matt personally goes in two days after carb loading every time to standardize things and prevent bad data from emerging.

If you cannot access a DEXA scan, you may need to use the skinfold caliper, hydrostatic weighing, or Bod Pod methods. Body circumference measurements and pictures are also helpful pieces of data to track your progress.

We strongly caution against bioimpedance, which puts a small amount of electrical current through your body to estimate how much fat you have. These devices include scales in which you stand on two metal pads or hold metal joysticks. Bioimpedance doesn't measure the whole body. It can also give massive fluctuations in readings within the same day, even with high-end devices, making it a poor tool to track progress and performance. Matt was once able to manipulate the results of a $500 bioimpedance scale by 70 percent in the same day. They're borderline worthless in our opinion.

Visit Chapter 4, The Five Epic Journeys You Can Take with Your Body, to see what various levels of body fat look like.

Five Basic Aesthetics Measurements for Under $50

If you don't have access to a DEXA, there are some inexpensive options. Anybody can use the five most important basic measurements to track their diet results, which combined cost less than $50.

1. Pictures

How you look can be a good indicator of your body fat, muscle mass, and health status. It goes along with other pieces of data, such as body composition measurements. You should take pictures in the same space with the same lighting and same angle at the same time of day.

2. Clothing Fit

Pay attention to how your clothes feel. Are they tighter or looser? If you're building muscle, then a tighter T-shirt around the chest, shoulders, and arms is a good sign. If you're losing weight, looser pants and tighter beltlines are telling you you're winning.

3. Tape Measurements

Tape measurements are arguably the second-best way to measure results. It's objective and you can track small changes. It's effective for tracking both muscle gain and fat loss.

Here are the areas we suggest measuring:

1. Neck
2. Shoulders
3. Arms: right and left
4. Shoulders
5. Chest
6. Ribs
7. Waist
8. Hips
9. Legs: right and left
10. Calves: right and left

Once you're used to it, it just takes two minutes to measure your whole body. You can use the Me Diet app to help track your gains.

4. Body Fat Calipers

Body fat calipers can be a good way of tracking your body fat by pinching your skinfolds. Always use a spring-loaded caliper, because without the spring, it's easy to either push too hard or not hard enough, introducing more human error. The nine sites include abdomen, biceps, calf, kidney, pectoral, quadricep, subscapula, suprailiac, and triceps.

5. Scale

The scale provides an excellent piece of data that should be correlated with other measurements and observations to gauge where you're at with your lean and fat mass.

If someone is over 250 pounds, the scale is probably going to be their best friend. This is because they can lose a lot of weight pretty fast.

Either way, it's critical to take into account and minimize sources of variability when you weigh yourself. Step on the scale first thing in the morning before you eat. Weigh yourself daily and learn to become unemotional about the scale.

It's totally normal to have a few pounds of weight fluctuation from shifts in glycogen, intestinal bulk (poop), salt, sodium, water retention, and more. If you don't take these normal variabilities into account, the measurements will mess with your head and discourage your efforts. Some people panic, dialing up their workouts and doing extreme dieting. Others quit and binge on cookies and ice cream. Know that the scale is just a tool with a lot of natural variety.

Power Move: Using Scale and Tape Measurements to Track Body Fat Changes

The scale by itself isn't a great tool, especially if you're building lean muscle mass (which we recommend). However, pairing the scale with tape measurements is an awesome system to track progress. The tape shows fat areas are going down, you're making epic gains, even when the scale says your weight didn't change.

When people are near their ultimate aesthetic goal, we often shoot for body recomposition, which means your weight stays the same while your body fat lowers and lean mass increases. If your weight is the same but the tape measurements are shrinking in your fattiest areas like hips and waist, you know you're losing body fat and gaining muscle.

Assessment Factor #3: Biofeedback Technologies

Biofeedback is a fast-growing space with many exciting new technologies emerging. These tracking technologies are unlocking new levels of optimization opportunity.

Sleep Tracking

Here's a short list of options:

Oura Ring

The Oura Ring tracks overnight heart rate, heart rate variability, body temperature, respiratory rates, and overnight movement. With these pieces of data, it estimates your sleep stages and calculates your recovery score. You may find that light exposure, electronic devices, and your stress levels influence your sleep quality.

Your overall sleep quality will affect your appetite, craving, energy levels, and more. Conversely, eating foods that don't agree with your body, eating too close to bedtime, or blood sugar problems can interfere with your sleep.

DREEM

The most direct measurement of sleep stages involves measuring your brain waves using an electroencephalogram (EEG). DREEM is a product that tracks EEG along with sound, movement, pulse, breathing disturbances, brain activity, and body temperature through a headband.

Fitness Tracking

Apple Watch, Biostrap, and Fitbit

These devices could help you track your nonexercise energy expenditure and overall activity levels. They also track steps, heart rate, and HRV, which are useful parameters.

Serious, hard-training athletes can use these technologies to give them objective feedback and see if their VO_2 max (a measurement of the cardio system) is improving. Runners and cyclists use these technologies to track their speed and power output. The tech all helps create motivating dopamine loops that drive performance.

Brain Optimization

Neurofeedback (brain training) technology accurately monitors and measures brain waves to help you increase mental resilience from home. You can access a wide variety of states with this, from calm and alert to Zen-master states.

The brain generates electrical signals, which this device can detect via its seven electroencephalography (EEG) sensors. It sends the brainwave data to your phone via Bluetooth, and its app analyzes whether your mind is relaxed or active. You can review the results to understand what is happening inside your head. This helps you create a plan to optimize your brain (i.e., whether you need to shift into parasympathetic or sympathetic mode).

There is one device that we recommend above all others. A company we've invested in has created the first medical-grade home unit. It's a game changer, and you can learn more at the link below. Best of all, it is dry (no goop in your hair!), and all you need is a mobile device to run it—no more lugging around expensive computers. This means you can train on a plane or a car-sharing ride. Go to www.BIOptimizers.com/book/neurofeedback to learn more.

The EmWave2: Heart Coherence Optimization

This handheld device has an integrated pulse sensor to measure your heart rhythm and guides you to breathe in and out every five seconds to determine the state of your nervous system. If you're stressed out, it will guide you through breathing techniques to synchronize your breathing and heart rate to reach a relaxed state of mind. It allows you to train your body to be in a state called *coherence*. You'll be a more resilient, grounded person when you develop the ability to live in this state.

Assessment Factor #4: Biomarkers

For health and performance optimization purposes, you're going to need to take snapshots of your biomarkers using blood and other medical tests. We suggest getting blood tests every three months during phases of transformation. If you're in homeostasis, then every six months is enough.

Keep in mind that blood tests are snapshots of a dynamic system. Each metabolite you test has its own natural fluctuations. Hopefully in the near future, we'll have access to constant data streams of all our key biomarkers.

Fasted vs. Non-Fasted Bloodwork

The standard way to test is fasted bloodwork, where you go get a blood draw in the morning before eating. Markers like glucose, cholesterol, triglycerides, and insulin tend to respond to meals, so you see numbers that have leveled off overnight. If you test them without fasting, these numbers will be elevated, and you should consider them as responses to meals.

However, HbA1c, kidney, liver, thyroid, blood cell counts, and many other markers are stable even after meals. It's becoming more common to do non-fasted bloodwork to track the response to foods.

Blood Sugar Optimization

Chronically elevated blood sugar levels accelerate aging and can lead to dangerous diseases like diabetes. This is why monitoring blood sugar levels is a good idea. Currently, there are two different technologies that can give you instant or near-instant glucose levels.

Snapshot Glucose Monitoring

The most common type of blood sugar testing is finger pricking. You get a reading within seconds. This option is readily available wherever home medical supplies are sold.

Constant Glucose Monitoring

This metabolic health tracker is a continuous glucose monitor (CGM) placed on your arm. It syncs to an app on your phone and uses machine learning to optimize your metabolic fitness. It tracks your blood glucose in real time so you can see how your body responds to the food you eat and different daily activities. It allows you to make smarter nutritional decisions and upgrade your diet.

The true power of the CGM feedback loop is in two things:

- A 24-hour view of your blood sugar levels
- Learning your blood sugar response from every meal

Running a CGM for one to two months will give you very powerful learnings. You'll know which foods you should avoid or minimize and which ones your body thrives on.

Advanced Metabolic Health Lab Tests

Men's health, performance, and aesthetics expert Paul Maximus, N.D., routinely uses the following lab tests:

General Screening

These are common screening tests you can get from your general practitioner:

- *Fasting glucose.* A measure of your insulin sensitivity and ability to handle carbs
- *Fasted insulin.** Gives a fuller picture of your blood sugar regulation than fasting glucose alone (for example, it is possible to have normal fasting glucose but very high insulin, which means that you are insulin resistant)
- *Cholesterol.* Assesses your metabolic health, risk of heart disease and Alzheimer's disease, and many other conditions
- *Liver function tests.* Watches for GGT* (gamma-glutamyl transferase), other liver enzymes, and some proteins in your blood (GGT is the best indicator of health and your oxidative stress level)
- *Kidney function tests.* Screen for any issues with your kidneys, including diabetes and hypertension
- *Complete blood count.* Screens for anemia, some nutrient deficiencies, blood disorders, and infections

*In a general checkup, your doctor will typically not order GGT or fasted insulin, so you will have to specifically request them.

Homeostatic Model Assessment (HOMA-IR)

HOMA-IR is calculated from fasting glucose and fasting insulin. It is used to assess beta (insulin-producing) cell function and insulin resistance. A low value means you're insulin sensitive, as you only need a small amount of insulin to keep your blood sugar in balance.

SpectraCell Micronutrient Test

This test checks for your micronutrient status over a three-to-six-month time window. Your blood is split into 30 different sample tubes to test for micronutrients like vitamin C, calcium, magnesium, chromium, and more. This test also looks at your metabolism, oxidative stress, and immune response.

Protein Unstable Lesion Signature (PULS)

PULS estimates your heart attack risk by measuring the traces of proteins that leak from heart lesions in the blood vessel walls, along with HDL, inflammatory proteins, and HbA1c. Based on this, the report estimates your heart age and likelihood of getting a heart attack in the next five years.

Dried Urine Test for Comprehensive Hormones (DUTCH)

DUTCH provides a very illuminating snapshot of your stress response, circadian rhythm, hormone levels, metabolism, and toxic hormone metabolites. It is a noninvasive urine test where you send in dried filter papers saturated with your urine samples. We recommend the DUTCH Complete, which includes both adrenal and sex hormones. The test also looks for neurotransmitters, vitamins, melatonin, and oxidative stress markers in your urine.

The four-point daily cortisol pattern assesses your stress response and circadian rhythm, which could also be abnormal due to inflammation. The ratio of stress hormones to prohormones (DHEA-S and pregnenolone) can tell whether your stress is stealing the resources from your sex hormone production, causing hormone imbalances.

Last, your toxic hormone metabolites and your hormone metabolism pattern may explain some hormonal symptoms such as hair loss, low libido, weight gain, or acne. Some toxic metabolites increase cancer risks. The DUTCH report also tells you which pathways are responsible for these hormonal issues, so you can address them naturally.

Assessment Factor #5: Gut Biome

The 100 trillion bacteria in your large intestine work like an extra organ that masterminds all aspects of your health. A rich and diverse microbiota full of friendly species will keep you lean, healthy, happy, and resilient. Conversely, lacking a diverse microbiome and having more unfriendly strains can keep you suboptimal or sick.[2]

Biome tests can assess the bacteria in your gut. They also tell you which foods are best for your good bacteria and which ones feed the bad. Understanding your bacteria can help you optimize your diet for the optimal microbiome. The key is to eat and live right for your microbiome.

P3-OM, Biome Breakthrough, and Cognibiotics are three of the most powerful solutions to optimize your gut health. We discuss the best gut biome test in Chapter 29.

Assessment Factor #6: Epigenetics

As we've said, your genes load the gun, while your environment pulls the (epigenetic) trigger. New, cutting-edge aging tests, like TruAge, can measure your epigenetic age. It's another powerful tool in your BIOptimization toolbox. Make sure to refer to Chapter 33 to learn which diets are helpful for each gene.

THE TESTING PHASE

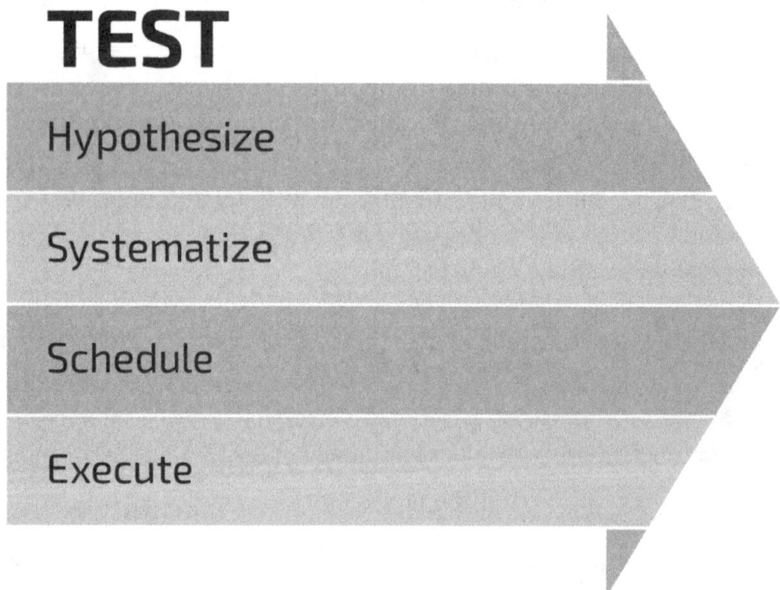

This important early data allows us to move on to the testing phase, where we follow an n = 1 scientific game plan to see which ways optimize your biology.

We recommend working with a knowledgeable coach to help you create a winning game plan and keep you accountable, plus troubleshoot as problems arise. Even the most self-motivated athletes achieve better results with a coach's support. See the Jedi Council discussion on page 259 to learn more. Or go to www.BIOptimizers.com/book/coaching.

Testing Factor #1: Hypothesize

Hypothesizing involves formulating the best game plan possible that will lead to the desired outcome. The changes you make could be in your exercise, supplement stack, diet, biohacking technologies, or lifestyle. An experienced coach can hypothesize based on preexisting science, their clinical experience, and your data.

Testing Factor #2: Systematize

An unfortunate—but guaranteed—way to fail is to do what you feel like doing, or to change your plans randomly. The lack of a system will cause confusion and prevent results. And trying too many changes at once makes it impossible to know which changes produce results.

Systematization is all about creating a great game plan. Make sure you have a systematized exercise, nutrition, and supplementation program. Systematize whatever approach you incorporate into your Biological Optimization journey.

Testing Factor #3: Schedule

Failing to plan is planning to fail. To ensure success, you must plan it into your schedule. For you to do this effectively, we recommend using your preferred calendar app (Google Calendar and Outlook are the most popular).

Success = plan and build a routine, and stick to it:

- Put your workouts in your schedule
- Plan your diet and prep your food for the week
- Create your supplement stack on paper and stick it on your fridge door
- Preload your pills into a weekly pill case when possible

Testing Factor #4: Execute

Executing the game plan is the most important part. Even a poorly executed plan is better than the greatest plan on earth that stays as an idea on paper. "Action over perfection" is a key mindset, especially for perfectionists. The goal is to just get started. Build momentum and don't stop. Don't worry, we will optimize and improve everything later.

THE OPTIMIZATION PHASE

During this phase, we optimize certain parameters for the best results. By monitoring the data, we can tweak the variables to improve results. The biological levers for optimization include diet structure, caloric intake, fasting, managing macros and minerals, supplements, exercise programming, and sleep.

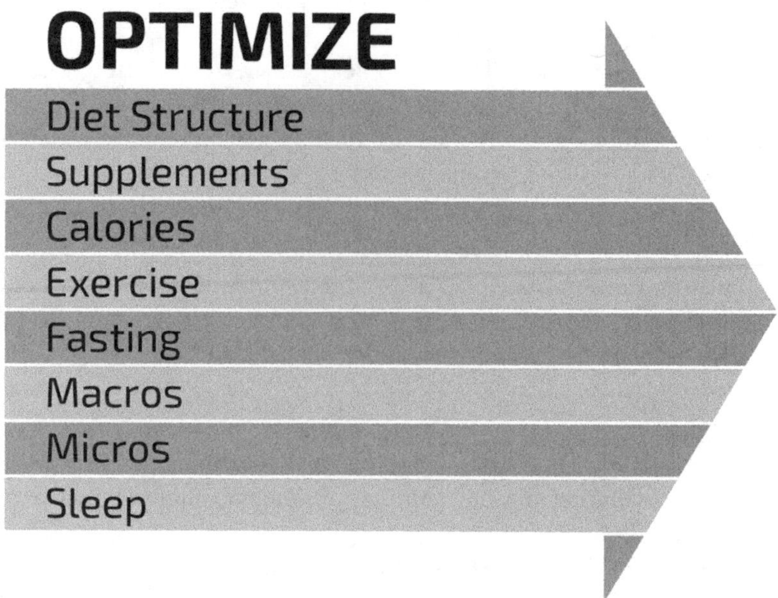

Optimize Diet Structure and Nutrition

Diet structure is the kind of diet you choose. Are you going to follow a ketogenic diet; a high-carb, low-fat diet; a paleo diet; or some other type?

What macronutrient composition is best for you? Typically, high protein, along with a caloric surplus, improves muscle anabolism during a muscle-building phase. It also preserves muscle tissue when your body operates in a caloric deficit.

Manipulating carbs and fats can also be important to help you achieve your goals. As we've noted, every diet works for a while, including high-carb, low-fat diets and high-fat, low-carb diets, as long as you're in a caloric deficit. However, the best macro balance for you may depend on your genetics and your environment, which is why we periodically reassess.

Matt tracked his calories and hunger on keto vs. when he was eating carbs. He found that a keto diet saves him from the insatiable cravings of the blood sugar roller coaster:

eat carbs → blood sugar spike → released insulin → low blood sugar → cravings

Keto helps keep blood sugar levels stable. For many people, keto definitely works best for craving control. If Matt hadn't tracked that data, he wouldn't know what was best for his body. This book will help you select the right diet structure for *you*.

Optimize Supplements

We discuss supplements extensively in this book. And that's not an accident. Supplements can help you maximize the results of your efforts, especially when optimized for your design.

Some supplements are beneficial on an ongoing basis, while others work better being cycled or front-loaded in high doses. It is essential to reassess the impact of your supplement protocol with data, as some supplements can throw off your systems and set you back.

Optimize Calories

Your caloric intake is a biological lever with a massive impact on your results in muscle building, fat loss, athletic performance, and—potentially—longevity. Gaining muscle mass requires a caloric surplus. Losing body fat requires a caloric deficit. If your goal is longevity, then a slight caloric deficit might be beneficial. If you're an athlete, then "food is fuel," as the saying goes, and you need to fuel your body for hard workouts and recovery.

Optimize Exercise

Exercise includes all types of movements we've covered, as well as resistance training. These have massive effects and impact on all three sides of the BIOptimization Triangle: aesthetics, performance, and health goals. We could write an entire book on the ultimate exercise system. To get free training programs, download our BIOptimized app.

The key to optimizing exercise is to track your key objective. Key metrics include:

- Adding lean muscle mass
- Losing body fat
- Increasing strength and power
- Increasing endurance
- Increasing ability and coordination

Our suggestion is to have *only one core focus at a time.* If you're in a complex sport like mixed martial arts, this might not be feasible. However, certain key factors can still be prioritized during each training cycle.

Tracking Your Stress

A parasympathetic nervous system state is usually about rest, recovery, and healing, whereas a sympathetic one is fight, flight, and freeze. You can measure sympathetic and parasympathetic activation with a heart rate variability measurement tool (more on this later in the chapter).

People who are stuck in parasympathetic could be in sloth mode. It's hard for them to wake up and get going, whereas some people are stuck in sympathetic hypervigilance. They are usually aggressive and stressed out, which leads to burnout.

Being in a prolonged caloric deficit is stressful to the body. So is increased training volume. Under these stresses, some people become more emotional or emotionally sensitive. Others will develop anger or aggression issues. Some people become dissociated and look glazed over. Burning out and being overly stressed usually leads to quitting. This is why it's important to track your stress levels.

Pay attention to and journal your emotional states. Are you getting short and angry with people? Are you more emotionally reactive? Do you get frustrated or more fatigued? Do you struggle with attention and focus? If you answered yes to any of these questions, it might be time for a diet break to help you reboot.

Optimize Your Feeding/Fasting Window

Your fasting protocol and feeding window are another optimization parameter to prioritize. Fasting overnight every day is important for autophagy and rejuvenation. You may find that extending your fasting window delivers more health benefits, such as fat loss, improved insulin sensitivity, and improved performance. Again, some people have genetics that help them thrive on fasting, whereas for others it's a stressor.

Optimize Macros

Optimizing macros is another powerful lever, especially when people are dieting or trying to gain lean muscle.

The best approach when dieting is to increase and maintain high protein levels while decreasing calories from fats and carbs. This has several benefits: you can prevent excess lean muscle loss by keeping your protein optimized, and your net caloric intake from food will lower because of the thermic effect of protein. Both of these are crucial for fat loss.

For muscle building, increasing protein can sometimes lead to better gains. For sports, optimizing for energy and on-field performance is the key. For some endurance sports, adding ketones can be a needle-moving upgrade. Ketones can also help optimize brain performance, especially during taxing times. You can think of them as another macro.

Hydration Levels

Water is your best friend, period. Being sufficiently hydrated is the biggest factor to implement any diet successfully. You want to drink what you might consider an excessive amount of water. Bodybuilders are very cognizant of staying hydrated and drinking water throughout the day to offset food cravings and hunger.

When Wade was running his clinic, he tested a group of clients in a friend's facility using an electro-interstitial water scan. He found that virtually everyone was dehydrated. He would see that various organs weren't fully hydrated.

When Matt was running his sleep-deprivation experiment, getting four to five hours of sleep in his 20s, he had to drink water every 20 minutes to stay awake. If he didn't have the water, he'd start crashing and nodding off. So, he became aware of how critical water is for his energy. It makes a huge difference.

Digestion

Optimal digestion is critical for your success, so pay close attention to it. Any digestive symptoms could be signs that some food doesn't agree with you. They could also indicate insufficient enzymes, dysbiosis, or more serious underlying problems.

Common digestive symptoms include:

- *Acid reflux and heartburn.* These are quite common after the age of 30 as hydrochloric acid levels in the stomach decrease (it does happen to younger people as well). Sometimes there are food triggers, but acid reflux and heartburn are usually because of low stomach acid. One exception is when it's caused by hiatal hernia, so you should rule that out.
- *Bloating and gas.* These are signs of gut dysbiosis, but they could also be due to lack of enzymes or food sensitivities. They mean your body struggles to break down some food, especially dairy, gluten, and high-fat meals. You can hack these with Gluten Guardian for gluten and dairy, and kApex for high-fat meals.
- *Bowel frequency.* A rule of thumb is typically one bowel movement per meal. If you eat three meals a day, usually it's three bowel movements. However, this can depend on the fiber content of the diet. If you're on a lower-fiber diet or eating significantly less, you may have fewer bowel movements.
  - Constipation could be a sign of poor diet or disrupted thyroid.
  - Quality of stool. Paul Chek considers stool quality one of the most important markers of health. It reflects your autonomic nervous system balance, digestive functions, and even mental health.[3] You want to shoot for types 3 or 4 on the Bristol stool chart.

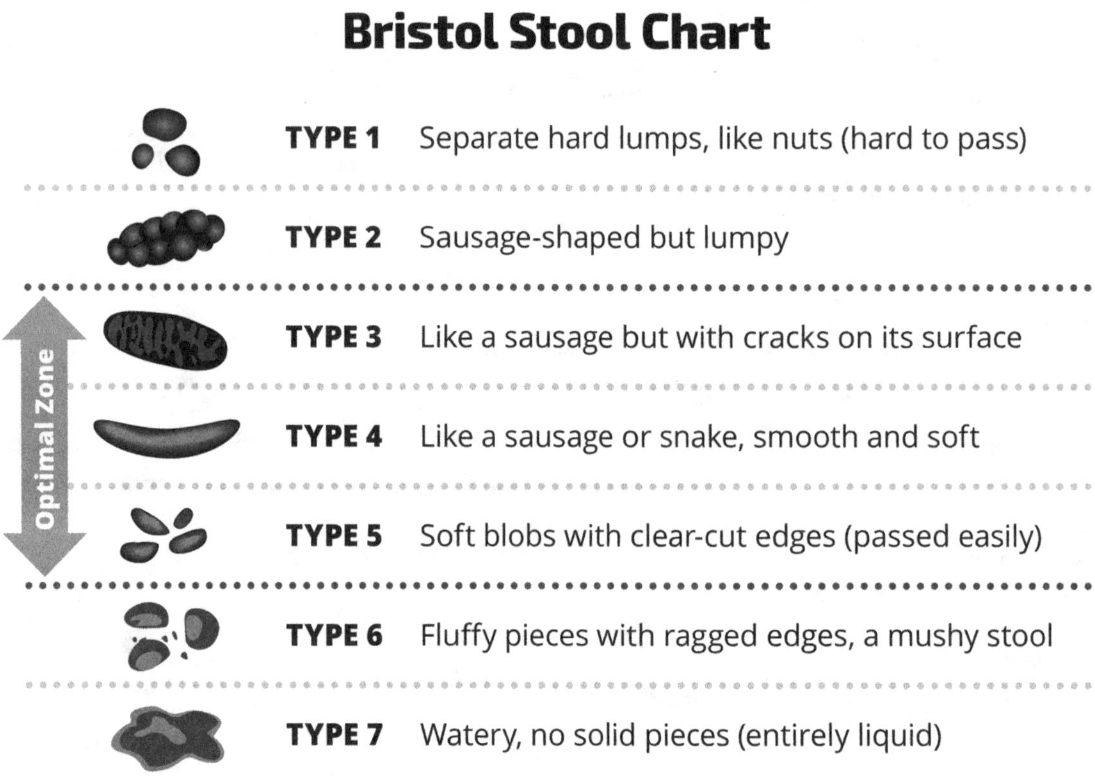

Bristol Stool Chart

TYPE 1	Separate hard lumps, like nuts (hard to pass)
TYPE 2	Sausage-shaped but lumpy
TYPE 3	Like a sausage but with cracks on its surface
TYPE 4	Like a sausage or snake, smooth and soft
TYPE 5	Soft blobs with clear-cut edges (passed easily)
TYPE 6	Fluffy pieces with ragged edges, a mushy stool
TYPE 7	Watery, no solid pieces (entirely liquid)

Optimal Zone

Optimize Micronutrients

Last, micronutrients, including trace minerals, vitamins, and other nutrients, are essential for your health, aesthetics, and performance. If you can't get optimal levels from your diet, you must supplement them. Unfortunately, it can be tough to get proper levels from our food supply. This is where getting the proper nutrient testing is key.

Cravings can also be related to low nutrient levels. Being low in important essential minerals can drive salty cravings. That's why we suggest incorporating sea salt, Magnesium Breakthrough, and potassium sources to help reduce salty snack seeking.

Listening to Your Skin and Nails

The skin is the largest detox organ, so if you have trouble metabolizing a particular food or if your food isn't agreeing with you, it tends to show up in your skin. Also, skin problems reflect gut inflammation, dysbiosis, and food sensitivities even when you have no digestive symptoms.[4]

When your blood sugar is too high, the skin ages quickly due to advanced glycation end products (AGEs). As we age, AGE molecules accumulate in the dermis and end up destroying the support cushion of the skin formed by elastin and collagen. Also, acne may be a sign of poor blood sugar and insulin control.[5] In fact, many bodybuilders struggle with acne from the insulinogenic and inflammatory effects of whey protein.

Going on a prolonged caloric deficit or having essential fat deficiencies can result in dry and dull skin, or flares of skin problems. If you're deficient in minerals, you may get lines in your fingernails, and your nails may become brittle. This can be due to a silica deficiency.

Optimize Sleep

Tracking sleep is critical for any diet and all aspects of health and performance. Sleep helps you burn fat, control your appetite, build and maintain muscle mass, and balance your hormones.[6, 7] The research is clear that sleep deprivation or excessive sleep (more than eight hours per day) are predictors of all-cause mortality.[8]

Sleep Study

Currently, no consumer devices can diagnose sleep problems. An in-depth diagnostic sleep study requires spending a night in a sleep lab hooked up to machines. The in-depth sleep tests are designed to diagnose sleep disorders, including central and obstructive sleep apnea, sleep-disordered breathing, narcolepsy, sleep behavior disorders, and chronic insomnia. If left untreated, sleep disorders will derail your diet results and affect all aspects of your health.

You should speak to your doctor about a sleep study if you suspect you may have a sleep disorder or can't seem to improve your sleeping habits in other ways. Check out the sleep chapter in our book *From Sick to Superhuman* for a detailed guide on sleep optimization.

THE NEVER-ENDING JOURNEY

The journey never ends. After you have implemented the Testing and Optimization phases for long enough to affect your physiology, it's time to reassess your body fat, biofeedback, bloodwork, and gut biome to see what changes are happening.

The data will show whether your hypothesis was good or not, and where you might need to refine or change it. Then you will follow the same process to test and optimize again. It's how you take your health, performance, and aesthetics to elite levels.

One of our core values at BIOptimizers is to test, learn, grow, and evolve. That core value is the force that drives the Biological Optimization Process. Humans are testing things, we're learning about ourselves, we're growing, and we're enjoying our results.

Successful BIOptimization requires knowledge, wisdom, discipline, and, often, problem-solving by experienced experts. Studies have also shown that accountability makes people 65 percent more likely to adhere and follow through with whatever diet and strategy they're using.[9]

This is why we offer our coaching to those who are serious about their journey into Biological Optimization. Visit www.BIOptimizers.com/book/coaching for more information.

As you can see, acquiring and keeping track of biofeedback is key to successful BIOptimization. Now let's deep dive in on how to work with biofeedback, understand its pros and cons, and avoid common pitfalls.

SUMMARY

Accurate, high-quality, data-driven feedback loops will multiply your learning speed and help you maximize your results.

Our experience and expertise have culminated in this three-phase feedback loop:

1. Assess the relevant data to get an accurate picture of where you are
2. Formulate a hypothesis or "game plan" and then test your new strategies, diets, exercise programs, and more
3. Optimize by tweaking parameters (diet, supplementation, exercise, technology, and sleep)

Assess

- Assessment Factor #1: Subjective Assessments
  - Subjective assessments are your own qualitative, self-reported assessment of your:
    - Psychological health
    - Energy levels
    - Mood
    - Appearance in the mirror
    - Appetite and cravings
    - Pain and any other symptoms
  - Objective assessments involve measuring data to see what's going on in your body, including measurable biofeedback such as:
    - Data from your Oura Ring or fitness trackers
    - Lab tests
    - Body composition measurements
    - And much more
- Assessment Factor #2: Body Fat
  - Lowering your body fat is one of the most powerful things you can do to improve your health and aesthetics and, in many cases, performance.
- Assessment Factor #3: Biofeedback
    - Biofeedback is a fast-growing space with many exciting new technologies emerging.
- Assessment Factor #4: Blood and Other Tests for Health Optimization
- Assessment Factor #5: Gut Biome
- Assessment Factor #6: Genetics

Test

- Testing Factor #1: Hypothesize
- Testing Factor #2: Systematize
- Testing Factor #3: Schedule
- Testing Factor #4: Execute

Optimize

- Diet structure and nutrition
- Supplements
- Calories
- Exercise
- Feeding and fasting window
- Macros
- Micronutrients
- Sleep

If you want to have an idea of the pinnacle of this process, Google "Bryan Johnson Blueprint." We applaud Bryan for doing what he's doing and sharing it with the world. He's running the ASSESS, TEST, OPTIMIZE process at the highest level. We share similar views with Bryan, and we are united in our goal to bring Biological Optimization to the world. It's one of our missions to make all of these processes faster, cheaper, and more powerful for you. We will not stop until BIOptimization is available and affordable to everyone on earth.

CHAPTER 33

NUTRIGENOMICS: CHOOSING THE PERFECT DIET FOR YOUR GENETICS

by Dr. Nattha Wannissorn, Ph.D., and Katrine Volynsky

Our client Tim (not his real name) was a health nut. He was up to date with his health and all the health trends.

When he started working with us, he was following an intermittent fasting regimen and doing hours of cardio every day. He was on a pescatarian diet and doing too much high-intensity interval training for his body to properly recover. As a result, he wasn't getting where he wanted to be. He was catabolic, losing muscle mass, tired, and couldn't sleep properly.

We found that he had the Mediterranean version of the PPARG gene, which made fasting a poor fit for him. People with this variant respond better to more frequent meals because there is food all year round in the Mediterranean. Fasting can be too stressful for someone with his genetics.

With his FUT2 gene, he was predisposed to problems with histamine and undermethylation. He also had compromises in the glutathione (GSH and GSMT) detoxification pathways, so he was more likely to store the heavy metal from the fish he was eating. These issues were creating a lot of oxidative stress. His mercury levels were off the charts. We focused on helping his body remove the heavy metal by supporting the compromised pathways, along with using binders and saunas.

Yet, he had genes that made him do well with saturated fats despite the health history of cardiovascular issues that had caused him to cut off red meat. So, we brought back some red meat and cut out the fish.

He also had genetic variants associated with making better gains by lifting heavier weights, so we adjusted his program.

He switched back to the higher-carb and more frequent feeding of the Mediterranean diet. He's now in the best shape of his life. He's got more muscle mass, he's the leanest ever, and he has more energy throughout the day.

In this chapter, you will learn:

- How to harness the power of nutrigenomics to make the right nutritional decisions
- Why your genes *are not* your destiny when you understand and work with them
- How to overcome bad genes with the right nutritional strategies and biohacks
- How to maximize your good genes and avoid genetic pitfalls when following each dietary pattern
- Pitfalls to avoid with nutrigenomics

The purpose of this chapter is to equip you with tools to move the movable levers in the context of your unchangeable genes. In most cases, you can make up for your genetic weaknesses and thrive despite them. This allows you to prioritize happiness, core values, and goals over your genes in the hierarchy of nutritional decisions.

Every diet produces different results for everyone, because everyone has different genes and genetic mutations. We're all genetically 0.1 percent different, but that's enough to make us all look different and respond differently to foods.

This book is about helping you understand your uniqueness and how to make the best of it. Inevitably, this involves understanding your genes and how they manifest.

Warning: this chapter is incredibly dense with science. If you don't care about the science and just want get the practical benefits of nutrigenomics, then go to: www.BIOptimizers.com/book/genes.

WHAT IS NUTRIGENOMICS?

Nutrigenomics is the study of how your genetic variants influence your body's response to nutrition and lifestyle choices.

However, it's not as simple as just using genes to predict the best diet for you because of this equation:

Your Health, Aesthetics, and Performance =
Genetics + Epigenetics + Microbiome + Exposome
(Exposomes include all health-related exposure,
including nutrition, fitness, and lifestyle.)

Your genes load the gun, while your epigenetics, microbiome, and exposome pull the trigger. This can turn your genes either off or on.

Understanding how the gun is loaded can be very helpful, but you also need to look at whether the gene is on or off.

One of the easiest ways to do this is to zoom in on an area of health, aesthetics, or performance that you want to improve. Then, look at genes that affect your nutrition in the categories of health, aesthetics, and performance. You want to start from your phenotype and look at genes that may explain it, given your current nutrition, lifestyle, and other exposomes.

You have more than 20,000 genes and 3 million genetic variants. Finding a variant responsible for your problem can be like finding a needle in a haystack. So don't go looking at your genetic variants without knowing your goals and your phenotype.

Katrine Volynsky, health researcher and nutrigenomic expert, uses the following steps:

Step 1: A very in-depth intake process that looks at:

- Symptoms
- Personality
- Environmental exposures
- Childhood history
- Food preferences
- Family history of health issues (especially on the maternal side, since everyone gets their mitochondria from their mothers)

Step 2: Lab tests to look at deeper-level phenotypes and biochemistry, such as:

- Organic acid test to look at how your body processes neurotransmitters and amino acids
- Micronutrient level tests, such as the SpectraCell test
- Gut tests for infections, dysbiosis, inflammation, and leaky gut

These pieces of information give you a snapshot of the outputs of your epigenetic and gut microbiome, which Katrine then uses to zoom in on the genetics.

Caveats of Reading Genes

Nutrigenomics is an emerging science. New discoveries are being made constantly. It's one of the most promising new branches of biological optimization, but we have much to learn.

Most nutrigenomic studies are "genome-wide association studies." They look for variants that are found more frequently in people who have a certain phenotype to "associate" the variants with the phenotype. However, although you'll find umbrellas along with rain, it doesn't mean umbrellas *cause* rain. Therefore, variants associated with a phenotype may not cause the phenotype.

More evidence, such as from biochemical studies of the protein or genetic studies in animals, is necessary to confirm that a variant causes a phenotype. Currently, only a small percentage of nutrigenomic genes come with this type of evidence.

In animals, you can delete genes to understand what they do or look at how the phenotypes transmit between generations. Biochemical studies can test enzymes or their mutants in test tubes to understand how the mutations affect the enzymes.

In humans, it's very difficult to confirm that a gene causes a disease, because it's unethical to manipulate genes or produce children based on their genetic combinations. Instead, human geneticists rely on looking at what genes are found most often among people with a certain phenotype, and studying genetic transmission in existing families.

In other words, if you have a variant associated with a condition, it doesn't necessarily mean that the variant causes the condition. It may indicate an increased risk. Either way, this means you shouldn't look at a problematic variant in a report and diagnose yourself with a bad gene.

Genome-wide association studies may also focus on specific ethnic groups or populations, which may not apply to you. In many cases, they'd have to focus on specific populations to make their findings statistically significant. Also, the lack of a bad variant in a gene doesn't mean that the gene is functioning perfectly.

If you're alive and functional, chances are that your genes aren't very bad. If you truly had bad genes, you'd have one of the awful genetic diseases or never make it to adulthood. The worst thing you can do is read a genetic report and believe you're doomed with bad genes.

As we noted, only a very small number of genes currently have sufficient evidence to prove causality in nutrigenomics. This doesn't mean that the rest of the genes aren't relevant—it only means that scientists haven't studied them.

Therefore, unless you're a geneticist, you should work with a practitioner who can put all of these pieces of information into context and help you determine what to do next.

HIERARCHY OF GENES TO ADDRESS IN NUTRIGENOMICS

The right way to address genes is to address them in the right hierarchy. Each lower tier of the pyramid prepares your biochemistry for the next tier above so you can minimize side effects and get better results.

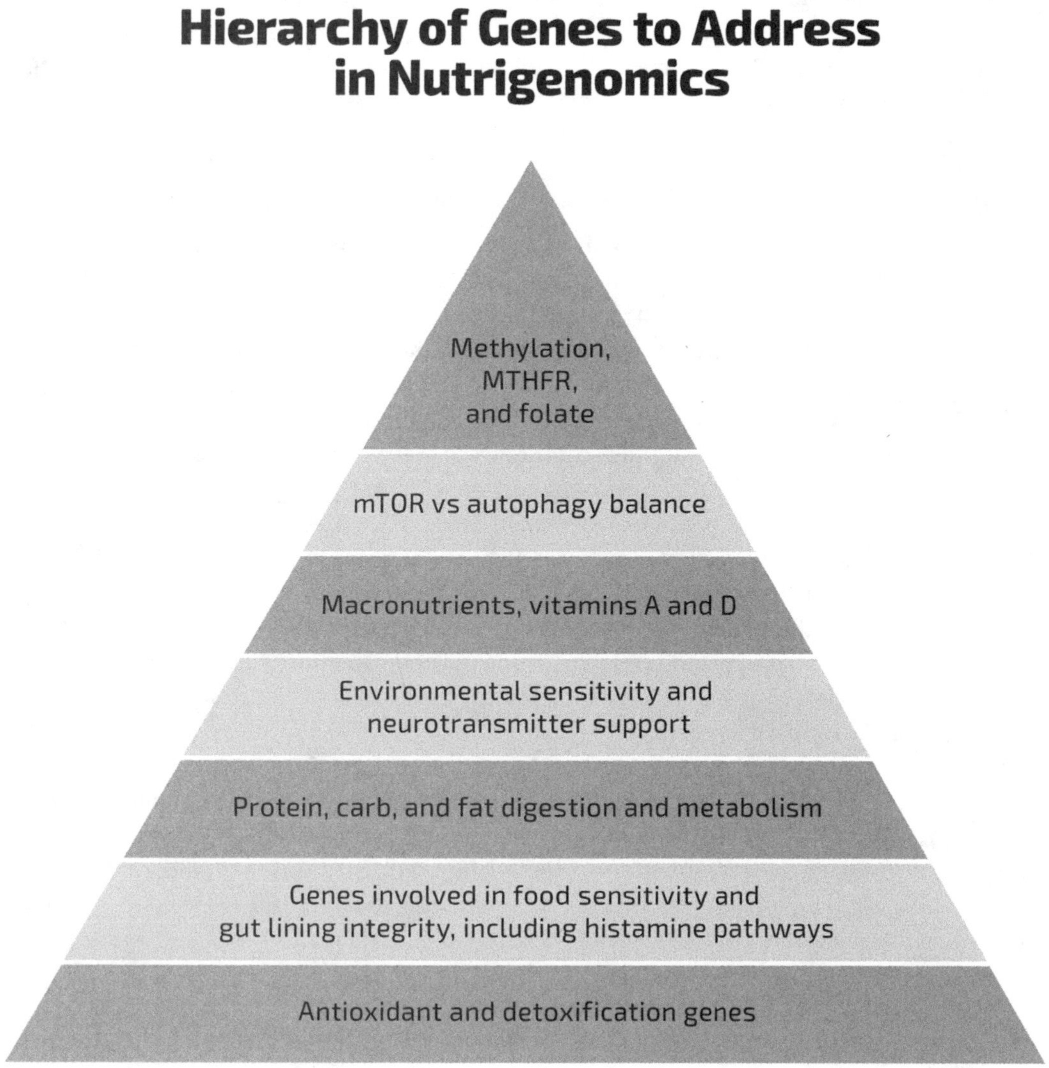

Lisa's Story

Lisa (not her real name) had a lot of problems with her hormones and weight. Estrogen dominance was causing premenstrual symptoms, including bad anxiety and panic attacks.

She was constantly cleansing her liver but gaining weight because she was listening to the wrong advice. Methylfolate was making her symptoms worse because she already had a weak COMT gene (see below).

The problem with these cleanses was that they pushed phase 1 of the detoxification, causing phase 2 and 3 to back up.

She was also fasting a lot, which made her estrogen dominance worse. We had to get her off the methylfolate and all the cleanses. Then, we supported phases 2 and 3 of the detoxification. She soon started to feel better and shed the weight.

This story demonstrates how the uninformed use of nutrigenomic information can backfire.

Your biochemistry involves thousands of enzymes and other types of proteins that work together in an interconnected web. When you have a genetic weakness in one of them, the rest of them adapt to keep you in homeostasis.

If you treat the weak gene and the rest of the biochemical web isn't ready for it, you may create biological chaos. This is why some people experience side effects when they introduce nutrigenomic treatments.

The best-studied genes in nutrigenomics are methylenetetrahydrofolate reductase (MTHFR) and the methylation pathways. Many uninformed people and even practitioners make the mistake of addressing these genes first.

For those who have preexisting inflammation, elevated oxidative stress, and nutrient deficiencies, abruptly increasing methylation can backfire. It can increase histamine and throw off neurotransmitters, causing inflammatory and neurological symptoms.

Let's now discuss each level of the Hierarchy of Genes pyramid from the bottom up.

Level 1: Antioxidant, Detoxification Genes, and Metal Balance Genes

Reactive oxygen species (ROS) are very combative molecules with an extra electron, such as bleach or hydrogen peroxide. If there is nothing to neutralize the extra electron, the reactive oxygen species can attack your cell membranes and DNA, causing damage and potentially killing the cells.

ROS might sound evil, but they're actually very important for life itself. Your mitochondria produce energy by moving electrons between cell membranes to create an electrical gradient. This process necessarily creates some ROS. That said, too much runaway ROS can damage the mitochondria and cause your energy production to grind to a halt, so you feel tired and brain fogged. And too much ROS contributes to every single human disease and suboptimal states.

Your immune cells use ROS to kill germs and communicate with one another. This is why runaway ROS from other sources, such as fried foods, toxic exposure, stress, and aging can cause inflammation throughout the body. Also, oxidative stress and inflammation make you sleepy at night and tired when you're sick. If you want to live a long, healthy life, minimizing inflammation is critical.

Your cells and mitochondria have their own checks and balances to neutralize the ROS. You also eat some antioxidants in your food, like in colorful fruits and vegetables. Some of these can directly neutralize the ROS, while others work as hormesis (beneficial stress). The hormetic ones create tiny amounts of oxidative stress inside your cells to gently nudge your own cellular antioxidant system.

Weak versions of antioxidant and detox genes are linked to a variety of diseases that relate to high toxicity, oxidative stress, and DNA damages. These include Parkinson's disease, heart disease, diabetes, cancers, and high blood pressure.[1]

In terms of BIOptimization, paying attention to these genes will help you maintain a healthy metabolism, hormone balance, and brain function. Oxidative stress ages your cells, so addressing these genes before you develop diseases is important if your goal is to maximize your health span and life span.

- NFE2L2 (NRF2) is your cell's project manager for antioxidant response and detoxification pathways. It turns on genes that encode antioxidant and detoxification enzymes at the right times.[2] Many biohacks and food-based antioxidants work by creating a small amount of oxidative stress to activate NRF2.

- SOD2 is a mitochondrial enzyme that neutralizes oxidative stress. The weaker version of SOD2 is linked to depression, cancer, Parkinson's disease, diabetes complications, and reduced stress resilience.[3, 4, 5, 6]
- NQO1 is a very important detoxification gene that inactivates many hydrocarbon toxins.[7] It also activates vitamin K and ubiquinone (CoQ10).[8, 9]
- PON1 is very important for detoxing many pesticides, drugs, and oxidized fats. The PON1 enzyme is also part of HDL (good cholesterol) particles and one of the reasons having high HDL is typically heart healthy.[10] Low-grade inflammation and omega-6 intake can inhibit PON1.[11]
- CAT (catalase) is an enzyme that helps break down hydrogen peroxide into oxygen and water. It is located in peroxisomes—small bags inside your cells that contain very oxidative enzymes. Low catalase levels are also associated with more gray hair.
- Glutathione is the most important cellular antioxidant, including in the liver and the brain. Variants that affect glutathione production in the GSTM1, GSTT1, GSTP1, GCLM, and GCLC genes may affect mercury detoxification, especially from fish consumption.[12]
- Detoxification genes aren't just important for removing very toxic substances. Your detox systems also process and remove food substances, including vitamins, polyphenols, and caffeine that are unfamiliar to your body.
- CYP1A2 helps with cholesterol synthesis, steroids, and fat molecules. It also converts omega-3 and omega-6 fats into other important molecules. More important, it's known as the caffeine-sensitivity gene because it encodes the main enzyme that breaks down caffeine.[13]
- Weak versions of CYP1A2 are associated with being a "slow caffeine metabolizer" and increased blood pressure from caffeine consumption, whereas people with the strong version of CYP1A2 can consume caffeine just fine and get more health benefits from the antioxidants in coffee.
- Cruciferous vegetables, chemicals in char from grilled meats, proton pump inhibitors, and cigarette smoking increase CYP1A2.[14]
- AhR is another cellular project manager that works closely with NRF2. It detects xenobiotics (chemicals unfamiliar to your body) and turns on other genes that help eliminate these substances. Both dioxins and cruciferous vegetables turn on AhR.[15]
- NAT1 and NAT2 activity may determine whether you're at a higher risk of getting cancer from eating red meat. These are enzymes that convert the heterocyclic aromatic amines in cooked red meat into DNA-damaging substances, which can cause cancers. Therefore, if you have strong versions of NAT1 and NAT2, you may want to watch your red meat consumption.
- CBS, when mutated, can lead to high or low ammonia levels. This gene is part of the sulfur/ammonia pathway. Individuals with a CBS mutation (elevated activity) often have high levels of taurine and ammonia and low cystathionine and homocysteine. This is due to rapid conversion, and if this is coupled with NOS mutations, it can exacerbate ammonia issues.
- High ammonia is extremely toxic and inflammatory to the body. When someone has ultra-high ammonia levels, we recommend going on a low protein diet where protein makes up about 10 percent of total caloric intake. For these individuals, we typically recommend a nutrition plan consisting of 70 to 80 percent fat, 10 to 20 percent carbohydrate, and 10 percent protein. *Gut health* must be addressed.[16, 17]

Level 2: Genes Involved in Food Sensitivity and Gut Lining Integrity, Including Histamine Pathways

As mentioned in a previous chapter, inflammation from food has both a genetic and environmental component. In many cases, you can build your resilience to reduce your inflammatory responses to a certain food so that you can occasionally enjoy it, or at least avoid getting sick from accidental exposure.

Most people are completely unaware of their food reactions unless something is really severe. So, knowing your genes may indicate that certain foods could be problematic, especially if you have some symptoms of inflammatory food reactions.

Harvard pediatric gastroenterologist Alessio Fasano, M.D., states that three things combined can lead to autoimmune diseases:[18]

1. Genetic predisposition
2. Leaky gut or intestinal permeability
3. Environmental or lifestyle triggers (such as stress, gluten consumption, infections, and toxic exposures)

Therefore, if you know that you have some genes contributing to a predisposition, you can work on your gut barrier and minimize the environmental or lifestyle triggers.

Genes that can make you more likely to react to foods include:

- *Immune cell antennas (receptors).* Your immune cells have more than 20,000 types of antennas (receptors) on their surfaces to detect specific patterns on foreign proteins. When an antenna picks up a foreign protein it recognizes, it can activate other immune cells and trigger inflammatory responses.
- *Tight-junction components.* Weak tight junctions may increase the risk of leaky gut and gut inflammation.
- *Immune cell project managers.* Also known as transcription factors, they can make your immune system more reactive to certain components.

Genes That Make Gluten Problematic

HLA-DQA1 and HLA-DQA2 genes provide instructions for making antennas outside of your immune cells. When these cells recognize antigens like gluten, they present it to the immune system. Everyone has a combination of these HLA-DQ variants, but only the DQ2.5, DQ8, 2.2, and DQ7 are problematic.

More than 95 percent of people with celiac disease have the HLA-DQ2.5, HLA-DQ8, and HLA-2.2 versions.[19] HLA-DQ7 may also predispose celiac disease, but it is rare. Gluten is typically incompletely digested, resulting in short peptides that these HLA-DQ receptors recognize.

However, not everyone with these celiac-linked HLA-DQ variants has celiac disease. About 30 percent of the U.S. population has these variants, and only about 3 percent of them develop celiac disease.[20] So, celiac disease isn't purely genetic; it's rather caused by a combination of multiple genes plus environmental factors.

An enzyme blend like Gluten Guardian is a useful defense especially when eating out at restaurants.

Some of these other genes encode other immune cell receptors and proteins that form tight junctions between our gut lining cells. Many of these genes are linked to Parkinson's and inflammatory bowel diseases.[21, 22]

Myosin 9B is an important protein for the gut barrier. Many variants inside this protein are linked to celiac disease and ulcerative colitis.[23] Having both myosin 9B variants and two copies of HLA-DQ2 can increase the risk for refractory celiac disease and enteropathy-associated lymphoma.[24]

Toll-like receptors (TLRs) recognize patterns on microbial cells and trigger immune responses. Certain variants in TLR receptors may increase the risk of autoimmune and allergic diseases.[25] These could make gluten and some other plant lectins especially problematic because they activate toll-like receptors.[26, 27]

Claudins are proteins that make the tight junction between our gut lining cells. Several variants in claudin genes are linked to inflammatory bowel disease.[28]

Mucins are gel-forming proteins that become the mucus covering the gut lining and other mucus-covered tissues. The mucus layer protects your gut barrier and feeds some good gut bacteria, so low mucin function can contribute to gut inflammation and leakiness.[29, 30] Weak mucin variants are linked to inflammation, leaky gut, bacterial toxins in the blood, and cancers of mucosal tissues.[31]

FOXP3 is a cellular project manager (transcription factor) that gets T cells to develop into regulatory T cells instead of the autoimmune-promoting Th17 cells. Regulatory T cells help your immune system ignore your own tissues and harmless proteins, such as in those who are not allegic to pollen and seafood.

In other words, FOXP3 and regulatory T cells help prevent allergies, autoimmunity, and all kinds of excess inflammation. Variants that affect FOXP3 are linked to autoimmune diseases, asthma, and cancer.[32] Low FOXP3 function may also be involved in food allergy and food-induced anaphylaxis.[33, 34]

GENES RELATED TO HISTAMINE BREAKDOWN

Histamine is made from the amino acid histidine when the enzyme histidine decarboxylase removes the carboxyl group. Some other amino acids can also be converted into amines in the same way and have similar effects as histamine. Both histamine and amines from other amino acids are found in high levels in fermented foods.

Although most people think of histamine as related to allergies, it actually has many other functions in your body. Histamine is an essential neurotransmitter for wakefulness and energy, as well as stomach acid production. It is also a signaling molecule that your immune cells use to communicate with each other, typically promoting inflammation.

Excess histamine in the gut wall can cause a leaky gut and other digestive issues such as diarrhea.[35, 36] Gene variants that reduce your ability to break down histamine can make you more sensitive to food or more prone to leaky gut. These genes are also linked to asthma, allergies, and histamine intolerance.[37] An overload of histamine can create uncontrollable itching.

ABP1 (also known as AOC1) produces the enzyme diamine oxidase, which deactivates histamine. It's made in the gut lining, kidneys, colon, thymus, and testicles.

Genes Related to Histamine Breakdown

Histidine

HISTIDINE DECARBOXYLASE

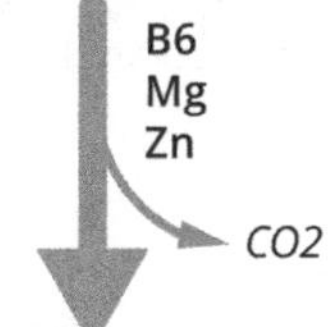

Histamine

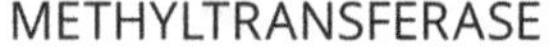

DIAMINE OXIDASE

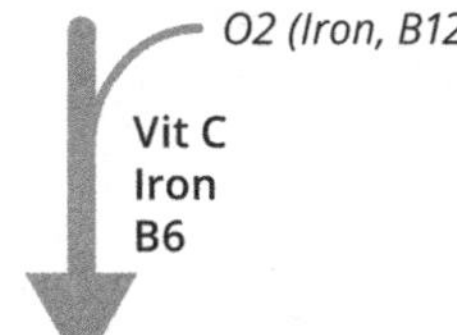

ALDEHYDE OXIDASE

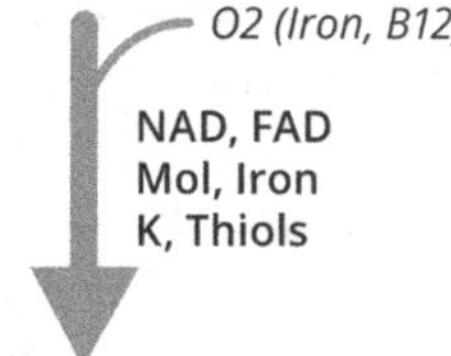

Methylhistamine

MONOAMINE OXIDASE

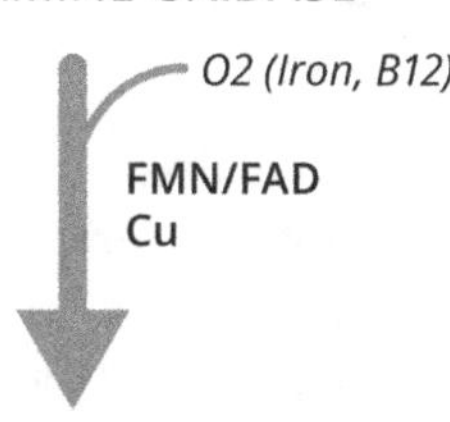

Methyl imidazole acetic acid

Imidazole acetic acid

(Systemic histamine)
Natural anti-histamines:
Vit E, Zn, Mg, Bioflavonoids

Diamine oxidase breaks down histamine outside of cells and is responsible for breaking down histamine in your food so you don't absorb too much of it.[38] The weak variant of ABP1 may reduce its function and thus your ability to break down histamine and inflammatory bowel disease.[39]

HNMT (histamine N-methyltransferase) deactivates histamine inside cells by methylating the histamine. It is produced in most bodily tissues. Variants that reduce HNMT activity can cause histamine intolerance and symptoms of allergic conditions.[40] Drugs that inhibit HNMT such as Benadryl and chloroquine can make low HNMT function worse.[41]

MAOB (monoamine oxidase) is produced in the liver and many other tissues, but its most important roles involve breaking down neurotransmitters in the brain. It also breaks down products of HNMT to help detoxify histamine.[42] Variants of MAOB are linked to:

- Fatigue[43]
- ADHD[44]
- Some mental health disorders[45]
- Parkinson's disease[46]
- Essential hypertension[47]

Cannabinoid receptors: CNR1 produces the CB1 receptors, which are mainly in your brain, whereas CNR2 produces CB2 receptors on white blood cells and gut. The endocannabinoid system, especially CNR2, inhibits the inflammatory response and histamine release. CB1 regulates gut inflammation and stress response. Therefore, having variants inside CB1 can predispose you to lectin and other types of food sensitivity.[48, 49]

Dairy and Lactose Intolerance Genes

LCT produces lactase, an enzyme that digests the milk sugar lactose. Many adults become lactose intolerant because their guts stop producing lactase by a certain age. Some genetic variants around this gene and the MCM6 gene are linked to continued lactase production into adulthood.[50] Using the lactase enzyme (as found in Gluten Guardian) is a useful hack that can allow people to eat dairy products without suffering.

LEVEL 3: PROTEIN, FAT, AND CARB DIGESTION AND METABOLISM

Once you address the antioxidant genes and food sensitivity, it's time to look at genes that influence your macronutrient digestion and metabolism of micronutrients. These genes will likely influence the dietary strategies that may work best for you.

PPAR (Peroxisome proliferator-activated receptors) are a family of cellular project managers (transcription factors) that manage genes related to protein and carb metabolism. They are also sensors that detect lipids and insulin. There are three types of PPARs: alpha, beta or delta, and gamma, which are produced in different tissues and have slightly different functions.[51]

PPAR-α mainly influences fatty acid metabolism. Activating PPAR-α lowers blood lipid levels while increasing good cholesterol (HDL).[52] Some variants in this gene may lower production of ketone bodies in ketosis and fasting, making them stressful for the body.

PPAR-***β*** helps with fat burning in muscles and the heart. It also controls blood glucose and cholesterol levels. Strong PPAR-***β*** is linked to endurance.[53]

PPAR-γ governs insulin sensitivity, along with the production of new fat cells, energy balance, and the production of fat molecules. It is the energy storage transcription factor. A strong version of PPAR-γ is linked to lowering the risk of diabetes, whereas the P12A variant is linked to increasing the risk of diabetes.[54, 55]

Those with the CC variant of this gene have a significantly increased risk of atherosclerosis and elevated blood lipid levels when saturated fats are present in the diet. Those with the GG and GC variants do not share this increased risk.[56, 57]

ACAT determines how your body converts protein and fat to cellular energy. We make our bodyweight in ATP (cellular energy) every day. This involves cholesterol balance in the cell and the ability to get energy from high protein and fat intake.[58]

LEVEL 4: ENVIRONMENTAL SENSITIVITY AND NEUROTRANSMITTER SUPPORT

Detoxification genes can make you more sensitive to certain environmental factors. Also, certain variants of ion channel genes, such as CACNA genes, can affect your sensitivity to electromagnetic exposure.[59]

Your nutrition influences these genes, and thus your overall well-being. Also, conversely, your neurotransmitter balance affects your food desires, trauma responses, and ability to stick to a nutritional strategy. This is why we look at neurotransmitter genes as part of nutrigenomics.

COMT is one of the most important genes in nutrigenomics. It helps degrade catecholamine neurotransmitters such as dopamine and norepinephrine. Also, it helps with hormone detoxification and certain nutrient pathways.

This gene determines your personality traits. Fast COMT makes you a warrior—someone who recovers from stress quickly because you break down stress neurotransmitters faster. On the other hand, slow COMT makes you a worrier because you break down catecholamine more slowly. B vitamins and magnesium are especially important to support healthy COMT function.

MAO genes produce the monoamine oxidase enzymes, which are also important for removing norepinephrine, dopamine, and serotonin from the brain. Low MAO-A gene can cause aggression.[60]

LEVEL 5: VITAMINS A AND D

Vitamins A and D work together. The receptors of these vitamins are cellular project managers (transcription factors). Every cell in your body has vitamin A receptors, and almost every cell has vitamin D receptors.

These vitamins affect your eye health, gut lining integrity, brain function, immune function, metabolism, and hormone balance. Also, thyroid hormone receptors and PPARs need to partner with vitamin A receptors to work correctly. This is why you should pay attention to your vitamin A and D variants.

Many genes are involved in vitamin A absorption, transport, and metabolism.[61] Some of them are involved in lipid metabolism, which explains why these are at a level to address before you address vitamin A itself.

One of the most important vitamin A genes is BCMO1, which converts beta-carotene to vitamin A. BCMO1 variants may reduce the conversion of beta-carotene into retinol (vitamin D) by 69 to 90 percent. About 45 percent of the population has BCMO1 variants that make it harder to produce vitamin A from plant carotenoids.[62]

Most people nowadays don't get enough vitamin D from the sun and need to supplement. Many SNPs in vitamin D receptors, vitamin D binding proteins, and vitamin D conversion enzymes can influence your response to vitamin D supplementation.[63]

Variants near the following genes affect the efficiency of your vitamin D supplementation on your blood 25-hydroxy vitamin D (25-OHD):

- VDR, which produces the vitamin D receptor
- CYP2R1, which produces an enzyme that activates vitamin D[64]
- CYP24A1, which produces an enzyme that deactivates vitamin D
- CYP27B1, which produces an enzyme that converts vitamin D to 25-OHD
- GC, which produces a protein that binds to vitamin D
- DHCR7, which produces an enzyme that moves vitamin D precursors toward cholesterol production

LEVEL 6: MTOR-VS.-AUTOPHAGY BALANCE

mTOR is your cell's nutrient sensor. Once you have an abundance of nutrients and calories, it puts your cells in an anabolic state. Most of the best bodybuilders in the world have the right mTOR mutation.

On the other hand, when nutrients and calories are scarce, your cells start to break down old cellular parts to reuse the building block. This is a rejuvenative process called *autophagy*.

To maximize all three sides of your BIOptimization Triangle, you need both the mTOR and autophagy pathways to be on at the right time. For example, mTOR helps you gain and retain muscles, but too much of it can cause cancers. On the other hand, not enough autophagy can contribute to inflammatory conditions and age-related health issues.[65]

The good news is that you can easily manipulate these pathways with nutrition and training once you understand your genetic weaknesses or strengths in these genes.

For example, if you have one of the elevated mTOR SNPs, then you may need to dial up your autophagy pathway more. If you have weak mTOR, then you may need to stimulate it more to be anabolic.

LEVEL 7: METHYLATION, MTHFR, AND FOLATE

The methylation and folate pathways are two of the most important in nutrigenomics. Methylation is so important for your neurotransmitters, hormones, and detoxification. Also, folate provides a backbone for your DNA. You need DNA for cell division, which is important for making your red blood cells and regenerating your gut lining. Low function of genes in this pathway can contribute to infertility, birth defects, mental health issues, chronic inflammation, and more.

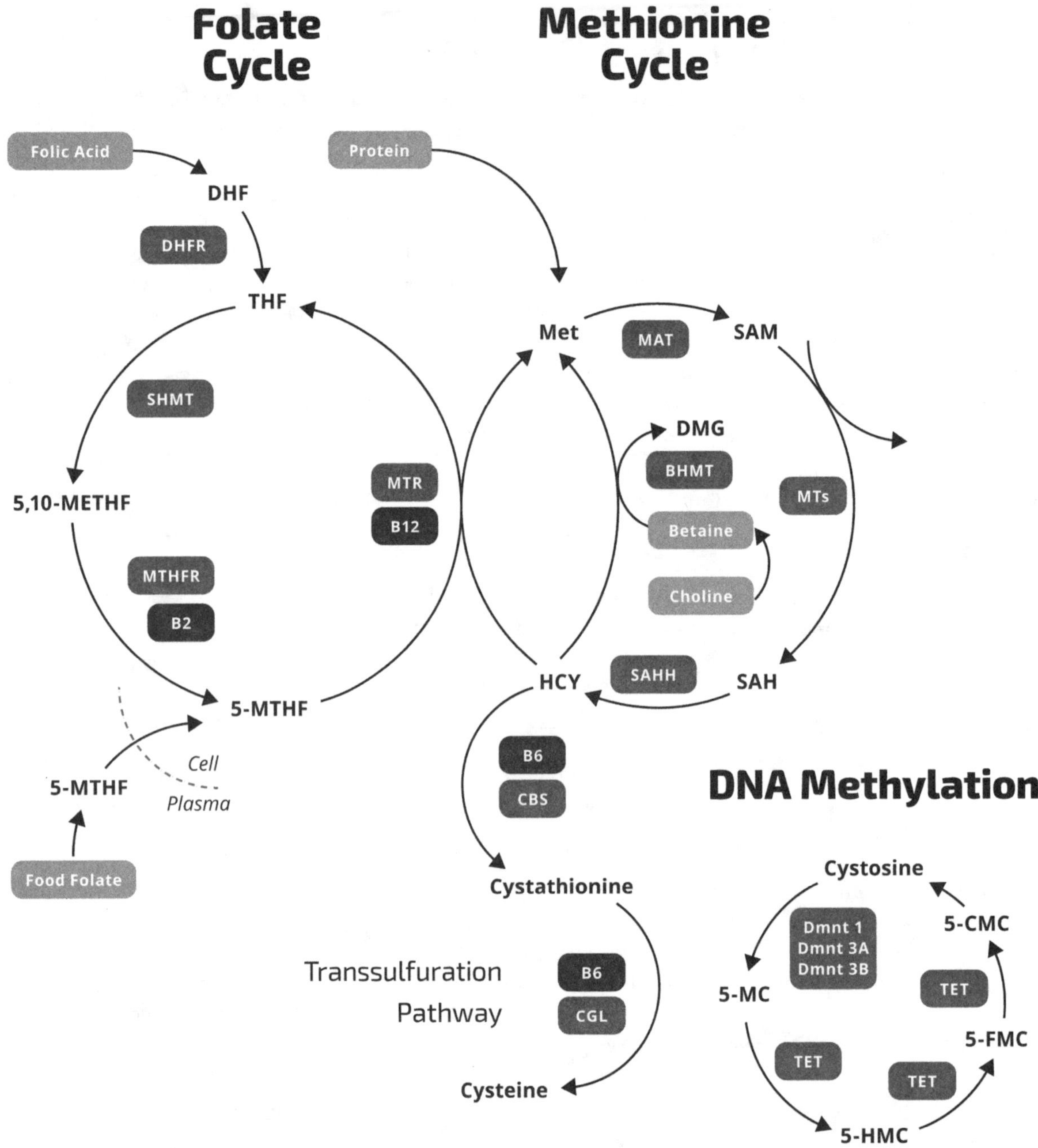

The MTHFR gene produces the enzyme that converts folate into methylfolate, the active form of folate. This gene is a bottleneck in the methylation cycle, so if you have reduced function of the gene, you may be at a higher risk of low folate function. However, there are other enzymes in this pathway, including MTHFD1, MTR, MTRR, and the methionine cycle, which can also compromise methylation.

Genes to Keep in Mind for Each Nutritional Goal and Strategy

In this book, we're not married to any particular diet. You may cycle through different nutritional strategies. Sometimes, a nutritional strategy or food may set off a genetic disruption particular to you.

For example, some diets may increase the risk of certain nutrient deficiencies, especially if you have specific variants. So, you want to test your genes and learn about strategies to address them.

The following are genes you need to keep in mind when you're on each of these dietary patterns.

Unsaturated, Plant-Based Fats vs. Saturated Animal Fats

ACSL1 is a cellular project manager that governs neuronal development. It also influences how well you metabolize saturated fats from animals. People with weak variants in this gene tend to develop higher fasting glucose and insulin resistance from eating a lot of saturated fats. So, if you have weak versions of ACSL1, focus on getting your fats from plant-based sources rather than animal sources.[66]

ADIPOQ is your red meat gene. It provides instructions for adiponectin, a hormone released in your gut when you eat food. Adiponectin also controls how much insulin is released. Certain versions of ADIPOQ influence the risk for metabolic diseases. If you have low adiponectin, saturated fat further reduces it—so you'll be at a higher risk for insulin resistance, heart disease, and colon cancers if you eat a lot of red meat and saturated fats. So, it will be critical to exercise, practice intermittent fasting (unless otherwise contraindicated), and use omega-3 to increase your adiponectin levels.[67, 68]

FTO is your hangry gene, which governs your ghrelin levels. The C variant of FTO can make you hungrier if you eat a lot of fat, especially saturated fat. Both the CC and CT variants of this gene tend to hold on to fat harder, and so you need less of it in the diet to compensate. The TT variant has an easier time of letting go of fat stores than other variants. People who have the C variant, especially homozygous (CC), tend to be hungry all the time. If you have this variant, it will be extra important to manage hunger and check your blood sugar levels.[69, 70] More effort may need to go into managing hunger.

LPL decides whether you'll store saturated fats as body fat or burn them as fuel, and it plays a role in how saturated fats are broken down for energy. Those with the GG variant of this gene break down saturated fats and use them for energy easily. The CG and CC variants of this gene, however, have less ability to tolerate saturated fats in the diet, since they can be easily converted into cholesterol.[71, 72]

APOC3 regulates blood triglyceride levels and LDL (bad) cholesterol. Saturated fats in the diet are the modulating factor of how strong a role this gene plays. Those with the CC variant of this gene have a significantly increased risk of atherosclerosis and elevated blood lipid levels when saturated fats are present in the diet. Those with the GG and GC variants do not share this increased risk.[73, 74]

APOA2 is the eat fat, get fat gene (satiation gene). The C variant increases appetite, and thus BMI, when saturated fats are included in the diet.[75, 76]

ApoE, especially the ApoE4 variant, is a known risk for Alzheimer's and bad response to high-saturated-fat diets. People with ApoE4 should avoid saturated fats or high-fat diets and stick to more plant-based diets.

Genes That Can Make You More Exhausted on Keto and Fasting

Aside from the fat metabolism genes above, you should also pay attention to these genes if you want to try a ketogenic diet or fasting. PPAR-alpha is important for getting into ketosis. People with strong PPAR-alpha tend to improve blood sugar on a low-carb diet. They also feel good on exogenous ketones. On the other hand, weak PPAR-alpha can make it harder to get into ketosis.[77, 78] It will also make it harder to reap benefits from fasting.

ACAT controls how your body converts protein and fat into cellular energy (ATP) in the mitochondria. If you are homozygous, your cholesterol may go up on keto and you are more likely to feel exhausted on keto since your body cannot use fats for fuel efficiently. Liver enzymes have to be monitored as well, since your body will have trouble processing fats.[79]

A CPT1A variant is found in many populations in cold climates—e.g., 81 percent of Canadians, 54 percent of Greenland Inuits, and 68 percent of one Northeast Siberian population. The weak variant reduces CPT1A enzyme by 20 percent, reducing blood ketones and sugar. So, people with this variant tend to have trouble entering ketosis and develop hypoglycemia in response to fasting.[80]

Power Move:
If you're exhausted trying to enter ketosis or become keto adapted, kApex can help boost your energy levels.

Plant-Based vs. Animal-Sourced Nutrients

The following genes mean you may need to supplement if you will be on a plant-based diet.

High copy number of AMY1 is a salivary starch predigestion enzyme. Vegetarians with more AMY1 will do better long term. Amylase production strongly influences how we metabolize starchy foods.[81]

BCMO1 weak variants are found in 45 percent of the population. These variants can reduce the conversion of beta-carotene into retinol, which may cause a vitamin A deficiency on a plant-based diet.[82]

Lactase (Lct1)-influencing variant located inside the MCM6 gene determines whether you should keep dairy in your diet.[83]

FUT2 influences your gut bacteria and vitamin B_{12}. It means you do better with more fiber but also need more B_{12}.[84, 85]

FADS1 and FADS2 genes produce enzymes that convert short-chain (plant-based) omega-3 and omega-6 fatty acids into long-chain ones. You need long-chain omega-3s like EPA and DHA either from animal sources or FADS1 and FADS2 conversions. These enzymes also convert plant-based omega-6 into arachidonic acid, which is important for muscle building, among other things. So, people who do well on plant-based diets tend to have strong versions of these genes. However, if you have the weak versions, you can simply supplement with the long-chain polyunsaturated fatty acids.[86, 87, 88]

PEMT gene produces an important enzyme for choline production, so vegetarians who have weak PEMT may not produce enough choline. The lack of choline, especially in perimenopausal and menopausal women who have low PEMT, can worsen methylation problems in vegetarians.[89, 90]

SHBG gene produces sex-hormone-binding globulin, a blood protein that binds to your sex hormones for transport. Blood SHBG levels may be low or high on a plant-based diet.[91] Either can worsen PMS for some women.[92] In premenopausal women, a variant of SHBG causes SHBG to rise in response to higher isoflavones (plant-based estrogens) in their diets, such as soy. The SHBG can bind to estrogen and make their menopausal symptoms worse.[93]

Goal-Specific Genetic Considerations

Fat Gain and Fat Loss Genes

Peter's Story

Peter (not his real name) was overweight and sluggish. He responded poorly to a ketogenic diet. His wife was ready to divorce him. He had a high-stress job and frequently worked late. On first evaluation, we found that he had thyroid issues and estrogen dominance, along with very slow COMT.

He decided to introduce a quercetin supplement to protect himself from COVID-19, which unfortunately inhibited his COMT even further. Here are the changes we made:

- Put him on thyroid medication
- Took him off quercetin
- Managed his stress with HRV, nootropics, and adaptogens
- Fixed his broken circadian rhythm
- Used a carb-cycling diet rather than a ketogenic one

Both your genes and your environment contribute to your body composition. Often, being fat, skinny, or muscular runs in the family. On the other hand, most people fail to tap into their genetic potential or weaknesses as they work to optimize their body composition.

Storing body fat can be an appropriate evolutionary response to many different types of stressors. It's one of the ways your body attempts to keep you alive.

Therefore, we often find that people who struggle to lose weight have problems with detoxification, circadian rhythm, micronutrients, and stress response genes more than genes in the present category of discussion. Also, some people gain fat just because they're not eating right for their genes. This is why it's important to look at the full picture rather than just treating for specific genes. That said, consider the following genes if you're working on fat loss.

GENES	POLY-MORPHISMS	ALLELES	DIET INTERACTIONS	DIETARY RESPONSES
FTO	rs1558902	A	High protein	Greater weight loss
FTO	rs1558902	A	Low fat	Fewer reductions in insulin and HOMA-IR
TCF7L2	rs7903146	T	High fat	Smaller weight loss and HOMA-IR
APOA5	rs964184	G	Low fat	Greater reduction in TC and LDL-c
GIPR	rs2287019	T	Low fat	Greater weight loss and greater decreases in glucose, insulin, and HOMA-IR
CETP	rs3764261	C	High fat	Larger increases in HDL-c and decreases in triglycerides
DHCR7	rs12785878	T	High protein	Greater decreases in insulin and HOMA-IR
LIPC	rs2070895	A	Low fat	Higher decreases in TC and LDL-c and a lower increase in HDL-c
PPM1K	rs1440581	C	High fat	Less weight loss and smaller decreases in insulin and HOMA-IR
TFAP2B	rs987237	G	High protein	Higher weight regains
IRS1	rs2943641	C	High carbohydrate	Greater decreases in insulin, HOMA-IR, and weight loss
PCSK7	rs236918	G	High carbohydrate	Higher decreases in insulin and HOMA-IR
MTNR1B	rs10830963	G	High protein	Lower weight loss in women
IL6	rs2069827	C	Mediterranean diet	Lower weight gains

FTO, fat mass and obesity associated; **TCF7L2**, transcription factor 7 like 2; **APOA5**, apolipoprotein A5; **GIPR**, gastric inhibitory polypeptide receptor; **CETP**, cholesteryl ester transfer protein; **DHCR7**, 7-dehydrocholesterol reductase; **LIPC**, lipase C, hepatic type; **PPM1K**, protein phosphatase, Mg^{2+}/Mn^{2+} dependent 1K; **TFAP2B**, transcription factor AP-2 beta; **IRS1**, insulin receptor substrate 1; **PCSK7**, proprotein convertase subtilisin/kexin type 7; **MTNR1B**, melatonin receptor 1B; **IL6**, interleukin-6; TC, total cholesterol; LDL-c, low-density lipoprotein cholesterol; HDL-c, high-density lipoprotein cholesterol; HOMA-IR, homeostasis model assessment of insulin resistance.

An FTO variant can predispose you for more weight loss with a high-protein diet, and less improvement of insulin sensitivity on a low-fat diet. However, a higher-protein diet with a variant of TFAP2B or MTNR1B can make you gain more weight or make it harder to lose fat.

Variants in the TCF7L2, APOC, LPL, PPM1K, and ADIPOQ can make it harder to lose fat on a high-fat diet.

Having variants in the APOA5 and GIPR gene means you'll do better with a low-fat diet.

Having the PCSK7 gene means you'll do better on a high-carb diet.

IL-6, a gene for the inflammatory cytokine, means you'll gain less weight on a Mediterranean diet.

Variants in circadian genes, including BMAL1, CLOCK, and MC4R, also influence blood sugar and fat loss efforts. These can make it harder to lose weight if you are a night owl or don't entrain your circadian rhythm correctly.[94] MC4R can increase appetite on a high-protein diet.[95]

Genes-Related Fitness Goals and Muscle Gain

Mitochondrial Biogenesis and Antioxidant Response Gene

Your mitochondria are the energy powerhouses of your cells. They strongly control your health, aesthetics, and performance. Healthy mitochondria allow you to train hard and recover from your training sessions with the desired gains.

Genes that influence your mitochondrial function may indicate that certain types of mitochondria support are more effective for you. The genes may also indicate whether endurance or power training is best.

Remember, though, your genes are not your destiny. Typically, having the "endurance" genes doesn't mean you are fated to do only endurance sports. You can have any fitness goals you want, including explosive, hypertrophy, and strength. But you may get more results with higher-rep and higher-volume training and need to put in extra effort if you want to excel at explosive, hypertrophy, or strength. Last, you can use nutritional interventions to support your weak genes or pathways.

PPARGC1A (PPARG coactivator 1 alpha) is a cellular project manager that works with PPARG and PPARA. Together, they manage mitochondrial fatty acid oxidation and the creation of new mitochondria.[96] Endurance training typically increases PPARGC1A levels. A variant in this gene impairs exercise-induced adaptation of fast-twitch fibers to slow-twitch fibers in response to endurance training.[97]

NRF2 is your cellular project manager for antioxidant genes. Exercise increases oxidative stress that activates NRF2, so NRF2 variants can affect your exercise response.[98] NRF2 also works with PPARGC1A and other cellular project managers to stimulate the generation of new mitochondria.[99] High-functioning variants of NRF2 improve endurance capacity in response to training and are associated with being an endurance athlete.[100, 101]

Fatigue/Endurance

NOS3 produces nitric oxide synthase 3. Nitric oxide produced by NOS3 relaxes the blood vessels and improves blood flow, which correlates with healthy blood pressure, stamina, and endurance. Variants of NOS3 affect blood pressure response to exercise.[102] Also, strong NOS3 is associated with being an elite endurance swimmer.[103]

PPARD is a cellular project manager in the same family as PPARA and PPARG. It's responsible for the shift from glucose (glycolytic) to fatty acid use as energy. Certain variants of PPARD correspond to greater reduction in cholesterol and triglycerides in response to training. Certain variants of PPARD correspond to better muscle mass gain in response to aerobic training.[104]

MCT1 or SLC16A1 transports lactic acid in both slow-twitch and fast-twitch muscle fibers. A weak variant in MCT1 may mean that you need more time to recover from glycolytic exercises, such as high-intensity interval training.[105]

Inflammation Response to Training

Exercise creates a small amount of inflammation that triggers your body to adapt, such as by building muscle mass. Now, some variants in inflammatory proteins and cytokines may increase soreness and the time you need to recover from exercise.[106]

If you have these variants in the TNF-alpha, IL-6, IL-10, and CRP genes, you may get more muscle damage from exercise.[107] Fortunately, you can mitigate a lot of the soreness nutritionally with omega-3 fatty acids and other recovery modalities.

Training Response

ACE produces an angiotensin-converting enzyme, which is responsible for activating angiotensin. Angiotensin constricts the blood vessels, which typically hinders athletic performance and recovery. There is a long version of ACE that is 287 base pairs longer than the short version. A small clinical study of 52 subjects found that the long version may contribute to up to 11 percent increase in peak power output in a strength-endurance exercise. On average, untrained subjects with the long version also had larger muscle cross-sectional area than those with the short version. The short version also depletes muscle glycogen faster than the long version.[108]

ACTN3 produces alpha-actinin-3, a protein that structures your fast-twitch muscle fibers. The majority of the population has the normal version that produces the protein, whereas the remaining minority has the absent variant that doesn't produce the protein at all. The normal version is associated with greater strength and less muscle damage from training and sports injury. Speed, power, and strength athletes have higher frequencies of the normal version than the general population,[109] whereas endurance athletes are 3.74 times more likely to have the absent version.[110]

MSTN produces myostatin, a protein that prevents muscle mass from growing out of control. It limits AKT1, a target of insulin-like growth factor-1 (IGF1). So, if your goal is to gain muscle, you want less myostatin. There is a variant that produces a weaker version of myostatin. This variant is 2.1 times more common among endurance athletes than nonathletes.[111]

ADRB2 produces a beta-2 adrenergic receptor, which takes signals from adrenaline. It affects your fight-or-flight response, which is important for exercise performance and fat burning.[112] ADRB2 variants may affect relative strength. A variant of ADRB2 may predispose you for endurance performance and higher weight.[113]

UCP2 and UCP3 produce uncoupling proteins, which cause your mitochondria to turn energy into heat rather than ATP. Certain variants of these genes make you more energy efficient with training experience, which means you'll burn fewer calories.[114]

Variants in genes related to vitamin D absorption, reception, and processing are associated with strength and lean body mass.[115] This makes sense because vitamin D is important for muscle strength, testosterone levels, and sports performance.[116]

AGT produces angiotensin, the hormone that increases blood pressure, body salt, and fluid balance. A variant of this gene may predispose people for power sports performance.[117]

Connective Tissue Genes Affecting Injury Risk

COL1A produces a type of collagen that is most abundant in your body. Variants inside this gene may influence ligament injury risk, especially anterior cruciate ligament (ACL) rupture.[118]

COL5A produces another type of collagen. It also determines collagen assembly and fiber width. Some variants of this gene cause Ehlers-Danlos syndrome, which leads to joint hypermobility and ACL rupture.[119]

Antiaging and Longevity

Aging encompasses many genes and cellular pathways. Both genes and lifestyle influence these pathways. See the hallmarks of aging below.

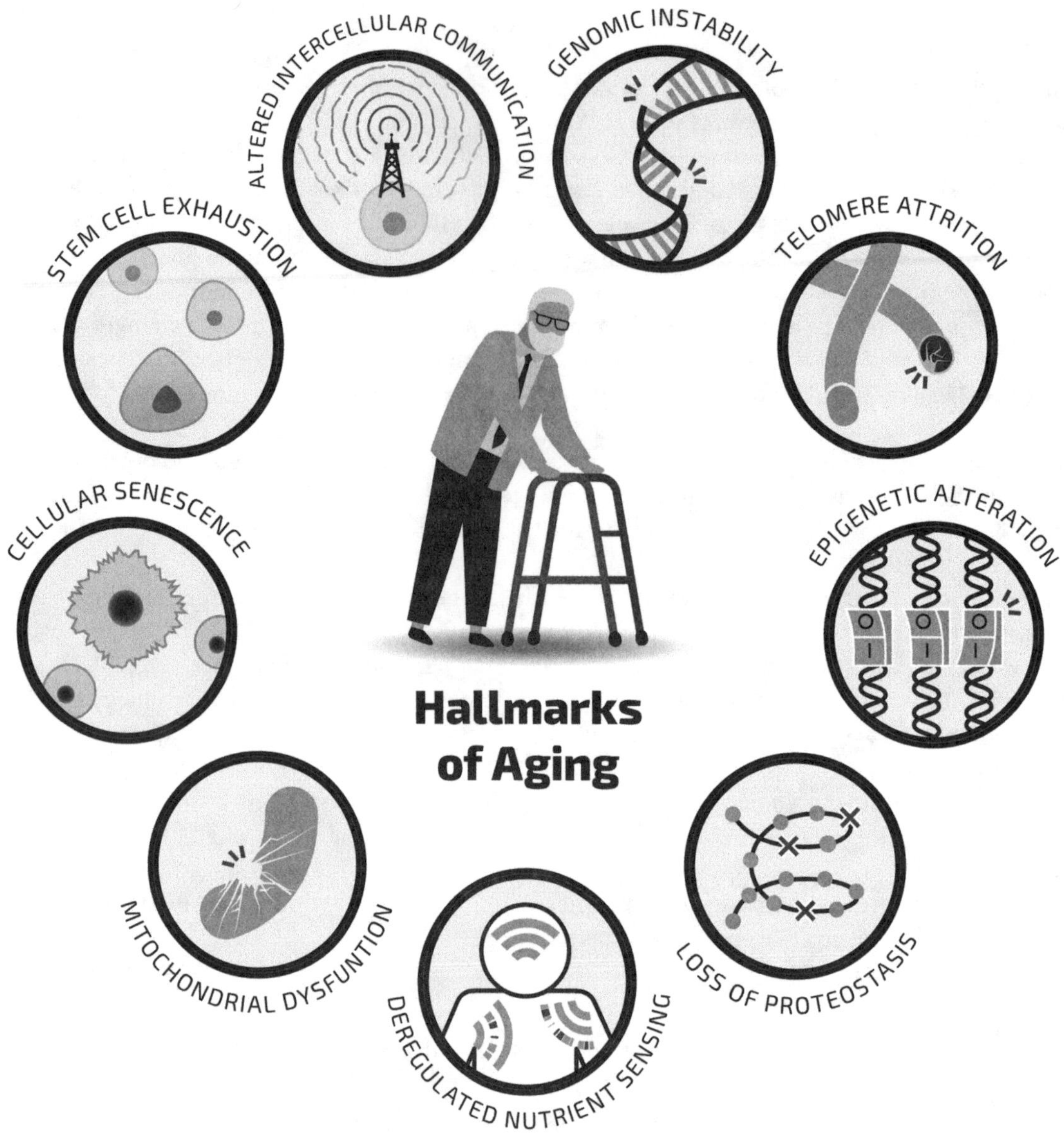

Hallmarks of aging[120]

The genes directly involved in the hallmarks of aging include:

- Cellular antioxidant genes, such as NRF2, SOD2, and catalase that protect your cellular components and DNA from damage
- Mitochondrial function genes, such as PPARGC1A and AMPK
- Genes such as MTHFR and MTHFD1, which produce enzymes in the methylation pathway that are important for epigenetic regulation
- DNA damage-repair genes
- Autophagy genes, which help renew cellular components and healthy immune function[121]
- Apoptosis genes that ensure cancer cells and virus-infected cells commit suicide[122]
- Genes that help proteins fold properly, such as heat shock proteins
- Nutrient-sensing genes, such as mTOR, sirtuins, and insulin signaling
- Inflammation genes, such as inflammatory cytokines (IL-6, CRP, and IL-1beta) and cellular project managers that manage immune responses, such as FOXO3 and NF-**κ**B

There are genes that are collaterally involved with aging, such as genes related to diet and lifestyle factors that increase oxidative stress and DNA damage.

Variants in these genes are linked to risk factors for diseases of aging. The good news is that you can manipulate most of these genes with nutrition, lifestyle, training, supplements, and biohacks. You want to home in on your genetic weak links and support those variants rather than inhibit them. Having the right nutrigenomic test and analysis can help you find these variants and address them accordingly.

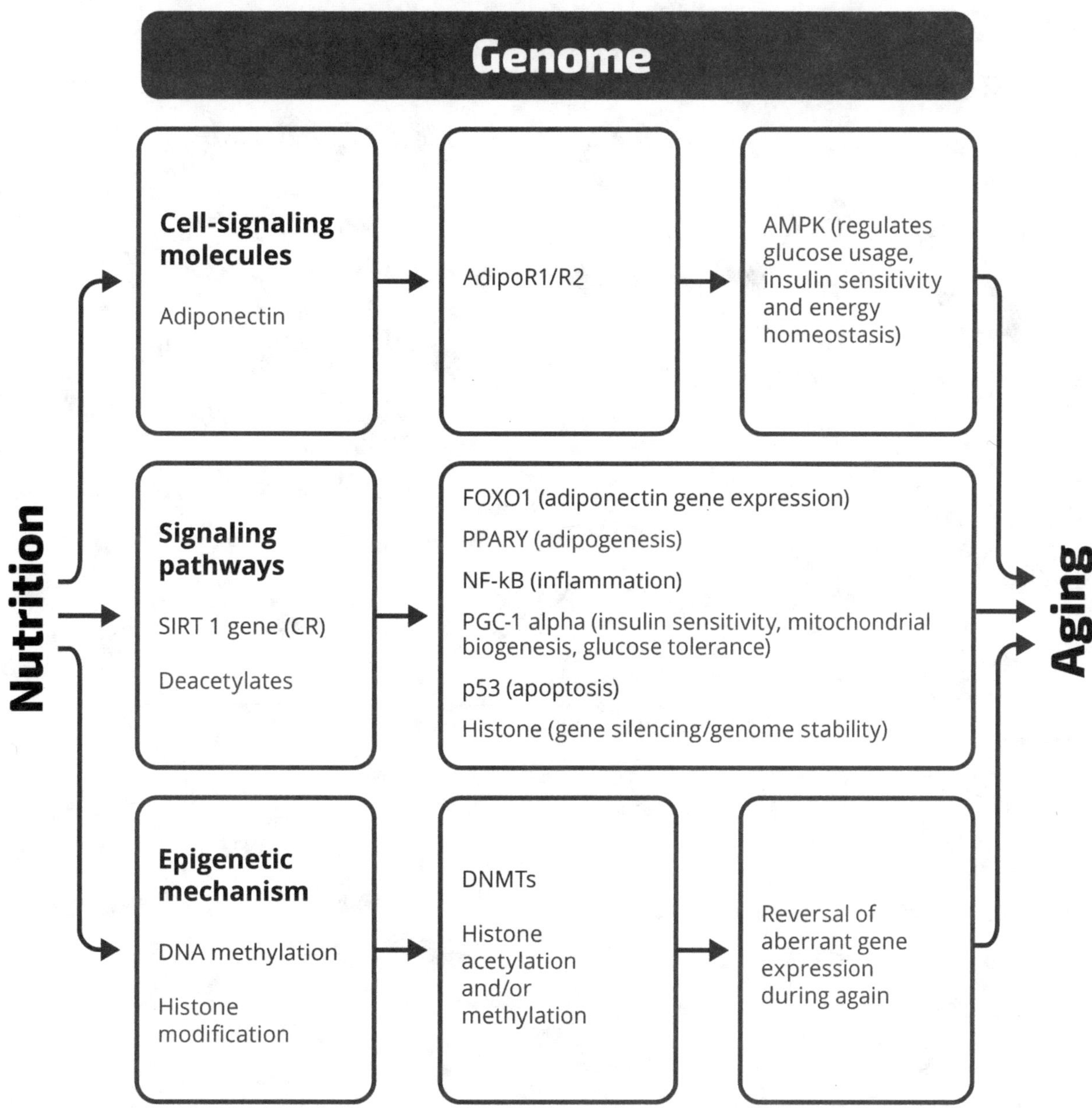

Adaptive responses to nutrition related to aging[123]

PUTTING THE BENEFITS OF THIS CHAPTER INTO YOUR LIFE

You have two options for benefiting from the information we've given you here. Either A, you find a nutrigenomic expert who has this knowledge and work with them, or B, you become a nutrigenomic expert yourself, which is a long, hard road.

We have worked with some of the best nutrigenomic experts in the world to create what we feel is the most beneficial health genetic system assembled. You can learn more here: www.BIOptimizers.com/book/genes.

Gratitude

Special thanks to Nattha Wannissorn, Ph.D., and Katrine Volynsky for helping assemble this chapter. We couldn't have done it without you.

Scientific Background and Glossary on Genetics

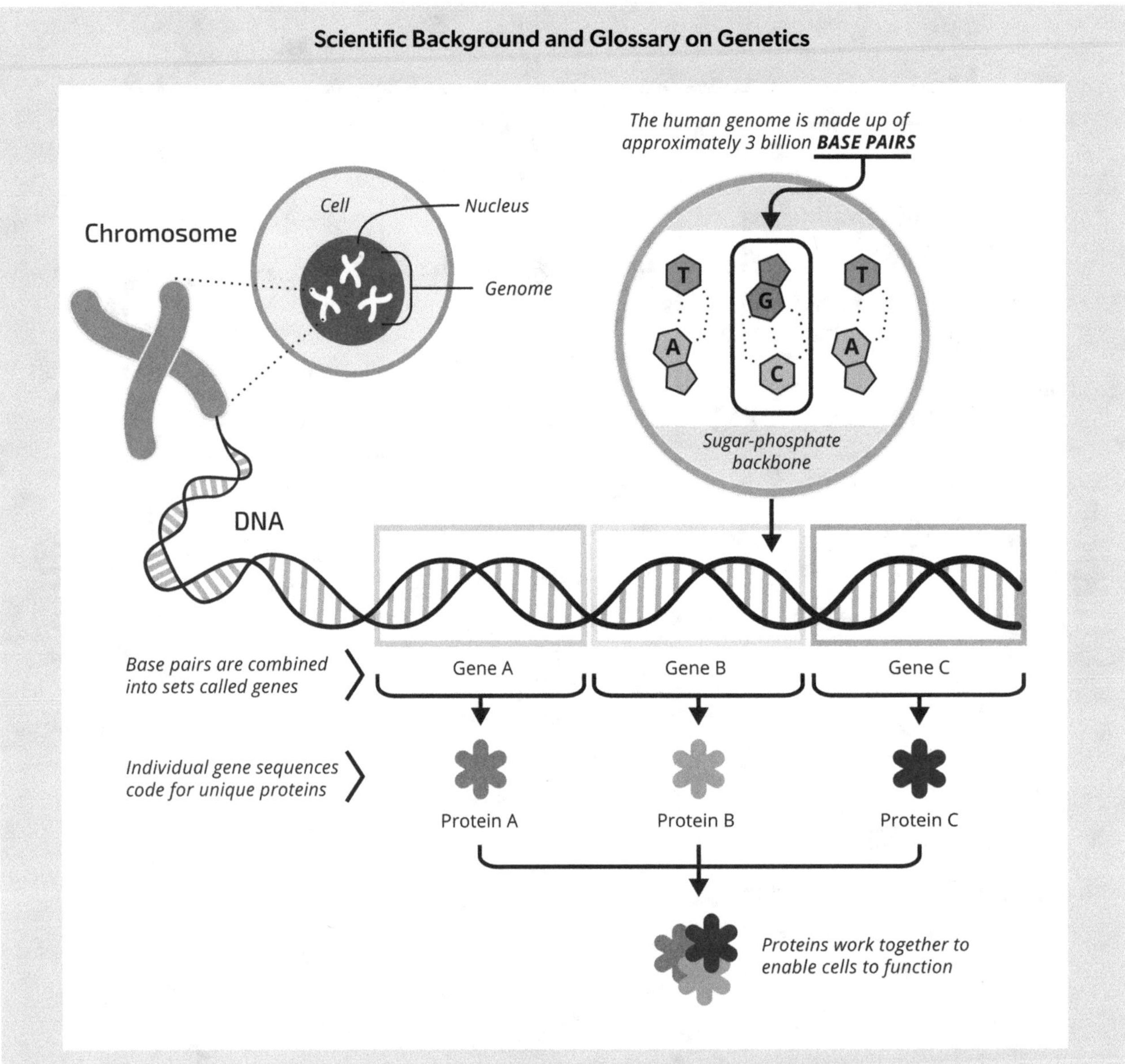

Human genome and gene readouts[124]

Your genome is made of 46 pieces of DNA, each packaged into a chromosome. Each chromosome is like a long scroll of recipes encoded with four letters or base pairs: A, C, G, and T. Each part of this recipe is a gene. The sequence of these letters is called your *genetic sequence.* In total, combining all 46 chromosomes, your genome is about 3 billion letters long and encodes about 20,000 recipes or genes. The 46 chromosomes come in pairs. Your father contributed 23 of them, and the other 23 are from your mother. One of the pairs is called the *sex chromosomes*—XX if you're biologically female and XY if you're biologically male. This is why genetic variants come in two letters—you get one copy of each gene (and thus variants) from each of your parents. One exception to this is if you're biologically male and the gene is on the X or Y chromosome; then you should have only one copy and one variant. The term *genetic variation* (also called variants, polymorphisms, or mutations) refers to the 0.1 percent of genetic difference between any two people who are not identical twins. These variations include the 3 million letters of differences.

A Note on Mutations

The word *mutation* often has a bad connotation in the mind of the public. However, there are good mutations—meaning they are beneficial for your health. There are certainly also bad mutations that could negatively impact your health. Our strategy is to become aware of the bad mutations and create a game plan to overcome their potential downside. Most of the 3 million genetic differences have very little to no effect on your health whatsoever. However, a small subset of these provide either some benefit or harmful effect.

Some terminology you may find in nutrigenomic reports and discussions is good to understand. *Genotype* refers to an individual's genetic constitution. Sometimes, it refers to specific combinations of genetic variants within an individual. *Phenotypes* are traits that result from the combined effects of your genetics, epigenetics, microbiome and diet, lifestyle, and environment. Phenotypes may be visible to the eye or detectable with technologies such as blood tests or a heart rate variability (HRV) response. These factors are what you have great control over.

An *allele* is a version of a gene, which may have one or more variations. Some genes can have multiple variations within them, and any specific combination of variations is called an allele.

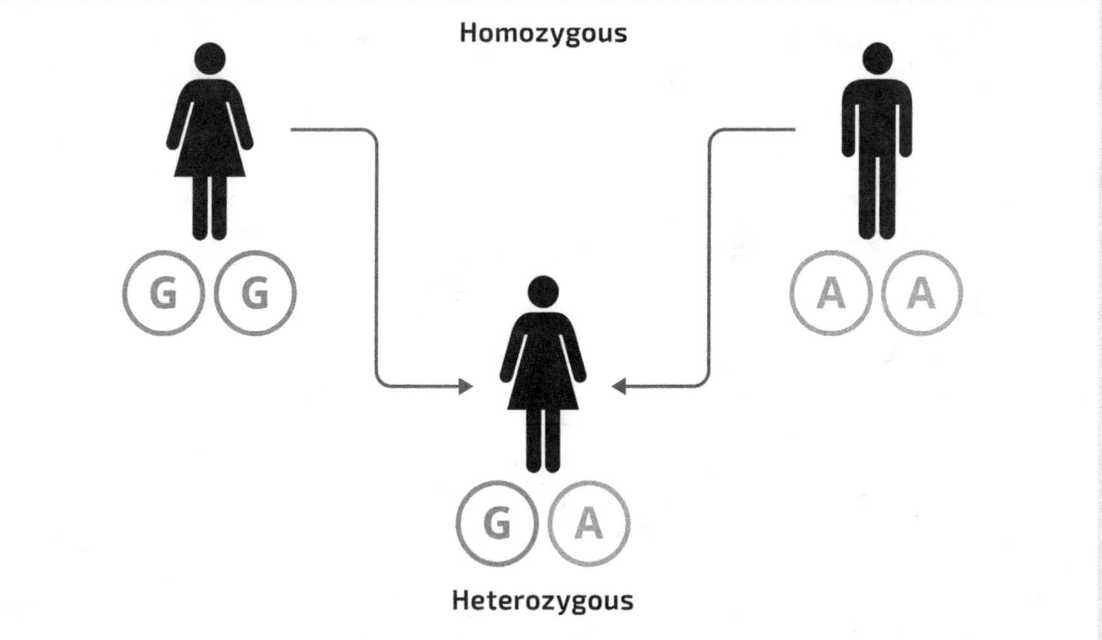

If you are *homozygous* for a gene, that means you have two copies of the same allele, whereas if you are heterozygous, that means you have two different alleles of the same gene.

Types of Genetic Variations

Your genes are like recipes embedded in the DNA strings of the four different nucleotide bases A, G, C, and T. The genetic sequence determines the gene products, such as enzymes and other proteins. Changes in the genetic sequence called *genetic variations* can affect the output of these gene recipes. Here are some of the most common types of genetic variations:[125]

- *Copy number variation* (CNV) refers to the variation of gene copy numbers on a stretch of DNA. The latter may also be called variable number tandem repeats.
- *Single nucleotide polymorphism* (SNP) refers to the difference in one base pair of DNA within the population.
- *Insertion/deletion* (indel) refers to the addition or subtraction, respectively, of a DNA sequence. Indels can be of any size from one to thousands of base pairs.

Of these, SNPs are easiest to test for, so they are most often discussed. However, CNVs and indels often have bigger biochemical impacts than SNPs because they are larger. Keep in mind that the research on how our genetic variations influence our metabolism and nutritional needs is still in its infancy. Also, your genes are static, but your life is dynamic. So, gene-based advice needs to be taken in the context of your health status and current nutritional needs.

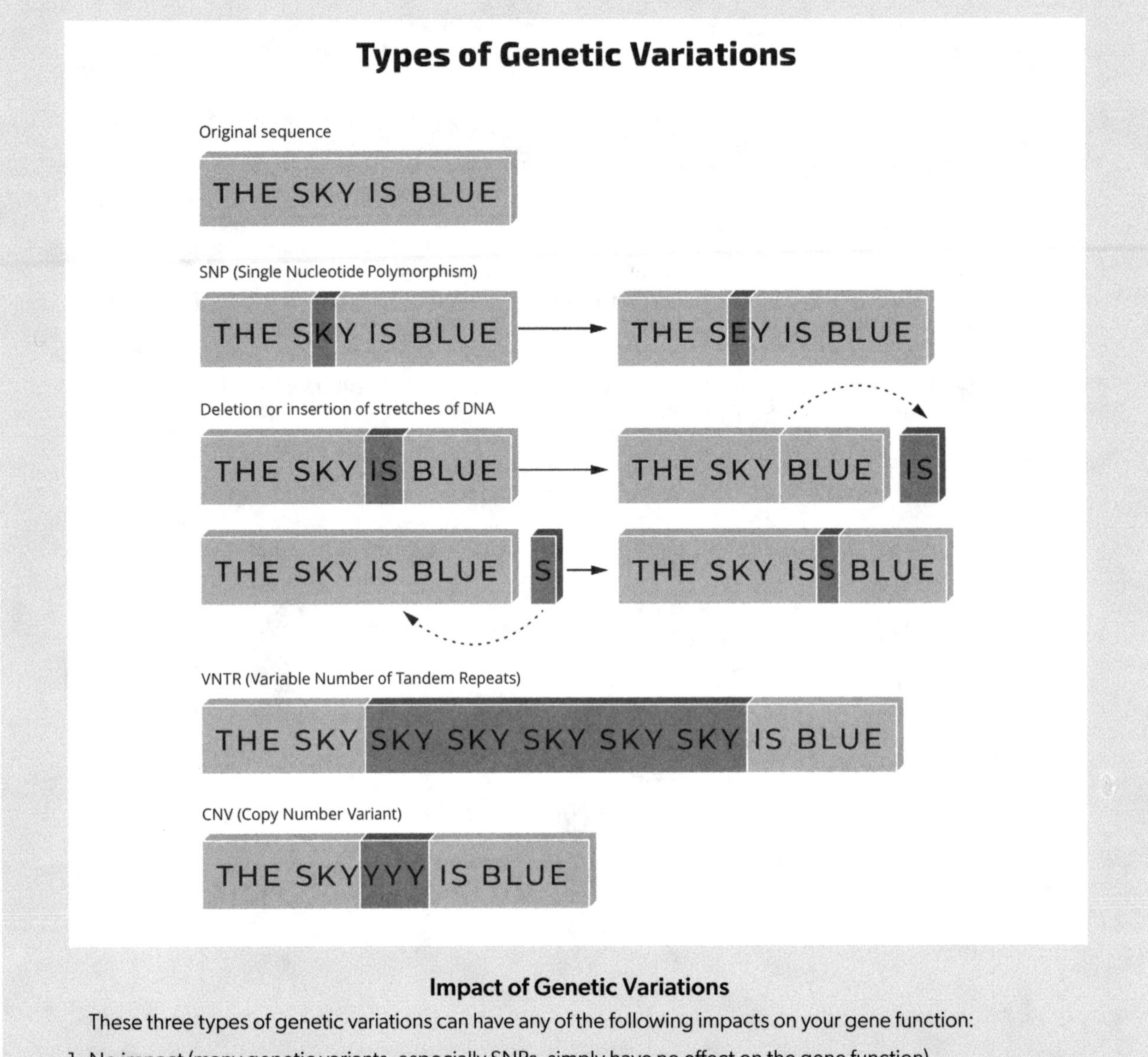

Impact of Genetic Variations

These three types of genetic variations can have any of the following impacts on your gene function:

1. No impact (many genetic variants, especially SNPs, simply have no effect on the gene function)
2. Reduction of function (the most common type of gene function change due to genetic variants)
3. Gain of function, such as by increasing protein production or protein activity
4. Creation of new function, or protein that functions in a completely different way

SUMMARY

Nutrigenomics is the study of how your genetic variants influence your body's response to nutrition and lifestyle choices.

The purpose of this chapter is to give you the tools you need to make up for any genetic weaknesses and thrive in spite of them. However, it's not as simple as just using genes to predict the best diet for you. That's because of this equation:

Your Health, Aesthetics, and Performance =
Genetics + Epigenetics + Microbiome + Exposome

You have over 20,000 genes and 3 million genetic variants. Finding a variant responsible for your problem can be like finding a needle in a haystack.

Katrine Volynsky, health researcher and nutrigenomic expert, uses the following steps:

Step 1: A very in-depth intake process that looks at:

- Symptoms
- Personality
- Environmental exposures
- Childhood history
- Food preferences
- Family history of health issues, especially on the maternal side, since everyone gets their mitochondria from their mother

Step 2: Lab tests to look at deeper-level phenotypes and biochemistry, such as:

- Organic acid test to look at how your body processes neurotransmitters and amino acids
- Micronutrient levels, such as with the SpectraCell test
- Gut tests for infections, dysbiosis, inflammation, and leaky gut

Caveats of reading genes:

- Nutrigenomics is an emerging science
- Most nutrigenomic studies are genome-wide association studies
- Variants associated with a phenotype may not *cause* the phenotype
- In humans, it's very difficult to confirm whether a gene causes a disease
- If you're alive and functional, chances are that your genes aren't very bad
- Unless you're a geneticist, you should work with a practitioner who can put all of these pieces of information into context and help you determine what to do next

Hierarchy of Genes to Address in Nutrigenomics

The right way to address genes is to do so according to the right hierarchy. The levels of the hierarchy are:

Level 1: Antioxidant, Detoxification Genes, and Metal Balance Genes

- Reactive oxygen species (ROS) are very combative molecules with an extra electron, such as bleach or hydrogen peroxide
- Too much ROS contributes to every single human disease and suboptimal states
- Your immune cells use ROS to kill germs and communicate with one another
- Your cells and mitochondria have their own checks and balances to neutralize the ROS
- Paying attention to these genes will help you maintain a healthy metabolism, hormone balance, and brain function
- NFE2L2 (NRF2) is your cell's project manager for antioxidant response and detoxification pathways
- SOD2 is a mitochondrial enzyme that neutralizes oxidative stress
- NQO1 is a very important detoxification gene that inactivates many hydrocarbon toxins
- PON1 is very important for detoxing many pesticides, drugs, and oxidized fats
- CAT (catalase) is an enzyme that helps break down hydrogen peroxide into oxygen and water
- Glutathione is the most important cellular antioxidant, including in the liver and the brain
- CYP1A2 helps with cholesterol synthesis, steroids, and fat molecules
- AhR is another cellular project manager that works closely with NRF2

- NAT1 and NAT2 activity may determine whether you're at a higher risk of getting cancer from eating red meat
- Mutations in CBS can lead to high or low ammonia levels

Level 2: Genes Involved in Food Sensitivity and Gut Lining Integrity, Including Histamine Pathways

- Most people are completely unaware of their food reactions, unless something is really severe
- A combination of three things can lead to autoimmune diseases:
  1. Genetic predisposition
  2. Leaky gut or intestinal permeability
  3. Environmental or lifestyle triggers (such as stress, gluten consumption, infections, and toxic exposures)
- Genes that can make you more likely to react to foods include:
  - Immune cell antennas (receptors)
  - Tight-junction components. Weak tight junctions may increase the risk of leaky gut and gut inflammation
  - Immune cell project managers (transcription factors) can make your immune system more reactive to certain componenets
- Genes that make gluten problematic:
  - HLA-DQA1 and HLA-DQA2 genes provide instructions for making antennas outside of your immune cells
  - Myosin 9B is an important protein for the gut barrier
  - Toll-like receptors (TLRs) recognize patterns on microbial cells and trigger immune responses
  - Claudins are proteins that make the tight junction between gut lining cells
  - Mucins are gel-forming proteins that become the mucus covering the gut lining and other mucus-covered tissues
  - FOXP3 is a cellular project manager (transcription factor) that gets T cells to develop into regulatory T cells instead of the autoimmune-promoting Th17 cells
- Genes related to histamine breakdown:
  - ABP1 (also known as AOC1) produces the enzyme diamine oxidase, which deactivates histamine
  - HNMT (histamine N-methyltransferase) deactivates histamine inside cells by methylating the histamine
  - MAOB (monoamine oxidase) is produced in the liver and many other tissues, but its most important roles involve breaking down neurotransmitters in the brain
  - Cannabinoid receptors
- Dairy and lactose intolerance genes:
  - LCT produces lactase, an enzyme that digests the milk sugar lactose

Level 3: Protein, Fat, and Carb Digestion and Metabolism

- PPAR (peroxisome proliferator-activated receptors) is a family of cellular project managers (transcription factors) that manage genes related to protein and carb metabolism
  - PPAR-α mainly influences fatty acid metabolism
  - PPAR-*β* helps with fat burning in muscles and the heart
  - PPAR-γ governs insulin sensitivity, along with the production of new fat cells, energy balance, and the production of fat molecules
- ApoA2 is the eat fat, get fat gene
- ApoE helps transport fat and cholesterol
- ACSL-1 gives you the ability to metabolize saturated fats
- PEMT makes choline in the liver, which is important for fat metabolism, especially in women

- AMY1 provides instructions for the enzyme amylase, which digests starches
- LPL helps to modulate whether saturated fats are stored as body fat or burned as fuel, and plays a role in how saturated fats are broken down for energy
- APOC3 controls triglyceride levels as well as LDL cholesterol, which is the more dangerous type
- ACAT determines how your body converts protein and fat to cellular energy

Level 4: Environmental Sensitivity and Neurotransmitter Support

- COMT is one of the most important genes in nutrigenomics. It helps degrade catecholamine neurotransmitters such as dopamine and norepinephrine.
- MAO genes produce the monoamine oxidase enzymes, which are also important for removing norepinephrine, dopamine, and serotonin from the brain

Level 5: Vitamins A and D

- One of the most important vitamin A genes is BCMO1, which converts beta-carotene to vitamin A
- Variants near the following genes affect the efficiency of vitamin D supplementation on 25-hydroxy vitamin D (25-OHD) in the blood:
    - VDR, which produces the vitamin D receptor
    - CYP2R1, which produces an enzyme that activates vitamin D
    - CYP24A1, which produces an enzyme that deactivates vitamin D
    - CYP27B1, which produces an enzyme that converts vitamin D to 25-OHD
    - GC, which produces a protein that binds to vitamin D
    - DHCR7, which produces an enzyme that moves vitamin D precursors toward cholesterol production

Level 6: mTOR-vs.-Autophagy Balance

- mTOR is your cell's nutrient sensor. Once you have an abundance of nutrients and calories, it puts your cells in an anabolic state.
- Autophagy is a rejuvenative process in which, when nutrients and calories are scarce, your cells break down old cellular parts to reuse them as building blocks

Level 7: Methylation, MTHFR, and Folate

- Methylation is important for your neurotransmitters, hormones, and detoxification
- Folate provides a backbone for your DNA
- The MTHFR gene produces the enzyme that converts folate into methylfolate, the active form of folate. This gene is a bottleneck in the methylation cycle.

Genes to Keep in Mind for Each Nutritional Goal and Strategy

- Sometimes, a nutritional strategy or food may set off a hidden genetic minefield
- The following are genes to keep in mind when you're on either an unsaturated-fat, plant-based dietary pattern or one significant in saturated animal fats:
    - ACSL1 is a cellular project manager that governs neuronal development
    - ADIPOQ is the red meat gene
    - FTO is the hangry gene that governs your ghrelin levels
    - LPL decides whether you'll store saturated fats as body fat or burn them as fuel, and plays a role in how saturated fats are broken down for energy
    - APOC3 regulates blood triglyceride levels and LDL (bad) cholesterol
    - APOA2 is the eat fat, get fat gene

    - ApoE, especially the ApoE4 variant, is a known risk for Alzheimer's and bad response to high-saturated-fat diets
- Genes that can make you more exhausted on keto and fasting:
    - PPAR-alpha is important for getting into ketosis
    - ACAT controls how your body converts protein and fat into cellular energy (ATP) in the mitochondria
    - A CPT1A variant is found in many populations in the cold climate
- Plant-based vs. animal-sourced nutrients:
    - High copy number of AMY1, which is a salivary starch predigestion enzyme
    - BCMO1 weak variants can reduce the conversion of beta-carotene into retinol, which may cause a vitamin A deficiency on a plant-based diet
    - Lactase (Lct1)-influencing variant located inside the MCM6 gene determines whether you should keep dairy in your diet
    - FUT2 influences your gut bacteria and vitamin B_{12}
    - FADS1 and FADS2 genes produce enzymes that convert short-chain (plant-based) omega-3 and omega-6 fatty acids into long-chain ones
    - PEMT gene produces an important enzyme for choline production, so vegetarians who have weak PEMT may not produce enough choline
    - SHBG gene produces sex-hormone binding globulin, a blood protein that binds to your sex hormones for transport
- Goal-specific genetic considerations:
    - Fat gain and fat loss genes
- Genes related to fitness goals and muscle gain:
    - Mitochondrial biogenesis and antioxidant response gene

        PPARGC1A (PPARG coactivator 1 alpha) is a cellular project manager that works with PPARG and PPARA

        NRF2 is your cellular project manager for antioxidant genes
    - Fatigue/Endurance:

        NOS3 produces nitric oxide synthase 3

        PPARD is a cellular project manager in the same family as PPARA and PPARG

        MCT1 or SLC16A1 transports lactic acid in both slow-twitch and fast-twitch muscle fibers
    - Inflammation response to training:

        If you have these variants in the TNF-alpha, IL-6, IL-10, and CRP genes, you may get more muscle damage from exercise
    - Training response:
        - ACE produces an angiotensin-converting enzyme, which is responsible for activating angiotensin
        - ACTN3 produces alpha-actinin-3, a protein that structures your fast-twitch muscle fibers
        - MSTN produces myostatin, a protein that prevents muscle mass from growing out of control
        - ADRB2 produces a beta-2 adrenergic receptor, which takes signals from adrenaline
        - UCP2 and UCP3 produce uncoupling proteins, which cause your mitochondria to turn energy into heat rather than ATP
        - Variants in genes related to vitamin D absorption, reception, and processing are associated with strength and lean body mass
        - AGT produces angiotensin, the hormone that increases blood pressure, body salt, and fluid balance
    - Connective tissue genes affecting injury risk:
        - COL1A produces a type of collagen that is most abundant in your body
        - COL5A produces another type of collagen. It also determines collagen assembly and fiber width

- Antiaging and longevity genes:
    - Cellular antioxidant genes such as NRF2, SOD2, and catalase that protect your cellular components and DNA from damage
    - Mitochondrial function genes, such as PPARGC1A and AMPK
    - Genes such as MTHFR and MTHFD1 that produce enzymes in the methylation pathway and are important for epigenetic regulation
    - DNA damage-repair genes
    - Autophagy genes, which help renew cellular components and healthy immune function
    - Apoptosis genes that ensure cancer cells and virus-infected cells commit suicide
    - Genes that help proteins fold properly, such as heat shock proteins
    - Nutrient-sensing genes, such as mTOR, sirtuins, and insulin signaling
    - Inflammation genes, such as inflammatory cytokines (IL-6, CRP, and IL-1beta) and cellular project managers that manage immune responses, such as FOXO3 and NF-κB

Putting the Benefits of This Chapter into Your Life

You have two options for benefiting from the information we've provided here:

1. You find a nutrigenomic expert that has this knowledge and work with them
2. You become a nutrigenomic expert yourself, which is a long, hard road
3. Use our Nutrigenomics Testing Kit at to: www.BIOptimizers.com/book/genes

CHAPTER 34

YOUR GENETICS ARE NOT YOUR DESTINY

The Story of Your Great-Great-Grandparents' Epigenetics

In this chapter, you'll learn:

- Why your genes are not your fate, how you are in control of your genetic expression, and how to turn your genes on and off through diet, exercise, sleep, supplementation, and more
- Why your parents' environment and your lifestyle choices determine your health, and how up to 14 generations of your family health history is part of your body today
- What epigenetics are and how to tip the epigenetic odds in your favor to optimize activation and take control of your health
- The main driver of most modern health issues, including why two out of three Americans struggle with weight and 97 percent struggle to lose it
- How your nervous system impacts your epigenetics through traumas and mental-emotional stress—and exactly how meditation can be used as a powerful tool to combat these responses
- The seven bioactive compounds in food that you should start including in your diet *now* to promote a healthy epigenome
- Why the "one pill for one disease" model sets you up to *fail*, even if it's seemingly natural or healthy—and how effects may persist through your children, grandchildren, and great-grandchildren's generations
- How physical exercise, both aerobic and resistance, positively influences your epigenetics, and why endurance exercise training is important
- What we can learn about epigenetics from pregnant Dutch women in World War II when all routes of food supply to the Netherlands were blocked
- That obesity is a direct effect only of making unhealthy lifestyle choices, right? *Wrong!* Obesity can be inherited via epigenetics both paternally and maternally.
- How to form the best habits to turn on your positive gene expressions and minimize the habits that turn on your bad genes
- How epigenetics happen: the bird's-eye view—and the eight steps that lead to genetic expression
- *Be advised:* This is one of the most science-dense chapters in this book. You don't need to understand all of the scientific nuances of genetics. If it's too much, just focus on the key takeaways and implement the practical Power Moves.

Access to the uncut version: We decided to cut more than 50 percent of this chapter, keeping only the most practical information for you. For the uncut version, go to: www.BIOptimizers.com/book/resources.

YOUR GENETICS ARE NOT YOUR FATE

To what extent, then, do our genes determine our fate? Study after study shows that although some traits are fully determined by genes, those are the exception and not the rule.

Let's start with the key takeaway of this chapter: you're in control of your genetic expression—a more empowering story has overturned the idea of genetic determinism. How? Through the foods you eat, the exercise you do, the sleep you get, your emotional health, the amout of sun exposure you get, the supplements you take, and many more factors. All of these constantly turn genes on and off.

The journey to optimal health is to build positive habits that turn on positive gene expression—and minimize the habits that turn on bad genes.

In the early 90s, researchers expected humans to have around 120,000 genes, given how complex our physiology is. To their surprise, the Human Genome Project found that we have between 20,000 and 25,000 genes—the same order of magnitude as roundworms (20,470).

However, our physiology is hundreds of times more complicated than that of roundworms. Those 25,000 genes aren't even enough to construct our brains. Given the few genes we have, there are two other key factors that make us human:

1. The human microbiome, which contains ~3.3 million genes[1] (See Chapter 6.)
2. Epigenetics is the way your genes express, depending on your environment. Your genes constantly turn on and off in real time in response to it.

WHAT IS EPIGENETICS?

Epigenetics is the set of factors that adjust levels of gene function without actually changing the genetic sequence.

Your genome is like 46 scrolls of recipes. In total, it has about 25,000 recipes for producing something in your cells, such as protein or RNA. Each recipe is a gene encoded in a language that consists of four letters: A, G, C, and T. So, your genetic sequence refers to the recipe sequence of these four letters, which is unique for each person.

Most of your genes encode instructions for producing something within your cells, such as proteins or RNA. Adjusting the level of gene readouts means your genes can produce more or fewer proteins or RNA as needed.

Some epigenetic phenomena are short-lived, lasting only a few seconds to a few minutes. Others could last years or a lifetime. Learning to optimize your epigenetic activation is how you truly take control of your health.

If epigenetic changes make their way into someone's egg or sperm, they can be inherited.

Signals that trigger the epigenetic phenomena can be external, such as nutrient status and traumas. Or they can be internal, such as your circadian rhythm. Many natural phenomena, such as growth and aging, occur through epigenetics. Your genes load the gun, while your environment pulls the trigger.

Here's a shocking finding from a recent experiment on roundworms: the epigenome was passed down for *14 generations.*

Here's what this means for you: the epigenetics of your parents, grandparents, great-grand-parents, great-great-grandparents—up to 14 generations back—are part of your body today.

Remember that epigenetic research is still very new and a rapidly growing field of research. So, this chapter cannot possibly offer comprehensive coverage of the subject. Our goal here is to empower you with knowledge you can use right now to change your gene expression. You have the power!

WHAT TO DO WITH YOUR EPIGENETICS

Epigenetics, not genetics, is likely the main driver of most modern health issues. Epigenetics is one of the key reasons why two out of three Americans struggle with weight and 97 percent struggle to lose it. The epigenetic marks that tell genes to hang on to weight may have started with our grandparents' or great-grandparents' exposures to an environment of scarcity.

Epigenetics also partly explains the rise of insulin resistance, diabetes, cancers, fertility problems, mental and cognitive problems, autoimmune diseases, and more.[2]

To date, very few therapies target epigenetics, aside from a few cancer drugs that have severe side effects. Because epigenetic mechanisms are used throughout your genome, it's nearly impossible to develop safe interventions to target specific epigenetics on your genes.

The goal of this book is to empower you to thrive despite any suboptimal epigenetics from your ancestors rather than experience the health decline that may come with them.

HOW TO TIP THE EPIGENETIC ODDS IN YOUR FAVOR

The best way to account for epigenetics is to combine genetic data with biofeedback such as lab tests and symptoms (see Chapter 34). Our kaizen process of BIOptimization takes into account epigenetic optimization (see Chapter 32).

The following can help you reverse or counteract many of the bad epigenetics and play up the good ones based on the latest science.

Optimize Your Mindset and Nervous System

Your mindset and the state of your nervous system can strongly influence your epigenetics.

According to Bruce Lipton, Ph.D., having loving, positive, and empowering thoughts can improve your epigenetics, whereas negative thoughts, such as the fixed belief that you cannot achieve your health goals, can program unhealthy epigenetic marks.[3]

Traumas and mental and emotional stresses program the stress epigenetics that can keep you from achieving your best health.[4] Most people, even those without post-traumatic stress disorder (PTSD), have hundreds of micro-traumas that can affect their health.

The good news is that you can address your traumas and overcome their negative epigenetic impacts. As coaches, we are trauma-informed and are equipped with many tools and a network of professionals to help our clients address these traumas. (See Chapter 11 for a list of resources to help you address your traumas.)

Power Move: Meditate

Practices such as mindfulness meditation, yoga, and tai chi have been proven to have a positive effect on epigenetics and well-being.

These emotional- and attention-regulatory practices have been shown to produce a greater state of self-awareness. They can also promote inner silence, which can be considered a powerful tool to combat the negative effects of stress-related symptoms.

The key is to find a meditation practice that resonates with you and make it part of your daily BIOptimized habits.

FIND AND FOLLOW THE DIET THAT WORKS FOR YOU

A high-carb, low-fat diet can be optimal for one person and fattening for another. The same is true for keto or any other diet.

Keto feels very good for Matt. It keeps him full, maximizes his cognitive function, and makes it easier for him to stay lean, while high-carb diets make him ravenous. The opposite is true for Wade—he feels awful on keto but amazing and even-keeled on high-carb, plant-based diets.

In short, a diet that doesn't work for your body can lead to bad epigenetics.

This is why one of the premises of this book is individualization and iteration based on your personal biofeedback.

OPTIMIZE YOUR GUT FLORA

It shouldn't be a surprise that your gut microbes influence your epigenetics. Your bacteria produce metabolites such as short-chain fatty acids, vitamins, amino acids, and more.

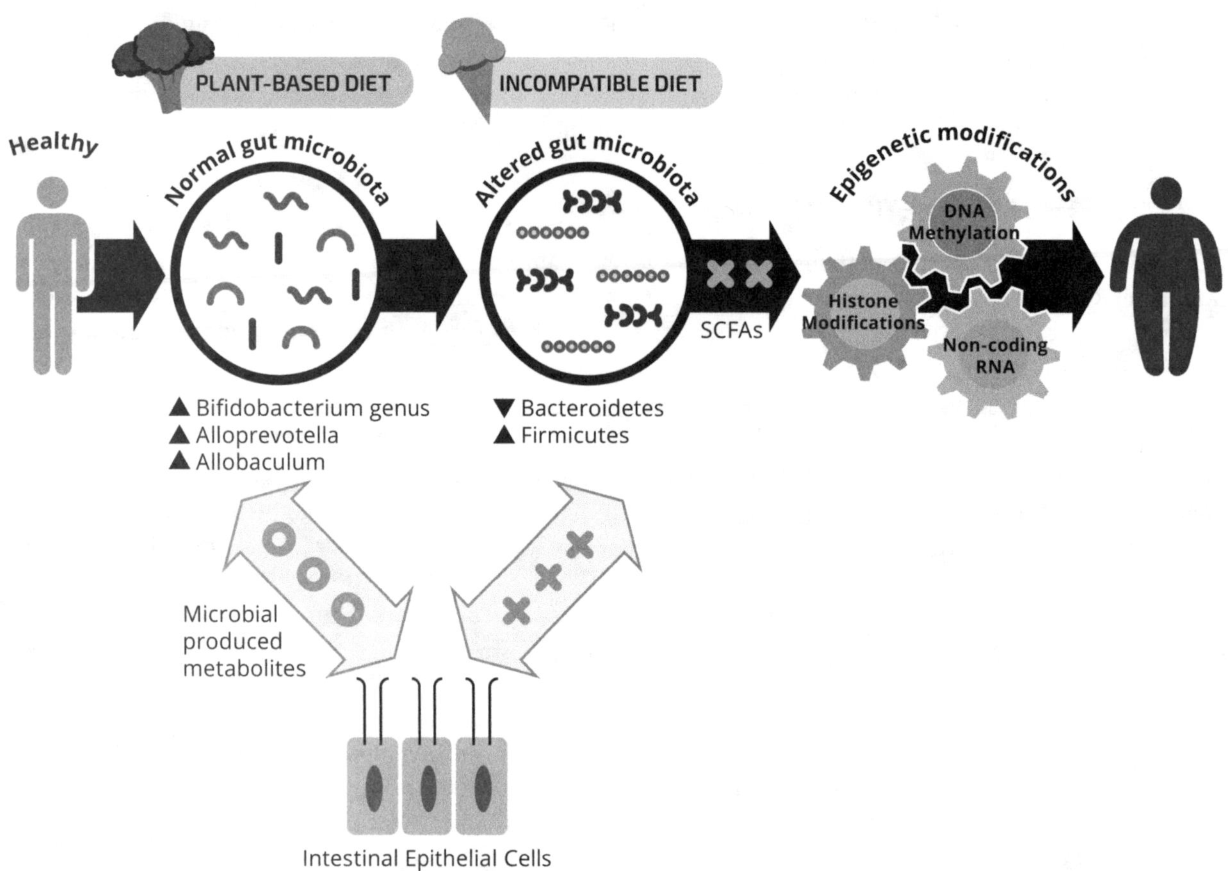

Caution: Physiologically incompatible diets can influence both the gut flora and epigenetics, leading to obesity.

For example, short-chain fatty acids—such as butyrate and propionate—inhibit the removal of acetyl groups from histones. They also reduce DNA methylation, thereby increasing expression of genes that prevent cancers (tumor suppressor genes).[5]

Through epigenetic changes and supporting mitochondrial health, short-chain fatty acids can powerfully reverse many metabolic problems caused by a modern lifestyle. They can also reduce diet-related inflammation and help seal a leaky gut.[6]

High-fiber diets and synbiotic supplements promote healthy gut bacteria composition and increase short-chain fatty acid production. This is why we formulate our probiotic supplements as synbiotics.[7]

To learn more about improving your gut flora, refer to Chapter 12.

Power Move: Eat Foods That Promote Healthy Epigenetics

Many bioactive compounds in food can promote a healthy epigenome. These include:[8]

- Sulforaphane and isothiocyanates in cruciferous vegetables
- EGCG from green tea
- Resveratrol in grapes, blueberries, and red wine
- Genistein found in soy
- Other plant polyphenols
- Vitamins B complex, C, D, folate, choline, and other methyl donors
- Selenium

Many promising studies have found that these compounds and nutrients can reverse the harmful epigenetic marks caused by pollution and endocrine disruption.

However, the effects of these compounds can be dose dependent. These substances also have a balancing effect on your entire epigenome, so their effects may not be targeted—they can create healthy epigenetic marks on one spot and unfavorable ones on another in your genome.

Therefore, it's generally safest to consume these compounds from foods rather than as isolated nutrients in high doses, especially in the long term . . . which brings us to the next point.

Watch for Physiological Imbalances when Introducing Supplements and Biohacks

One of the reasons overall human health is declining is that we've introduced interventions using the myopic "one pill for one disease" model.

This model eventually fails because biology always works like an intricate network. Everything (even seemingly natural or healthy) has a ripple effect on your physiology, microbiome, and epigenome. The effects may also be passed to your children, grandchildren, and great-grandchildren for generations.

For example, as mentioned earlier, folic acid fortification may increase the overall risk of cancers and metabolic problems in future generations.

The Selenium and Vitamin E Cancer Prevention Trial (SELECT) enrolled over 35,000 middle-aged men. The trial tested the hypothesis of whether vitamin E and selenium, which have antioxidant properties, could prevent cancers.

For ethical reasons, the trial terminated three years early. Men in the supplement group were developing prostate cancers at a 17 percent higher rate than the placebo group.[9]

Given how large the trial was, this is a statistically significant and medically accepted finding. It's a prime example of why you need to be mindful of your biology when introducing supplements and biohacks. It shows consequences of increasing a dosage past optimal levels.

Folate is another good example of an important nutrient that must be monitored.

Power Move: Optimize Your Folate

Low folate can increase the risk for many types of cancers, potentially through abnormal methylation of cancer genes.

On the other hand, excessive folic acid intake can result in high unmetabolized folic acid in the blood, known as *unmetabolized folic acid syndrome*. The syndrome has been clearly linked to prostate cancers and potentially to other types as well.[10]

The good news is that you can supplement safely with folate by using safer forms such as methylfolate. Also, be sure to take it in balance with other B vitamins and methyl acceptors.

The safest forms of folate are from food sources, such as chicken liver, vegetables, and whole-food supplements.

EXAMPLES OF HOW YOUR EPIGENETICS AFFECT YOUR HEALTH AND RESPONSES TO NUTRITIONAL INTERVENTIONS

Epigenetic research has discovered many examples of how prenatal (or even preconception) exposure can affect lifelong health and nutritional responses.

This section is not an exhaustive list of how epigenetics operate, but our examples can give you an idea of what epigenetics can do.

Power Move: Move, Baby, Move!

Physical exercise, both aerobic and resistance, can positively influence your epigenetics.

Endurance exercise training induces a number of adaptations in skeletal muscle, the most important of which is an increase in mitochondria with an improvement in respiratory capacity.

Some epigenetic modifications that possibly occur due to physical exercise can have a positive effect on restoring the genomic stability in cells with carcinogenic (cancer-causing) potential.

There are numerous rapid mRNA and mitochondrial improvements to repeated high-intensity interval training sessions. Increases in mitochondrial proteins occur within five days following three sessions of high-intensity interval training.

HOW EPIGENETIC ALTERATIONS ACCUMULATE

If we send "bad signals," meaning signals that don't help our health, negative changes in the genome accumulate over time and have been correlated with the decline observed in aging cells. This is a very important factor for all aspiring parents. You have an opportunity to become healthier and pass on its advantages to your children.

Alterations to gene expression patterns are an important influencer of aging. Aging can cause changes to our epigenome, eventually compromising your cells' function. Remember that your cells are your body's building blocks—the bricks that create your walls. Your epigenome is a record of the chemical changes to your DNA, and these changes can be passed down to your children via epigenetic inheritance.

IN UTERO FAMINE AND GROWTH RESTRICTION CAN PREDISPOSE YOU TO BROKEN METABOLISM

During World War II, the Dutch went through eight months of famine before they were liberated.

Many Dutch women were pregnant throughout this period. The children who were born from these pregnancies ended up with significantly higher rates of obesity, high cholesterol, and heart diseases. They also had shorter life spans than their siblings and other Dutch people whose mothers hadn't starved through pregnancy.[11]

A DNA methylation study examined the DNA of these individuals compared to their siblings. By the time technologies that detected DNA methylation became available, these Dutch people were in their 70s and 80s, so any changes in epigenetic marks would have been lifelong.

The study found that the Dutch who went through in utero starvation had a different methylation pattern. They had more methylation on genes that controlled energy metabolism, carb and fat metabolism, insulin production, and cholesterol levels.[12]

The methylation marks silenced the genes, predisposing these individuals to obesity, poor blood sugar control, metabolic problems, and high cholesterol.

Consistent with this, a mouse study found that a low-protein diet during pregnancy and breastfeeding increased belly fat and insulin resistance in offspring. The offspring's epigenetics expected a nutrient-poor environment, so they had more neuropeptide Y. As a result, they easily gained fat.[13]

Evolutionarily, it made sense that the epigenetics of the Dutch children remembered what their mothers went through and stayed prepared for another famine. The end of World War II didn't reverse the methylation patterns, unfortunately.

Power Move: Build a Gratitude Practice

Feelings of gratitude and love have been shown to positively affect your epigenetics.

The hormones the brain releases when experiencing feelings of love include positive hormones such as oxytocin and dopamine, which are made in the pituitary gland and secreted into the bloodstream. This causes cells to function optimally, creating that look of being in love, or a "glowing" appearance.

It may take time to wire your brain to default to gratitude, especially during challenging times. However, as you hardwire your brain for gratitude, you will be able to create a new baseline of happiness.

There are many ways to make this a daily habit. From gratitude apps to WhatsApp groups to gratitude journals such as *The Five Minute Journal* by Intelligent Change, it's never been simpler and easier to incorporate this power move into your life.

INSULIN RESISTANCE AND ABNORMAL LIPID METABOLISM

In rodents, high-fat diets cause insulin resistance, fatty liver, and obesity. On the other hand, some people reverse insulin resistance, fatty liver, and obesity by shifting from low-fat to high-fat diets.

Humans are obviously not rodents, but we may extrapolate the results of high-fat diets in mice to what you may observe when you eat a diet that is physiologically incompatible. For example, the effects of high-fat diets in rodents are similar to those we see from prolonged junk food diets in humans.

Pregnant rats fed with high-fat and high-sugar diets give birth to offspring that have higher fasting blood glucose and lipid homeostasis. In humans, obese pregnant mothers increase the risk of obesity, type 2 diabetes, heart disease, nonalcoholic fatty liver, and kidney issues in their children.[14]

HOW DOES EPIGENETICS HAPPEN?

As we've seen, the term *genetic expression* refers to anything that influences gene function. It can include the entire process, from when the genetic recipe is read to how fast a gene product is destroyed.

Your cells have numerous ways to coordinate gene expression and adjust it to the environment. Some of these, such as methylation, have been studied for a long time. However, many others have only been discovered in the past few years, and scientists are still discovering more ways epigenetics happen, including:

- DNA methylation
- Chemical tags added to histone tails
- DNA packaging
- Histone swapping
- RNA splicing
- Regulatory RNAs and MicroRNA (miRNA)
- Messenger RNA (mRNA) stability
- Protein stability

SUMMARY

You are in control of your genetic expression. You control the foods you eat, the exercise you do, the sleep you get, your emotional health, the amount of sun exposure you get, the supplements you take, and many more habits. These habits constantly turn your genes on and off.

The main goal is to form habits that will turn positive gene expression on and to minimize the habits that turn on bad genes.

Epigenetics refers to anything that adjusts gene function without actually changing the genetic sequence. Learning to optimize your epigenetic activation is how you take control of your health.

Epigenetics is one of the key reasons why two out of three Americans struggle with weight and 97 percent of them struggle to lose it.

The best way to account for epigenetics is to combine genetic data with biofeedback such as lab tests and monitoring symptoms. The following can help you reverse or counteract many of the bad epigenetics and play up the good ones based on the latest science:

- Optimize your mindset and nervous system
- Find and follow the diet that works for you
- Optimize your gut flora
- Pay attention to physiologic balances when introducing supplements and biohacks

Epigenetic research has discovered many examples of how prenatal—or even preconception—exposure can affect lifelong health and nutritional responses.

If epigenetic changes make their way into egg or sperm, they can be inherited. In utero famine and growth restriction can predispose you to a broken metabolism. Obesity can be inherited via epigenetics from both the mother and father.

Epigenetics happens by:

- DNA methylation
- Chemical tags added to histone tails
- DNA packaging
- Histone swapping
- RNA splicing
- Regulatory RNAs
- mRNA stability
- Protein stability

You can also help improve your epigenetics by completing Power Moves such as:

- Optimizing your folate
- Meditating and other spiritual practices
- Eating the right diet for your body type
- Exercising
- Optimized supplementation
- Creating a gratitude practice

CONCLUSION

MANIFESTING YOUR DREAM BODY

Now that you've read the book from start to finish:

- You'll never be confused about nutrition and diets again. You now understand how to build the best diets for you, and how to evolve them based on your goals, for the rest of your life.
- You'll never fall prey to diet marketing lies again.
- You have a wide variety of effective nutritional strategies to lose excess body fat and reach your ideal weight.
- You know how to avoid regaining fat and how to stay slim forever.
- You know how to build as much lean muscle as you want.
- You know how to optimize your nutrition to maximize your life span and health span (we call this your BioSpan).
- You know how to eat for maximum athletic performance.
- You know the best nutritional strategies to optimize your mental performance.

CREATING THE VISION

It all starts with a vision. What do you want your body to be? What do you want it to look like? What do you want it to feel like? Move like?

Don't let poor genetics and previous struggles stop you from dreaming *big*. One of the core messages we want you to get from this book is that you are in control of your body. The future of your body is in your hands. By applying the strategies in this book, making them habits, and living the BIOptimized lifestyle, you can manifest your dream body.

Start with the End in Mind by Wade T. Lightheart

Start with the end in mind. For me, that was, "Hey, I want to compete in the Mr. Universe contest."

Well, to compete at the Mr. Universe contest, I had to win a national championship. To win a national championship, I had to win a provincial championship. To win a provincial championship, I had to win a local contest. And to win a local contest, I needed to get some muscle and learn how to get lean.

Then, I created a feedback loop that measured my weekly progress. I hired Scott Abel, one of the greatest bodybuilding coaches of all time. My success went to the next level. And after a few years, I stood on stage at the Mr. Universe contest in India.

And it all starts in your mind. Where the mind goes, the body will follow. However, a great vision isn't enough. Millions of people have big visions, but they are simply dreamers who take little action. To become a creator and a manifester, you need a compelling vision and to take the right actions over time.

The formula for success is vision plus the right actions applied over time.

CYCLING THROUGH THE FIVE GOALS AND BECOMING THE MAIN CHARACTER IN YOUR BIOPTIMIZATION STORY

Become the protagonist in the movie *My Biological Optimization Story*. Earlier in the book, we laid out five epic quests you can take with your body.

There's a lot of fun and enjoyment in creating new goals and challenges. We've gone from being obsessed with muscle building because we were insecure, wanted to attract girls, and craved respect from guys. Wade followed his passion with competitive bodybuilding. Matt became obsessed with mixed martial arts and self-defense.

In our 30s, our goals shifted again. We had enough lean body mass. Then we focused on improving our cognitive performance. We started doing neurofeedback and using nootropics (like Nootopia).

We also focused on taking our health to its pinnacle. That's really where BIOptimizers started—we engaged in the Biological Optimization Process. We built a great Jedi Council and started looking at our health data: bloodwork, genetics, biomarkers, and biofeedback, and we systematically optimized things that needed to be fixed.

Now in our 40s and 50s, we continue to double down on the Biological Optimization Process and brain optimization. Now our primary goal is to maximize our longevity and quality of life.

CONQUERING THE FOES IN YOUR MIND

The one thing that holds people back is how they view themselves and what they believe is possible. Our identities are forged over time by our genetics, peer groups, friends, family, and the media. When the evidence demonstrates that your identity isn't working for you, it's time to create a new one. To achieve a new outcome, you have to create a new identity.

Creating a New Identity

Wade had a conversation with a super-successful friend of his. He asked Garrett what the journey was to get to his stunning 25-million-dollar home in San Diego.

Garrett replied, "I was running on the Pacific Coast Highway, looking at all the massive mansions. I asked myself, 'Who is the person I have to become to make that normal? Who is the person that I need to become?'"

Meditate and contemplate on who this new version of you is. What does your day look like? What's your lifestyle? What are your key habits? What's your mindset around health? How does that new body feel?

HEALTH IS THE ULTIMATE WEALTH

Good investors constantly manage and rebalance their portfolios based on market conditions. They're investing in things that they believe will compound over time. Ultimately, what is their goal? They're seeking a better quality of life. Investors believe that wealth will improve quality of life by providing independence and freedom.

What's the value of your money if your health is compromised? If you don't invest in your health today, your golden years are going to be more like the grueling years.

In our opinion, nothing adds more high-quality living than the BIOptimized lifestyle. Most of the most powerful health upgrades are free: walking, sun, exercise, drinking water, sleeping, spiritual practices, and being happy. Just like in investing, each healthy habit compounds your return on investment, which gets bigger and bigger with every new upgrade. Biological Optimization is the greatest investment you'll ever make.

TRULY LIVING LIFE TO THE FULLEST

So, what we're striving for at BIOptimizers is to give you the tools to optimize your aesthetics, performance (both mental and physical), and health.

We envision making 100 the new 50. That's the goal we're holding in mind and believe is possible. As a company, our aim is to help the world's life span go beyond 100 years and to add 10 points to the average person's IQ.

With all the innovations today in aging, brain optimization, genetics, cybernetics, nutrition, and peptides, longevity is going to improve exponentially over the next few decades. BIOptimizers is here to lead the charge.

When you're BIOptimized, you can enjoy your great-grandchildren. Maybe you want to jump out of planes or surf 10-foot waves when you're 80 years old. Maybe you want to build spaceships and go to Mars. Or maybe you just want to enjoy a simple and joyful life with your family and loved ones. The BIOptimized lifestyle will help you live those dreams.

THE DECISION: MAKING THE UNBREAKABLE COMMITMENT

We believe that one of the biggest differences between people who are living healthy lifestyles and those who struggle to follow them is an Unbreakable Commitment.

The Unbreakable Commitment is *the decision* that you will pursue health forever, no matter what. It's a core part of your life.

Goals are powerful, but the Unbreakable Commitment is 100 times more powerful. As trainers, we would get clients who came in with short-term goals, achieved them, and lost motivation. They'd go right back to their old habits.

Someone who's made the decision to pursue and develop health for the rest of their life doesn't stop. When Matt got shot a few years ago, he was in the gym training with a cast on. When Wade travels and is under extreme conditions, he still makes time to go to the gym.

We've burnt out more times than we can remember and kept going. Matt tore his Achilles tendon and kept training. Wade gained 42 pounds of fat and water after competing and got back on track. We kept training at home under severe lockdowns. Nothing stops us. And nothing will stop you once you make the Unbreakable Commitment.

Will we waver in our motivation sometimes? Of course—we're human. Will we drift away from our ideal standards at times? Of course—we're human. If we gain a little bit of weight, we get back on track with a weight loss cycle. If our health gets compromised because we push ourselves too hard and too long, we make the adjustments and get back on track. We're always recalibrating.

The Unbreakable Commitment is your North Star. It goes back to getting that clear vision of where you want to be a year from now—and 5 years, 50 years. What kind of person do you want to be when you're 100 or 150 years old?

Once you make the Unbreakable Commitment, you'll always course correct. Your internal GPS tells you when to turn around and get back on track.

EMBARK ON THE ULTIMATE BIOLOGICAL ADVENTURE

Turn biological optimization into an adventure. Make it fun.

With the tools in this book, you can now do things with your body that you maybe didn't think possible. You can build lean muscle mass, burn body fat, become more athletic, feel better, and activate your brain. It's truly an awesome feeling of empowerment when you master these processes.

Now is the time—right here, right now—to make that Unbreakable Commitment to yourself . . . that you will pursue biological optimization as long as your heart beats.

Enjoy the journey!

ENDNOTES

Preface

1. "Survey: Nutrition Information Abounds, But Many Doubt Food Choices," *Food Insight*, accessed April 30, 2023, http://www.foodinsight.org/press-releases/survey-nutrition-information-abounds-many-doubt-food-choices.
2. Stuart Wolpert, "Dieting Does Not Work, UCLA Researchers Report," UCLA, accessed July 19, 2021, https://newsroom.ucla.edu/releases/Dieting-Does-Not-Work-UCLA-Researchers-7832.
3. Nicholas Seltzer, "The evolution of tribalism: A social-ecological model of cooperation and inter-group conflict under pastoralism," Journal of Artificial Societies and Social Simulation 22, no. 2 (March 2019): 6. https://www.jasss.org/22/2/6.html.
4. Gardner et al., "Effect of low fat vs low carbohydrate diet on 12-month weight loss in overweight adults with genotype patter or insulin secretion: The DIETFITS randomized clinical trial," *JAMA* 319, no. 7 (2018): 667–679. https://doi.org/10.1001/jama.2018.0245.
5. T. Mann, "Why Do Dieters Regain Weight?" American Psychological Association, accessed October 24, 2020, https://www.apa.org/science/about/psa/2018/05/calorie-deprivation.
6. Strohacker et al., "Consequences of weight cycling: An increase in disease risk?" *International Journal of Exercise Science* 2, no. 3 (2009): 191–201. https://www.ncbi.nlm.nih.gov/pmc/articles/PMC4241770.

Chapter 1

1. Kelly D. Brownell and Mark S. Gold, eds., *Food and Addiction: A Comprehensive Handbook* (New York, NY: Oxford University Press, 2012).
2. Gearhardt et al., "The addiction potential of hyperpalatable foods," *Current Drug Abuse Reviews* 4, no. 3 (2011): 140–145. https://doi.org/10.2174/1874473711104030140.
3. Lenoir et al., "Intense sweetness surpasses cocaine reward," *PLoS One* 2, no. 8 (2007): e698. https://doi.org/10.1371/journal.pone.0000698.
4. Inam et al., "Effects of sugar rich diet on brain serotonin, hyperphagia and anxiety in animal models of both genders," *Pakistan Journal of Pharmaceutical Sciences* 29, no. 3 (2016): 757–763. https://pubmed.ncbi.nlm.nih.gov/27166525.
5. Luo et al., "Differential effects of fructose versus glucose on brain and appetitive responses to food cues and decisions for food rewards," *Proceedings of the National Academy of Sciences of the United States of America* 112, no. 20 (2015): 6509–6514. https://doi.org/10.1073/pnas.1503358112.
6. J. Rodin, "Insulin levels, hunger, and food intake: an example of feedback loops in body weight regulation," *Health Psychology* 4, no. 1 (1985): 1–4. https://pubmed.ncbi.nlm.nih.gov/3894001/.
7. Hägele et al., "High orange juice consumption with or in-between three meals a day differently affects energy balance in healthy subjects," *Nutrition & Diabetes* 8, no, 1 (2018): 19. https://www.ncbi.nlm.nih.gov/pmc/articles/PMC5916905/.
8. James H. Hollis and Richard D. Mattes, "Effect of increased dairy consumption on appetitive ratings and food intake," *Obesity* 15, no. 6 (2007): 1520–1526. https://pubmed.ncbi.nlm.nih.gov/17557989/.
9. Fothergill et al., "Persistent metabolic adaptation 6 years after 'The Biggest Loser' competition," *Obesity (Silver Spring)* 24, no. 8 (2016): 1612–1619. https://doi.org/10.1002/oby.21538.
10. M. M. Manore, "Dietary recommendations and athletic menstrual dysfunction," *Sports Medicine* 32, no. 14 (2002): 887–901. https://doi.org/10.2165/00007256-200232140-00002.
11. Mohamad et al., "A concise review of testosterone and bone health," *Clinical Interventions in Aging* 11 (2016): 1317–1324. https://doi.org/10.2147/CIA.S115472.
12. Anderson et al., "Long-term weight-loss maintenance: a meta-analysis of US studies," *The American Journal of Clinical Nutrition* 74, no. 5 (2001): 579–584. https://doi.org/10.1093/ajcn/74.5.579.
13. Fantus et al., "The association between popular diets and serum testosterone among men in the United States," *Journal of Urology* 203, no. 2 (2020): 398–404. doi:10.1097/JU.0000000000000482.
14. J. Whittaker and K. Wu, "Low-fat diets and testosterone in men: Systematic review and meta-analysis of intervention studies," *Journal of Steroid Biochemistry and Molecular Biology* 210 (2021): 105878. doi:10.1016/j.jsbmb.2021.105878.
15. Cangemi et al., "Long-term effects of calorie restriction on serum sex-hormone concentrations in men," *Aging Cell* 9, no. 2 (2010): 236–242. doi:10.1111/j.1474-9726.2010.00553.x.
16. A. Schwartz and E. Doucet, "Relative changes in resting energy expenditure during weight loss: a systematic review," *Obesity Reviews: An Official Journal of the International Association for the Study of Obesity* 11, no. 7 (2010): 531–547. https://doi.org/10.1111/j.1467-789X.2009.00654.x.
17. M. J. Müller, J. Enderle, and A. Bosy-Westphal, "Changes in energy expenditure with weight gain and weight loss in humans," *Current Obesity Reports* 5, no. 4 (2016): 413–423. doi:10.1007/s13679-016-0237-4.
18. Fothergill et al., "Persistent metabolic adaptation 6 years after 'The Biggest Loser' competition," *Obesity (Silver Spring)* 24, no. 8 (2016): 1612–1619. doi:10.1002/oby.21538.
19. Anderberg et al., "The stomach-derived hormone ghrelin increases impulsive behavior," *Neuropsychopharmacology* 41, no. 5 (2016): 1199–1209. doi:10.1038/npp.2015.297.

20. M. Perello and S. L. Dickson, "Ghrelin signalling on food reward: a salient link between the gut and the mesolimbic system," *Journal of Neuroendocrinology* 27, no. 6 (2015): 424–434. doi:10.1111/jne.12236.
21. The Endocrine Society, "'Hunger hormone' ghrelin affects monetary decision making: High ghrelin levels in healthy females predict more impulsive choices, researchers say," *ScienceDaily*, last modified March 21, 2021, www.sciencedaily.com /releases/2021/03/210321215443.htm.
22. MacLean et al., "The role for adipose tissue in weight regain after weight loss," *Obesity Reviews: An Official Journal of the International Association for the Study of Obesity* 16, Suppl 1 (2015): 45–54. https://doi.org/10.1111/obr.12255.
23. M. Lafontan, "Fat cells: afferent and efferent messages define new approaches to treat obesity," *Annual Review of Pharmacology and Toxicology* 45 (2005): 119–146. doi:10.1146/annurev.pharmtox.45.120403.095843.
24. Jackman et al., "Weight regain after sustained weight reduction is accompanied by suppressed oxidation of dietary fat and adipocyte hyperplasia," *American Journal of Physiology-Regulatory, Integrative and Comparative Physiol*ogy 294, no. 4 (2008): R1117–R1129. doi:10.1152/ajpregu.00808.2007.
25. Rossmeislová et al., "Weight loss improves the adipogenic capacity of human preadipocytes and modulates their secretory profile," *Diabetes* 62, no. 6 (2013): 1990–1995. doi:10.2337/db12-0986.
26. M. A. van Baak and E. C. M. Mariman, "Mechanisms of weight regain after weight loss—the role of adipose tissue," *National Review of Endocrinology* 15, no. 5 (2019): 274–287. doi:10.1038/s41574-018-0148-4.
27. "Your Belly Fat Could be Making You Hungrier," *Medical Xpress*, last modified April 16, 2008, https://medicalxpress.com /news/2008-04-belly-fat-hungrier.html.
28. Vink et al., "The effect of rate of weight loss on long-term weight regain in adults with overweight and obesity," *Obesity (Silver Spring)* 24, no. 2 (2016): 321–327. doi:10.1002/oby.21346.
29. D. Willoughby, S. Hewlings, and D. Kalman, "Body composition changes in weight loss: strategies and supplementation for maintaining lean body mass, a brief review," *Nutrients* 10, no. 12 (2018): 1876. doi:10.3390/nu10121876.
30. R. Preidt, "Fast Weight Loss May Mean Muscle Loss," WebMD, accessed August 10, 2021. https://www.webmd.com/diet /news/20140529/fast-weight-loss-may-mean-muscle-loss.

Chapter 2

1. T. L. Fazzino, K. Rohde, and D. K. Sullivan, "Hyper-palatable foods: development of a quantitative definition and application to the US food system database," *Obesity (Silver Spring)* 27, no. 11 (2019): 1761–1768. https://doi.org/10.1002/oby.22639.
2. Hägele et al., "High orange juice consumption with or in-between three meals a day differently affects energy balance in healthy subjects," *Nutrition & Diabetes* 8, no. 1 (2018): 19.
3. Q. Xiao, M. Garaulet, and F. Scheer, "Meal timing and obesity: interactions with macronutrient intake and chronotype," *International Journal of Obesity (2005)* 43, no. 9 (2019): 1701–1711.
4. Brewer et al., "Can mindfulness address maladaptive eating behaviors? why traditional diet plans fail and how new mechanistic insights may lead to novel interventions," *Frontiers in Psychology* 9 (2018): 1418. https://doi.org/10.3389/fpsyg.2018.01418.
5. A. L. Simmons, J. J. Schlezinger, and B. E. Corkey, "What are we putting in our food that is making us fat? Food additives, contaminants, and other putative contributors to obesity," *Current Obesity Reports* 3, no. 2 (2014): 273–285. https://doi.org/10.1007 /s13679-014-0094-y.
6. Linus Pauling Institute, "Micronutrient Inadequacies in the US Population: an Overview," Oregon State University, accessed October 23, 2020, https://lpi.oregonstate.edu/mic/micronutrient-inadequacies/overview.
7. C. D. Davis, "The gut microbiome and its role in obesity," *Nutrition Today* 51, no. 4 (2016), 167–174. https://doi.org/10.1097 /NT.0000000000000167.
8. Gearhardt et al., "The addiction potential of hyperpalatable foods," *Current Drug Abuse Reviews* 4, no. 3 (2011): 140–145. https://doi .org/10.2174/1874473711104030140.
9. Inam et al., "Effects of sugar rich diet on brain serotonin, hyperphagia and anxiety in animal model of both genders," *Pakistan Journal of Pharmaceutical Sciences* 29, no. 3 (2016): 757–763.

Chapter 3

1. Field et al., "Relationship of a large weight loss to long-term weight change among young and middle-aged US women," *International Journal of Obesity and Related Metabolic Disorders* 25, no. 8 (2001): 1113–1121. https://doi.org/10.1038/sj.ijo.0801643.
2. S. Sarlio-Lähteenkorva, A. Rissanen, and J. Kaprio, "A descriptive study of weight loss maintenance: 6 and 15 year follow-up of initially overweight adults," *International Journal of Obesity and Related Metabolic Disorders* 24, no. 1 (2000): 116–125. https://doi .org/10.1038/sj.ijo.0801094.
3. S. B. Votruba, S. Blanc, and D. A. Schoeller, "Pattern and cost of weight gain in previously obese women," *American Journal of Physiology-Endocrinology and Metabolism* 282, no. 4 (2002): E923–E930. https://doi.org/10.1152/ajpendo.00265.2001.
4. B. Wansink and P. Chandon, "Meal size, not body size, explains errors in estimating the calorie content of meals" [retracted in: *Ann Intern Med.* 170, no. 2 (2019): 138], *Annals of Internal Medicine* 145, no. 5 (2006): 326–332. doi:10.7326/0003-4819-145-5-200609050-00005.
5. R. Leproult and E. Van Cauter, "Effect of 1 week of sleep restriction on testosterone levels in young healthy men," *JAMA* 305, no. 21 (2011): 2173–2174. https://doi.org/10.1001/jama.2011.710.
6. Nedeltcheva et al., "Insufficient sleep undermines dietary efforts to reduce adiposity," *Annals of Internal Medicine* 153, no. 7 (2010): 435–441. https://doi.org/10.7326/0003-4819-153-7-201010050-00006.
7. Morselli et al., "Role of sleep duration in the regulation of glucose metabolism and appetite," *Best Practice & Research Clinical endocrinology & metabolism* 24 no. 5 (2010): 687–702. https://doi.org/10.1016/j.beem.2010.07.005.
8. Asociación RUVID, "Dopamine regulates the motivation to act, study shows," *ScienceDaily*, last modified January 10, 2013, accessed July 27, 2021, www.sciencedaily.com/releases/2013/01/130110094415.htm.

9. C. Liu and P. S. Kaeser, "Mechanisms and regulation of dopamine release," *Current Opinion in Neurobiology* 57 (2019):46–53. doi:10.1016/j.conb.2019.01.001.
10. Butryn et al., "Consistent self-monitoring of weight: a key component of successful weight loss maintenance," *Obesity* (Silver Spring) 15, no. 12 (2007): 3091–3096. doi:10.1038/oby.2007.368.
11. Wing et al., "A self-regulation program for maintenance of weight loss," *New England Journal of Medicine* 355, no. 15 (2006): 1563–1571. doi:10.1056/NEJMoa061883.
12. Newbold et al., "Developmental exposure to endocrine disruptors and the obesity epidemic," *Reproductive Toxicology* (Elmsford, N.Y.) 23, no. 3 (2007): 290–296. https://doi.org/10.1016/j.reprotox.2006.12.010.
13. Diamanti-Kandarakis et al., "Endocrine-disrupting chemicals: an Endocrine Society scientific statement," *Endocrine Reviews* 30, no. 4 (2009): 293–342. https://doi.org/10.1210/er.2009-0002.
14. A. Bansal, J. Henao-Mejia, and R. A. Simmons, "Immune system: an emerging player in mediating effects of endocrine disruptors on metabolic health," *Endocrinology* 159, no. 1 (2018): 32–45. https://doi.org/10.1210/en.2017-00882.
15. P. Riccio, and R. Rossano, "Undigested Food and gut microbiota may cooperate in the pathogenesis of neuroinflammatory diseases: a matter of barriers and a proposal on the origin of organ specificity," *Nutrients* 11, no. 11 (2019): 2714. https://doi.org/10.3390/nu11112714.
16. A. Lerner, and T. Matthias, "Changes in intestinal tight junction permeability associated with industrial food additives explain the rising incidence of autoimmune disease," *Autoimmunity Reviews* 14, no. 6 (2015): 479–489. https://doi.org/10.1016/j.autrev.2015.01.009.
17. Brooke-Taylor et al., "Systematic review of the gastrointestinal effects of A1 compared with A2 β-Casein," *Advances in Nutrition* 8, no. 5 (2017): 739–748. https://doi.org/10.3945/an.116.013953.
18. Gagliardi et al., "Rebuilding the gut microbiota ecosystem," *International Journal of Environmental Research and Public Health* 15, no. 8 (2018): 1679. https://doi.org/10.3390/ijerph15081679.
19. Scripps Research Institute, "A chemical clue to how life started on Earth: Every living thing stems from the same limited set of 20 amino acids, and now scientists may know why," *ScienceDaily*, last modified August 1, 2019, accessed July 27, 2021, www.sciencedaily.com/releases/2019/08/190801093310.htm.
20. Adarme-Vega et al., "Microalgal biofactories: a promising approach towards sustainable omega-3 fatty acid production," *Microbial Cell Factories* 11, no. 96 (2012). https://doi.org/10.1186/1475-2859-11-96.
21. R. L. Weinsier, Y. Schutz, and D. Bracco, "Reexamination of the relationship of resting metabolic rate to fat-free mass and to the metabolically active components of fat-free mass in humans," *American Journal of Clinical Nutrition* 55 (1992): 790–794. https://doi.org/10.1093/ajcn/55.4.790.
22. de Brito et al., "Ability to sit and rise from the floor as a predictor of all-cause mortality," *European Journal of Preventive Cardiology* 21, no. 7 (2012), 892–898. https://doi.org/10.1177/2047487312471759.

Chapter 4

1. Bergland et al., "Mobility as a predictor of all-cause mortality in older men and women: 11.8 year follow-up in the Tromsø study," *BMC Health Services Research* 17, no. 1 (2017): 22. doi:10.1186/s12913-016-1950-0.
2. Kouri et al., "Fat-free mass index in users and nonusers of anabolic-androgenic steroids," *Clinical Journal of Sport Medicine* 5, no. 4 (1995): 223–228. https://doi.org/10.1097/00042752-199510000-00003.
3. Fontana et al., "Visceral fat adipokine secretion is associated with systemic inflammation in obese humans," *Diabetes* 56, no. 4 (2007): 1010–1013. https://doi.org/10.2337/db06-1656.
4. Pettersson-Pablo et al., "Body fat percentage is more strongly associated with biomarkers of low-grade inflammation than traditional cardiometabolic risk factors in healthy young adults—the Lifestyle, Biomarkers, and Atherosclerosis study," *Scandinavian Journal of Clinical and Laboratory Investigation* 79, no. 3 (2019): 182–187. https://doi.org/10.1080/00365513.2019.1576219.
5. T. A. Salthouse, "When does age-related cognitive decline begin?" *Neurobiology of Aging* 30, no. 4 (2009): 507–514. https://doi.org/10.1016/j.neurobiolaging.2008.09.023.
6. "Goldman's dilemma," Wikipedia.org, last modified September 21, 2022, accessed August 3, 2021, https://en.wikipedia.org/wiki/Goldman%27s_dilemma.
7. A. Nagesh, "Apparently We're All Going to Live Forever by 2029." *Kurzweil*, last modified May 9, 2016, https://www.kurzweilai.net/metro-apparently-were-all-going-to-live-forever-by-2029.
8. "Prescription Drugs," Georgetown University Health Policy Institute, https://hpi.georgetown.edu/rxdrugs/.
9. "The Health of Millennials," BlueCross BlueShield, last modified April 24, 2019, accessed August 2, 2021, https://www.bcbs.com/the-health-of-america/reports/the-health-of-millennials.

Chapter 5

1. "What Percent Of Players Walk Out A Casino @ Loser?" Vegas Message Board, accessed September 14, 2021, https://www.vegasmessageboard.com/forums/index.php?threads/what-percent-of-players-walk-out-a-casino-loser.94782/.
2. W. Mischel and E. B. Ebbesen, "Attention in delay of gratification," *Journal of Personality and Social Psychology* 16, no. 2 (1970): 329–337. https://doi.org/10.1037/h0029815.
3. "PTSD," National Center for PTSD, n.d., https://www.ptsd.va.gov/understand/common/common_adults.asp.
4. L. E. Burke, J. Wang, and M. A. Sevick, "Self-monitoring in weight loss: a systematic review of the literature," *Journal of the American Dietetic Association* 111, no. 1 (2011): 92–102. https://doi.org/10.1016/j.jada.2010.10.008.
5. Hollis et al., "Weight loss during the intensive intervention phase of the weight-loss maintenance trial," *American Journal of Preventive Medicine* 35, no. 2 (2008): 118–126. https://doi.org/10.1016/j.amepre.2008.04.013.

Chapter 6

1. "Short-Bowel Syndrome in Dogs and Cats," VetFolio, n.d., retrieved August 1, 2022, https://www.vetfolio.com/learn/article/short-bowel-syndrome-in-dogs-and-cats.
2. Ursell et al., "Defining the human microbiome," *Nutrition Reviews* 70, Suppl 1 (2012): S38–S44. doi:10.1111/j.1753-4887.2012.00493.x.
3. Beal et al., "Global trends in dietary micronutrient supplies and estimated prevalence of inadequate intakes," *PLoS One* 12, no. 4 (2017): e0175554. doi:10.1371/journal.pone.0175554.

Chapter 7

1. Cigolini et al., "Moderate alcohol consumption and its relation to visceral fat and plasma androgens in healthy women," *International Journal of Obesity and Related Metabolic Disorders* 20, no. 3 (1996): 206–212. https://doi.org/10.1001/jama.2011.1590.
2. L. Tappy, "Thermic effect of food and sympathetic nervous system activity in humans," *Reproduction, Nutrition, Development* 36, no. 4 (1996): 391–397. https://doi.org/10.1051/rnd:19960405.
3. Bray et al., "Effect of protein overfeeding on energy expenditure measured in a metabolic chamber," *The American Journal of Clinical Nutrition* 101, no. 3 (2015): 496–505. https://doi.org/10.3945/ajcn.114.091769.
4. A. Leaf and J. Antonio, "The effects of overfeeding on body composition: the role of macronutrient composition—a narrative review," *International Journal of Exercise Science* 10, no. 8 (2017): 1275–1296. https://www.ncbi.nlm.nih.gov/pubmed/29399253.
5. N. Nagai, N. Sakane, and T. Moritani. "Metabolic responses to high-fat or low-fat meals and association with sympathetic nervous system activity in healthy young men," *Journal of Nutritional Science and Vitaminology* 51, no. 5 (2005): 355–360. https://doi.org/10.3177/jnsv.51.355.
6. Calcagno et al., "The thermic effect of food: a review," *Journal of the American College of Nutrition* 38, no. 6 (2019): 547–551. https://doi.org/10.1080/07315724.2018.1552544.
7. E. T. Poehlman, C. L. Melby, and S. F. Badylak, "Relation of age and physical exercise status on metabolic rate in younger and older healthy men," *Journal of Gerontology* 46, no. 2 (1991): B54–B58. https://doi.org/10.1093/geronj/46.2.b54.
8. Barnard et al., "The effects of a low-fat, plant-based dietary intervention on body weight, metabolism, and insulin sensitivity," *The American Journal of Medicine* 118, no. 9 (2005): 991–997. https://doi.org/10.1016/j.amjmed.2005.03.039.
9. Wu et al., "Mechanisms controlling mitochondrial biogenesis and respiration through the thermogenic coactivator PGC-1," *Cell* 98, no. 1 (1999): 115–124. https://doi.org/10.1016/S0092-8674(00)80611-X.
10. Lehman et al., "Peroxisome proliferator-activated receptor gamma coactivator-1 promotes cardiac mitochondrial biogenesis," *The Journal of Clinical Investigation* 106, no. 7 (2000): 847–856. https://doi.org/10.1210/er.2006-0037.
11. St-Pierre et al., "Bioenergetic analysis of peroxisome proliferator-activated receptor gamma coactivators 1alpha and 1beta (PGC-1alpha and PGC-1beta) in muscle cells," *The Journal of Biological Chemistry* 278, no. 29 (2003): 26597–26603. https://doi.org/10.1074/jbc.M301850200.
12. MacDougall et al., "Muscle performance and enzymatic adaptations to sprint interval training," *Journal of Applied Physiology* 84, no. 6 (1998): 2138–2142. https://doi.org/10.1152/jappl.1998.84.6.2138.
13. Burgomaster et al., "Similar metabolic adaptations during exercise after low volume sprint interval and traditional endurance training in humans," *The Journal of Physiology* 586, no. 1 (2008): 151–160. https://doi.org/10.1113/jphysiol.2007.142109.
14. Falcone et al., "Caloric expenditure of aerobic, resistance, or combined high-intensity interval training using a hydraulic resistance system in healthy men," *Journal of Strength and Conditioning Research* 29, no. 3 (2015): 779–785. https://doi.org/10.1519/JSC.0000000000000661.
15. Wingfield et al., "The acute effect of exercise modality and nutrition manipulations on post-exercise resting energy expenditure and respiratory exchange ratio in women: a randomized trial," *Sports Medicine Open* 1, no. 1 (2015): 11. https://doi.org/10.1186/s40798-015-0010-3.
16. Wingfield et al., "The acute effect of exercise modality."
17. Lemmer et al., "Effect of strength training on resting metabolic rate and physical activity: age and gender comparisons," *Medicine and Science in Sports and Exercise* 33, no. 4 (2001): 532–541. https://doi.org/10.1097/00005768-200104000-00005.
18. Lamon et al., "The effect of acute sleep deprivation on skeletal muscle protein synthesis and the hormonal environment," *Physiological Reports* 9 no. 1 (January 2021): e14660. https://doi.org/10.14814/phy2.14660.
19. Hanlon et al., "Sleep restriction enhances the daily rhythm of circulating levels of endocannabinoid 2-arachidonoylglycerol," *Sleep* 39, no. 3 (2016): 653–664. https://doi.org/10.5665/sleep.5546.
20. Pilz et al., "Effect of vitamin D supplementation on testosterone levels in men," *Hormone and Metabolic Research* 43, no. 3 (2011): 223–225. https://doi.org/10.1055/s-0030-1269854.
21. K. P. Dzik and J. J. Kaczor, "Mechanisms of vitamin D on skeletal muscle function: oxidative stress, energy metabolism and anabolic state," *European Journal of Applied Physiology* 119, no. 4 (2019): 825–839. https://doi.org/10.1007/s00421-019-04104-x.
22. Gordon et al., "Relationship between vitamin D and muscle size and strength in patients on hemodialysis," *Journal of Renal Nutrition* 17, no. 6 (2007): 397–407. https://doi.org/10.1053/j.jrn.2007.06.001.
23. Salles et al., "1,25(OH)2-vitamin D3 enhances the stimulating effect of leucine and insulin on protein synthesis rate through Akt/PKB and mTOR mediated pathways in murine C2C12 skeletal myotubes," *Molecular Nutrition & Food Research* 57, no. 12 (2013): 2137–2146. https://doi.org/10.1002/mnfr.201300074.
24. Straetemans et al., "Effect of growth hormone treatment on energy expenditure and its relation to first-year growth response in children." *European Journal of Applied Physiology* 119, no. 2 (2019): 409–418. https://doi.org/10.1007/s00421-018-4033-6.
25. "Growth Hormone as a Determinant of Weight Regulation," ClinicalTrials.gov, last modified January 1, 2016, accessed August 27, 2021, https://clinicaltrials.gov/ct2/show/NCT00355784.
26. J. A. Chromiak and J. Antonio, "Use of amino acids as growth hormone-releasing agents by athletes," *Nutrition* 18, no. 7–8 (2002): 657–661. https://doi.org/10.1016/s0899-9007(02)00807-9.

27. M. P. K. J. Engelen and N. E. P. Deutz, "Is β-hydroxy β-methylbutyrate an effective anabolic agent to improve outcome in older diseased populations?" *Current Opinion in Clinical Nutrition and Metabolic Care* 21, no. 3 (2018): 207–213. https://doi.org/10.1097/MCO.0000000000000459.

28. P. Imbeault, I. Dépault, and F. Haman, "Cold exposure increases adiponectin levels in men," *Metabolism: Clinical and Experimental* 58, no. 4 (2009): 552–559. https://doi.org/10.1016/j.metabol.2008.11.017.

29. Wei et al., "Adiponectin is required for maintaining normal body temperature in a cold environment," *BMC Physiology* 17, no. 1 (2017): 8. https://doi.org/1010.1186/s12899-017-0034-7.

30. Acosta et al., "Physiological responses to acute cold exposure in young lean men," *PloS One* 13, no. 5 (2018): e0196543. https://doi.org/10.1371/journal.pone.0196543.

31. Mills et al., "Accumulation of succinate controls activation of adipose tissue thermogenesis," *Nature* 560, no. 7716 (2018): 102–106. https://doi.org/10.1038/s41586-018-0353-2.

32. L. Sidossis and S. Kajimura, "Brown and beige fat in humans: thermogenic adipocytes that control energy and glucose homeostasis." *The Journal of Clinical Investigation* 125, no. 2 (2015): 478–486. https://doi.org/10.1172/JCI78362.

33. University of Florida, "Exercise In Cold Water May Increase Appetite, UF Study Finds," *ScienceDaily*, accessed August 27, 2021, https://www.sciencedaily.com/releases/2005/05/050504225732.htm.

34. J. Berg, J. Tymoczko, and L. Stryer, "Each Organ Has a Unique Metabolic Profile," in *Biochemistry*, 5th ed. (New York: W. H. Freeman and Company, 2001), 851–854.

35. P. Robb, "Cross crawl: neurological disorganisation," *Head Back to Health* (blog), last modified October 2011, http://www.headbacktohealth.com/Cross_crawl.html.

36. Cramer et al., "Yoga for depression: a systematic review and meta-analysis," *Depression and Anxiety* 30, no. 11 (2013): 1068–1083. https://doi.org/10.1002/da.22166.

37. M. Hagins and A. Rundle, "Yoga improves academic performance in urban high school students compared to physical education: A randomized controlled trial," *Mind, Brain, and Education* 10, no. 2 (2016): 105–116. https://doi.org/10.1111/mbe.12107.

38. Hagins et al., "A randomized controlled trial comparing the effects of yoga with an active control on ambulatory blood pressure in individuals with prehypertension and stage 1 hypertension," *Journal of Clinical Hypertension* 16, no. 1 (2014): 54202162. https://doi.org/10.1111/jch.12244.

39. Demartini et al., "The effect of a single yoga class on interoceptive accuracy in patients affected by anorexia nervosa and in healthy controls: a pilot study," *Eating and Weight Disorders* 26, no. 5 (2021): 142720211435. ttps://doi.org/doi:10.1007/s40519-020-00950-3.

40. M. Apfelbaum, J. Bostsarron, and D. Lacatis, "Effect of caloric restriction and excessive caloric intake on energy expenditure," *The American Journal of Clinical Nutrition* 24, no. 12 (1971): 1405–1409. https://doi.org/10.1093/ajcn/24.12.1405.

41. Wang et al., "Gut microbiota mediates the anti-obesity effect of calorie restriction in mice," *Scientific Reports* 8, no. 1 (2018): 13037. https://doi.org/10.1038/s41598-018-31353-1.

42. Murray et al., "Cheat meals: A benign or ominous variant of binge eating behavior?" *Appetite* 130 (2018): 274–278. https://doi.org/10.1016/j.appet.2018.08.026.

43. Davoodi et al., "Calorie shifting diet versus calorie restriction diet: a comparative clinical trial study," *International Journal of Preventive Medicine* 5, no. 4 (2014): 447–456. https://pubmed.ncbi.nlm.nih.gov/24829732/.

44. Byrne et al., "Intermittent energy restriction improves weight loss efficiency in obese men: the MATADOR study," *International Journal of Obesity* 42, no. 2 (2018): 129–138. https://doi.org/10.1038/ijo.2017.206.

45. Lichtman et al., "Discrepancy between self-reported and actual caloric intake and exercise in obese subjects," *The New England Journal of Medicine* 327, no. 27 (1992): 1893–1898. https://doi.org/10.1056/NEJM199212313272701.

Chapter 8

1. Byrne et al., "Intermittent energy restriction."

2. Byrne et al., "Intermittent energy restriction."

3. K. A. Varady, "Intermittent versus daily calorie restriction: which diet regimen is more effective for weight loss?" *Obesity Reviews* 12, no. 7 (2011): e593–e601. https://doi.org/10.1111/j.1467-789X.2011.00873.x.

4. Hartman et al., "Augmented growth hormone (GH) secretory burst frequency and amplitude mediate enhanced GH secretion during a two-day fast in normal men," *The Journal of Clinical Endocrinology and Metabolism* 74, no. 4 (1992): 757–765. https://doi.org/10.1210/jcem.74.4.1548337.

5. Levine et al., "Low protein intake is associated with a major reduction in IGF-1, cancer, and overall mortality in the 65 and younger but not older population," *Cell Metabolism* 19, no. 3 (2014): 407–417. https://doi.org/10.1016/j.cmet.2014.02.006.

6. T. A. Wehr, "Photoperiodism in humans and other primates: evidence and implications," *Journal of Biological Rhythms* 16, no. 4 (2001): 348–364. doi: 10.1177/074873001129002060.

7. Mariné-Casadó et al., "The Exposure to different photoperiods strongly modulates the glucose and lipid metabolisms of normoweight Fischer 344 rats," *Frontiers in Physiology* 9 (2018): 416. https://doi.org/10.3389/fphys.2018.00416.

8. Larkin et al., "Effect of photoperiod on body weight and food intake of obese and lean Zucker rats," *Life Sciences* 49, no. 10 (1991): 735–745. https://doi.org/10.1016/0024-3205(91)90106-l.

9. Geldenhuys et al., "Ultraviolet radiation suppresses obesity and symptoms of metabolic syndrome independently of vitamin D in mice fed a high-fat diet," *Diabetes* 63, no. 11 (2014): 3759–3769. https://doi.org/10.2337/db13-1675.

10. Wu et al., "Vitamin D supplementation and glycemic control in type 2 diabetes patients: A systematic review and meta-analysis," *Metabolism: Clinical and Experimental*, 73 (2017): 67–76. https://doi.org/10.1016/j.metabol.2017.05.006.

11. A. Gibert-Ramos, A. Crescenti, and M. J. Salvadó, "Consumption of cherry out of season changes white adipose tissue gene expression and morphology to a phenotype prone to fat accumulation," *Nutrients*, 10, no. 8 (2018). https://doi.org/10.3390/nu10081102.

Chapter 9

1. Sørensen, et al., "Effect of Sensory Perception of Foods on Appetite and Food Intake: A Review of Studies on Humans," *Nature News*, last modified September 26, 2003, https://www.nature.com/articles/0802391.
2. Sørensen, et al., "Effect of Sensory Perception."
3. F. Bellisle and J. Le Magnen, "The analysis of human feeding patterns the edogram," *Appetite* 1, no. 2 (1980): 141–150. https://doi.org/10.1016/S0195-6663(80)80018-3.
4. F. Bellisle and J. Le Magnen, "The structure of meals in humans: eating and drinking patterns in lean and obese subjects,: *Physiology & Behavior* 27, no. 4 (1981): 649–658. https://doi.org/10.1016/0031-9384(81)90237-7.
5. Rolls et al., "Variety in meal enhances food intake in man," *Physiology & Behavior* 26, no. 2 (1981): 215–221. https://doi.org/10.1016/0031-9384(81)90014-7.
6. B. J. Rolls, E. A. Rowe, and E. T. Rolls, "How sensory properties of foods affect human feeding behavior," *Physiology & Behavior* 29, no. 3 (1982): 409–417. https://doi.org/10.1016/0031-9384(82)90259-1.
7. B. J. Rolls, P. M. Van Duijvenvoorde, and E. T. Rolls, "Pleasantness changes and food intake in a varied four-course meal," *Appetite* 5, no. 4 (1984): 337–348. https://doi.org/10.1016/s0195-6663(84)80006-9.
8. S. L. Berry, W. W. Beatty, and R. C. Klesges, "Sensory and social influences on ice cream consumption by males and females in a laboratory setting," *Appetite* 6, no. 1 (1985): 41–45. https://doi.org/10.1016/s0195-6663(85)80049-0.
9. J. Alcock, C. C. Maley, and C. A. Aktipis, "Is eating behavior manipulated by the gastrointestinal microbiota? Evolutionary pressures and potential mechanisms," *BioEssays: News and Reviews in Molecular, Cellular and Developmental Biology* 36, no. 10 (2014): 940–949. https://doi.org/10.1002/bies.201400071.

Chapter 10

1. "The 4 Types of Hunger," *Westwind Counselling* (blog), last modified August 4, 2016, https://www.westwindcounselling.ca/post/2016/08/04/the-4-types-of-hunger.
2. Nedeltcheva et al., "Insufficient sleep undermines dietary efforts to reduce adiposity," *Annals of Internal Medicine* 153, no. 7 (2010): 435–441. https://doi.org/10.7326/0003-4819-153-7-201010050-00006.
3. Morselli et al., "Role of sleep duration in the regulation of glucose metabolism and appetite," *Best Practice & Research Clinical endocrinology & metabolism* 24, no. 5 (2010): 687–702. https://doi.org/10.1016/j.beem.2010.07.005.
4. Bosy-Westphal et al, "Influence of partial sleep deprivation on energy balance and insulin sensitivity in healthy women," *Obesity Facts* 1, no. 5 (2008): 266–273. https://doi.org/10.1159/000158874.
5. K. Spiegel, R. Leproult, and E. Van Cauter, "Impact of sleep debt on metabolic and endocrine function," *Lancet (London, England)* 354, no. 9188 (1999): 1435–1439. https://doi.org/10.1016/S0140-6736(99)01376-8.
6. McNeil et al., "Short sleep duration is associated with a lower mean satiety quotient in overweight and obese men," *European Journal of Clinical Nutrition* 67, no. 12 (2013): 1217–1230. https://doi.org/10.1038/ejcn.2013.204.
7. J. A. Greenberg and A. Geliebter, "Coffee, Hunger, and Peptide YY," *Journal of the American College of Nutrition* 31, no. 3 (2012): 160–166. https://doi.org/10.1080/07315724.2012.
8. K. Efthimia et al., "The role of peptide yy in appetite regulation and obesity," *The Journal of Physiology* 587, no. 1 (2009): 19–25. https://doi.org/10.1113/jphysiol.2008.164269.
9. A. Alkhatib and R. Atcheson, "Yerba maté (ilex paraguariensis) metabolic, satiety, and mood state effects at rest and during prolonged exercise," *Nutrients* 9, no. 8 (2017): 882. doi: https://doi.org/10.3390/nu9080882.
10. Cheung et al., "Association between hedonic hunger and glycemic control in non-obese and obese patients with type 2 diabetes," *Journal of Diabetes Investigation* 9, no. 5 (2018): 1135–1143. https://doi.org/10.1111/jdi.12800.
11. Mendes-Soares et al., "Model of personalized postprandial glycemic response to food developed for an Israeli cohort predicts responses in Midwestern American individuals," *The American Journal of Clinical Nutrition* 110, no. 1 (2019): 63–75. https://doi.org/10.1093/ajcn/nqz028.
12. Schubert et al., "Acute exercise and hormones related to appetite regulation: A meta-analysis," *Sports Medicine* 44 (2014): 387–403. https://doi.org/10.1007/s40279-013-0120-3.
13. Corney et al., "Immediate pre-meal water ingestion decreases voluntary food intake in lean young males," *European Journal of Nutrition* 55, no. 2 (2016): 815–819. https://doi.org/10.1007/s00394-015-0903-4.
14. V. A. K. Vij and A. S. Joshi, "Effect of excessive water intake on body weight, body mass index, body fat, and appetite of overweight female participants," *Journal of Natural Science, Biology, and Medicine* 5, no. 2 (2014): 340–344. https://doi.org/10.4103/0976-9668.136180.
15. J. E. Flood and B. J. Rolls, "Soup preloads in a variety of forms reduce meal energy intake," *Appetite* 49, no. 3 (2007): 626–634. https://doi.org/10.1016/j.appet.2007.04.002.
16. Holt et al., "A satiety index of common foods," *European Journal of Clinical Nutrition* 49, no. 9 (1995): 675–690. https://pubmed.ncbi.nlm.nih.gov/7498104/.
17. L. Chambers, K. McCrickerd, and M. R. Yeomans, "Optimising Foods for Satiety," *Trends in Food Science & Technology* 41, no. 2 (2015): 149–160. https://doi.org/10.1016/j.tifs.2014.10.007.
18. L. B. Sørensen and A. Astrup, "Eating dark and milk chocolate: A randomized crossover study of effects on appetite and energy intake," *Nutrition & Diabetes* 1 (2011): e21. https://doi.org/10.1038/nutd.2011.17.
19. M. Mansour et al., "Ginger consumption enhances the thermic effect of food and promotes feelings of satiety without affecting metabolic and hormonal parameters in overweight men: a pilot study," *Metabolism* 61, no. 10 (2012): 1347–1352. https://doi.org/10.1016/j.metabol.2012.03.016.
20. Almiron-Roig et al., "Factors that determine energy compensation: a systematic review of preload studies," *Nutrition Reviews* 71, no. 7 (2013): 458–473. https://doi.org/10.1111/nure.12048.

21. Robinson et al., "A systematic review and meta-analysis examining the effect of eating rate on energy intake and hunger," *The American Journal of Clinical Nutrition* 100, no. 1 (2014): 123–151. https://doi.org/10.3945/ajcn.113.081745.
22. Eweis et al., "Carbon dioxide in carbonated beverages induces ghrelin release and increased food consumption in male rats: implications on the onset of obesity," *Obesity Research & Clinical Practice* 11, no. 5 (2017): 534–543. https://doi.org/10.1016/j.orcp.2017.02.001.
23. Gray et al., "Omega-3 Fatty acids: A review of the effects on adiponectin and leptin and potential implications for obesity management," *European Journal of Clinical Nutrition* 67, no. 12 (2013): 1234–1242. https://doi.org/10.1038/ejcn.2013.197.
24. Parra et al., "A diet rich in long chain omega-3 fatty acids modulates satiety in overweight and obese volunteers during weight loss," *Appetite* 51, no. 3 (2008): 676–680. https://doi.org/10.1016/j.appet.2008.06.003.
25. Groesz et al., "What is eating you? Stress and the drive to eat," *Appetite* 58, no. 2 (2012): 717–721. https://doi.org/10.1016/j.appet.2011.11.028.
26. B. Scheibehenne, P. M. Todd, and B. Wansink, "Dining in the dark. the importance of visual cues for food consumption and satiety," *Appetite* 55, no. 3 (2010): 710–713. https://doi.org/10.1016/j.appet.2010.08.002.
27. B. Wansink and K. van Ittersum, "Portion size me: plate-size induced consumption norms and win-win solutions for reducing food intake and waste," *Journal of Experimental Psychology: Applied* 19, no, 4 (2013): 320–332. https://doi.org/10.1037/a0035053.
28. B. Wansink, K. van Ittersum, and J. E. Painter, "Ice cream illusions bowls, spoons, and self-served portion sizes," *American Journal of Preventive Medicine* 31, no. 3 (2006): 240–243. https://doi.org/10.1016/j.amepre.2006.04.003.
29. Vartanian et al., "Self-Reported overeating and attributions for food intake," *Psychology & Health* 32, no. 4 (2017): 483–492. https://doi.org/10.1080/08870446.2017.1283040.
30. C. H. Hsieh, "The effects of auricular acupressure on weight loss and serum lipid levels in overweight adolescents," *The American Journal of Chinese Medicine* 38, no. 4 (2010): 675–682. https://doi.org/10.1142/S0192415X10008147.
31. Suen et al., "Self-Administered auricular acupressure integrated with a smartphone app for weight reduction: randomized feasibility trial," *JMIR MHealth and UHealth* 7, no. 5 (2019): e14386. https://doi.org/10.2196/14386.
32. Hewagalamulage et al., "Stress, cortisol, and obesity: a role for cortisol responsiveness in identifying individuals prone to obesity," *Domestic Animal Endocrinology* 56, Suppl (2016): S112–120. https://doi.org/10.1016/j.domaniend.2016.03.004.
33. Church et al., "Naturally thin you: Weight loss and psychological symptoms after a six-week online clinical EFT (emotional freedom techniques) course," *Explore* 14, No. 2 (2018): 131–136. https://doi.org/10.1016/j.explore.2017.10.009.

Chapter 11

1. Gardner et al., "Adverse childhood experiences are associated with an increased risk of obesity in early adolescence: a population-based prospective cohort study," *Pediatric Research* 86, no. 4 (2019): 522–528. https://doi.org/10.1038/s41390-019-0414-8.
2. Girgenti et al., "Molecular and cellular effects of traumatic stress: implications for PTSD," *Current Psychiatry Reports* 19, no. 11 (2017): 85. https://doi.org/10.1007/s11920-017-0841-3.
3. P. Stapleton, T. Sheldon, and B. Porter, "Clinical benefits of emotional freedom techniques on food cravings at 12-months follow-up: A randomized controlled trial," *Energy Psychology Journal* 4, no. 1 (2012). https://doi.org/10.9769/EPJ.2012.4.1.PS.TS.BP.
4. Stapleton et al., "Portion perfection and Emotional Freedom Techniques to assist bariatric patients post surgery: A randomised control trial," *Heliyon* 6, no. 6 (2020): e04058. https://doi.org/10.1016/j.heliyon.2020.e04058.
5. Church et al., "Naturally Thin You: Weight loss and psychological symptoms after a six-week online clinical EFT (emotional freedom techniques) course," *Explore: The Journal of Science and Healing*, 14 no. 2 (2018): 131-136. doi:10.1016/j.explore.2017.10.009.
6. D. Church and A. J. Brooks, "The effect of a brief EFT (Emotional Freedom Techniques) self-intervention on anxiety, depression, pain and cravings in healthcare workers," *Journal of Ayurveda and Integrative Medicine* 9, no. 5 (2010): 40–43. https://eftinternational.org/scientific-articles/the-effect-of-a-brief-eft-self-intervention-on-anxiety-depression-pain-and-cravings-in-health-care-workers/.
7. D. Church, G. Yount, and A. J. Brooks, "The effect of emotional freedom techniques on stress biochemistry: a randomized controlled trial," *The Journal of Nervous and Mental Disease* 200, no. 10 (2012): 891–896. https://doi.org/10.1097/NMD.0b013e31826b9fc1.
8. P. G. Swingle, L. Pulos, and M. K. Swingle, "Neurophysiological indicators of EFT treatment of post-traumatic stress," *Subtle Energies & Energy Medicine Journal Archives* 15, no. 1 (2004). https://journals.sfu.ca/seemj/index.php/seemj/article/view/377.
9. Kamiński et al., "Novelty-sensitive dopaminergic neurons in the human substantia nigra predict success of declarative memory formation," *Current Biology* 28, no. 9 (2018): 1333–1343.e4. https://doi.org/10.1016/j.cub.2018.03.024.
10. Krebs et al., "Novelty increases the mesolimbic functional connectivity of the substantia nigra/ventral tegmental area (SN/VTA) during reward anticipation: Evidence from high-resolution fMRI," *Neuroimage* 58, no. 2 (2011): 647–655. https://doi.org/10.1016/j.neuroimage.2011.06.038.
11. R. M. Krebs, B. H. Schott, and E. Düzel, "Personality traits are differentially associated with patterns of reward and novelty processing in the human substantia nigra/ventral tegmental area," *Biological Psychiatry* 65, no. 2 (2009): 103–110. https://doi.org/10.1016/j.biopsych.2008.08.019.
12. Heck et al., "Investigation of 17 candidate genes for personality traits confirms effects of the HTR2A gene on novelty seeking," *Genes, Brain, and Behavior* 8, no. 4 (2009): 464–472. https://doi.org/10.1111/j.1601-183X.2009.00494.x.
13. E. Thomson, "Carbs are essential for effective dieting and good mood, Wurtman says," *MIT News*, last modified February 20, 2004, accessed August 30, 2021, https://news.mit.edu/2004/carbs.
14. M. P. Yeager, P. A. Pioli, and P. M. Guyre, "Cortisol exerts bi-phasic regulation of inflammation in humans," *Dose Response* 9, no. 3 (2011): 332–347. https://doi.org/10.2203/dose-response.10-013.
15. R. Coccurello and M. Maccarrone, "Hedonic eating and the 'delicious circle': from lipid-derived mediators to brain dopamine and back," *Frontiers in Neuroscience* 12 (2018): 271. https://doi.org/10.3389/fnins.2018.00271.
16. H. Whiteman, "Loneliness a Bigger Killer than Obesity," MedicalNewsToday, last modified August 6, 2017, https://www.medicalnewstoday.com/articles/318723.

Chapter 13

1. Kolaczynski et al., "Responses of leptin to short-term fasting and refeeding in humans: a link with ketogenesis but not ketones themselves," *Diabetes* 45, no. 11 (1996): 1511–1515. https://doi.org/10.2337/diab.45.11.1511.
2. Byrne, et al., "Intermittent energy restriction."
3. J. Cooper, K. Polonsky, and D. Schoeller, "Serum leptin levels in obese males during over- and underfeeding," Obesity 17, no. 12 (2009): 2149–2154. https://doi.org/10.1038/oby.2009.149.
4. Davoodi et al., "Calorie shifting diet."

Chapter 14

1. N. D. Volkow, G.-J. Wang, and R. D. Baler, "Reward, dopamine and the control of food intake: implications for obesity," *Trends in Cognitive Sciences* 15, no. 1 (2011): 37–46. https://doi.org/10.1016/j.tics.2010.11.001.
2. F. S. Radhakishun, J. M. van Ree, and B. H. Westerink, "Scheduled eating increases dopamine release in the nucleus accumbens of food-deprived rats as assessed with on-line brain dialysis," *Neuroscience Letters* 85, no. 3 (1988): 351–356. https://doi .org/10.1016/0304-3940(88)90591-5.
3. Manfredi et al., "A Systematic review of genetic polymorphisms associated with binge eating disorder," *Nutrients* 13, no. 3 (2021). https://doi.org/10.3390/nu13030848.
4. Romer et al., "Dopamine genetic risk is related to food addiction and body mass through reduced reward-related ventral striatum activity," *Appetite* 133 (2019): 24–31. https://doi.org/10.1016/j.appet.2018.09.010.
5. E. M. Schulte, C. M. Grilo, and A. N. Gearhardt, "Shared and unique mechanisms underlying binge eating disorder and addictive disorders," *Clinical Psychology Review* 44 (2016): 125. https://doi.org/10.1016/j.cpr.2016.02.001.
6. "Comorbidity," National Eating Disorders Collaboration, last modified September 14, 2017, https://nedc.com.au/eating-disorders /eating-disorders-explained/types/comorbidity/.
7. Hagger et al., "Ego depletion and the strength model of self-control: a meta-analysis," *Psychological Bulletin* 136, no. 4 (2010): 495–525. https://doi.org/10.1037/a0019486.
8. A. A. Gibson and A. Sainsbury, "Strategies to improve adherence to dietary weight loss interventions in research and real-world settings," *Behavioral Sciences* 7, no. 3 (2017): 44. https://doi.org/10.3390/bs7030044.
9. C. S. Bickel, J. M. Cross, and M. M. Bamman, "Exercise dosing to retain resistance training adaptations in young and older adults," *Medicine & Science in Sports & Exercise* 43, no. 7 (2011): 1177–1187. https://doi.org/10.1249/MSS.0b013e318207c15d.

Chapter 15

1. de Brito et al., "Ability to sit and rise from the floor."
2. G. Lyon, "High-quality protein is essential for healthier muscles," *Arla Food Ingredients* (blog), last modified March 22, 2018, https:// www.arlafoodsingredients.com/the-whey-and-protein-blog/health/high-quality-protein-is-essential-for-healthier-muscles/.
3. R. R. Wolfe, "The underappreciated role of muscle in health and disease," *The American Journal of Clinical Nutrition* 84, no. 3 (2006): 475–482. https://doi.org/10.1093/ajcn/84.3.475.
4. Iraki et al., "Nutrition recommendations for bodybuilders in the off-season: a narrative review," *Sports* 7, no. 7 (2019): 154. https:// doi.org/10.3390/sports7070154.
5. Garthe et al., "Effect of nutritional intervention on body composition and performance in elite athletes," *European Journal of Sport Science* 13 (2013): 295–303. https://doi.org/10.1080/17461391.2011.643923.
6. Layman et al., "Defining meal requirements for protein to optimize metabolic roles of amino acids," *American Journal of Clinical Nutrition* 101, no. 6 (2015): 1330S–1338S. https://doi.org/10.3945/ajcn.114.084053.
7. Norton, "Leucine: The Anabolic Trigger," Bodybuilding, accessed May 18, 2021. https://www.bodybuilding.com/fun/layne39.htm.
8. Serwinski, "Leucine Threshold for Building Muscle," *The Strong Kitchen*, last modified March 31, 2019. https://thestrongkitchen. com/blog/post/leucine-threshold-for-building-muscle
9. Loenneke et al., "Per meal dose and frequency of protein consumption is associated with lean mass and muscle performance," *Clinical Nutrition* 35, no. 6 (2016): 1506–1511. https://doi.org/10.1016/j.clnu.2016.04.002.
10. E. R. Helms, A. A. Aragon, and P. J. Fitschen, "Evidence-based recommendations for natural bodybuilding contest preparation: nutrition and supplementation," *Journal of the International Society of Sports Nutrition* 11 (2014): 20. https://doi.org/10.1186/1550-2783-11-20.
11. Mata et al., "Carbohydrate availability and physical performance: physiological overview and practical recommendations," *Nutrients* 11, no. 5 (2019): 1084. https://doi.org/10.3390/nu11051084.
12. Kerksick et al., "International society of sports nutrition position stand: nutrient timing," *Journal of the International Society of Sports Nutrition* 14 (2017): 33. https://doi.org/10.1186/s12970-017-0189-4.
13. Fujita et al., "Effect of insulin on human skeletal muscle protein synthesis is modulated by insulin-induced changes in muscle blood flow and amino acid availability," *The American Journal of Physiology-Endocrinology and Metabolism* 291, no. 4 (2006): E745–E754. https://doi.org/10.1152/ajpendo.00271.2005.
14. van Loon et al., "Ingestion of Protein hydrolysate and amino acid–carbohydrate mixtures increases postexercise plasma insulin responses in men," *The Journal of Nutrition* 130, no. 10 (2000): 2508–2513. https://doi.org/10.1093/jn/130.10.2508.
15. Dorgan et al., "Effects of dietary fat and fiber on plasma and urine androgens and estrogens in men: a controlled feeding study," *The American Journal of Clinical Nutrition* 64, no. 6 (1996): 850–855. https://doi.org/10.1093/ajcn/64.6.850.
16. Riechman et al., "Statins and dietary and serum cholesterol are associated with increased lean mass following resistance training," *The Journals of Gerontology: Series A* 62, no. 10 (2007): 1164–1171. https://doi.org/10.1093/gerona/62.10.1164.
17. T. P. B. De Luccia, "Use of the testosterone/cortisol ratio variable in sports," *The Open Sports Sciences Journal* 9 (2016): 104–113. https://doi.org/10.2174/1875399X01609010104.
18. B. Tachtsis, D. Camera, and O. Lacham-Kaplan, "Potential roles of n-3 PUFAs during skeletal muscle growth and regeneration," *Nutrients* 10, no. 3 (2018): 309. https://doi.org/10.3390/nu10030309.

19. De Souza et al., "Effects of arachidonic acid supplementation on acute anabolic signaling and chronic functional performance and body composition adaptations," *PLoS One* 11, no. 5 (2016): e0155153. https://doi.org/10.1371/journal.pone.0155153.
20. K. B. Jouris, J. L. McDaniel, and E. P. Weiss, "The effect of omega-3 fatty acid supplementation on the inflammatory response to eccentric strength exercise," *Journal of Sports Science & Medicine* 10, no. 3 (2011): 432–438. https://pubmed.ncbi.nlm.nih.gov/24150614/.
21. Iraki et al., "Nutrition recommendations for bodybuilders in the off-season: a narrative review." *Sports* 7, no. 7 (2019): 154. https://doi.org/10.3390/sports7070154.
22. Huang et al., "Effects of omega-3 fatty acids on muscle mass, muscle strength and muscle performance among the elderly: a meta-analysis," *Nutrients* 12, no. 12 (2020): 3739. https://doi.org/10.3390/nu12123739.
23. L. T. Rossato, B. J. Schoenfeld, and E. P. de Oliveira, "Is there sufficient evidence to supplement omega-3 fatty acids to increase muscle mass and strength in young and older adults?" *Clinical Nutrition* 39, no. 1 (2020): P23–32. https://doi.org/10.1016/j.clnu.2019.01.0.
24. F. Wüest, "90% of People Quit After 3 Months of Hitting the Gym, Here's How to Be the Exception," Lifehack, last modified June 10, 2022, https://www.lifehack.org/649556/90-of-people-quit-after-3-months-of-hitting-the-gym-heres-how-to-be-the-exception.

Chapter 16

1. Chung et al., "Do exercise-associated genes explain phenotypic variance in the three components of fitness? a systematic review & meta-analysis," *PloS One* 16, no. 10 (October 2021): e0249501. https://doi.org/10.1371/journal.pone.0249501.
2. Kouri et al., "Fat-free mass index in users and nonusers of anabolic-androgenic steroids," *Clinical Journal of Sport Medicine* 5, no. 4 (1995): 223–228. https://doi.org/10.1097/00042752-199510000-00003.

Chapter 17

1. Ackland et al., "Current status of body composition assessment in sport: review and position statement on behalf of the ad hoc research working group on body composition health and performance, under the auspices of the I.O.C. Medical Commission," *Sports Medicine* 42, no. 3 (2012): 227–249. https://doi.org/10.2165/11597140-000000000-00000.
2. Meyer et al., "Body composition for health and performance: a survey of body composition assessment practice carried out by the Ad Hoc Research Working Group on Body Composition, Health and Performance under the auspices of the IOC Medical Commission," *British Journal of Sports Medicine* 47, no. 16 (2013): 1044–1053. https://doi.org/10.1136/bjsports-2013-092561.
3. Table taken from A. Jeukendrup and M. Gleeson, *Sport Nutrition, 2nd Edition* (Champaign, IL: Human Kinetics, 2009). Soccer numbers updated from Wittich et al., "Body composition of professional football (soccer) players determined by dual X-ray absorptiometry," *Journal of Clinical Densitometry* 4, no. 1 (2001): 51–55. https://doi.org/10.1385/jcd:4:1:51.
4. Luo et al., "Fasting before or after wound injury accelerates wound healing through the activation of pro-angiogenic SMOC1 and SCG2," *Theranostics* 10, no. 8 (2020): 3779–3792. https://doi.org/10.7150/thno.44115.
5. Jeong et al., "Intermittent fasting improves functional recovery after rat thoracic contusion spinal cord injury," *Journal of Neurotrauma* 28, no. 3 (2011): 479–492. https://doi.org/10.1089/neu.2010.1609.
6. E. A. Fulgrave, "Enzyme Therapy and Sports Injuries," *Annals of the New York Academy of Science*s 68 (1957): 192.
7. Anthony Cichoke, *Enzymes & Enzyme Therapy* (New York: McGraw Hill 2000), 143.
8. G.M.M.J. Kerkhoffs et al., "A double blind, randomised, parallel group study on the efficacy and safety of treating acute lateral ankle sprain with oral hydrolytic enzymes," *British Journal of Sports Medicine* 38 no.4 (2004): 431–435. doi: 10.1136/bjsm.2002.004150.
9. A. L. Lichtman, "Traumatic injury in athletes," *International Record of Medicine and General Practice Clinics* 170, no. 6 (1957): 322–326.

Chapter 18

1. Eric R. Braverman, *The Edge Effect: Achieve Total Health and Longevity with the Balanced Brain Advantage* (New York, NY: Union Square & Co., 2011), Kindle edition.
2. A. Huberman, "Maximizing Productivity, Physical & Mental Health with Daily Tools," July 12, 2021, in Huberman Lab, podcast, MP3 audio, https://www.youtube.com/watch?v=aXvDEmo6uS4.
3. Bhanumathy et al., "Nootropic activity of Celastrus paniculatus seed," *Pharmaceutical Biology* 48, no. 3 (2010): 324–327. https://doi.org/10.3109/13880200903127391.
4. Mori et al., "Effects of Hericium erinaceus on amyloid β(25-35) peptide-induced learning and memory deficits in mice," *Biomedical Research* 32, no. 1 (2011): 67–72. https://doi.org/10.2220/biomedres.
5. D. Tomen, "Lion's Mane," *Nootropics Expert* (blog), accessed April 30, 2023, https://nootropicsexpert.com/lions-mane/.
6. Brown et al., "A randomized, double-blind, placebo-controlled trial of pregnenolone for bipolar depression," *Neuropsychopharmacology* 39, no. 12 (2014): 2867–2873. https://doi.org/10.1038/npp.2014.138.
7. Vojtechovsky et al., "The influence of centrophenoxine (lucidril) on learning and memory in alcoholics," *International Journal of Psychobiology* 1, no. 1 (1970): 49–56. https://psycnet.apa.org/record/1972-11088-001.
8. K. Patel, "Centrophenoxine," Examine, last modifed September 28, 2022, https://examine.com/supplements/centrophenoxine/.
9. Chung et al., "Administration of phosphatidylcholine increases brain acetylcholine concentration and improves memory in mice with dementia," *Journal of Nutrition* 125, no. 6 (1995): 1484–1489. https://doi.org/10.1093/jn/125.6.1484.
10. "What Is Phosphatidylcholine and How Can It Benefit Your Health?" BodyBio, last modified December 28, 2020, https://bodybio.com/blogs/blog/what-is-phosphatidylcholine.
11. K. Patel, "Huperzine A," Examine, last modified September 28, 2022, https://examine.com/supplements/huperzine-a/.
12. "Huperzine A," *ScienceDirect*, accessed April 30, 2023, https://www.sciencedirect.com/topics/medicine-and-dentistry/huperzine-a.

13. Elston et al., "Aniracetam does not alter cognitive and affective behavior in adult C57BL/6J mice," *PLoS One* 9, no. 8 (2014): e104443. https://doi.org/10.1371/journal.pone.0104443.
14. C. R. Lee and P. Benfield, "An overview of its pharmacodynamic and pharmacokinetic properties, and a review of its therapeutic potential in senile cognitive disorders," *Drugs & Aging* 4, no. 3 (1994): 257–273. https://doi.org/10.2165/00002512-199404030-00007.
15. K. Patel, "Oxiracetam," Examine, last modified September 28, 2022, https://examine.com/supplements/oxiracetam/.
16. K. Patel, "Oxiracetam."
17. K. Patel, "Nefiracetam," Examine, last modified September 28, 2022, https://examine.com/supplements/nefiracetam/.
18. Yamada et al., "Improvement by nefiracetam of β-amyloid-(1-42)-induced learning and memory impairments in rats," *British Journal of Pharmacology* 126, no. 1 (1999): 235–244. https://doi.org/10.1038/sj.bjp.0702309.
19. A. I. Savchenko, N. S. Zakharova, and I. N. Stepanov. "[The phenotropil treatment of the consequences of brain organic lesions]," *Zh Nevrol Psikhiatr Im S S Korsakova* 105, no. 12 (2005): 22–26. https://pubmed.ncbi.nlm.nih.gov/16447562/.
20. K. Patel, "Phenylpiracetam," Examine, last modified September 28, 2022, https://examine.com/supplements/phenylpiracetam/.
21. K. Patel, "N-Phenylacetyl-L-Prolylglycine Ethyl Ester," Examine, last modified November 17, 2022, https://examine.com/supplements/noopept/.
22. K. Patel, "N-Phenylacetyl-L-Prolylglycine Ethyl Ester."
23. K. Patel, "CDP-Choline," Examine, last modified September 28, 2022, https://examine.com/supplements/cdp-choline/#hem-memory.
24. K. Patel, "Phosphatidylserine," Examine, last modified September 28, 2022, https://examine.com/supplements/phosphatidylserine/#hem-cognition.
25. G. Van De Walle, "Tyrosine: Benefits, Side Effects and Dosage," Healthline, last modified February 1, 2018, https://www.healthline.com/nutrition/tyrosine.
26. "Schizandrol-A: The Stimulant Of The Body And Mind," *NutriAvenue*, last modified May 5, 2019, https://www.nutriavenue.com/schizandrol-a-the-stimulant-of-the-body-and-mind/.
27. J. V. Higdon and B. Frei, "Coffee and health: a review of recent human research," *Critical Reviews in Food Science and Nutrition* 46, no. 2 (2006): 101–123. https://doi.org/10.1080/10408390500400009.
28. K. Patel, "Higenamine," Examine, last modified September 28, 2022, https://examine.com/supplements/higenamine/.
29. Cansev et al., "Oral uridine-5′-monophosphate (UMP) increases brain CDP-choline levels in gerbils," *Brain Research* 1058, no. 1–2 (2005): 101–108. https://doi.org/10.1016/j.brainres.2005.07.054.
30. "Uridine Monophosphate Guide: Effects, Dosage, & More (2022)," *Nanotech Project* (blog), December 18, 2021, https://nanotechproject.org/uridine-monophosphate/.
31. Fernandes et al., "N-Acetylcysteine in depressive symptoms and functionality: a systematic review and meta-analysis," *Journal of Clinical Psychiatry* 77, no. 4 (2016): e457–e466. https://doi.org/10.4088/JCP.15r09984.
32. J. Lefton, "What Is N-Acetylcysteine? Benefits, uses, side effects of NAC supplements," *Verywell Health* (blog), last modified September 19, 2022, https://www.verywellhealth.com/the-benefits-of-n-acetylcysteine-89416#toc-dosage.
33. N. Craven, "Cholecalciferol Vitamin D3 Dosage," *ScriptSave WellRx* (blog), June 22, 2021, https://www.wellrx.com/news/cholecalciferol-vitamin-d3-dosage/.
34. E. Sydenham, A. D. Dangour, and W. S. Lim, "Omega 3 fatty acid for the prevention of cognitive decline and dementia," *Cochrane Database of Systematic Reviews* no. 6 (2012): CD005379. https://doi.org/10.1002/14651858.CD005379.pub3.
35. Chew et al., "Effect of omega-3 fatty acids, lutein/zeaxanthin, or other nutrient supplementation on cognitive function: the areds2 randomized clinical trial," *The Journal of the American Medical Association* 314, no. 8 (2015): 791–801. https://doi.org/10.1001/jama.2015.9677.
36. Tully et al., "Low serum cholesteryl ester-docosahexaenoic acid levels in Alzheimer's disease: a case-control study," *British Journal of Nutrition* 89, no. 4 (2003): 483–489. https://doi.org/10.1079/BJN2002804.

Chapter 19

1. E. J. Masoro, "Calorie Restriction, Aging and Longevity," In *Calorie Restriction, Aging and Longevity*, ed. A. V. R. S. Everitt, D. G. le Couteur, and R. de Cabo (Springer Science+Business Media: 2010). [Google Scholar]
2. L. M. Redman and E. Ravussin, "Caloric restriction in humans: impact on physiological, psychological, and behavioral outcomes," *Antioxidants & Redox Signaling* 14, no. 2 (2011): 275–287. https://doi.org/10.1089/ars.2010.3253.
3. L. Jiang, "Alexis Carrel's Immortal Chick Heart Tissue Cultures (1912–1946)," The Embryo Project Encyclopedia, last modified July 3, 2018, https://embryo.asu.edu/pages/alexis-carrels-immortal-chick-heart-tissue-cultures-1912-1946.
4. Pifferi et al., "Caloric restriction increases lifespan but affects brain integrity in grey mouse lemur primates," *Communications Biology* 1, no. 30 (2018). https://doi.org/10.1038/s42003-018-0024-8.
5. Mattison et al., "Dietary restriction in aging nonhuman primates," *Interdisciplinary Topics in Gerontology and Geriatrics* 35 (2007): 137–158. https://doi.org/10.1159/000096560.
6. R. Weindruch, "Caloric restriction and aging," *Scientific American* 274 (1996): 46–52. https://doi.org/10.1038/scientificamerican0196-46.
7. Pifferi et al., "Caloric restriction."
8. C. W. Bales and W. E. Kraus, "Caloric restriction: implications for human cardiometabolic health," *Journal of Cardiopulmonary Rehabilitation and Prevention* 33, no. 4 (2013): 201–208. https://doi.org/10.1097/HCR.0b013e318295019e.
9. D. Buettner, "Hara Hachi Bu: Enjoy Food and Lose Weight With This Simple Japanese Phrase," BlueZones, last modified December 2018, https://www.bluezones.com/2017/12/hara-hachi-bu-enjoy-food-and-lose-weight-with-this-simple-phrase/.
10. S. F. Jackson, "Celebrate Healthy Living," Walk Kansas, week 6, 2020, https://www.midway.k-state.edu/family-consumer-science/docs/walkks/2020/Week%206%20Newsletter.pdf.

11. Y. Kagawa, "Impact of Westernization on the nutrition of Japanese: changes in physique, cancer, longevity and centenarians," *Preventive Medicine* 7, no. 2 (1978): 205–217. https://doi.org/10.1016/0091-7435(78)90246-3.
12. Kraus et al., "2 years of calorie restriction and cardiometabolic risk (CALERIE): exploratory outcomes of a multicentre, phase 2, randomised controlled trial," *The Lancet Diabetes & Endocrinology* 7, no. 9 (2019): 673–683. https://doi.org/10.1016/S2213-8587(19)30151-2.
13. Romashkan et al., "Safety of two-year caloric restriction in non-obese healthy individuals," *Oncotarget* 7, no. 15 (2016): 19124–19133. https://doi.org/10.18632/oncotarget.8093.
14. Redman et al., "Metabolic slowing and reduced oxidative damage with sustained caloric restriction support the rate of living and oxidative damage theories of aging," *Cell Metabolism* 27, no. 4 (2018): 805–815.e4. https://doi.org/10.1016/j.cmet.2018.02.019.
15. Hofer et al., "Caloric restriction mimetics in nutrition and clinical trial," *Frontiers in Nutrition* 8 (2021): 717343. https://doi.org/10.3389/fnut.2021.717343.
16. S. C. Fang, Y. L. Wu, and P. S. Tsai, "Heart rate variability and risk of all-cause death and cardiovascular events in patients with cardiovascular disease: a meta-analysis of cohort studies," *Biological Research for Nursing* 22, no. 1 (2020): 45–56. https://doi.org/10.1177/1099800419877442.
17. A. B. Shreiner, J. Y. Kao, and V. B. Young, "The gut microbiome in health and in disease," *Current Opinion in Gastroenterology* 31, no. 1 (2015): 69–75. https://doi.org/10.1097/MOG.0000000000000139.
18. Lemstra et al., "Weight loss intervention adherence and factors promoting adherence: a meta-analysis," *Patient Preference and Adherence* 10 (2016): 1547–1559. https://doi.org/10.2147/PPA.S103649.
19. V. Morhenn, L. E. Beavin, P. J. Zak, "Massage increases oxytocin and reduces adrenocorticotropin hormone in humans," *Alternative Therapies in Health and Medicine* 18 no. 6 (2012): 11–18. https://www.ncbi.nlm.nih.gov/pubmed/23251939.
20. Y. H. Lee, B. N. Park, and S. H. Kim, "The effects of heat and massage application on autonomic nervous system," *Yonsei Medical Journal* 52, no. 6 (2011): 982–989. https://doi.org/10.3349/ymj.2011.52.6.982.

Chapter 20

1. Cunnane et al., "Can ketones help rescue brain fuel supply in later life? Implications for cognitive health during aging and the treatment of Alzheimer's disease," *Frontiers in Molecular Neuroscience* 9 (2016): 53. https://doi.org/10.3389/fnmol.2016.00053.
2. M. Gasior, M. A. Rogawski, and A. L. Hartman, "Neuroprotective and disease-modifying effects of the ketogenic diet," *Behavioural Pharmacology* 17, no. 5–6 (2006): 431–439. https://doi.org/10.1097/00008877-200609000-00009.
3. E. C. S. Bostock, K. C. Kirkby, and B. V. M. Taylor, "The current status of the ketogenic diet in psychiatry," *Frontiers in Psychiatry* 8 (2017): 43. https://doi.org/10.3389/fpsyt.2017.00043.
4. V. M. Gershuni, S. L. Yan, and V. Medici, "Nutritional ketosis for weight management and reversal of metabolic syndrome," *Current Nutrition Reports* 7, no. 3 (2018): 97–106. https://doi.org/10.1007/s13668-018-0235-0.
5. Gibson et al., "Do ketogenic diets really suppress appetite? A systematic review and meta-analysis," *Obesity Reviews* 16, no. 1 (2015): 64–76. https://doi.org/10.1111/obr.12230.
6. Sumithran et al., "Ketosis and appetite-mediating nutrients and hormones after weight loss," *European Journal of Clinical Nutrition* 67, no. 7 (2013): 759–764. https://doi.org/10.1038/ejcn.2013.90.
7. Westman et al., "Low-carbohydrate nutrition and metabolism," *The American Journal of Clinical Nutrition* 86, no. 2 (2007): 276–284. https://doi.org/10.1093/ajcn/86.2.276.
8. S. A. Masino and D. N. Ruskin, "Ketogenic diets and pain," *Journal of Child Neurology* 28, no. 8 (2013): 993–1001. https://doi.org/10.1177/0883073813487595.
9. Iikuni et al., "Leptin and Inflammation," *Current Immunology Reviews* 4, no. 2 (2008): 70–79. https://doi.org/10.2174/157339508784325046.
10. Cani et al., "Metabolic endotoxemia initiates obesity and insulin resistance," *Diabetes* 56, no. 7 (2007): 1761–1772. https://doi.org/10.2337/db06-1491.
11. López-Armad et al., "Mitochondrial dysfunction and the inflammatory response," *Mitochondrion* 13, no. 2 (2013): 106–118. https://doi.org/10.1016/j.mito.2013.01.003.
12. Masino and Ruskin, "Ketogenic diets and pain."
13. Ruth et al., "Consuming a hypocaloric high fat low carbohydrate diet for 12 weeks lowers C-reactive protein, and raises serum adiponectin and high density lipoprotein-cholesterol in obese subjects," *Metabolism: Clinical and Experimental* 62, no. 12 (2013): 1779–1787. https://doi.org/10.1016/j.metabol.2013.07.006.
14. V. J. Miller, F. A. Villamena, and J. S. Volek, "Nutritional ketosis and mitohormesis: potential implications for mitochondrial function and human health," *Journal of Nutrition and Metabolism* 2018 (2018): 5157645. https://doi.org/10.1155/2018/5157645.
15. A. Paoli, "Ketogenic diet for obesity: friend or foe?" *International Journal of Environmental Research and Public Health* 11, no. 2 (2014): 2092–2107. https://doi.org/10.3390/ijerph110202092.
16. I. Partsalaki, A. Karvela, and B. E. Spiliotis, "Metabolic impact of a ketogenic diet compared to a hypocaloric diet in obese children and adolescents," *Journal of Pediatric Endocrinology & Metabolism* 25, no. 7–8 (2012): 697–704. https://doi.org/10.1515/jpem-2012-0131.
17. Gomez-Arbelaez et al., "Resting metabolic rate of obese patients under very low calorie ketogenic diet," *Nutrition & Metabolism* 15 (2018): 18. https://doi.org/10.1186/s12986-018-0249-z.
18. Bagherniya et al., "The effect of fasting or calorie restriction on autophagy induction: A review of the literature," *Ageing Research Reviews* 47 (2018): 183–197. https://doi.org/10.1016/j.arr.2018.08.004.
19. R. E. Mistlberger, "Circadian food-anticipatory activity: formal models and physiological mechanisms," *Neuroscience and Biobehavioral Reviews* 18, no. 2 (1994): 171–195. https://doi.org/10.1016/0149-7634(94)90023-x.

20. Brehm et al., "A randomized trial comparing a very low carbohydrate diet and a calorie-restricted low fat diet on body weight and cardiovascular risk factors in healthy women," *The Journal of Clinical Endocrinology and Metabolism* 88, no. 4 (2003): 1617–1623. https://doi.org/10.1210/jc.2002-021480.

21. Campbell et al., "Intermittent energy restriction attenuates the loss of fat free mass in resistance trained individuals. a randomized controlled trial," *Journal of Functional Morphology and Kinesiology* 5, no. 1 (2020): 19. https://doi.org/10.3390/jfmk5010019.

22. Campbell et al., "Intermittent energy restriction."

23. Falchi et al., "Low copy number of the salivary amylase gene predisposes to obesity," *Nature Genetics* 46, no. 5 (2014): 492–497. https://doi.org/10.1038/ng.2939.

24. Clemente et al., "A selective sweep on a deleterious mutation in CPT1A in Arctic populations," *American Journal of Human Genetics* 95, no. 5 (2014): 584–589. https://doi.org/10.1016/j.ajhg.2014.09.016.

25. A V. Contreras, N. Torres, and A. R. Tovar, "PPAR-α as a key nutritional and environmental sensor for metabolic adaptation," *Advances in Nutrition* 4, no. 4 (2013): 439–452. https://doi.org/10.3945/an.113.003798.

26. Takenaka et al., "Human-specific SNP in obesity genes, adrenergic receptor beta2 (ADRB2), Beta3 (ADRB3), and PPAR γ2 (PPARG), during primate evolution," *PloS One* 7, no. 8 (2012): e43461. https://doi.org/10.1371/journal.pone.0043461.

27. Brondani et al., "The presence of at least three alleles of the ADRB3 Trp64Arg (C/T) and UCP1 -3826A/G polymorphisms is associated with protection to overweight/obesity and with higher high-density lipoprotein cholesterol levels in Caucasian-Brazilian patients with type 2 diabetes," *Metabolic Syndrome and Related Disorders* 12, no. 1 (2014): 16–24. https://doi.org/10.1089/met.2013.0077.

28. Smith et al., "Apolipoprotein A-II polymorphism: relationships to behavioural and hormonal mediators of obesity," *International Journal of Obesity* 36, no. 1 (2012): 130–136. https://doi.org/10.1038/ijo.2011.24.

29. Ellulu et al., "Obesity and inflammation: the linking mechanism and the complications," *Archives of Medical Science* 13, no. 4 (2017): 851–863. https://doi.org/10.5114/aoms.2016.58928.

30. He et al., "Effects of cow's milk beta-casein variants on symptoms of milk intolerance in Chinese adults: a multicentre, randomised controlled study," *Nutrition Journal* 16, no. 1 (2017): 72. https://doi.org/10.1186/s12937-017-0275-0.

31. Tucker et al., "Dairy consumption and insulin resistance: the role of body fat, physical activity, and energy intake," *Journal of Diabetes Research* 2015 (2015): 206959. https://doi.org/10.1155/2015/206959.

32. Rohr et al., "Negative effects of a high-fat diet on intestinal permeability: a review," *Advances in Nutrition* 11, no. 1 (2020): 77–91. https://doi.org/10.1093/advances/nmz061.

33. Myhrstad et al., "Dietary fiber, gut microbiota, and metabolic regulation-current status in human randomized trials," *Nutrients* 12, no. 3 (2020). https://doi.org/10.3390/nu12030859.

34. C. Burdette and M. Heck, "IgY Max Increases Beneficial Flora, Improves Gut Integrity," PR Newswire, last modified June 29, 2016, https://www.prnewswire.com/news-releases/igy-max-increases-beneficial-flora-improves-gut-integrity-300292061.html.

35. Costantini et al., "Impact of omega-3 fatty acids on the gut microbiota," *International Journal of Molecular Sciences* 18, no. 12 (2017). https://doi.org/10.3390/ijms18122645.

36. Cândido et al., "Impact of dietary fat on gut microbiota and low-grade systemic inflammation: mechanisms and clinical implications on obesity," *International Journal of Food Sciences and Nutrition* 69, no. 2 (2018): 125–143. https://doi.org/10.1080/09637486.2017.1343286.

37. Lang et al., "Impact of individual traits, saturated fat, and protein source on the gut microbiome," *mBio* 9, no. 6 (2018). https://doi.org/10.1128/mBio.01604-18.

38. Wolters et al., "Dietary fat, the gut microbiota, and metabolic health—A systematic review conducted within the MyNewGut project," *Clinical Nutrition* 38, no. 6 (2019): 2504–2520. https://doi.org/10.1016/j.clnu.2018.12.024.

39. Carvalho et al., "Impact of trans-fats on heat-shock protein expression and the gut microbiota profile of mice," *Journal of Food Science* 83, no. 2 (2018): 489–498. https://doi.org/10.1111/1750-3841.13997.

40. Ge et al., "Effect of industrial trans-fatty acids-enriched diet on gut microbiota of C57BL/6 mice." *European Journal of Nutrition* 58, no. 7 (2019): 2625–2638. https://doi.org/10.1007/s00394-018-1810-2.

41. Rohr et al., "Negative effects of a high-fat diet on intestinal permeability: a review," *Advances in Nutrition* 11, no. 1, 77–91. https://doi.org/10.1093/advances/nmz061.

42. E. Bourdua-Roy, "Blood Tests for Patients on Low Carb," Diet Doctor, last modified June 17, 2022, https://www.dietdoctor.com/low-carb/for-doctors/lab-tests.

43. Volek et al., "Comparison of energy-restricted very low-carbohydrate and low-fat diets on weight loss and body composition in overweight men and women," *Nutrition & Metabolism* 1, no. 1 (2004): 13. https://doi.org/10.1186/1743-7075-1-13.

44. "Testosterone levels in athletes on carnivore diet. 'N=1' of Paul Saladino and Shawn Baker," The New Neander's *Physiological Literacy* (blog), May 23, 2019, https://nneandersphysiologicalliteracy.wordpress.com/2019/05/23/testosterone-levels-in-athletes-on-carnivore-diet-n1-of-paul-saladino/.

45. Bergman et al., "Effects of fasting on insulin action and glucose kinetics in lean and obese men and women," *American Journal of Physiology. Endocrinology and Metabolism* 293, no. 4 (2007): E1103–E1111. https://doi.org/10.1152/ajpendo.00613.2006.

46. Cox et al., "Nutritional ketosis alters fuel preference and thereby endurance performance in athletes," *Cell Metabolism* 24, no. 2 (2016): 256–268. https://doi.org/10.1016/j.cmet.2016.07.010.

47. Brietzke et al., "Ketogenic diet as a metabolic therapy for mood disorders: Evidence and developments," *Neuroscience and Biobehavioral Reviews* 94 (2018): 11–16. https://doi.org/10.1016/j.neubiorev.2018.07.020.

48. Saben et al., "Maternal metabolic syndrome programs mitochondrial dysfunction via germline changes across three generations," *Cell Reports* 16, no. 1 2016: 1–8. https://doi.org/10.1016/j.celrep.2016.05.065.

49. D'Andrea Meira et al., "Ketogenic diet and epilepsy: what we know so far," *Frontiers in Neuroscience* 13 (2019): 5. https://doi.org/10.3389/fnins.2019.00005.

50. Brenton et al, "Pilot study of a ketogenic diet in relapsing-remitting MS," *Neurology(R) Neuroimmunology & Neuroinflammation* 6, no. 4 (2019): e565. https://doi.org/10.1212/NXI.0000000000000565.

51. D. Włodarek, "Role of Ketogenic diets in neurodegenerative diseases (Alzheimer's disease and Parkinson's disease)," *Nutrients* 11, no. 1 (2019). https://doi.org/10.3390/nu11010169.
52. Nielsen et al., "Plasticity in mitochondrial cristae density allows metabolic capacity modulation in human skeletal muscle," *The Journal of Physiology* 595, no. 9 (2017): 2839–2847. https://doi.org/10.1113/JP273040.
53. Cox et al., "Nutritional ketosis alters fuel preference."
54. "The Great Ketogenic Experiment—Full Transcript," *Ben Greenfield Fitness* (blog), September 2, 2013, https://bengreenfieldfitness.com/podcast/low-carb-Ketogenic-diet-podcasts/great-Ketogenic-experiment-full-transcript/.
55. J. Alcock, C. C. Maley, and C. A. Aktipis, "Is eating behavior manipulated by the gastrointestinal microbiota? Evolutionary pressures and potential mechanisms," *BioEssays: News and Reviews in Molecular, Cellular and Developmental Biology* 36, no. 10 (2014): 940–949. https://doi.org/10.1002/bies.201400071.
56. W. Masood, P. Annamaraju, and K. R. Uppaluri, "Ketogenic Diet," in *StatPearls* [Internet] (Treasure Island, FL: StatPearls Publishing, 2022). https://pubmed.ncbi.nlm.nih.gov/29763005/.

Chapter 21

1. David et al., "Diet rapidly and reproducibly alters the human gut microbiome," *Nature* 505 (2014): 559–563. https://doi.org/10.1038/nature12820.
2. David et al., "Diet rapidly and reproducibly alters the human gut microbiome."
3. Wu et al., "Linking long-term dietary patterns with gut microbial enterotypes," *Science* 334, no. 6052 (2011): 105–108. https://doi.org/10.1126/science.1208344.
4. Turnbaugh et al., "The effect of diet on the human gut microbiome: a metagenomic analysis in humanized gnotobiotic mice," *Science Translational Medicine* 1, no. 6 (2009): 6ra14. https://doi.org/10.1126/scitranslmed.3000322.
5. Muegge et al., "Diet drives convergence in gut microbiome functions across mammalian phylogeny and within humans," *Science* 332, no. 6032 (2011): 970–974. https://doi.org/10.1126/science.1198719.
6. David et al., "Diet rapidly and reproducibly alters the human gut microbiome."
7. "Dietary Fibre," BetterHealth Channel, accessed April 23, 2023, https://www.betterhealth.vic.gov.au/health/healthyliving/fibre-in-food.
8. "Only 1 in 10 Adults Get Enough Fruits or Vegetables," CDC Newsroom, November 16, 2017, https://www.cdc.gov/media/releases/2017/p1116-fruit-vegetable-consumption.html.
9. S. B. Eaton SB, "The ancestral human diet: what was it and should it be a paradigm for contemporary nutrition?" *Proceedings of the Nutrition Society* 65, no. 1 (2006): 1–6. https://doi.org/10.1079/pns2005471.
10. Wegh et al., "Postbiotics and their potential applications in early life nutrition and beyond," *International Journal of Molecular Science* 20, no. 19 (2019): 4673. https://doi.org/10.3390/ijms20194673.
11. Martin et al., "The influence of the gut microbiome on host metabolism through the regulation of gut hormone release," *Frontiers in Physiology* 10 (2019): 428. https://doi.org/10.3389/fphys.2019.00428.
12. L. Galland. "The gut microbiome and the brain," *Journal of Medicinal Food* 17, no. 12 (2014): 1261–1272. https://doi.org/10.1089/jmf.2014.7000.
13. Ridlon et al., "Bile acids and the gut microbiome," *Current Opinion in Gastroenterology* 30, no. 3 (2014): 332–338. https://doi.org/10.1097/MOG.0000000000000057.
14. Nagengast et al., "The effect of a natural high-fibre diet on faecal and biliary bile acids, faecal pH and whole-gut transit time in man. A controlled study," *European Journal of Clinical Nutrition* 47, no. 9 (1993): 631–639. https://pubmed.ncbi.nlm.nih.gov/8243428/.
15. A. Clark and N. Mach, "The crosstalk between the gut microbiota and mitochondria during exercise," *Frontiers in Physiology* 8 (2017): 319. https://doi.org/10.3389/fphys.2017.00319.
16. Furusawa et al., "Commensal microbe-derived butyrate induces the differentiation of colonic regulatory T cells," *Nature* 504 (2013): 446–450. https://doi.org/10.1038/nature12721.
17. Peng et al., "Effects of butyrate on intestinal barrier function in a Caco-2 cell monolayer model of intestinal barrier," *Pediatric Research* 61, no. 1 (2007): 37–41. https://doi.org/10.1203/01.pdr.0000250014.92242.f3.
18. Roshanravan et al., "Effect of butyrate and insulin supplementation on glycemic status, lipid profile and glucagon-like peptide 1 level in patients with type 2 diabetes: A randomized double-blind, placebo-controlled trial," *Hormone and Metabolic Research* 49, no. 11 (2017): 886–891. https://doi.org/10.1055/s-0043-119089.
19. Gao et al., "Butyrate improves insulin sensitivity and increases energy expenditure in mice," *Diabetes* 58, no. 7 (2009): 1509–1517. https://doi.org/10.2337/db08-1637.
20. Wu et al., "Effects of the intestinal microbial metabolite butyrate on the development of colorectal cancer," *Journal of Cancer* 9, no. 14 (2018): 2510–2517. https://doi.org/10.7150/jca.25324.
21. Szentirmai et al., "Butyrate, a metabolite of intestinal bacteria, enhances sleep," *Scientific Reports* 9, no. 1 (2019): 7035. https://doi.org/10.1038/s41598-019-43502-1.
22. Murray et al., "Dietary tributyrin, an HDAC inhibitor, promotes muscle growth through enhanced terminal differentiation of satellite cells," *Physiological Reports* 6, no. 10 (2018): e13706. https://doi.org/10.14814/phy2.13706.
23. Anderson et al., "Health benefits of dietary fiber," *Nutrition Reviews* 67, no. 4 (2009): 188–205. https://doi.org/10.1111/j.1753-4887.2009.00189.x.
24. Anderson et al., "Health benefits of dietary fiber."
25. Cordain et al., "Plant-animal subsistence ratios and macronutrient energy estimations in worldwide hunter-gatherer diets," *The American Journal of Clinical Nutrition* 71, no. 3 (2000): 682–692. https://doi.org/10.1093/ajcn/71.3.682.
26. Clarys et al., "Comparison of nutritional quality of the vegan, vegetarian, semi-vegetarian, pesco-vegetarian and omnivorous diet," *Nutrients* 6, no. 3 (2014): 1318–1332. https://doi.org/10.3390/nu6031318.

27. Beane et al., "Effects of dietary fibers, micronutrients, and phytonutrients on gut microbiome: a review," *Applied Biological Chemistry* 64, no. 36 (2021). https://doi.org/10.1186/s13765-021-00605-6.
28. C. Leitzmann, "Characteristics and Health Benefits of Phytochemicals," *Forschende Komplementärmedizin* 23, no. 2 (2016): 69–74. https://doi.org/10.1159/000444063.
29. A. Devrim-Lanpir et al., "Vegan vs. omnivore diets paradox: A whole-metagenomic approach for defining metabolic networks during the race in ultra-marathoners- a before and after study design," *PloS ONE* 16, no. 9 (2021): e0255952. https://doi.org/10.1371/journal.pone.0255952.
30. Schüpbach et al., "Micronutrient status and intake in omnivores, vegetarians and vegans in Switzerland," *European Journal of Nutrition* 56, no. 1 (2017): 283–293. https://doi.org/10.1007/s00394-015-1079-7.
31. Forster et al., "Macrophage-derived insulin-like growth factor-1 is a key neurotrophic and nerve-sensitizing factor in pain associated with endometriosis," *FASEB Journal* 33, no. 10 (2019): 11210–11222. https://doi.org/10.1096/fj.201900797R.
32. M. S. Lewitt, M. S. Dent, and K. Hall, "The insulin-like growth factor system in obesity, insulin resistance and type 2 diabetes mellitus," *Journal of Clinical Medicine* 3, no. 4 (2014): 1561–1574. https://doi.org/10.3390/jcm3041561.
33. Allen et al., "The associations of diet with serum insulin-like growth factor I and its main binding proteins in 292 women meat-eaters, vegetarians, and vegans," *Cancer Epidemiology, Biomarkers & Prevention* 11, no. 11 (2002): 1441–1448. https://pubmed.ncbi.nlm.nih.gov/12433724/.
34. Catany Ritter et al., "Impact of elimination or reduction of dietary animal proteins on cancer progression and survival: protocol of an online pilot cohort study," *JMIR Research Protocols* 5, no. 3 (2016): e157. https://doi.org/10.2196/resprot.5804.
35. B. Morton, "How a Vegan Diet Affects My Endometriosis," Endometriosis.net, last modified December 2021, https://endometriosis.net/living/diet-vegan.
36. Medawar et al., "The effects of plant-based diets on the body and the brain: a systematic review," *Translational Psychiatry* 9, no. 1 (2019): 226. https://doi.org/10.1038/s41398-019-0552-0.
37. Schüpbach et al., "Micronutrient status and intake."
38. Kristensen et al., "Intake of macro- and micronutrients in Danish vegans," *Nutrition Journal* 14, no. 115 (2015). https://doi.org/10.1186/s12937-015-0103-3.
39. T. Decsi and K. Kennedy, "Sex-specific differences in essential fatty acid metabolism," *American Journal of Clinical Nutrition* 94, no. 6 Suppl (2011): 1914S–1919S. https://doi.org/10.3945/ajcn.110.000893.
40. Ameur et al., "Genetic adaptation of fatty-acid metabolism: a human-specific haplotype increasing the biosynthesis of long-chain omega-3 and omega-6 fatty acids," *American Journal of Human Genetics* 90, no. 5 (2012): 809–820. https://doi.org/10.1016/j.ajhg.2012.03.014.
41. H. Tallima and R. El Ridi, "Arachidonic acid: Physiological roles and potential health benefits—A review," *Journal of Advanced Research* 11 (2017): 33–41. https://doi.org/10.1016/j.jare.2017.11.004.
42. Tallima and El Ridi, "Arachidonic acid."
43. Mele et al., "Involvement of arachidonic acid and the lipoxygenase pathway in mediating luteinizing hormone-induced testosterone synthesis in rat leydig cells," *Endocrine Research* 23, no. 1–2 (1997): 15–26. https://doi.org 10.1080/07435809709031839.
44. H. Kawashima, "Intake of arachidonic acid-containing lipids in adult humans: dietary surveys and clinical trials," *Lipids in Health and Disease* 18, no. 101 (2019). https://doi.org/10.1186/s12944-019-1039-y.
45. Ameur et al., "Genetic adaptation of fatty-acid metabolism."
46. M. G. Mehedint and S. H. Zeisel, "Choline's role in maintaining liver function: new evidence for epigenetic mechanisms," *Current Opinion in Clinical Nutrition and Metabolic Care* 16 no. 3 (2013): 339–345. https://doi.org/10.1097/MCO.0b013e3283600d46.
47. Lombard et al., "Carnitine status of lactoovovegetarians and strict vegetarian adults and children," *American Journal of Clinical Nutrition* 50, no. 2 (1989): 301–306. https://doi.org/10.1093/ajcn/50.2.301.
48. Chung et al., "Tannins and human health: a review," *Critical Reviews in Food Science and Nutrition* 38, no. 6 (1998): 421–464. https://doi.org/10.1080/10408699891274273.
49. V. Ganji and C. V. Kies, "Zinc bioavailability and tea consumption. Studies in healthy humans consuming self-selected and laboratory-controlled diets," *Plant Foods for Human Nutrition* 46, no. 3 (1994): 267–276. https://doi.org/10.1007/BF01088999.
50. E. A. Prystai, C. V. Kies, and J. A. Driskell, "Calcium, copper, iron, magnesium and zinc utilization of humans as affected by consumption of black, decaffeinated black and green teas," *Nutrition Research* 19, no. 2 (1999): 167–177. https://doi.org/10.1016/S0271-5317(98)00181-X.
51. N. M. Delimont, M. D. Haub, and B. L. Lindshield, "The impact of tannin consumption on iron bioavailability and status: a narrative review," *Current Developments in Nutrition* 1, no. 2 (2017): 1–12. https://doi.org/10.3945/cdn.116.000042.
52. W. Chai and M. Liebman, "Effect of different cooking methods on vegetable oxalate content," *Journal of Agricultural and Food Chemistry* 53, no. 8 (2005): 3027–3030. https://doi.org/10.1021/jf048128d.
53. Iguacel et al., "Vegetarianism and veganism compared with mental health and cognitive outcomes: a systematic review and meta-analysis," *Nutrition Reviews* 79, no. 4 (2021): 361–381. doi:10.1093/nutrit/nuaa030.
54. P. G. Brady, A. M. Vannier, and J. G. Banwell, "Identification of the dietary lectin, wheat germ agglutinin, in human intestinal contents," *Gastroenterology* 75, no. 2 (1978): 236–239. https://doi.org/10.1016/0016-5085(78)90409-2.
55. B. Tchernychev and M. Wilchek, "Natural human antibodies to dietary lectins," *FEBS Letters* 397, no. 2–3 (1996): 139–142. https://doi.org/10.1016/s0014-5793(96)01154-4.
56. L. C. Dolan, R. A. Matulka, and G. A. Burdock, "Naturally occurring food toxins," *Toxins (Basel)* 2, no. 9 (2010): 2289–2332. https://doi.org/10.3390/toxins2092289.
57. Audi et al., "Ricin poisoning: a comprehensive review," *JAMA* 294, no. 18 (2005): 2342–2351. https://doi.org/10.1001/jama.294.18.2342.
58. Kregiel et al, "Saponin-Based, Biological-Active Surfactants from Plants," in *Application and Characterization of Surfactants*, ed. Reza Najjar (IntechOpen, 2017). https://doi.org/10.5772/68062.
59. M. Samtiya, R. E. Aluko, and T. Dhewa, "Plant food anti-nutritional factors and their reduction strategies: an overview," *Food Production, Processing and Nutrition* 2, no. 6 (2020). https://doi.org/10.1186/s43014-020-0020-5.

60. S. Magge and A. Lembo, "Low-FODMAP diet for treatment of irritable bowel syndrome," *Gastroenterology and Hepatology* 8, no. 11 (2012): 739–745. https://www.ncbi.nlm.nih.gov/pmc/articles/PMC3966170/.
61. R. Pawlak, J. Berger, and I. Hines, "Iron status of vegetarian adults: a review of literature," *American Journal of Lifestyle Medicine* 12, no. 6 (2016): 486–498. https://doi.org/10.1177/1559827616682933.
62. Pawlak, Berger, and Hines, "Iron status of vegetarian adults."
63. H. A. Roth-Bassell and F. M. Clydesdale, "The influence of zinc, magnesium, and iron on calcium uptake in brush border membrane vesicle," *Journal of the American Nutrition Association* 10, no. 1 (1991): 44–49. https://doi.org/10.1080/07315724.1991.10718125.
64. M. Maares and H. Haase, "A guide to human zinc absorption: general overview and recent advances of in vitro intestinal models," *Nutrients* 12, no. 3 (2020): 762. https://doi.org/10.3390/nu12030762.
65. J. Winkler and S. Ghosh, "Therapeutic potential of fulvic acid in chronic inflammatory diseases and diabetes," *Journal of Diabetes Research* 2018 (2018): 5391014. https://doi.org/10.1155/2018/5391014.
66. A. M. Uwitonze and M. S. Razzaque, "Role of magnesium in vitamin d activation and function," *Journal of the American Osteopathic Association* 118, no. 3 (2018): 181–189. doi:10.7556/jaoa.2018.037.
67. Shahbazi et al., "Anti-Inflammatory and immunomodulatory properties of fermented plant foods," *Nutrients* 13, no. 5 (2021): 1516. https://doi.org/10.3390/nu13051516.
68. Shahbazi et al., "Anti-Inflammatory and immunomodulatory properties of fermented plant foods."
69. Shahbazi et al., "Probiotics in treatment of viral respiratory infections and neuroinflammatory disorders," *Molecules* 25, no. 21 (2020): 4891. https://doi.org/10.3390/molecules25214891.
70. Olivares et al., "Dietary deprivation of fermented foods causes a fall in innate immune response. Lactic acid bacteria can counteract the immunological effect of this deprivation," *Journal of Dairy Research* 73, no. 4 (2006): 492–498. https://doi.org/10.1017/S0022029906002068.
71. Clemente et al., "The impact of the gut microbiota on human health: an integrative view," *Cell* 148, no. 6 (2012): 1258–1270. https://doi.org/10.1016/j.cell.2012.01.035.
72. A. C. Brown and A. Valiere, "Probiotics and medical nutrition therapy," *Nutrition in Clinical Care* 7, no. 2 (2004): 56–68. https://pubmed.ncbi.nlm.nih.gov/15481739/.
73. M. F. Hsu and B. H. Chiang, "Stimulating effects of Bacillus subtilis natto-fermented Radix astragali on hyaluronic acid production in human skin cells," *Journal of Ethnopharmacology* 125, no. 3 (2009), 474–481. https://doi.org/10.1016/j.jep.2009.07.011.
74. Küllenberg de Gaudry et al., "Milk A1 β-casein and health-related outcomes in humans: a systematic review," *Nutritional Reviews* 77, no. 5 (2019): 278–306. https://doi.org/10.1093/nutrit/nuy063.
75. Joint WHO/FAO/UNU Expert Consultation, "Protein and amino acid requirements in human nutrition," *World Health Organization Technical Report Series* no. 935 (2007): 1–265, back cover. https://pubmed.ncbi.nlm.nih.gov/18330140/.
76. Tujioka et al., "Effect of the quality of dietary amino acids composition on the urea synthesis in rats," *Journal of Nutritional Science and Vitaminology* 57, no. 1 (2011): 48–55. https://doi.org/10.3177/jnsv.57.48.
77. Berrazaga et al., "The role of the anabolic properties of plant- versus animal-based protein sources in supporting muscle mass maintenance: a critical review," *Nutrients* 11, no. 8 (2019): 1825. https://doi.org/10.3390/nu11081825.
78. J. Gangwisch, "Seasonal variation in metabolism: evidence for the role of circannual rhythms in metabolism?" *Hypertension Research* 36 (2013): 392–393. https://doi.org/10.1038/hr.2012.229.
79. Gangwisch, "Seasonal variation in metabolism."
80. K. Norman and S. Klaus, "Veganism, aging and longevity: new insight into old concepts," *Current Opinion in Clinical Nutrition and Metabolic Care* 23, no. 2 (2020): 145–150. https://doi.org/10.1097/MCO.0000000000000625.
81. Tomova et al., "The effects of vegetarian and vegan diets on gut microbiota," *Frontiers in Nutrition* 6: 47. https://doi.org/10.3389/fnut.2019.00047.
82. Tantamango-Bartley et al., "Vegetarian diets and the incidence of cancer in a low-risk population," *Cancer Epidemiology, Biomarkers & Prevention* 22, no. 2 (2013): 286–294. https://doi.org/10.1158/1055-9965.EPI-12-1060.
83. Huang et al., "Vegetarian diets and weight reduction: a meta-analysis of randomized controlled trials," *Journal of General Internal Medicine* 31, no. 1 (2016): 109–116. https://doi.org/10.1007/s11606-015-3390-7.
84. M. Cappel, D. Mauger, and D. Thiboutot, "Correlation between serum levels of insulin-like growth factor 1, dehydroepiandrosterone sulfate, and dihydrotestosterone and acne lesion counts in adult women," *Archives of Dermatology* 141, no. 3 (2005): 333–338. https://doi.org/10.1001/archderm.141.3.333.
85. Iguacel et al., "Vegetarianism and veganism compared with mental health and cognitive outcomes: a systematic review and meta-analysis," *Nutrition Reviews* 79, no. 4 (2021): 361–381. https://doi.org/10.1093/nutrit/nuaa030.
86. Iguacel et al., "Vegetarianism and veganism compared with mental health."

Chapter 22

1. Gong et al., "Plant lectins activate the nlrp3 inflammasome to promote inflammatory disorders," *Journal of Immunology* 198, no. 5 (2017): 2082–2092. https://doi.org/10.4049/jimmunol.1600145.
2. A. P. Simopoulos, "The importance of the omega-6/omega-3 fatty acid ratio in cardiovascular disease and other chronic diseases," *Experimental Biology and Medicine (Maywood)* 233, no. 6 (2008): 674–688. https://doi.org/10.3181/0711-MR-311.
3. Kumar Singh et al., "Beneficial effects of dietary polyphenols on gut microbiota and strategies to improve delivery efficiency," *Nutrients* 11, no. 9 (2019): 2216. https://doi.org/10.3390/nu11092216.
4. Yeomans et al., "Palatability: response to nutritional need or need-free stimulation of appetite?" *British Journal of Nutrition* 92, no. S1 (2004): S3–S14. https://doi.org/10.1079/BJN20041134.
5. Simopoulos, "The importance of the omega-6/omega-3 fatty acid ratio."
6. Patterson et al., "Health implications of high dietary omega-6 polyunsaturated fatty acids," *Journal of Nutrition and Metabolism* 2012 (2012): 539426. https://doi.org/10.1155/2012/539426.

7. A. Lerner, Y. Shoenfeld, and T. Matthias, "Adverse effects of gluten ingestion and advantages of gluten withdrawal in nonceliac autoimmune disease," *Nutrition Reviews* 75, no. 12 (2017): 1046–1058. https://doi.org/10.1093/nutrit/nux054.
8. Konijeti et al., "Efficacy of the autoimmune protocol diet for inflammatory bowel disease," *Inflammatory Bowel Disease* 23, no. 11 (2017): 2054–2060. https://doi.org/10.1097/MIB.0000000000001221.
9. R. D. Abbott, A. Sadowski, and A. G. Alt, "Efficacy of the autoimmune protocol diet as part of a multi-disciplinary, supported lifestyle intervention for Hashimoto's thyroiditis," *Cureus* 11, no. 4 (2019): e4556. https://doi.org/10.7759/cureus.4556.
10. Harvard T. H. Chan School of Public Health, "Diet Review: Paleo Diet for Weight Loss," The Nutrition Source, last modified October 28, 2019, https://www.hsph.harvard.edu/nutritionsource/healthy-weight/diet-reviews/Paleo-diet.
11. "Chemicals in Meat Cooked at High Temperatures and Cancer Risk," National Cancer Institute, last modified July 11, 2017, https://www.cancer.gov/about-cancer/causes-prevention/risk/diet/cooked-meats-fact-sheet.

Chapter 23

1. Deborah et al., "Interaction effects of selected pesticides on soil enzymes," *Toxicology International* 20, no. 3 (2013): 195–200. https://doi.org/10.4103/0971-6580.121665.
2. Woods et. al., "Religiosity is associated with affective and immune status in symptomatic HIV-infected gay men," *Journal of Psychosomatic Research* 46, no. 2 (1999): 165–176. https://doi.org/10.1016/s0022-3999(98)00078-6.
3. Xu et al., "Light-harvesting chlorophyll pigments enable mammalian mitochondria to capture photonic energy and produce ATP," *Journal of Cell Science* 127, Pt 2 (2014): 388–399. https://doi.org/10.1242/jcs.134262.
4. Xu et al., "Light-harvesting chlorophyll pigments."
5. "Amino Acid Deficiency," *ScienceDirect Topics*, accessed April 30, 2023, https://www.sciencedirect.com/topics/pharmacology-toxicology-and-pharmaceutical-science/amino-acid-deficiency.
6. E. E. Groopman, R. N. Carmody, and R. W. Wrangham, "Cooking increases net energy gain from a lipid-rich food," *American Journal of Physical Anthropology* 156, no. 1 (2015): 11–18. https://doi.org/10.1002/ajpa.22622.
7. M. F. Ullah, "Sulforaphane (SFN): an isothiocyanate in a cancer chemoprevention paradigm," *Medicines (Basel)* 2, no. 3 (2015): 141–156. https://doi.org/10.3390/medicines2030141.
8. Li et al., "Sulforaphane, a dietary component of broccoli/broccoli sprouts, inhibits breast cancer stem cells," *Clinical Cancer* 16, no. 9 (2010): 2580–2590. https://doi.org/10.1158/1078-0432.CCR-09-2937.
9. P. C. Evans, "The influence of sulforaphane on vascular health and its relevance to nutritional approaches to prevent cardiovascular disease," *The EPMA Journal* 2, no. 1 (2011): 9–14. https://doi.org/10.1007/s13167-011-0064-3.
10. Axelsson et al., "Sulforaphane reduces hepatic glucose production and improves glucose control in patients with type 2 diabetes," *Science Translational Medicine* 9, no. 394 (2017): eaah4477. https://doi.org/10.1126/scitranslmed.aah4477.
11. Xu et al., "Sulforaphane ameliorates glucose intolerance in obese mice via the upregulation of the insulin signaling pathway," *Food & Function* 9, no. 9 (2018): 4695–4701. https://doi.org/10.1039/c8fo00763b.
12. Jiménez-Osorio et al., "Natural NRF2 activators in diabetes," *Clinica Chimica Acta* 448 (2015): 182–192. https://doi.org/10.1016/j.cca.2015.07.009.

Chapter 24

1. R. A. Brewer, V. K. Gibbs, and D. L. Smith, Jr., "Targeting glucose metabolism for healthy aging." *Nutrition and Healthy Aging* 4, no. 1 (2016): 31–46. https://doi.org/10.3233/NHA-160007.
2. Myhrstad et al., "Dietary fiber, gut microbiota, and metabolic regulation—current status in human randomized trials," *Nutrients* 12, no. 3 (2020). https://doi.org/10.3390/nu12030859.
3. Zafar et al., "Low-glycemic index diets as an intervention for diabetes: a systematic review and meta-analysis," *The American Journal of Clinical Nutrition* 110, no. 4 (2019): 891–902. https://doi.org/10.1093/ajcn/nqz149.
4. J. A. Bittencourt, *The Power of Carbohydrates, Proteins, and Lipids*, 4th ed. (CreateSpace Independent Publishing Platform: 2018).
5. Zeevi et al., "Personalized nutrition by prediction of glycemic responses," *Cell* 163, no. 5 (2015): 1079–1094. https://doi.org/10.1016/j.cell.2015.11.001.

Chapter 25

1. "Micronutrient Facts," Centers for Disease Control and Prevention, last modified December 3, 2021, https://www.cdc.gov/nutrition/micronutrient-malnutrition/micronutrients/index.html.

Chapter 26

1. "Nutrition," *Encyclopedia Britannica*, https://www.britannica.com/science/nutrition.
2. "Dirt Poor: Have Fruits and Vegetables Become Less Nutritious?" *Scientific American*, last modified April 27, 2011, https://www.scientificamerican.com/article/soil-depletion-and-nutrition-loss/.
3. Kopittke et al., "Global changes in soil stocks of carbon, nitrogen, phosphorus, and sulphur as influenced by long-term agricultural production," *Global Change Biology* 23, no. 6 (2017): 2509-2519. doi: 10.1111/gcb.13513.
4. K. Harding, "Drank too much water, woman dies," *The Globe and Mail*, last modified January, 15, 2007, https://www.theglobeandmail.com/news/world/drank-too-much-water-woman-dies/article1069137/.

Chapter 27

1. V. J. Drake, "Micronutrient Inadequacies in the US Population: An Overview," Linus Pauling Institute, last modified November 2017. https://lpi.oregonstate.edu/mic/micronutrient-inadequacies/overview.
2. E. Gaffney-Stomberg, "The impact of trace minerals on bone metabolism—biological trace element research," *Biological Trace Element Research* 188 (2019): 26–34. https://doi.org/10.1007/s12011-018-1583-8.
3. C. Castillo-Durán and F. Cassorla, "Trace minerals in human growth and development," *Journal of Pediatric Endocrinology and Metabolism* 12, no. 5 (1999): 589–602. https://doi.org/10.1515/JPEM.1999.12.5.589.
4. Herrmann et al., "Vitamin B-12 status, particularly holotranscobalamin II and methylmalonic acid concentrations, and hyperhomocysteinemia in vegetarians," *The American Journal of Clinical Nutrition* 78, no. 1 (2003): 131–136. https://doi.org/10.1093/ajcn/78.1.131.

Chapter 28

1. M. Tiwari, "Science behind human saliva," *Journal of Natural Science, Biology, and Medicine* 2, no. 1 (2011), 53–58. https://doi.org/10.4103/0976-9668.82322.
2. Fábián et al., "Salivary defense proteins: their network and role in innate and acquired oral immunity," *International Journal of Molecular Sciences* 13, no, 4 (2012): 4295–4320. https://doi.org/10.3390/ijms13044295.
3. H. J. Alberts, R. Thewissen, and L. Raes, "Dealing with problematic eating behaviour. The effects of a mindfulness-based intervention on eating behaviour, food cravings, dichotomous thinking and body image concern," *Appetite* 58, no. 3 (2012): 847–851. doi:10.1016/j.appet.2012.01.009.
4. H. J. Alberts et al., "Coping with food cravings. Investigating the potential of a mindfulness-based intervention," *Appetite* 55, no. 1 (2010): 160–163. doi:10.1016/j.appet.2010.05.044.
5. M. Beshara, A. D. Hutchinson, and C. Wilson, "Does mindfulness matter? Everyday mindfulness, mindful eating and self-reported serving size of energy dense foods among a sample of South Australian adults," *Appetite* 67 (2013): 25–29. doi:10.1016/j.appet.2013.03.012.
6. Dalen et al., "Pilot study: Mindful Eating and Living (MEAL): weight, eating behavior, and psychological outcomes associated with a mindfulness-based intervention for people with obesity," *Complementary Therapies in Medicine* 18, no, 6 (2010): 260–264. doi:10.1016/j.ctim.2010.09.008.
7. J. Mathieu, "What should you know about mindful and intuitive eating?" [published correction appears in *Journal of the American Dietetic Association* 110, no. 3 (Mar 2010): 475], *Journal of the American Dietetic Association* 109, no. 12 (2009): 1982–1987. doi:10.1016/j.jada.2009.10.023.
8. Okubo et al., "The relationship of eating rate and degree of chewing to body weight status among preschool children in Japan: a nationwide cross-sectional study," *Nutrients* 11, no. 1 (2018): 64. doi:10.3390/nu11010064.
9. Y. Zhu and J. H. Hollis, "Increasing the number of chews before swallowing reduces meal size in normal-weight, overweight, and obese adults," *Journal of the Academy of Nutrition and Dietetics* 114, no. 6 (2014): 926–931. doi:10.1016/j.jand.2013.08.020.
10. Y. Hamada, H. Kashima, and N. Hayashi, "The number of chews and meal duration affect diet-induced thermogenesis and splanchnic circulation," *Obesity* (Silver Spring) 22, no. 5 (2014): E62–E69. doi:10.1002/oby.20715.
11. J. Wright and L. Lenard, *Why Stomach Acid Is Good for You: Natural Relief from Heartburn, Indigestion, Reflux and GERD* (Lanham, MD: M. Evans, 2001).
12. Van Such et al., "Extent of diagnostic agreement among medical referrals," *Journal of Evaluation in Clinical Practice* 23, no. 4 (2017): 870–874. doi:10.1111/jep.12747.
13. J. Keller and P. Layer, "The pathophysiology of malabsorption," *Viszeralmedizin* 30, no. 3 (2014): 150–154. https://doi.org/10.1159/000364794.
14. V. Urdaneta and J. Casadesús, "Interactions between bacteria and bile salts in the gastrointestinal and hepatobiliary tracts," *Frontiers of Medicine* 4 (2017): 163. https://doi.org/10.3389/fmed.2017.00163.
15. Ridlon et al., "Consequences of bile salt biotransformations by intestinal bacteria," *Gut Microbes* 7, no. 1 (2016): 22–39. https://doi.org/10.1080/19490976.2015.1127483.
16. Levine et al., "Low protein intake is associated with a major reduction in IGF-1, cancer, and overall mortality in the 65 and younger but not older population," *Cell Metabolism* 19, no. 3 (2014): 407–417. https://doi.org/10.1016/j.cmet.2014.02.006.
17. S. Chakrabarti, F. Jahandideh, and J. Wu, "Food-derived bioactive peptides on inflammation and oxidative stress," *BioMed Research International* 2014, no. 608979 (2014) https://doi.org/10.1155/2014/608979.
18. K. de Punder and L. Pruimboom, "The dietary intake of wheat and other cereal grains and their role in inflammation," *Nutrients* 5, no. 3 (2013): 771–787. https://doi.org/10.3390/nu5030771.
19. N. E. Diether and B. P. Willing, "Microbial fermentation of dietary protein: an important factor in diet–microbe–host interaction," *Microorganisms* 7, no. 1 (2019). https://doi.org/10.3390/microorganisms7010019.
20. Evenepoel et al., "Evidence for impaired assimilation and increased colonic fermentation of protein, related to gastric acid suppression therapy," *Alimentary Pharmacology & Therapeutics* 12, no. 10 (1998): 1011–1019. https://doi.org/10.1046/j.1365-2036.1998.00377.x.
21. Kris Verburgh, *The Longevity Code: Slow Down the Aging Process and Live Well for Longer: Secrets from the Leading Edge of Science* (New York, NY: The Experiment, LLC, 2019) Kindle Edition.
22. Vojdani et al., "Heat shock protein and gliadin peptide promote development of peptidase antibodies in children with autism and patients with autoimmune disease," *Clinical and Diagnostic Laboratory Immunology* 11, no. 3 (2004): 515–524. https://doi.org/10.1128/CDLI.11.3.515-524.2004.
23. Brooke-Taylor et al., "Systematic review of the gastrointestinal effects of A1 compared with A2 β-Casein," *Advances in Nutrition* 8, no. 5 (2017): 739–748. https://doi.org/10.3945/an.116.013953.
24. Parada Venegas et al., "Short chain fatty acids (scfas)-mediated gut epithelial and immune regulation and its relevance for inflammatory bowel diseases," *Frontiers in Immunology* 10 (2019): 277. https://doi.org/10.3389/fimmu.2019.00277.

Chapter 29

1. J. Hodgkin, "What does a worm want with 20,000 genes?" *Genome Biology* 2, no. 11 (2001): comment2008.1. https://doi.org/10.1186/gb-2001-2-11-comment2008.
2. M. Pertea and S. L. Salzberg, "Between a chicken and a grape: estimating the number of human genes," *Genome Biology* 11, no. 5 (2010): 206. https://doi.org/10.1186/gb-2010-11-5-206.
3. R. Sender, S. Fuchs, and R. Milo, "Revised estimates for the number of human and bacteria cells in the body," *PLoS Biology* 14, no. 8 (2016): e1002533. https://doi.org/10.1371/journal.pbio.1002533.
4. Tierney et al., "The landscape of genetic content in the gut and oral human microbiome," *Cell Host & Microbe* 26, no. 2 (2019): 283–295.e8. https://doi.org/10.1016/j.chom.2019.07.008.
5. A. B. Shreiner, J. Y. Kao, and V. B. Young, "The gut microbiome in health and in disease," *Current Opinion in Gastroenterology* 31, no. 1 (2015): 69–75. https://doi.org/10.1097/MOG.0000000000000139.
6. Anwar et al., "Gut Microbiome: A New Organ System in Body," in *Parasitology and Microbiology Research*, ed. G. A. B. Pacheco and A. A. Kamboh (Rijeka: IntechOpen, 2020). https://doi.org/10.5772/intechopen.89634.
7. J. Alcock, C. C. Maley, and C. A. Aktipis, "Is eating behavior manipulated by the gastrointestinal microbiota? Evolutionary pressures and potential mechanisms," *BioEssays: News and Reviews in Molecular, Cellular and Developmental Biology* 36, no. 10 (2014): 940–949. https://doi.org/10.1002/bies.201400071.
8. "NIH Human Microbiome Project defines normal bacterial makeup of the body," National Institutes of Health, last modified June 13, 2012, https://www.nih.gov/news-events/news-releases/nih-human-microbiome-project-defines-normal-bacterial-makeup-body.
9. "NIH Human Microbiome Project defines normal bacterial makeup of the body," National Institutes of Health, last modified June 13, 2012, https://www.nih.gov/news-events/news-releases/nih-human-microbiome-project-defines-normal-bacterial-makeup-body.
10. L. J. Wilkins, M. Monga, and A. W. Miller, "Defining Dysbiosis for a Cluster of Chronic Diseases," *Scientific Reports* 9, no. 1 (2019): 12918. https://doi.org/10.1038/s41598-019-49452-y.
11. P. J. Wisniewski, R. A. Dowden, and S. C. Campbell, "Role of dietary lipids in modulating inflammation through the gut microbiota," *Nutrients* 11, no. 1 (2019). https://doi.org/10.3390/nu11010117.
12. Boutagy et al., "Metabolic endotoxemia with obesity: Is it real and is it relevant?" *Biochimie* 124 (2016): 11–20. https://doi.org/10.1016/j.biochi.2015.06.020.
13. C. B. de La Serre, G. de Lartigue, and H. E. Raybould, "Chronic exposure to low dose bacterial lipopolysaccharide inhibits leptin signaling in vagal afferent neurons," *Physiology & Behavior* 139 (2015): 188–194. https://doi.org/10.1016/j.physbeh.2014.10.032.
14. M. He and B. Shi, "Gut microbiota as a potential target of metabolic syndrome: the role of probiotics and prebiotics," *Cell & Bioscience* 7 (2017): 54. https://doi.org/10.1186/s13578-017-0183-1.
15. Le Chatelier et al., "Richness of human gut microbiome correlates with metabolic markers," *Nature* 500 (2013): 541–546. https://doi.org/10.1038/nature12506.
16. Ridaura et al., "Gut microbiota from twins discordant for obesity modulate metabolism in mice," *Science* 341, no. 6150 (2013): 1241214. https://doi.org/10.1126/science.1241214.
17. Castaner et al., "The gut microbiome profile in obesity: a systematic review," *International Journal of Endocrinology* 2018 (2018): 4095789. https://doi.org/10.1155/2018/4095789.
18. A. C. Gomes, C. Hoffmann, and J. F. Mota, "The human gut microbiota: Metabolism and perspective in obesity," *Gut Microbes* 9, no. 4 (2018): 308–325. https://doi.org/10.1080/19490976.2018.1465157.
19. Jumpertz et al., "Energy-balance studies reveal associations between gut microbes, caloric load, and nutrient absorption in humans," *The American Journal of Clinical Nutrition* 94, no. 1 (2011): 58–65. https://doi.org/10.3945/ajcn.110.010132.
20. Clarke et al., "The gut microbiota and its relationship to diet and obesity: new insights," *Gut Microbes* 3, no. 3 (2012): 186–202. https://doi.org/10.4161/gmic.20168.
21. A. Chaix and A. Zarrinpar, "The effects of time-restricted feeding on lipid metabolism and adiposity," *Adipocyte* 4, no. 4 (2015): 319–324. https://doi.org/10.1080/21623945.2015.1025184.
22. S. R. Knowles, E. A. Nelson, and E. A. Palombo, "Investigating the role of perceived stress on bacterial flora activity and salivary cortisol secretion: a possible mechanism underlying susceptibility to illness," *Biological Psychology* 77, no. 2 (2008): 132–137. https://doi.org/10.1016/j.biopsycho.2007.09.010.
23. Dill-McFarland et al., "Close social relationships correlate with human gut microbiota composition," *Scientific Reports* 9, no. 1 (2019): 703. https://doi.org/10.1038/s41598-018-37298-9.
24. Moeller et al., "Social behavior shapes the chimpanzee pan-microbiome," *Science Advances* 2, no. 1 (2016): e1500997. https://doi.org/10.1126/sciadv.1500997.
25. Karl et al., "Effects of psychological, environmental and physical stressors on the gut microbiota," *Frontiers in Microbiology* 9 (2018): 2013. https://doi.org/10.3389/fmicb.2018.02013.
26. Benedict et al., "Gut microbiota and glucometabolic alterations in response to recurrent partial sleep deprivation in normal-weight young individuals," *Molecular Metabolism* 5, no. 12 (2016): 1175–1186. https://doi.org/10.1016/j.molmet.2016.10.003.
27. Poroyko et al., "Chronic sleep disruption alters gut microbiota, induces systemic and adipose tissue inflammation and insulin resistance in mice," *Scientific Reports* 6 (2016): 35405. https://doi.org/10.1038/srep35405.
28. Y. Litvak, M. X. Byndloss, and A. J. Bäumler, "Colonocyte metabolism shapes the gut microbiota," *Science* 362, no. 6418 (2018). https://doi.org/10.1126/science.aat9076.
29. M. Y. Zeng, N. Inohara, and G. Nuñez, "Mechanisms of inflammation-driven bacterial dysbiosis in the gut," *Mucosal Immunology* 10, no. 1 (2017): 18–26. https://doi.org/10.1038/mi.2016.75.
30. Zheng et al., "Gut microbiome remodeling induces depressive-like behaviors through a pathway mediated by the host's metabolism," *Molecular Psychiatry* 21, no. 6 (2016): 786–796. https://doi.org/10.1038/mp.2016.44.
31. Bercik et al., "The intestinal microbiota affect central levels of brain-derived neurotropic factor and behavior in mice," *Gastroenterology* 141, no. 2 (2011): 599–609, 609.e1–3. https://doi.org/10.1053/j.gastro.2011.04.052.

32. R. K. McNamara and F. E. Lotrich, "Elevated immune-inflammatory signaling in mood disorders: a new therapeutic target?" *Expert Review of Neurotherapeutics* 12, no. 9 (2012): 1143–1161. https://doi.org/10.1586/ern.12.98.

33. Kelley et al., "Cytokine-induced sickness behavior," *Brain, Behavior, and Immunity* 17, Suppl. 1 (2003): S112–8. https://doi.org/10.1016/s0889-1591(02)00077-6.

34. McNamara and Lotrich, "Elevated immune-inflammatory signaling."

35. Y.-K. Kim and S. W. Jeon, "Neuroinflammation and the immune-kynurenine pathway in anxiety disorders," *Current Neuropharmacology* 16, no. 5 (2018): 574–582. https://doi.org/10.2174/1570159X15666170913110426.

36. A. Evrensel, B. Ö. Ünsalver, and M. E. Ceylan, "Immune-kynurenine pathways and the gut microbiota-brain axis in anxiety disorders," *Advances in Experimental Medicine and Biology* 1191 (2020): 155–167. https://doi.org/10.1007/978-981-32-9705-0_10.

37. D'Mello et al., "Probiotics improve inflammation-associated sickness behavior by altering communication between the peripheral immune system and the brain," *The Journal of Neuroscience: The Official Journal of the Society for Neuroscience* 35, no. 30 (2015): 10821–10830. https://doi.org/10.1523/JNEUROSCI.0575-15.2015.

38. McBurney et al., "Establishing what constitutes a healthy human gut microbiome: state of the science, regulatory considerations, and future directions," *The Journal of Nutrition* 149, no. 11 (2019): 1882–1895. https://doi.org/10.1093/jn/nxz154.

39. C. D. Davis, "The Gut Microbiome and Its Role in Obesity," *Nutrition Today* 51, no. 4 (2016): 167–174. https://doi.org/10.1097/NT.0000000000000167.

40. Hehemann et al., "Transfer of carbohydrate-active enzymes from marine bacteria to Japanese gut microbiota," *Nature* 464, no. 7290 (2010): 908–912. https://doi.org/10.1038/nature08937.

41. Hollants et al., "What we can learn from sushi: a review on seaweed-bacterial associations," *FEMS Microbiology Ecology* 83, no. 1 (2013): 1–16. https://doi.org/10.1111/j.1574-6941.2012.01446.x.

42. J. Alcock, C. C. Maley, and C. A. Aktipis, "Is eating behavior manipulated by the gastrointestinal microbiota? Evolutionary pressures and potential mechanisms," *BioEssays: News and Reviews in Molecular, Cellular and Developmental Biology* 36, no. 10 (2014): 940–949. https://doi.org/10.1002/bies.201400071.

43. Alcock, Maley, and Aktipis, "Is eating behavior manipulated?"

44. Alcock, Maley, and Aktipis, "Is eating behavior manipulated?"

45. David et al., "Diet rapidly and reproducibly alters the human gut microbiome," *Nature* 505, no. 7484 (2014): 559–563. https://doi.org/10.1038/nature12820.

46. Bermudez-Brito et al., "Probiotic mechanisms of action," *Annals of Nutrition and Metabolism* 61, no. 2 (2012): 160–174. https://doi.org/10.1159/000342079.

47. P. Hemarajata and J. Versalovic, "Effects of probiotics on gut microbiota: mechanisms of intestinal immunomodulation and neuromodulation," *Therapeutic Advances in Gastroenterology* 6, no. 1 (2013): 39–51. https://doi.org/10.1177/1756283X12459294.

48. U. Vyas and N. Ranganathan, "Probiotics, prebiotics, and synbiotics: gut and beyond," *Gastroenterology Research and Practice*, 2012 (2012): Article ID 872716. https://doi.org/10.1155/2012/872716.

49. Śliżewska et al., "The effect of synbiotic preparations on the intestinal microbiota and her metabolism in broiler chickens," *Scientific Reports* 10, no. 1 (2020): 4281. https://doi.org/10.1038/s41598-020-61256-z.

50. P. Markowiak and K. Śliżewska, "Effects of probiotics, prebiotics, and synbiotics on human health," *Nutrients* 9, no. 9 (2017). https://doi.org/10.3390/nu9091021.

51. M. Y. Zeng, N. Inohara, and G. Nuñez, "Mechanisms of inflammation-driven bacterial dysbiosis in the gut," *Mucosal Immunology* 10, no. 1 (2017): 18–26. https://doi.org/10.1038/mi.2016.75.

52. Wang et al., "Infection-induced intestinal dysbiosis is mediated by macrophage activation and nitrate production," *mBio* 10, no. 3 (2019). https://doi.org/10.1128/mBio.00935-19.

53. R. Ambekar, "Effect of a Nutritious Drink Fortified with Immune Egg in Improving the Weight and Enhancing the Well-Being of Subjects," unpublished study (1998).

54. Clemente et al., "The impact of the gut microbiota on human health: an integrative view," *Cell* 148, no. 6 (2012): 1258–1270. https://doi.org/10.1016/j.cell.2012.01.035.

55. A. C. Brown and A. Valiere, "Probiotics and medical nutrition therapy," *Nutrition in Clinical Care: An Official Publication of Tufts University* 7, no. 2 (2004): 56–68.

56. M. F. Hsu and B. H. Chiang, "Stimulating effects of Bacillus subtilis natto-fermented Radix astragali on hyaluronic acid production in human skin cells," *Journal of Ethnopharmacology* 125, no. 3 (2009): 474–481. https://doi.org/10.1016/j.jep.2009.07.011.

57. Wastyk et al., "Gut-microbiota-targeted diets modulate human immune status," *Cell* 184, no. 16 (2021): 4137–4153.e14 . doi:10.1016/j.cell.2021.06.019.

58. P. Riccio and R. Rossano, "Undigested food and gut microbiota may cooperate in the pathogenesis of neuroinflammatory diseases: a matter of barriers and a proposal on the origin of organ specificity," *Nutrients* 11, no. 11 (2019). https://doi.org/10.3390/nu11112714.

59. Ke et al., "Orlistat-induced gut microbiota modification in obese mice," *Evidence-Based Complementary and Alternative Medicine: eCAM* (2020): 9818349. https://doi.org/10.1155/2020/9818349.

60. Vidal-Lletjós et al., "Dietary protein and amino acid supplementation in inflammatory bowel disease course: what impact on the colonic mucosa?" *Nutrients* 9, no. 3 (2017):310. https://doi.org/10.3390/nu9030310.

61. J. J. Majnarich and T. J. O'Brien, Strain of lactobacillus Plantarum, U.S. Patent 5,895,758, filed June 10, 1997, and issued April 20, 1999. https://patentimages.storage.googleapis.com/07/37/a2/a23677f5a63019/US5895758.pdf

62. C. M. C. Chapman, G. R. Gibson, and I. Rowland, "Health benefits of probiotics: are mixtures more effective than single strains?" *European Journal of Nutrition* 50, no. 1 (2011): 1–17. https://doi.org/10.1007/s00394-010-0166-z.

63. Chang et al., "Multiple strains probiotics appear to be the most effective probiotics in the prevention of necrotizing enterocolitis and mortality: An updated meta-analysis," *PloS One* 12, no. 2 (2017): e0171579. https://doi.org/10.1371/journal.pone.0171579.

64. Yu et al., "Urinary and fecal metabonomics study of the protective effect of chaihu-shu-gan-san on antibiotic-induced gut microbiota dysbiosis in rats," *Scientific Reports* 7 (2017): 46551. https://doi.org/10.1038/srep46551.

65. Liang et al., "Chaihu-Shugan-San decoction modulates intestinal microbe dysbiosis and alleviates chronic metabolic inflammation in NAFLD rats via the NLRP3 inflammasome pathway," *Evidence-Based Complementary and Alternative Medicine: eCAM* 2018 (2018): 9390786. https://doi.org/10.1155/2018/9390786.

66. Lu et al., "Microbiota influence the development of the brain and behaviors in C57BL/6J mice," *PloS One* 13, no. 8 (2018): e0201829. https://doi.org/10.1371/journal.pone.0201829.

67. Lu et al., "Microbiota influence."

68. Allen et al., "Mitochondria and mood: mitochondrial dysfunction as a key player in the manifestation of depression," *Frontiers in Neuroscience* 12 (2018): 386. https://doi.org/10.3389/fnins.2018.00386.

69. Attanzio et al., "Oxidative stress and cognitive function: focus on the interplay between immune and nervous system in neurodegenerative diseases," *Oxidative Medicine and Cellular Longevity*, Special Issue (November 1, 2019). https://www.hindawi.com/journals/omcl/si/963124/.

70. Fukuda et al., "A potential biomarker for fatigue: Oxidative stress and anti-oxidative activity," *Biological Psychology* 118 (2016): 88–93. https://doi.org/10.1016/j.biopsycho.2016.05.005.

71. P. Schönfeld and L. Wojtczak, "Short- and medium-chain fatty acids in energy metabolism: the cellular perspective," *Journal of Lipid Research* 57, no. 6 (2016): 943–954.https://doi.org/10.1194/jlr.R067629.

72. Chambers et al., "Role of Gut Microbiota-Generated Short-Chain Fatty Acids in Metabolic and Cardiovascular Health," *Current Nutrition Reports* 7, no. 4 (2018): 198–206. https://doi.org/10.1007/s13668-018-0248-8.

73. Peng et al., "Effects of butyrate on intestinal barrier function in a Caco-2 cell monolayer model of intestinal barrier," *Pediatric Research* 61, no. 1 (2007): 37–41. https://doi.org/10.1203/01.pdr.0000250014.92242.f3.

74. Braniste et al., "The gut microbiota influences blood-brain barrier permeability in mice," *Science Translational Medicine* 6, no. 263 (2014): 263ra158. https://doi.org/10.1126/scitranslmed.3009759.

75. Bourassa et al., "Butyrate, neuroepigenetics and the gut microbiome: Can a high fiber diet improve brain health?" *Neuroscience Letters* 625 (2016): 56–63. https://doi.org/10.1016/j.neulet.2016.02.009.

76. Liu et al., "Psychotropic effects of Lactobacillus plantarum PS128 in early life-stressed and naïve adult mice." *Brain Research* 1631 (2016): 1–12. https://doi.org/10.1016/j.brainres.2015.11.018.

77. Bravo et al., "Ingestion of Lactobacillus strain regulates emotional behavior and central GABA receptor expression in a mouse via the vagus nerve," *Proceedings of the National Academy of Sciences of the United States of America* 108, no. 38 (2011): 16050–16055. https://doi.org/10.1073/pnas.1102999108.

78. Ohland et al., "Effects of Lactobacillus helveticus on murine behavior are dependent on diet and genotype and correlate with alterations in the gut microbiome," *Psychoneuroendocrinology* 38, no. 9 (2013): 1738–1747. https://doi.org/10.1016/j.psyneuen.2013.02.008.

79. Wang et al., "Lactobacillus fermentum NS9 restores the antibiotic induced physiological and psychological abnormalities in rats," *Beneficial Microbes* 6, no. 5 (2015): 707–717. https://doi.org/10.3920/BM2014.0177.

80. Takada et al., "Probiotic Lactobacillus casei strain Shirota relieves stress-associated symptoms by modulating the gut-brain interaction in human and animal models," *Neurogastroenterology and Motility: The Official Journal of the European Gastrointestinal Motility Society* 28, no. 7 (2016): 1027–1036. https://doi.org/10.1111/nmo.12804.

81. Sowndhararajan et al., "An overview of neuroprotective and cognitive enhancement properties of lignans from Schisandra chinensis," *Biomedicine & Pharmacotherapy* 97 (2018): 958–968. https://doi.org/10.1016/j.biopha.2017.10.145.

82. Feng et al., "Nine traditional Chinese herbal formulas for the treatment of depression: an ethnopharmacology, phytochemistry, and pharmacology review," *Neuropsychiatric Disease and Treatment* 12 (2016): 2387–2402. https://doi.org/10.2147/NDT.S114560.

83. M.-J. R. Howes, R. Fang, and P. J. Houghton, "Effect of Chinese herbal medicine on Alzheimer's disease," *International Review of Neurobiology* 135 (2017): 29–56. https://doi.org/10.1016/bs.irn.2017.02.003.

84. Ohland et al., "Effects of Lactobacillus helveticus on murine behavior are dependent on diet and genotype and correlate with alterations in the gut microbiome," *Psychoneuroendocrinology* 38, no. 9 (2013): 1738–1747. https://doi.org/10.1016/j.psyneuen.2013.02.008.

85. Wang et al., "Effect of probiotics on central nervous system functions in animals and humans: a systematic review," *Journal of Neurogastroenterology and Motility* 22, no. 4 (2016): 589–605. https://doi.org/10.5056/jnm16018.

86. M. Dehhaghi, H. Kazemi Shariat Panahi, and G. J. Guillemin, "Microorganisms, tryptophan metabolism, and kynurenine pathway: a complex interconnected loop influencing human health status," *International Journal of Tryptophan Research: IJTR* 12 (2016): 1178646919852996. https://doi.org/10.1177/1178646919852996.

87. Ohland et al., "Effects of Lactobacillus helveticus on murine behavior are dependent on diet and genotype and correlate with alterations in the gut microbiome," *Psychoneuroendocrinology* 38, no. 9 (2013): 1738–1747. https://doi.org/10.1016/j.psyneuen.2013.02.008.

88. Howes, Fang, and Houghton, "Effect of Chinese herbal medicine on Alzheimer's disease."

89. B.-H. Lee and Y.-K. Kim, "The roles of BDNF in the pathophysiology of major depression and in antidepressant treatment," *Psychiatry Investigation* 7, no. 4 (2010): 231–235. https://doi.org/10.4306/pi.2010.7.4.231.

90. Kumar et al., "Amyloid-β peptide protects against microbial infection in mouse and worm models of Alzheimer's disease," *Science Translational Medicine* 8, no. 340 (2016): 340ra72. https://doi.org/10.1126/scitranslmed.aaf1059.

91. Mushtaq et al., "Alzheimer's disease and type 2 diabetes via chronic inflammatory mechanisms," *Saudi Journal of Biological Sciences* 22, no. 1 (2015): 4–13. https://doi.org/10.1016/j.sjbs.2014.05.003.

92. Davari et al., "Probiotics treatment improves diabetes-induced impairment of synaptic activity and cognitive function: behavioral and electrophysiological proofs for microbiome-gut-brain axis," *Neuroscience* 240 (2013): 287–296. https://doi.org/10.1016/j.neuroscience.2013.02.055.

93. Howes, Fang, and Houghton, "Effect of Chinese herbal medicine on Alzheimer's disease."

94. G. Chen and X. Guo, "Neurobiology of Chinese herbal medicine on major depressive disorder," *International Review of Neurobiology* 135 (2017): 77–95. https://doi.org/10.1016/bs.irn.2017.02.005/.

95. Qiu et al., "Changes in regional cerebral blood flow with Chaihu-Shugan-San in the treatment of major depression," *Pharmacognosy Magazine* 10, no. 40 (2014): 503–508. https://doi.org/10.4103/0973-1296.141775.

96. Bercik et al., "The anxiolytic effect of Bifidobacterium longum NCC3001 involves vagal pathways for gut-brain communication," *Neurogastroenterology and Motility: The Official Journal of the European Gastrointestinal Motility Society* 23, no. 12 (2011): 1132–1139. https://doi.org/10.1111/j.1365-2982.2011.01796.x.

97. Bravo et al., "Ingestion of Lactobacillus strain regulates emotional behavior and central GABA receptor expression in a mouse via the vagus nerve," *Proceedings of the National Academy of Sciences of the United States of America* 108, no. 38 (2011): 16050–16055. https://doi.org/10.1073/pnas.1102999108.

98. Breit et al., "Vagus nerve as modulator of the brain-gut axis in psychiatric and inflammatory disorders," *Frontiers in Psychiatry* 9 (2018): 44. https://doi.org/10.3389/fpsyt.2018.00044.

99. Le Barz et al., "Probiotics as complementary treatment for metabolic disorders," *Diabetes & Metabolism Journal* 39, no. 4 (2015): 291–303. https://doi.org/10.4093/dmj.2015.39.4.291.

100. Kadooka et al., "Effect of Lactobacillus gasseri SBT2055 in fermented milk on abdominal adiposity in adults in a randomised controlled trial," *British Journal of Nutrition* 110, no. 9 (2013): 1696–1703. https://doi.org/10.1017/S0007114513001037.

101. Kim et al., "Lactobacillus gasseri BNR17 supplementation reduces the visceral fat accumulation and waist circumference in obese adults: a randomized, double-blind, placebo-controlled trial," *Journal of Medicinal Food* 21, no. 5 (2018): 454–461. https://doi.org/10.1089/jmf.2017.3937.

102. Sanchez et al., "Effect of Lactobacillus rhamnosus CGMCC1.3724 supplementation on weight loss and maintenance in obese men and women," *British Journal of Nutrition* 111, no. 8 (2014): 1507–1519. https://doi.org/10.1017/S0007114513003875.

103. Li et al., "Lactobacillus plantarum helps to suppress body weight gain, improve serum lipid profile and ameliorate low-grade inflammation in mice administered with glycerol monolaurate," *Journal of Functional Foods* 53 (2019): 54–61. https://doi.org/10.1016/j.jff.2018.12.015.

104. Zoetendal et al., "Mucosa-associated bacteria in the human gastrointestinal tract are uniformly distributed along the colon and differ from the community recovered from feces," *Applied and Environmental Microbiology* 68, no. 7 (2002): 3401–3407. https://doi.org/10.1128/aem.68.7.3401-3407.2002.

Chapter 30

1. Fond et al., "Fasting in mood disorders: neurobiology and effectiveness. A review of the literature," *Psychiatry Research* 209, no. 3 (2013): 253–258. https://doi.org/10.1016/j.psychres.2012.12.018.

2. A. J. Brown, "Low-carb diets, fasting and euphoria: Is there a link between ketosis and gamma-hydroxybutyrate (GHB)?" *Medical Hypotheses* 68, no. 2 (2007): 268–271. https://doi.org/10.1016/j.mehy.2006.07.043.

3. A. G. Roseberry, "Acute fasting increases somatodendritic dopamine release in the ventral tegmental area," *Journal of Neurophysiology* 114, no. 2 (2015): 1072–1082. https://doi.org/10.1152/jn.01008.2014.

4. Alirezaei et al., "Short-term fasting induces profound neuronal autophagy," *Autophagy* 6, no. 6 (2010): 702–710. https://doi.org/10.4161/auto.6.6.12376.

5. T. J. Horton and J. O. Hill, "Prolonged fasting significantly changes nutrient oxidation and glucose tolerance after a normal mixed meal," *Journal of Applied Physiology* 90, no. 1 (2001): 155–163. https://doi.org/10.1152/jappl.2001.90.1.155.

6. Pavlica et al., "Uticaj trodnevnog gladovanja na psihofizicku sposobnost mladih ljudi [The effect of a 3-day fast on psychophysical functions in young people]," *Vojnosanit Pregl* 47, no. 4 (1990): 254–258. Serbian. https://pubmed.ncbi.nlm.nih.gov/2238509/.

7. M. P. Mattson, V. D. Longo, and M. Harvie, "Impact of intermittent fasting on health and disease processes," *Ageing Research Reviews* 39 (2017): 46–58. https://doi.org/10.1016/j.arr.2016.10.005.

8. L. Adda, S. A. Melhem, and J. Pol, "Le jeûne réduit l'inflammation associée aux maladies inflammatoires chroniques sans altérer la réponse immunitaire aux infections aiguës [Fasting reduces inflammation associated with chronic inflammatory diseases without affecting the immune response to acute infections]," *Med Sci* (Paris) 36, no. 6–7 (2020): 665–668. French. https://doi.org/10.1051/medsci/2020119.

9. Mesnage et al., "Changes in human gut microbiota composition are linked to the energy metabolic switch during 10 d of Buchinger fasting," *Journal of Nutritional Science* 8 (2019): e36. https://doi.org/10.1017/jns.2019.33.

10. C. Ozkul, M. Yalinay, and T. Karakan, "Structural changes in gut microbiome after Ramadan fasting: a pilot study," *Beneficial Microbes* 11, no. 3 (2020): 227–233. https://doi.org/10.3920/BM2019.0039.

11. Mohammadzadeh et al., "The interplay between fasting, gut microbiota, and lipid profile," *The International Journal of Clinical Practice* 75, no. 10 (2021): e14591. https://doi.org/10.1111/ijcp.14591.

12. Mesnage et al., "Changes in human gut microbiota composition."

13. C. von Loeffelholz and A. L. Birkenfeld, "Non-Exercise Activity Thermogenesis in Human Energy Homeostasis." [Updated Nov 25, 2022] In *Endotext* [Internet], ed. Feingold et al. (South Dartmouth, MA: MDText.com, Inc.; 2000-). https://www.ncbi.nlm.nih.gov/books/NBK279077/.

14. Mesnage et al., "Changes in human gut microbiota composition."

15. Lahdimawan et al., "Effect of Ramadan fasting on endorphin and endocannabinoid level in serum, PBMC, and macrophage," *International Journal of Pharmaceutical Science Invention* 2, no. 3 (2013): 46–54. https://www.ijpsi.org/Papers/Vol2(3)/Version-1/J234654.pdf

16. E.C. Lloyd, A. M. Haase, and B. Verplanken, "Anxiety and the development and maintenance of anorexia nervosa: protocol for a systematic review," *Systematic Reviews* 7, no. 14 (2018). https://doi.org/10.1186/s13643-018-0685-x.

17. Kolaczynski et al., "Responses of leptin to short-term fasting and refeeding in humans: a link with ketogenesis but not ketones themselves," *Diabetes* 45, no. 11 (1996): 1511–1515. https://doi.org/10.2337/diab.45.11.1511.

18. Zauner et al., "Resting energy expenditure in short-term starvation is increased as a result of an increase in serum norepinephrine," *The American Journal of Clinical Nutrition* 71, no. 6 (2000): 1511–1515. https://doi.org/10.1093/ajcn/71.6.1511.
19. Beaumont et al., "The Acute Effect of Intermittent Fasting on Resting Energy Expenditure in College-Aged Males," Western Kentucky University, n.d., https://digitalcommons.wku.edu/cgi/viewcontent.cgi?article=3058&context=ijesab.
20. Nymo et al., "Timeline of changes in adaptive physiological responses, at the level of energy expenditure, with progressive weight loss," *British Journal of Nutrition* 120, no. 2 (2018): 141–149. https://doi.org/10.1017/S0007114518000922.
21. Nørrelund et al., "The protein-retaining effects of growth hormone during fasting involve inhibition of muscle-protein breakdown," *Diabetes* 50, no. 1 (2001): 96–104. https://doi.org/10.2337/diabetes.50.1.96.
22. Welton et al., "Intermittent fasting and weight loss: Systematic review," *Family Physician* 66, no. 2 (2020): 117–125. https://www.ncbi.nlm.nih.gov/pmc/articles/PMC7021351/.
23. Loeffelholz and Birkenfeld, "Non-Exercise Activity Thermogenesis."
24. Hollstein et al., "Metabolic response to fasting predicts weight gain during low-protein overfeeding in lean men: further evidence for spendthrift and thrifty metabolic phenotypes," *The American Journal of Clinical Nutrition* 110, no. 3 (2019): 593–604. https://doi.org/10.1093/ajcn/nqz062.

Chaper 31

1. Farré et al, "Intestinal permeability, inflammation and the role of nutrients," *Nutrients* 12, no. 4 (2020). https://doi.org/10.3390/nu12041185.
2. Ordiz et al., "EB 2017 Article: Interpretation of the lactulose:mannitol test in rural Malawian children at risk for perturbations in intestinal permeability," *Experimental Biology and Medicine* 243, no. 8 (2018): 677–683. https://doi.org/10.1177/1535370218768508.
3. Ordiz et al., "EB 2017 Article: Interpretation of the lactulose:mannitol test."
4. Fasano et al., "Zonulin, a newly discovered modulator of intestinal permeability, and its expression in coeliac disease," *The Lancet* 355, no. 9214 (2000): 1518–1519. https://doi.org/10.1016/S0140-6736(00)02169-3.
5. Barbaro et al., "Serum zonulin and its diagnostic performance in non-coeliac gluten sensitivity," *Gut* 69, no. 11 (2020): 1966–1974. https://doi.org/10.1136/gutjnl-2019-319281.
6. M. Camilleri, "Leaky gut: mechanisms, measurement and clinical implications in humans," *Gut* 68, no. 8 (2019): 1516–1526. https://doi.org/10.1136/gutjnl-2019-318427.
7. T. Suzuki, "Regulation of the intestinal barrier by nutrients: The role of tight junctions," *Animal Science Journal* 91, no. 1 (2020): e13357. https://doi.org/10.1111/asj.13357.
8. M. Sykes, "Immune tolerance: mechanisms and application in clinical transplantation," *Journal of Internal Medicine* 262, no. 3 (2007): 288–310. https://doi.org/10.1111/j.1365-2796.2007.01855.x.
9. Amouzegar et al., "The prevalence, incidence and natural course of positive antithyroperoxidase antibodies in a population-based study: Tehran thyroid study," *PloS One* 12, no. 1 (2017): e0169283. https://doi.org/10.1371/journal.pone.0169283.
10. A. Vojdani, A. Afar, and E. Vojdani., "Reaction of lectin-specific antibody with human tissue: possible contributions to autoimmunity," *Journal of Immunology Research* (2020): Article ID 1438957. https://doi.org/10.1155/2020/1438957.
11. D. A. Vignali, L. W. Collison, and C. J. Workman, "How regulatory T cells work," *Nature Reviews Immunology* 8, no. 7 (2008): 523–532. https://doi.org/10.1038/nri2343.
12. O. J. Harrison and F. M. Powrie, "Regulatory T cells and immune tolerance in the intestine," *Cold Spring Harbor Perspectives in Biology* 5, no. 7 (2013). https://doi.org/10.1101/cshperspect.a018341.
13. Y. Togashi, K. Shitara, and H. Nishikawa, "Regulatory T cells in cancer immunosuppression—implications for anticancer therapy," *Nature Reviews Clinical Oncology* 16, no. 6 (2019): 356–371. https://doi.org/10.1038/s41571-019-0175-7.
14. Fisher et al., "The role of vitamin D in increasing circulating T regulatory cell numbers and modulating T regulatory cell phenotypes in patients with inflammatory disease or in healthy volunteers: A systematic review," *PloS One* 14, no. 9 (2019): e0222313. https://doi.org/10.1371/journal.pone.0222313.
15. Bollinger et al., "Sleep-dependent activity of T cells and regulatory T cells," *Clinical and Experimental Immunology* 155, no. 2 (2009): 231–238. https://doi.org/10.1111/j.1365-2249.2008.03822.x.
16. K. de Punder and L. Pruimboom, "Stress induces endotoxemia and low-grade inflammation by increasing barrier permeability," *Frontiers in Immunology* 6 (2015): 223. https://doi.org/10.3389/fimmu.2015.00223.
17. Kelly et al., "Breaking down the barriers: the gut microbiome, intestinal permeability and stress-related psychiatric disorders," *Frontiers in Cellular Neuroscience* 9 (2015): 392. https://doi.org/10.3389/fncel.2015.00392.
18. M. F. Cusick, J. E. Libbey, and R. S. Fujinami, "Molecular mimicry as a mechanism of autoimmune disease," *Clinical Reviews in Allergy & Immunology* 42, no. 1 (2012): 102–111. https://doi.org/10.1007/s12016-011-8294-7.
19. A. Vojdani, "Antibodies as predictors of complex autoimmune diseases," *International Journal of Immunopathology and Pharmacology* 21, no. 2 (2008): 267–278. https://doi.org/10.1177/039463200802100203.
20. E. Untersmayr, "The influence of gastric digestion on the development of food allergy," *Revue Francaise D'allergologie* 55, no. 7 (2015): 444–447. https://doi.org/10.1016/j.reval.2015.09.004.
21. A. Vojdani, "Lectins, agglutinins, and their roles in autoimmune reactivities," *Alternative Therapies in Health and Medicine* 21, Suppl. 1 (2015): 46–51. https://pubmed.ncbi.nlm.nih.gov/25599185/.
22. Monetini et al., "Antibodies to bovine beta-casein in diabetes and other autoimmune diseases," *Hormone and Metabolic Research* 34, no. 8 (2002): 455–459. https://doi.org/10.1055/s-2002-33595.
23. Mu et al., "Leaky gut as a danger signal for autoimmune diseases," *Frontiers in Immunology* 8 (2017): 598. https://doi.org/10.3389/fimmu.2017.00598.
24. M. D. Rosenblum, K. A. Remedios, and A. K. Abbas, "Mechanisms of human autoimmunity," *Journal of Clinical Investigation* 125, no. 6 (2015): 2228–2233. https://doi.org/10.1172/JCI78088.

25. P. Zhang and Q. Lu, "Genetic and epigenetic influences on the loss of tolerance in autoimmunity," *Cellular & Molecular Immunology* 15, no. 6 (2018): 575–585. https://doi.org/ 10.1038/cmi.2017.137.

26. Institute for Quality and Efficiency in Health Care (IQWiG), "Food allergies: Anaphylactic reactions (anaphylaxis)," National Library of Medicine, last modified May 7, 2020, https://www.ncbi.nlm.nih.gov/books/NBK453101/.

27. F.-D. Popescu, "Cross-reactivity between aeroallergens and food allergens," *World Journal of Methodology* 5, no. 2 (2015): 31–50. https://doi.org/10.5662/wjm.v5.i2.31.

28. Vojdani et al., "Antibodies against molds and mycotoxins following exposure to toxigenic fungi in a water-damaged building," *Archives of Environmental Health* 58, no. 6 (2003), 324–336. https://pubmed.ncbi.nlm.nih.gov/14992307/.

29. Popescu, "Cross-reactivity."

30. Hilger et al., "Allergic cross-reactions between cat and pig serum albumin. Study at the protein and DNA levels," *Allergy* 52, no. 2 (1997): 179–187. https://doi.org/10.1111/j.1398-9995.1997.tb00972.x.

31. Price et al., "Oral allergy syndrome (pollen-food allergy syndrome)," *Dermatitis* 26, no. 2 (2015): 78–88. https://doi.org/10.1097/DER.0000000000000087.

32. Y. Özogul and F. Özogul, "Chapter 1. Biogenic Amines Formation, Toxicity, Regulations in Food," in *Biogenic Amines in Food* (London: Royal Society of Chemistry, 2019): 1–17.

33. L. Maintz and N. Novak, "Histamine and histamine intolerance," *The American Journal of Clinical Nutrition* 85, no. 5 (2007): 1185–1196. https://doi.org/10.1093/ajcn/85.5.1185.

34. Lopes et al., "Differential effect of plant lectins on mast cells of different origins," *Brazilian Journal of Medical and Biological Research* 38, no. 6 (2005): 935–941. https://doi.org/10.1590/s0100-879x2005000600016.

35. "IgY Max increases beneficial flora and improves gut integrity," *Nutraceutical Business Review*, n.d., accessed July 29, 2022, https://nutraceuticalbusinessreview.com/news/article_page/IgY_Max_increases_beneficial_flora_and_improves_gut_integrity/119301.

36. Wegh et al., "Postbiotics and their potential applications in early life nutrition and beyond," *International Journal of Molecular Sciences* 20, no. 19 (2019): 4673. https://doi.org/10.3390/ijms20194673.

37. D. Meyer, D. and M. Stasse-Wolthuis, "The bifidogenic effect of inulin and oligofructose and its consequences for gut health," *European Journal of Clinical Nutrition* 63, no. 11 (2009): 1277–1289. https://doi.org/10.1038/ejcn.2009.64.

38. P. Hill, J. G. Muir, and P. R. Gibson, "Controversies and recent developments of the low-FODMAP diet," *Gastroenterology & Hepatology* 13, no. 1 (2017): 36–45. https://pubmed.ncbi.nlm.nih.gov/28420945/.

39. Marum et al., "A low fermentable oligo-di-mono saccharides and polyols (FODMAP) diet reduced pain and improved daily life in fibromyalgia patients," *Scandinavian Journal of Pain* 13 (2016): 166–172. https://doi.org/10.1016/j.sjpain.2016.07.004.

40. Kortlever et al., "Low-FODMAP diet is associated with improved quality of life in IBS patients—a prospective observational study," *Nutrition in Clinical Practice* 34, no. 4 (2019): 623–630. https://doi.org/10.1002/ncp.10233.

41. Donnachie et al., "Incidence of irritable bowel syndrome and chronic fatigue following GI infection: a population-level study using routinely collected claims data," *Gut* 67, no. 6 (2018): 1078–1086. https://doi.org/10.1136/gutjnl-2017-313713.

42. K. B. Woodford, "Casomorphins and gliadorphins have diverse systemic effects spanning gut, brain and internal organs," *International Journal of Environmental Research and Public Health* 18, no. 15 (2021): 7911. https://doi.org/10.3390/ijerph18157911.

43. N. Sharon and H. Lis, "Lectins as cell recognition molecules," *Science* 246, no. 4927 (1989): 227–234. https://doi.org/10.1126/science.2552581.

44. P. G. Brady, A. M. Vannier, and J. G. Banwell, "Identification of the dietary lectin, wheat germ agglutinin, in human intestinal contents," *Gastroenterology* 75, no. 2 (1978): 236–239. https://pubmed.ncbi.nlm.nih.gov/669209/.

45. Lavelle et al., "The identification of plant lectins with mucosal adjuvant activity," *Immunology* 102, no. 1 (2001): 77–86. https://doi.org/10.1046/j.1365-2567.2001.01157.x.

46. B. Tchernychev and M. Wilchek, "Natural human antibodies to dietary lectins," *FEBS Letters* 397, nos. 2–3 (1996): 139–142. https://doi.org/10.1016/s0014-5793(96)01154-4.

47. Cordain et al., "Modulation of immune function by dietary lectins in rheumatoid arthritis," *British Journal of Nutrition* 83, no. 3 (2000): 207–217. https://doi.org/10.1017/s0007114500000271.

48. A. Fasano, "Leaky gut and autoimmune diseases," *Clinical Reviews in Allergy & Immunology* 42, no. 1 (2012): 71–78. https://doi.org/10.1007/s12016-011-8291-x.

49. L. C. Dolan, R. A. Matulka, and G. A. Burdock, "Naturally occurring food toxins," *Toxins* 2, no. 9 (2010): 2289–2332. https://doi.org/10.3390/toxins2092289.

50. Audi et al., "Ricin poisoning: a comprehensive review," *JAMA* 294, no. 18 (2005): 2342–2351. https://doi.org/10.1001/jama.294.18.2342.

51. Audi et al., "Ricin poisoning."

52. "Celiac Disease." Johns Hopkins Medicine, n.d., accessed July 29, 2022, https://www.hopkinsmedicine.org/health/conditions-and-diseases/celiac-disease.

53. J. R. Biesiekierski and J. Iven, "Non-coeliac gluten sensitivity: piecing the puzzle together," *United European Gastroenterology Journal* 3, no. 2 (2015): 160–165. https://doi.org/10.1001/10.1177/2050640615578388.

54. Barbaro et al., "Serum zonulin."

55. J.-C. Caubet and J. Wang, "Current understanding of egg allergy," *Pediatric Clinics of North America* 58, no. 2 (2011): 427–443, xi. https://doi.org/10.1016/j.pcl.2011.02.014.

56. Pablos-Tanarro et al., "Sensitizing and eliciting capacity of egg white proteins in BALB/c mice as affected by processing," *Journal of Agricultural and Food Chemistry* 65, no. 22 (2017): 4500–4508. https://doi.org/10.1021/acs.jafc.7b00953.

57. Davoodi et al., "Health-related aspects of milk proteins," *Iranian Journal of Pharmaceutical Research* 15, no. 3 (2016): 573–591. https://pubmed.ncbi.nlm.nih.gov/27980594/.

58. Ziauddeen et al., "Effects of the mu-opioid receptor antagonist GSK1521498 on hedonic and consummatory eating behaviour: a proof of mechanism study in binge-eating obese subjects," *Molecular Psychiatry* 18, no. 12 (2013): 1287–1293. https://doi.org/10.1038/mp.2012.154.

59. Salehi et al., "The insulinogenic effect of whey protein is partially mediated by a direct effect of amino acids and GIP on β-cells," *Nutrition & Metabolism* 9, no. 1 (2012): 48. https://doi.org/10.1186/1743-7075-9-48.
60. D. J. Drucker, "The biology of incretin hormones," *Cell Metabolism* 3, no. 3 (2006): 153–165. https://doi.org/10.1016/j.cmet.2006.01.004.
61. Chia et al., "A1 beta-casein milk protein and other environmental pre-disposing factors for type 1 diabetes," *Nutrition & Diabetes* 7, no. 5 (2017): e274. https://doi.org/10.1038/nutd.2017.16.
62. T. F. Malik and K. K. Panuganti, "Lactose Intolerance," in *StatPearls* [Internet] (Treasure Island, FL: StatPearls Publishing, 2022). https://pubmed.ncbi.nlm.nih.gov/30335318/.
63. A. S. Precetti, M. P. Oria, and S. S. Nielsen, "Presence in bovine milk of two protease inhibitors of the plasmin system," *Journal of Dairy Science* 80, no. 8 (1997): 1490–1496. https://doi.org/10.3168/jds.S0022-0302(97)76077-6.
64. J. J. Rackis, W. J. Wolf, and E. C. Baker, "Protease inhibitors in plant foods: content and inactivation," *Advances in Experimental Medicine and Biology* 199 (1986): 299–347. https://doi.org/10.1007/978-1-4757-0022-0_19.
65. Rolland-Fourcade et al., "Epithelial expression and function of trypsin-3 in irritable bowel syndrome," *Gut* 66, no. 10 (2017): 1767–1778. http://dx.doi.org/10.1136/gutjnl-2016-312094.
66. Van Spaendonk et al., "Regulation of intestinal permeability: The role of proteases," *World Journal of Gastroenterology* 23, no. 12 (2017): 2106–2123. https://doi.org/10.3748/wjg.v23.i12.2106.
67. W. Chai and M. Liebman, "Effect of different cooking methods on vegetable oxalate content," *Journal of Agricultural and Food Chemistry* 53, no. 8 (2005): 3027–3030. https://doi.org/10.1021/jf048128d.
68. H.-W. Baenkler, "Salicylate intolerance: pathophysiology, clinical spectrum, diagnosis and treatment," *Deutsches Arzteblatt International* 105, no. 8 (2008): 137–142. https://doi.org/10.3238/arztebl.2008.0137.
69. Kregiel et al, "Saponin-Based, Biological-Active Surfactants from Plants," in *Application and Characterization of Surfactants*, ed. Reza Najjar (IntechOpen, 2017). https://doi.org/10.5772/68062.
70. M. Samtiya, R. E. Aluko, and T. Dhewa, "Plant food anti-nutritional factors and their reduction strategies: an overview," *Food Production, Processing and Nutrition* 2, no. 1 (2020): 1–14. https://doi.org/10.1186/s43014-020-0020-5.
71. M. Bedard, "Over 50% of U.S. Homes and 85% of Commercial Buildings Have Water Damage and Mold," Mold Safe Solutions, last modified April 27, 2016, accessed July 29, 2022, https://moldsafesolutions.com/over-50-of-u-s-homes-and-85-of-commercial-buildings-have-water-damage-and-mold/.
72. Kritas et al., "Impact of mold on mast cell-cytokine immune response," *Journal of Biological Regulators and Homeostatic Agents* 32, no. 4 (2018): 763–768. https://pubmed.ncbi.nlm.nih.gov/30043558/.
73. I. Alassane-Kpembi, P. Pinton, and I. P. Oswald, "Effects of Mycotoxins on the Intestine," *Toxins* 11, no. 3 (2019): 159. https://doi.org/10.3390/toxins11030159.
74. A. C. A. Onbaşı, "Mycotoxins: The Hidden Danger in Foods," in *Mycotoxins and Food Safety*, ed. Suna Sabuncuoğlu (IntechOpen, 2019).
75. J. V. Martino, J. Van Limbergen, and L. E. Cahill, "The role of carrageenan and carboxymethylcellulose in the development of intestinal inflammation," *Frontiers in Pediatrics* 5 (2017): 96. https://doi.org/10.3389/fped.2017.00096.
76. A. Lerner and T. Matthias, "Changes in intestinal tight junction permeability associated with industrial food additives explain the rising incidence of autoimmune disease," *Autoimmunity Reviews* 14, no. 6 (2015): 479–489. https://doi.org/10.1016/j.autrev.2015.01.009.
77. Jerschow et al., "Dichlorophenol-containing pesticides and allergies: results from the US National Health and Nutrition Examination Survey 2005–2006," *Annals of Allergy, Asthma & Immunology* 109, no. 6 (2012): 420–425. https://doi.org/10.1016/j.anai.2012.09.005.
78. Cordeiro et al., "Barriers and Negative Nudges: Exploring Challenges in Food Journaling," *Proceedings of the SIGCHI Conference on Human Factors in Computing Systems* 2015 (2015): 1159–1162. https://doi.org/10.1145/2702123.2702155.
79. Valenta et al., "Food allergies: the basics," *Gastroenterology* 148, no. 6 (2015): 1120–31.e4. https://doi.org/10.1053/j.gastro.2015.02.006.
80. Burton et al., "Allergen-specific IgG antibody signaling through FcγRIIb promotes food tolerance," *The Journal of Allergy and Clinical Immunology* 141, no. 1 (2018): 189–201.e3. https://doi.org/10.1016/j.jaci.2017.03.045.
81. J. Gocki and Z. Bartuzi, "Role of immunoglobulin G antibodies in diagnosis of food allergy," *Postepy Dermatologii I Alergologii* 33, no. 4 (2016): 253–256. https://doi.org/10.5114/ada.2016.61600.
82. Bentz et al., "Clinical relevance of IgG antibodies against food antigens in Crohn's disease: a double-blind cross-over diet intervention study," *Digestion* 81, no. 4 (2010): 252–264. https://doi.org/10.1159/000264649.
83. Uzunısmaıl et al., "The effects of provocation by foods with raised IgG antibodies and additives on the course of Crohn's disease: a pilot study," *The Turkish Journal of Gastroenterology* 23, no. 1 (2012): 19–27. https://doi.org/10.4318/tjg.2012.0332.
84. Aydinlar et al., "IgG-based elimination diet in migraine plus irritable bowel syndrome," *Headache* 53, no. 3 (2013): 514–525. https://doi.org/10.1111/j.1526-4610.2012.02296.x.
85. Guo et al., "The value of eliminating foods according to food-specific immunoglobulin G antibodies in irritable bowel syndrome with diarrhoea," *The Journal of International Medical Research* 40, no. 1 (2012): 204–210. https://doi.org/10.1177/147323001204000121.
86. Gocki and Bartuzi, "Role of immunoglobulin G antibodies."
87. Gocki and Bartuzi, "Role of immunoglobulin G antibodies."
88. Vojdani, "Antibodies as predictors."
89. M. Carter, "Evaluating the Clinical Relevance of Food Sensitivity Tests: A Single-Subject Experiment," *Alternative Medicine Review* (blog), n.d., accessed July 29, 2022, https://altmedrev.com/blog/resource/evaluating-the-clinical-relevance-of-food-sensitivity-tests-a-single-subject-experiment/.
90. Sajadieh et al., "Increased heart rate and reduced heart-rate variability are associated with subclinical inflammation in middle-aged and elderly subjects with no apparent heart disease," *European Heart Journal* 25, no. 5 (2004): 363–370. https://doi.org/10.1016/j.ehj.2003.12.003.

91. Park et al., "Association between resting heart rate and inflammatory markers (white blood cell count and high-sensitivity C-reactive protein) in healthy Korean people," *Korean Journal of Family Medicine* 38, no. 1 (2017): 8–13. https://doi.org/10.4082/kjfm.2017.38.1.8.
92. Kim et al., "Stress and heart rate variability: a meta-analysis and review of the literature," *Psychiatry Investigation* 15, no. 3 (2018): 235–245. https://doi.org/10.30773/pi.2017.08.17.
93. S.-C. Fang, Y.-L. Wu, and P.-S. Tsai, "Heart rate variability and risk of all-cause death and cardiovascular events in patients with cardiovascular disease: a meta-analysis of cohort studies," *Biological Research for Nursing* 22, no. 1 (2020): 45–56. https://doi.org/10.1177/1099800419877442.
94. "Case study: The effects of diet on heart rate variability," *Elite HRV* (blog), n.d., accessed 29 July 2022, https://elitehrv.com/case-study-the-effects-of-diet-on-heart-rate-variability.

Chapter 32

1. de Zambotti et al., "The sleep of the ring: comparison of the ŌURA sleep tracker against polysomnography," *Behavioral Sleep Medicine* 17, no. 2 (2019): 124–136. https://doi.org/10.1080/15402002.2017.1300587.
2. A. B. Shreiner, J. Y. Kao, and V. B. Young, "The gut microbiome in health and in disease," *Current Opinion in Gastroenterology* 31, no. 1 (2015): 69–75. https://doi.org/10.1097/MOG.0000000000000139.
3. P. Chek, "Lessons from the toilet," *Chek Institute* (blog), accessed April 30, 2023, https://chekinstitute.com/blog/lessons-from-the-toilet/.
4. Salem et al., "The gut microbiome as a major regulator of the gut-skin axis," *Frontiers in Microbiology* 9 (2018): 1459. https://doi.org/10.3389/fmicb.2018.01459.
5. A. Pappas, "The relationship of diet and acne: A review," *Dermato-Endocrinology* 1, no. 5 (2009): 262–267. https://doi.org/10.4161/derm.1.5.10192.
6. Cooper et al., "Sleep deprivation and obesity in adults: a brief narrative review," *BMJ Open Sport & Exercise Medicine* 4, no. 1 (2018): e000392. https://doi.org/10.1136/bmjsem-2018-000392.
7. Chen et al., "Relationship between sleep and muscle strength among Chinese university students: a cross-sectional study," *Journal of Musculoskeletal & Neuronal Interactions* 17, no. 4 (2017): 327–333. https://www.ncbi.nlm.nih.gov/pubmed/29199194.
8. Cappuccio et al., "Sleep duration and all-cause mortality: a systematic review and meta-analysis of prospective studies," *Sleep* 33, no. 5 (2010): 585–592. https://doi.org/10.1093/sleep/33.5.585.
9. Lemstra et al., "Weight loss intervention adherence and factors promoting adherence: a meta-analysis," *Patient Preference and Adherence* 10 (2016): 1547–1559. https://doi.org/10.2147/PPA.S103649.

Chapter 33

1. N. Li, H.-Q. Huang, and G.-S. Zhang, "Association between SOD2 C47T polymorphism and lung cancer susceptibility: a meta-analysis," *Tumour Biology: The Journal of the International Society for Oncodevelopmental Biology and Medicine* 35, no. 2 (2014): 955–959. doi:10.1007/s13277-013-1127-y.
2. Saha et al., "An overview of Nrf2 signaling pathway and its role in inflammation," *Molecules* 25, no. 22 (2020). https://doi.org/10.3390/molecules25225474.
3. da Cruz Jung et al., "Superoxide imbalance triggered by Val16Ala-SOD2 polymorphism increases the risk of depression and self-reported psychological stress in free-living elderly people," *Molecular Genetics & Genomic Medicine* 8, no. 2 (2020): e1080. doi:10.1002/mgg3.1080.
4. Li, Huang, and Zhang, "Association between SOD2 C47T polymorphism and lung cancer susceptibility."
5. Wu et al., "Association of SOD2 p.V16A polymorphism with Parkinson's disease: A meta-analysis in Han Chinese," *Journal of the Formosan Medical Association = Taiwan Yi Zhi* 120, 1 Pt 2 (2021): 501–507. https://doi.org/10.1016/j.jfma.2020.06.023.
6. Flekac et al., "Gene polymorphisms of superoxide dismutases and catalase in diabetes mellitus," *BMC Medical Genetics* 9 (2008): 30. https://doi.org/10.1186/1471-2350-9-30.
7. P. Talalay and A. T. Dinkova-Kostova, "Role of nicotinamide quinone oxidoreductase 1 (NQO1) in protection against toxicity of electrophiles and reactive oxygen intermediates," *Methods in Enzymology* 382 (2004): 355–364. https://doi.org/10.1016/S0076-6879(04)82019-6.
8. Tan et al., "Thyroid function and the risk of Alzheimer disease: the Framingham Study," *Archives of Internal Medicine* 168, no. 14 (2008): 1514–1520. https://doi.org/10.1001/archinte.168.14.1514.
9. D. Ross and D. Siegel, "Functions of NQO1 in cellular protection and CoQ10 metabolism and its potential role as a redox sensitive molecular switch," *Frontiers in Physiology* 8 (2017): 595. https://doi.org/10.3389/fphys.2017.00595.
10. Razavi et al., "Associations between high density lipoprotein mean particle size and serum paraoxonase-1 activity," *Journal of Research in Medical Sciences: The Official Journal of Isfahan University of Medical Sciences* 17 no. 11 (2012): 1020–1026. https://www.ncbi.nlm.nih.gov/pmc/articles/PMC3702082/.
11. Rasic-Milutinovic et al., "Lower serum paraoxonase-1 activity is related to linoleic and docosahexanoic fatty acids in type 2 diabetic patients," *Archives of Medical Research* 43, no. 1 (2012): 75–82. https://doi.org/10.1016/j.arcmed.2011.12.008.
12. de Oliveira et al., "Genetic polymorphisms in glutathione (GSH-) related genes affect the plasmatic Hg/whole blood Hg partitioning and the distribution between inorganic and methylmercury levels in plasma collected from a fish-eating population," *BioMed Research International* (2014): 940952. https://doi.org/10.1155/2014/940952.
13. Guessous et al., "Caffeine intake and CYP1A2 variants associated with high caffeine intake protect non-smokers from hypertension," *Human Molecular Genetics* 21, no. 14 (2012): 3283–3292. https://doi.org/10.1093/hmg/dds137.
14. A. Gunes and M.-L. Dahl, "Variation in CYP1A2 activity and its clinical implications: influence of environmental factors and genetic polymorphisms," *Pharmacogenomics* 9, no. 5 (2008): 625–637. https://doi.org/10.2217/14622416.9.5.625.
15. C. Köhle and K. W. Bock, "Activation of coupled Ah receptor and Nrf2 gene batteries by dietary phytochemicals in relation to chemoprevention," *Biochemical Pharmacology* 72, no. 7 (2006): 795–805. https://doi.org/10.1016/j.bcp.2006.04.017.

16. D. W. Al-Sadeq and G. K. Nasrallah, "The spectrum of mutations of homocystinuria in the MENA region," *Genes* 11, no. 3 (2020). https://doi.org/10.3390/genes11030330.
17. Said et al., "A common mutation in the CBS gene explains a high incidence of homocystinuria in the Qatari population," *Human Mutation* 27, no. 7 (2006): 719. https://doi.org/10.1002/humu.9436.
18. A. Fasano. "Zonulin and its regulation of intestinal barrier function: the biological door to inflammation, autoimmunity, and cancer," *Physiological Reviews* 91, no. 1 (2011): 151–175. https://doi.org/10.1152/physrev.00003.2008.
19. Sapone et al., "Spectrum of gluten-related disorders: consensus on new nomenclature and classification," *BMC Medicine* 10 (2012): 13. https://doi.org/10.1186/1741-7015-10-13.
20. "Celiac Disease Tests," National Institute of Diabetes and Digestive and Kidney Diseases, last modified February 2021, https://www.niddk.nih.gov/health-information/professionals/clinical-tools-patient-management/digestive-diseases/celiac-disease-health-care-professionals.
21. Grondin et al., "Mucins in intestinal mucosal defense and inflammation: learning from clinical and experimental studies," *Frontiers in Immunology* 11 (2020): 2054. https://doi.org/10.3389/fimmu.2020.02054.
22. Gorecki et al., "Single nucleotide polymorphisms associated with gut homeostasis influence risk and age-at-onset of Parkinson's disease," *Frontiers in Aging Neuroscience* 12 (2020): 603849. https://doi.org/10.3389/fnagi.2020.603849.
23. Prager et al., "Myosin IXb variants and their pivotal role in maintaining the intestinal barrier: a study in Crohn's disease," *Scandinavian Journal of Gastroenterology* 49, no. 10 (2014): 1191–1200. https://doi.org/10.3109/00365521.2014.928903.
24. Wolters et al., "The MYO9B gene is a strong risk factor for developing refractory celiac disease," *Clinical Gastroenterology and Hepatology: The Official Clinical Practice Journal of the American Gastroenterological Association* 5, no. 12 (2007): 1399–1405, 1405.e1–e2. https://doi.org/10.1016/j.cgh.2007.08.018.
25. S. C. Corr and L. A. J. O'Neill, "Genetic variation in Toll-like receptor signalling and the risk of inflammatory and immune diseases," *Journal of Innate Immunity* 1, no. 4 (2009): 350–357. https://doi.org/10.1159/000200774.
26. S. Moossavi, "Gliadin is an uncatalogued Toll-like receptor ligand," *Journal of Medical Hypotheses and Ideas* 8, no. 1 (2014): 44–47. https://doi.org/10.1016/j.jmhi.2013.09.001.
27. R. Ricci-Acevedo, M.-C. Roque-Barreira, and N. J. Gay, "Targeting and recognition of toll-like receptors by plant and pathogen lectins," *Frontiers in Immunology* 8 (2017): 1820. https://doi.org/10.3389/fimmu.2017.01820.
28. Söderman et al., "Analysis of single nucleotide polymorphisms in the region of CLDN2-MORC4 in relation to inflammatory bowel disease," *World Journal of Gastroenterology* 19, no. 30 (2013): 4935–4943. https://doi.org/10.3748/wjg.v19.i30.4935.
29. Liu et al., "The role of MUC2 mucin in intestinal homeostasis and the impact of dietary components on MUC2 expression," *International Journal of Biological Macromolecules* 164 (2020): 884–891. https://doi.org/10.1016/j.ijbiomac.2020.07.191.
30. Y. S. Kim and S. B. Ho, "Intestinal goblet cells and mucins in health and disease: recent insights and progress," *Current Gastroenterology Report* 12, no. 5 (2010): 319–330. https://doi.org/10.1007/s11894-010-0131-2.
31. Moehle et al., "Aberrant intestinal expression and allelic variants of mucin genes associated with inflammatory bowel disease," *Journal of Molecular Medicine (Berlin)* 84, no. 12 (2006): 1055–1066. https://doi.org/10.1007/s00109-006-0100-2.
32. Z. Xie and J. Yin, "FOXP3 is associated with food-induced anaphylaxis," *Journal of Allergy and Clinical Immunology* 143, no. 2 (2019): Supplement. https://doi.org/10.1016/j.jaci.2018.12.4.
33. Krogulska et al., "Decreased FOXP3 mRNA expression in children with atopic asthma and IgE-mediated food allergy," *Annals of Allergy, Asthma & Immunology* 115, no. 5 (2015): 415–421. https://doi.org/10.1016/j.anai.2015.08.015.
34. Xie and Yin, "FOXP3 is associated with food-induced anaphylaxis."
35. M. Camilleri, "The leaky gut: mechanisms, measurement and clinical implications in humans," *Gut* 68, no. 8 (2019): 1516–1526. https://doi.org/10.1136/gutjnl-2019-318427.
36. Fabisiak et al., "Targeting histamine receptors in irritable bowel syndrome: a critical appraisal," *Journal of Neurogastroenterology and Motility* 23, no. 3 (2017): 341–348. https://doi.org/10.5056/jnm16203.
37. Szczepankiewicz et al., "Polymorphisms of two histamine-metabolizing enzymes genes and childhood allergic asthma: a case control study," *Clinical and Molecular Allergy* 8 (2010): 14. https://doi.org/10.1186/1476-7961-8-14.
38. W. J. Schnedl and D. Enko, "Histamine intolerance originates in the gut," *Nutrients* 13, no. 4 (2021): 1262. https://doi.org/10.3390/nu13041262.
39. Ayuso et al., "Genetic variability of human diamine oxidase: occurrence of three nonsynonymous polymorphisms and study of their effect on serum enzyme activity," *Pharmacogenetics and Genomics* 17, no. 9 (2007): 687–693. https://doi.org/10.1097/FPC.0b013e328012b8e4.
40. Kennedy et al., "Association of the histamine N-methyltransferase C314T (Thr105Ile) polymorphism with atopic dermatitis in Caucasian children," *Pharmacotherapy* 28, no. 12 (2008): 1495–1501. https://doi.org/10.1592/phco.28.12.1495.
41. Heidari et al., "Mutations in the histamine N-methyltransferase gene, HNMT, are associated with nonsyndromic autosomal recessive intellectual disability," *Human Molecular Genetics* 24, no. 20 (2015): 5697–5710. https://doi.org/10.1093/hmg/ddv286.
42. R. W. Schayer, "The metabolism of histamine in various species," *British Journal of Pharmacology and Chemotherapy* 11, no. 4 (1956): 472–473. https://doi.org/10.1111/j.1476-5381.1956.tb00020.x.
43. T. Wang, J. Yin, A. H. Miller, and C. Xiao, "A systematic review of the association between fatigue and genetic polymorphisms," *Brain, Behavior, and Immunity* 62 (2017): 230–244. https://doi.org/10.1016/j.bbi.2017.01.007.
44. A. Karmakar et al., "Monoamine oxidase B gene variants associated with attention deficit hyperactivity disorder in the Indo-Caucasoid population from West Bengal," *BMC Genetics* 17, no. 1 (2016): 92. https://doi.org/10.1186/s12863-016-0401-6.
45. S. E. Bergen et al., "Polymorphisms in SLC6A4, PAH, GABRB3, and MAOB and modification of psychotic disorder features," *Schizophrenia Research* 109, no. 1–3 (2009): 94–97. https://doi.org/10.1016/j.schres.2009.02.009.
46. C. B. Do et al., "Web-based genome-wide association study identifies two novel loci and a substantial genetic component for Parkinson's disease," *PLoS Genetics* 7, no. 6 (2011): e1002141. https://doi.org/10.1371/journal.pgen.1002141.
47. J. L. Royo et al., "Monoamino oxidase alleles correlate with the presence of essential hypertension among hypogonadic patients," *Molecular Genetics & Genomic Medicine* 8, no. 1 (2020): e1040. https://doi.org/10.1002/mgg3.1040.

48. Massa et al., "The endogenous cannabinoid system protects against colonic inflammation," *Journal of Clinical Investigation* 113, no. 8 (2004): 1202–1209. https://doi.org/10.1172/JCI19465.

49. Beins et al., "Cannabinoid receptor 1 signalling modulates stress susceptibility and microglial responses to chronic social defeat stress," *Translational Psychiatry* 11, no. 1 (2021): 164. https://doi.org/10.1038/s41398-021-01283-0.

50. Joslin et al., "Association of the lactase persistence haplotype block with disease risk in populations of European descent," *Frontiers in Genetics* 11 (2020). https://doi.org/10.3389/fgene.2020.558762.

51. B. Grygiel-Górniak, "Peroxisome proliferator-activated receptors and their ligands: nutritional and clinical implications—a review," *Nutrition Journal* 13, no. 17 (2014). https://doi.org/10.1186/1475-2891-13-17.

52. van Raalte et al., "Peroxisome proliferator-activated receptor (PPAR)-alpha: a pharmacological target with a promising future," *Pharmaceutical Research* 21, no. 9 (2004): 1531–1538. https://doi.org/10.1023/b:pham.0000041444.06122.8d. PMID: 15497675.

53. I. I. Ahmetov and O. N. Fedotovskaya, "Chapter Six—Current progress in sports genomics," *Advances in Clinical Chemistry* 70 (2015): 247–314. https://doi.org/10.1016/bs.acc.2015.03.003.

54. Sarhangi et al., "PPARG (Pro12Ala) genetic variant and risk of T2DM: a systematic review and meta-analysis," *Scientific Reports* 10 (2020): 12764. https://doi.org/10.1038/s41598-020-69363-7.

55. Florez et al., "Effects of the type 2 diabetes-associated PPARG P12A polymorphism on progression to diabetes and response to troglitazone," *The Journal of Clinical Endocrinology & Metabolism* 92, no. 4 (2007): 1502–1509. https://doi.org/10.1210/jc.2006-2275.

56. Malalla et al., "Sequence analysis and variant identification at the APOC3 gene locus indicates association of rs5218 with BMI in a sample of Kuwaiti's," *Lipids in Health Disease* 18, no. 1 (2019): 224. https://doi.org/10.1186/s12944-019-1165-6.

57. M. Hassan, "Triglycerides do matter," *Global Cardiology Science & Practice* 2014, no. 4 (2014): 241–244. https://doi.org/10.5339/gcsp.2014.38.

58. A. D. Marais, "Familial hypercholesterolaemia," *Clinical Biochemist Reviews* 25, no. 1 (2004): 49–68. https://www.ncbi.nlm.nih.gov/pmc/articles/PMC1853359/.

59. O. García-Minguillán and C. Maestú, "30 Hz, could it be part of a window frequency for cellular response?" *International Journal of Molecular Sciences* 22, no. 7 (2021): 3642. https://doi.org/10.3390/ijms22073642.

60. J. Volavka, R. Bilder, and K. Nolan, "Catecholamines and aggression: the role of COMT and MAO polymorphisms," *Annals of the New York Academy of Sciences* 1036 (2004): 393–398. https://doi.org/10.1196/annals.1330.023.

61. P. Borel and C. Desmarchelier, "Genetic variations associated with vitamin A status and vitamin A bioavailability," *Nutrients* 9, no. 3 (2017): 246. https://doi.org/10.3390/nu9030246.

62. Leung et al., "Two common single nucleotide polymorphisms in the gene encoding beta-carotene 15,15′-monoxygenase alter beta-carotene metabolism in female volunteers," *FASEB Journal* 23, no. 4 (2009): 1041–1053. https://doi.org/10.1096/fj.08-121962.

63. Barry et al., "Genetic variants in CYP2R1, CYP24A1, and VDR modify the efficacy of vitamin D3 supplementation for increasing serum 25-hydroxyvitamin D levels in a randomized controlled trial," *Journal of Clinical Endocrinology and Metabolism* 99, no. 10 (2014): e2133–e2137. https://doi.org/10.1210/jc.2014-1389.

64. Cheng et al., "Genetic evidence that the human CYP2R1 enzyme is a key vitamin D 25-hydroxylase," *PNAS* 101, no. 20 (2004): 7711–7715. https://doi.org/10.1073/pnas.0402490101.

65. M. Qian, X. Fang, and X. Wang, " Autophagy and inflammation," *Clinical and Translational Medicine* 6, no. 1 (2017): 24. https://doi.org/10.1186/s40169-017-0154-5.

66. Phillips et al., "Gene-nutrient interactions with dietary fat modulate the association between genetic variation of the ACSL1 gene and metabolic syndrome," *Journal of Lipid Research* 51, no. 7 (2010): 1793–1800. https://doi.org/10.1194/jlr.M003046.

67. Guo et al., "Association between adiponectin polymorphisms and the risk of colorectal cancer," *Genetic Testing and Molecular Biomarkers* 19, no. 1 (2015): 9–13. https://doi.org/10.1089/gtmb.2014.0238.

68. Cui et al., "Association between adiponectin gene polymorphism and environmental risk factors of type 2 diabetes mellitus among the Chinese population in Hohhot," *BioMed Research International* 2020: Article ID 6383906. https://doi.org/10.1155/2020/6383906.

69. Benedict et al., "Fat mass and obesity-associated gene (FTO) is linked to higher plasma levels of the hunger hormone ghrelin and lower serum levels of the satiety hormone leptin in older adults," *Diabetes* 63, no. 11 (2014): 3955–3959. https://doi.org/10.2337/db14-0470.

70. Fang et al., "Variant rs9939609 in the FTO gene is associated with body mass index among Chinese children," *BMC Medical Genetics* 22, no. 11 (2010): 136. https://doi.org/10.1186/1471-2350-11-136.

71. Al-Bustan et al., "Genetic association of LPL rs1121923 and rs258 with plasma TG and VLDL levels," *Scientific Reports* 9, no. 1 (2019): 5572. https://doi.org/10.1038/s41598-019-42021-3.

72. Kelishadi et al., "Relationship of lipoprotein lipase gene variants & fasting triglyceride levels in a pediatric population: The CASPIAN-III study," *Advances in Clinical and Experimental Medicine* 26, no. 1 (2017): 77–82. https://doi.org/10.17219/acem/61003.

73. Malalla et al., "Sequence analysis and variant identification at the APOC3 gene."

74. Hassan, "Triglycerides do matter."

75. Corella et al., "Association between the APOA2 promoter polymorphism and body weight in Mediterranean and Asian populations: replication of a gene-saturated fat interaction," *International Journal of Obesity* 35, no. 5 (2011): 666–675. https://doi.org/10.1038/ijo.2010.187.

76. Domínguez-Reyes et al., "Interaction of dietary fat intake with APOA2, APOA5 and LEPR polymorphisms and its relationship with obesity and dyslipidemia in young subjects," *Lipids in Health and Disease* 14, no. 106 (2015). https://doi.org/10.1186/s12944-015-0112-4.

77. Bougarne et al., "Molecular actions of PPARα in lipid metabolism and inflammation," *Endocrine Reviews* 39, no. 5 (2018): 760–802. https://doi.org/10.1210/er.2018-00064.

78. B. Grygiel-Górniak, "Peroxisome proliferator-activated receptors."

79. Marais, "Familial hypercholesterolaemia."

80. Rajakumar et al., "Carnitine palmitoyltransferase IA polymorphism P479L is common in Greenland Inuit and is associated with elevated plasma apolipoprotein A-I," *Journal of Lipid Research* 50, no. 6 (2009): 1223–1228. https://doi.org/10.1194/jlr.P900001-JLR200.

81. D. Shin and K. W. Lee, "Dietary carbohydrates interact with AMY1 polymorphisms to influence the incidence of type 2 diabetes in Korean adults," *Scientific Reports* 11 (2021): 16788. https://doi.org/10.1038/s41598-021-96257-z.

82. Leung et al., "Two common single nucleotide polymorphisms."

83. Friedrich et al., "Several different lactase persistence associated alleles and high diversity of the lactase gene in the admixed Brazilian population," *PLoS One* 7, no. 9 (2012): e46520. https://doi.org/10.1371/journal.pone.0046520.

84. Hazra et al., "Common variants of FUT2 are associated with plasma vitamin B12 levels," *Nature Genetics* 40, no. 10 (2008): 1160–1162. https://doi.org/10.1038/ng.210.

85. Giampaoli et al., "Can the FUT2 non-secretor phenotype associated with gut microbiota increase the children susceptibility for type 1 diabetes? A mini review," *Frontiers in Nutrition* 7 (2020): 606171. https://doi.org/10.3389/fnut.2020.606171.

86. R. A. Mathias, V. Pani, and F. H. Chilton, "Genetic variants in the FADS gene: Implications for dietary recommendations for fatty acid intake," *Current Nutrition Reports* 3, no. 2 (2014): 139–148. https://doi.org/10.1007/s13668-014-0079-1..

87. C. Glaser, J. Heinrich, and B. Koletzko, "Role of FADS1 and FADS2 polymorphisms in polyunsaturated fatty acid metabolism," *Metabolism* 59, no. 7 (2010): 993–999. https://doi.org/10.1016/j.metabol.2009.10.022.

88. Lattka et al., "Do FADS genotypes enhance our knowledge about fatty acid related phenotypes?" *Clinical Nutrition* 29, no. 3 (2010): 277–287. https://doi.org/10.1016/j.clnu.2009.11.005.

89. Ivanov et al., "Genetic variants in phosphatidylethanolamine N-methyltransferase and methylenetetrahydrofolate dehydrogenase influence biomarkers of choline metabolism when folate intake is restricted," *Journal of the Academy of Nutrition and Dietetics* 109, no. 2 (2009): 313–318. https://doi.org/10.1016/j.jada.2008.10.046.

90. A. B. Ganz, K. C. Klatt, and M. A. Caudill, "Common genetic variants alter metabolism and influence dietary choline requirements," *Nutrients* 9, no. 8 (2017): 837. https://doi.org/10.3390/nu9080837.

91. H. V. Thomas, G. K. Davey, and T. J. Key, "Oestradiol and sex hormone-binding globulin in premenopausal and post-menopausal meat-eaters, vegetarians and vegans," *British Journal of Cancer* 80, no. 9 (1999): 1470–1475. https://doi.org/10.1038/sj.bjc.6690546.

92. Barnard et al., "Diet and sex-hormone binding globulin, dysmenorrhea, and premenstrual symptoms," *Obstetrics & Gynecology* 95, no. 2 (2000): 245–250. https://doi.org/10.1016/s0029-7844(99)00525-6.

93. Low et al., "Implications of gene-environment interaction in studies of gene variants in breast cancer: an example of dietary isoflavones and the D356N polymorphism in the sex hormone-binding globulin gene," *Cancer Research* 66, no. 18 (2006): 8980–8983. https://doi.org/10.1158/0008-5472.CAN-06-2432.

94. Garaulet et al., "CLOCK gene is implicated in weight reduction in obese patients participating in a dietary programme based on the Mediterranean diet," *International Journal of Obesity* 34, no. 3 (2010): 516–523. https://doi.org/10.1038/ijo.2009.255.

95. Huang et al., "Dietary protein modifies the effect of the MC4R genotype on 2-year changes in appetite and food craving: The POUNDS Lost Trial," *Journal of Nutrition* 147, no. 3 (2017): 439–444. https://doi.org/10.3945/jn.116.242958.

96. R. B. Vega, J. M. Huss, and D. P. Kelly, "The coactivator PGC-1 cooperates with peroxisome proliferator-activated receptor alpha in transcriptional control of nuclear genes encoding mitochondrial fatty acid oxidation enzymes," *Molecular and Cellular Biology* 20, no. 5 (2000): 1868–1876. https://doi.org/10.1128/MCB.20.5.1868-1876.2000.

97. Steinbacher et al., "The Single Nucleotide Polymorphism Gly482Ser in the PGC-1α Gene Impairs Exercise-Induced Slow-Twitch Muscle Fibre Transformation in Humans," *PLoS ONE* 10, no. 4 (2015): e0123881. https://doi.org/10.1371/journal.pone.0123881.

98. Vargas-Mendoza et al., "Antioxidant and adaptative response mediated by Nrf2 during physical exercise," *Antioxidants* (Basel) 8, no. 6 (2019): 196. https://doi.org/10.3390/antiox8060196.

99. B. M. Spiegelman, "Transcriptional control of mitochondrial energy metabolism through the PGC1 coactivators," *Novartis Foundation Symposium* 287 (2007): 60–63; discussion 63-69. https://pubmed.ncbi.nlm.nih.gov/18074631/.

100. He et al., "NRF2 genotype improves endurance capacity in response to training," *International Journal of Sports Medicine* 28, no. 9 (2007): 717–721. https://doi.org/10.1055/s-2007-964913.

101. Eynon et al., "Interaction between SNPs in the NRF2 gene and elite endurance performance," *Physiological Genomics* 41, no. 1 (2010): 78–81. https://doi.org/10.1152/physiolgenomics.00199.2009.

102. Trapé et al., "NOS3 Polymorphisms can influence the effect of multicomponent training on blood pressure, nitrite concentration and physical fitness in prehypertensive and hypertensive older adult women," *Frontiers in Physiology* 12 (2021). https://doi.org/10.3389/fphys.2021.566023.

103. Zmijewski et al., "The NOS3 G894T (rs1799983) and -786T/C (rs2070744) polymorphisms are associated with elite swimmer status," *Biology of Sport* 35, no. 4 (2018): 313–319. https://doi.org/10.5114/biolsport.2018.76528.

104. Leońska-Duniec et al., "The polymorphisms of the PPARD gene modify post-training body mass and biochemical parameter changes in women," *PLoS ONE* 13, no. 8 (2018): e0202557. https://doi.org/10.1371/journal.pone.0202557.

105. Cupeiro et al., "MCT1 genetic polymorphism influence in high intensity circuit training: A pilot study," *Journal of Science and Medicine in Sport* 13, no. 5 (2010): 526–530. https://doi.org/10.1016/j.jsams.2009.07.004.

106. Pereira et al., "Interaction between cytokine gene polymorphisms and the effect of physical exercise on clinical and inflammatory parameters in older women: study protocol for a randomized controlled trial," *Trials* 13, no. 134 (2012). https://doi.org/10.1186/1745-6215-13-134.

107. Yamin et al., "IL6 (-174) and TNFA (-308) promoter polymorphisms are associated with systemic creatine kinase response to eccentric exercise," *European Journal of Applied Physiology* 104, no. 3 (2008): 579–586. https://doi.org/10.1007/s00421-008-0728-4.

108. P. Valdivieso et al., "The metabolic response of skeletal muscle to endurance exercise is modified by the ACE-I/D gene polymorphism and training state," *Frontiers in Physiology* 8 (2017): 993. https://doi.org/10.3389/fphys.2017.00993.

109. C. Pickering and J. Kiely, "ACTN3: More than just a gene for speed," *Frontiers in Physiology* 8 (2017). https://doi.org/10.3389/fphys.2017.01080.

110. Eynon et al., "The ACTN3 R577X polymorphism across three groups of elite male European athletes," *PLoS One* 7, no. 8 (2012): e43132. https://doi.org/10.1371/journal.pone.0043132.

111. Moore et al., "Obesity gene variant and elite endurance performance," *Metabolism* 50, no. 12 (2001): 1391–1392. https://doi.org/10.1053/meta.2001.28140.
112. V. Sarpeshkar and D. Bentley, "Adrenergic-β2 receptor polymorphism and athletic performance," *Journal of Human Genetics* 55 (2010): 479–485. https://doi.org/10.1038/jhg.2010.42.
113. Moore et al., "Obesity gene variant."
114. Dhamrait et al., "Variation in the uncoupling protein 2 and 3 genes and human performance," *Journal of Applied Physiology* 112, no. 7 (2012): 1122–1127. https://doi.org/10.1152/japplphysiol.00766.2011.
115. Krasniqi et al., "Association between polymorphisms in vitamin D pathway-related genes, vitamin D status, muscle mass and function: a systematic review," *Nutrients* 13, no. 9 (2021): 3109. https://doi.org/10.3390/nu13093109.
116. G. D. Abrams, D. Feldman, and M. R. Safran, "Effects of vitamin D on skeletal muscle and athletic performance," *Journal of the American Academy of Orthopaedic Surgeons* 26, no. 8 (2018): 278–285. https://sogacot.org/effects-of-vitamin-d-on-skeletal-muscle-and-athletic-performance/.
117. Gomez-Gallego et al., "The C allele of the AGT Met235Thr polymorphism is associated with power sports performance," *Applied Physiology, Nutrition, and Metabolism* 34, no. 6 (2009): 1108–1111. https://doi.org/10.1139/H09-108.
118. Stepien-Slodkowska et al., "Is the combination of COL1A1 gene polymorphisms a marker of injury risk?" *Journal of Sport Rehabilitation* 26, no. 3 (2017): 234–238. https://doi.org/10.1123/jsr.2015-0151.
119. Stepien-Slodkowska et al., "Is the combination of COL1A1 gene polymorphisms a marker of injury risk?"
120. López-Otín et al., "The hallmarks of aging," *Cell* 153, no. 6 (2013): 1194–1217. https://doi.org/10.1016/j.cell.2013.05.039.
121. H. W. Virgin and B. Levine, "Autophagy genes in immunity," *Nature Immunology* 10, no. 5 (2009): 461–470. https://doi.org/10.1038/ni.1726.
122. Virgin and Levine, "Autophagy genes in immunity."
123. Alam et al., "Relationship of nutrigenomics and aging: Involvement of DNA methylation," *Journal of Nutrition & Intermediary Metabolism* 16 (2019): 100098. https://doi.org/10.1016/j.jnim.2019.100098.
124. Philibert et al., "Methylation array data can simultaneously identify individuals and convey protected health information: an unrecognized ethical concern," *Clinical Epigenetics* 6, 28 (2014). https://doi.org/10.1186/1868-7083-6-28.
125. Philibert et al., "Methylation array data."

Chapter 34

1. Qin et al., "A human gut microbial gene catalogue established by metagenomic sequencing," *Nature* 464, no. 7285 (2010): 59–65. https://doi.org/10.1038/nature08821.
2. A. Moosavi and A. Motevalizadeh Ardekani, "Role of epigenetics in biology and human diseases," *Iranian Biomedical Journal* 20, no. 5 (2016): 246–258. https://doi.org/10.22045/ibj.2016.01.
3. C. Gustafson, "Bruce Lipton, PhD: The jump from cell culture to consciousness," *Integrative Medicine (Encinitas)* 16, no. 6 (2017): 44–50. https://www.ncbi.nlm.nih.gov/pmc/articles/PMC6438088/.
4. Youssef et al., "The effects of trauma, with or without PTSD, on the transgenerational DNA methylation alterations in human offsprings," *Brain Sciences* 8, no. 5 (2018): 83. https://doi.org/10.3390/brainsci8050083.
5. Sarkar et al., "Histone deacetylase inhibitors reverse CpG methylation by regulating DNMT1 through ERK signaling," *Anticancer Research* 31, no. 9 (2011): 2723–2732. https://pubmed.ncbi.nlm.nih.gov/21868513/.
6. Y. Silva, A. Bernardi, and R. L. Frozza, "The role of short-chain fatty acids from gut microbiota in gut-brain communication," *Frontiers in Endocrinology* 11 (2020). https://doi.org/10.3389/fendo.2020.00025.
7. K. R. Pandey, S. R. Naik, and B. V. Vakil, "Probiotics, prebiotics and synbiotics—a review," *Journal of Food Science and Technology* 52, no. 12 (2015): 7577–7587. https://doi.org/10.1007/s13197-015-1921-1.
8. Li et al., "Prenatal epigenetics diets play protective roles against environmental pollution," *Clinical Epigenetics* 11, no. 82 (2019). https://doi.org/10.1186/s13148-019-0659-4.
9. Klein et al., "Vitamin E and the risk of prostate cancer: The Selenium and Vitamin E Cancer Prevention Trial (SELECT)," *JAMA* 306, no. 14 (2011): 1549–1556. https://doi.org/10.1001/jama.2011.1437.
10. Pieroth et al., "Folate and its impact on cancer risk," *Current Nutrition Reports* 7, no. 3 (2018): 70–84. https://doi.org/10.1007/s13668-018-0237-y.
11. R. C. Painter, T. J. Roseboom, and O. P. Bleker, "Prenatal exposure to the Dutch famine and disease in later life: an overview," *Reproductive Toxicology* 20, no. 3 (2005): 345–352. https://doi.org/10.1016/j.reprotox.2005.04.005.
12. Tobi et al., "DNA methylation as a mediator of the association between prenatal adversity and risk factors for metabolic disease in adulthood," *Science Advances* 4, no. 1 (2018). https://doi.org/10.1126/sciadv.aao4364.
13. Han et al., "Maternal low-protein diet up-regulates the neuropeptide Y system in visceral fat and leads to abdominal obesity and glucose intolerance in a sex-and time-specific manner," *FASEB Journal* 26, no. 8 (2012): 3528–3536. https://doi.org/10.1096/fj.12-203943.
14. Glastras et al., "Maternal obesity increases the risk of metabolic disease and impacts renal health in offspring," *Bioscience Reports* 38, no. 2 (2018): BSR20180050. https://doi.org/10.1042/BSR20180050.

INDEX

A

B

C

D

E

F

G

M

R

S

T

U

V

W

Y

Z

ACKNOWLEDGMENTS

This book has been a Herculean effort and would not have been possible without the help of many people, including our parents, Normand, Yolande, Gary and Nancy, Dr. Nattha Wannisorn, Ph.D., Monia Advić, Katrine Volynsky, Tony Flores, Nina Ricci, Sophie Nethery, Quentin Matheson, Hay House, Todd Herman, Scott Hoffman, Steve Troha, our entire BioLab research team and BIOptimizers.

Also this book could never have been written without the influence of our mentors and coaches, including: Scott Abel, Kevin Weiss, Arnold Schwarzenegger, Tom Platz, Dr. David Hawkins, Dawson Church, Layne Norton, Paramahansa Yogananda, Sri Yukteswar, Dr. Mauro DiPasquale, Dr. Dom D'Agostino, Leo Costa Jr., Dr. Michael O'Brien, Dr. Edward Howell, Ben Pakulski, Sebastian Junger, Charles Poliquin, Dr. Steven Read, Alandra Napali Kai, Clayten Stedmann, David Hall, Paul Chek, Dorian Yates, Bill Pearl, Stu Mittleman, Dr. Cory Holly, Dr. Michael Colgan, Dr. Udo Erasamus, Paul and Patricia Bragg, countless clients, colleagues, and all of the researchers that are working to find the truths about health and nutrition.

And last, but certainly not least, we want to acknowledge YOU for trusting us with your health. We want to acknowledge you for being on the path and wanting to learn, grow and evolve. Now that you are equipped with new paradigms, go into the world and spread the message. Help others awaken to the power of BIOptimized health.

ABOUT THE AUTHORS

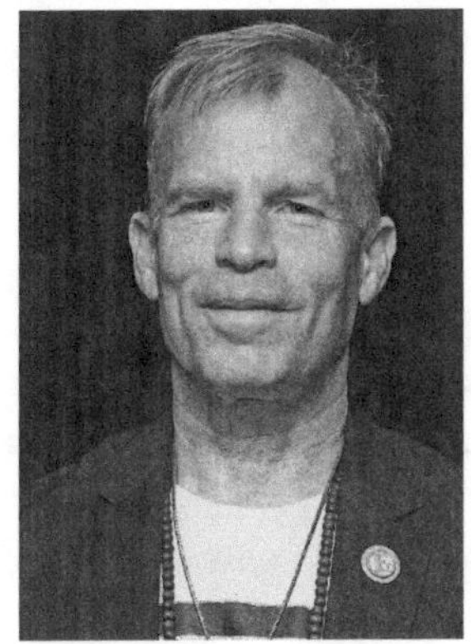

WADE T. LIGHTHEART

Just over 25 years ago, after more than a decade of dieting and training, I won several bodybuilding titles and built a reputation as someone who was always ripped. I captured my first two bodybuilding titles in 1997 at age 25. Despite this early success, I retired after the 1998 National Canadian Championships due to growing concerns regarding rampant drug use and extreme dieting in the sport. Over the next four years, I went from being a hard-partying and meat-consuming bodybuilder to living a drug- and alcohol-free vegetarian lifestyle. I began a practice of daily meditation and built a successful personal training business in Vancouver, B.C., the "fitness Capital of Canada." My client base was the talk of the local gym I trained at in Kitsilano, the most body-conscious neighborhood in one of the fittest cities in the world. I took on dozens of clients from every walk of life: a hairstylist, a banker, flight attendants, fitness competitors, models, cheerleaders, up-and-coming singers and actors, realtors, computer programmers, doctors, brokers, a few members of a notorious bike gang, people of all sexual persuasions, old, young, and everything in between.

These were fun times wherein I began to learn about different bodies, diet strategies, and the psychology and physiology of physiques in every shape and size. Many of my deepest friendships and greatest learning experiences grew from these client relationships. I consider myself extremely fortunate to have had so many people trust me with one of the deepest and most personal issues people struggle with their entire lives: maintaining a healthy and aesthetically pleasing body. A body that looks good, feels amazing, and can sustain high performance in a complex, fast-moving world.

In 2002, defying conventional bodybuilding theory, I returned to competitive bodybuilding as a drug-free vegetarian, captured my first Canadian National title, and competed at the IFBB Mr. Universe. Despite this triumph, in 2004 I retired from competition again, citing major digestive issues following the IFBB Mr. Universe. After learning about enzymes and probiotics from Dr. Michael O'Brien, I corrected my digestive issues and returned to competition in 2007, capturing two more Canadian National titles, and going on to compete at the INBA Natural Olympia.

Renewed with a deep desire to help others live a healthy and high-performance lifestyle, Matt Gallant and I co-founded BIOptimizers in 2004, with a mission to end physical suffering by moving people from sick to superhuman. Over the past 20 years, Matt and I have helped over 250,000 people across the world live healthier lives. We've co-authored several books and fitness programs, including *Freaky Big Naturally, Elite Exercise Performance, The Complete Physique Muscle Mastery System*, and *From Sick to Superhuman: The Ultimate Biological Optimization Blueprint.* I also wrote *Hydration Breakthrough for Athletes, Vital Power, Staying Alive in a Toxic World, The Wealthy Backpacker*, and the *84 Days Awesome Health Course*. In 2007, I began touring the globe as an international health and motivational speaker.

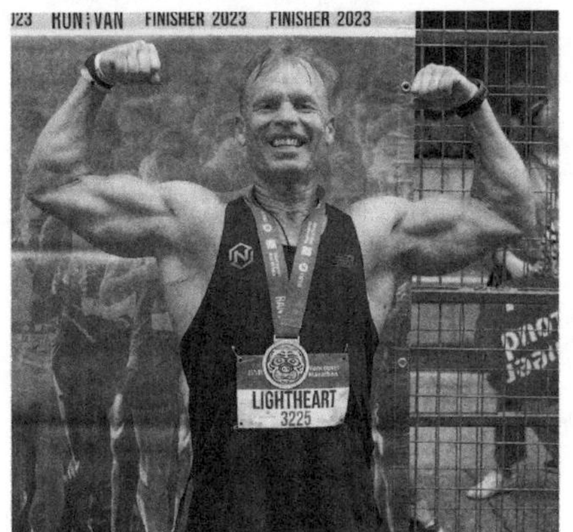

In 2022, at the age of 50, I returned to competitive bodybuilding and won the Open Men's and Grand Master's Categories at the INBA Ironman International, qualifying me as a professional bodybuilder. Four months later, I competed at the PNBA Natural Olympia. Immediately following that contest, I once again defied conventional bodybuilding philosophy by taking up endurance running. Six months later, I successfully ran my first marathon in four hours.

Now, here's the shocking part: Matt and I follow almost completely different strategies to maintain lean, healthy bodies. For years we engaged in spirited shouting debates with each other in the gym and over meals . . . arguing and citing research from the smartest code crackers in the world of diet and fitness. Matt is a keto advocate, which has produced amazing results for him and most of his clients. I am a dedicated plant-based eater, which has helped me and many of my clients stay ripped over the years. Between the two of us, we have tried almost every single dietary strategy: keto, paleo, vegan, vegetarian, carnivore, zone, time-restricted eating, fasting, feasting, raw food dieting, and virtually every variation of those. We've seen dozens of diet trends and fads come and go, and the diet tribes rise and fall. As you may have guessed, we're both extremely passionate about helping people get fit, be healthy, and stay in shape for life. While neither of us possess outstanding physical genetics, we do share a tenacious and fierce determination to achieve our goals and more importantly, to help others.

Together we have built a meta-mind of knowledge and experience stemming from insightful conversations and personal experimentation. Both Matt and I believe we've identified and systematized the key components to lifelong diet success. None of that would have happened, though, if we hadn't spent decades in the trenches working one-on-one with real people to help them solve their diet and fitness challenges.

This book aims to deliver the most comprehensive and strategic guide to nutrition ever written. Our goal is to give you the last diet book you'll ever need to read. We are sharing what we believe is the grand unifying theory of dieting so you will never be stuck in another dietary argument on social media with someone you've never met from another "diet tribe." Most of all, the book teaches you exactly how to choose the right dietary strategy to reach virtually any goal you desire. God willing, the strategies in this book will help you extend your life. If you apply the principles in this book, you will almost certainly live a higher quality life. This book is the beginning of the end of the diet wars.

Wade T. Lightheart, CSNA
President and co-founder of BIOptimizers
3-Time National Natural Bodybuilding Champion

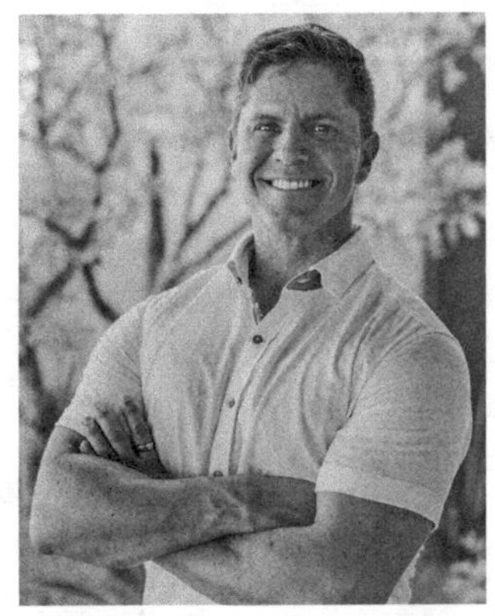

MATT GALLANT

My name is Matt Gallant, kinesiologist, health researcher, and co-founder of BIOptimizers.

I was born in a small village in New Brunswick, Canada, near the city of Moncton (where Wade grew up).

There are 3 key experiences that shaped my destiny.

The first experience was with my grandfather. He was the victim of a hit-and-run at the age of 75. It destroyed his hips and legs, and he was never able to walk normally again. My father built an apartment for him in our home, so I got to spend time with him almost every day.

I saw his health decline rapidly over the following years. For the last five years of his life, he was in so much pain that he prayed for death multiple times a day. The cocktail of painkillers and other pharmaceuticals didn't work anymore. It was a very impactful experience as a young teenager. This really showed me the value of health span (which we talk about greatly in this book).

My first dieting experience came after my uncle told me I looked fat when I was 15 years old. I weighed 190 pounds and my body fat was pretty high. It was a jarring experience and motivated me to start running every day, and I followed the Atkins Diet. I went from 190 pounds to 147 pounds in six months. It was an empowering experience to see how much the body could change.

The second experience that marked me was going to the beach and seeing two bodybuilders. I was 16 years old and I wanted to look like that. That was the beginning of a passion for physical aesthetics. Since that time, I've been able to add over 40 lbs of lean muscle mass to my frame (despite having horrible genetics).

Back then I felt small and weak. After seeing those muscular bodybuilders on the beach, I got bit by the bodybuilding bug. It became an obsession. It's all I cared about. I started lifting weights twice a day and followed the Anabolic Diet. I went from 147 pounds to 235 pounds without using drugs. And yes, I did add some bodyfat but I built a tremendous amount of muscle mass.

When I was 19 years old, I decided to compete. I did it on my own and the whole experience was a disaster. I lost 64 pounds in 14 weeks. I lost a tremendous amount of lean muscle mass and didn't look the way I wanted on stage. That was the end of my bodybuilding journey. I've always loved the power to change my body in different ways. It's one of the wonders of being human.

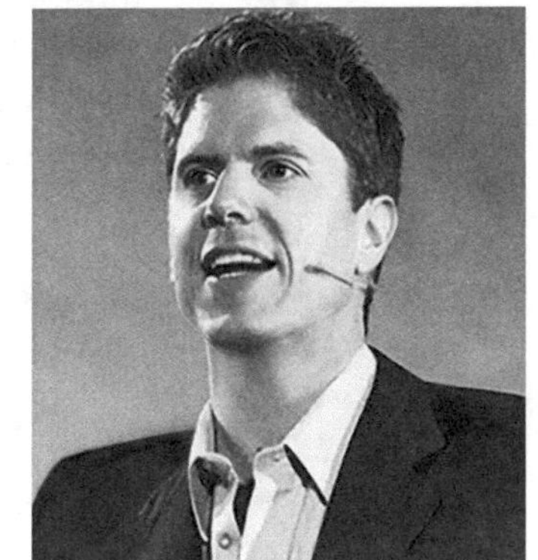

The third destiny shaping experience was helping my best friend lose 191 pounds in 18 months when I was 19. Before this, he was a 20-year-old who weighed 400 pounds and had never had a date.

I coached him for a year and a half and he became a new man. Not just physically, but mentally, and emotionally. He got married shortly after. That impacted me so much that I knew this is what I wanted to do for a living. I wanted to help more people change not just how they look, but how they feel, and help them upgrade themselves.

I got my bachelor's degrees in the science of physical activity and kinesiology and started helping hundreds of people. I became one of the busiest trainers in Moncton and then in Vancouver, spending up to 80 hours a week in the gym. I have been blessed to train professional athletes in multiple sports and become close friends with many of the top minds in health and fitness.

My next obsession was with hand-to-hand combat and self-defense. I started training with the legendary Christophe Clugston for many years. This was where I truly learned the keys and secrets to physical performance. His genius around optimizing and maximizing performance is truly world-class. I became a self-defense instructor and enjoyed it immensely.

Then in 2001, I met Wade and we became close friends. We were both trainers and both shared a deep passion for health and fitness. We shared all of our knowledge, experience, and insights with each other. We argued passionately about which diet was best.

Wade and I have built a deep meta-mind of knowledge and experience that has helped both of us become better versions of ourselves on multiple levels.

I had such great results with the ketogenic diet that I became a keto zealot. I thought I had found the holy grail of nutrition. However, after putting all my clients on a keto diet, several of them didn't feel well or look healthy.

Being a hardcore self-experimenter, I've tried almost every type of diet: multiple diets of ketogenic diets from Atkins to cyclical keto, the cycle diet, raw food diet, IIFYM, and zone diet (in my opinion, a scam), virtually every type of fasting strategy, various types of bodybuilding diets, and on and on.

As I tried various diet types, I realized that they all worked to some degree. I started to see the similarities between them. It took many years, but I started to realize that certain diets worked better for certain people.

In 2004, Wade and I decided to start a business together. That was the genesis of BIOptimizers. Our focus at that time was to help people build muscle naturally. Our book *Freaky Big Naturally* was quite successful.

Also, around that same time, we met Dr. Michael O'Brien, who taught us that you could produce extraordinary results when you give the body the right "workers" (enzymes and probiotics) and feed the body the right nutrients. We did his 90-day protocol and the rest is history. I got on his protocol and dropped over 40 pounds and completely changed my health.

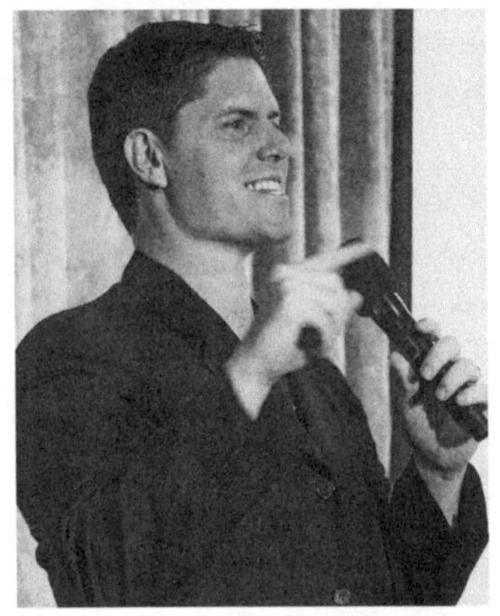

Over the years our passion shifted to health and biological optimization and that's why in 2014 we rebranded to BIOptimizers.

We knew our destiny was to share this amazing information, products, and protocols with the world so everyone can experience what BIOptimized health is. Most people have never experienced how good it feels to be BIOptimized.

Over the next few years, we tested, optimized, and perfected the protocols with thousands of clients from around the world. The results were outstanding.

Our clinical experience led us to develop a whole suite of digestive solutions to truly fix and optimize digestion and health. At BIOptimizers, we have continued to develop best-in-class formulas that can help you improve almost every aspect of your health. We now have best-in-class solutions for sleep, digestion, nootropics, and much more.

My passion and purpose for helping others experience biological optimization have only gotten stronger in the last three decades and are still growing stronger.

Our goal is to keep innovating on every key component of your health. We will not stop driving forward and, God willing, we aim to make biological optimization affordable and available to everyone on Earth.

We will create one best-in-class solution after another. This is my dharma and I'm ALL IN on helping you become the healthiest version of yourself.

God bless.

Matt Gallant, Bachelor of Science of Physical Activity
CEO and co-founder of BIOptimizers
Kinesiologist

Hay House Titles of Related Interest

YOU CAN HEAL YOUR LIFE, the movie, starring Louise Hay & Friends
(available as an online streaming video)
www.hayhouse.com/louise-movie

THE SHIFT, the movie,
starring Dr. Wayne W. Dyer
(available as an online streaming video)
www.hayhouse.com/the-shift-movie

***

BEYOND LONGEVITY: A Proven Plan for Healing Faster, Feeling Better, and Thriving at Any Age, by Jason Prall

EAT FOR ENERGY: How to Beat Fatigue, Supercharge Your Mitochondria, and Unlock All-Day Energy, by Ari Whitten

FAST LIKE A GIRL: A Woman's Guide to Using the Healing Power of Fasting to Burn Fat, Boost Energy, and Balance Hormones, by Dr. Mindy Pelz

MEDICAL MEDIUM LIFE-CHANGING FOODS: Save Yourself and the Ones You Love with the Hidden Healing Powers of Fruits & Vegetables, by Anthony William

All of the above are available at your local bookstore,
or may be ordered by contacting Hay House (see next page).

***

We hope you enjoyed this Hay House book. If you'd like to receive our online catalog featuring additional information on Hay House books and products, or if you'd like to find out more about the Hay Foundation, please contact:

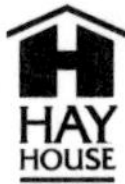

Hay House, Inc., P.O. Box 5100, Carlsbad, CA 92018-5100
(760) 431-7695 or (800) 654-5126
(760) 431-6948 (fax) or (800) 650-5115 (fax)
www.hayhouse.com® • www.hayfoundation.org

Published in Australia by: Hay House Australia Pty. Ltd., 18/36 Ralph St., Alexandria NSW 2015
Phone: 612-9669-4299 • *Fax:* 612-9669-4144
www.hayhouse.com.au

Published in the United Kingdom by: Hay House UK, Ltd., The Sixth Floor, Watson House, 54 Baker Street, London W1U 7BU
Phone: +44 (0)20 3927 7290 • *Fax:* +44 (0)20 3927 7291
www.hayhouse.co.uk

Published in India by: Hay House Publishers India, Muskaan Complex, Plot No. 3, B-2, Vasant Kunj, New Delhi 110 070
Phone: 91-11-4176-1620 • *Fax:* 91-11-4176-1630
www.hayhouse.co.in

NOTES

NOTES

NOTES

NOTES